Medical Microbiology: A Guide to Microbial Infections (Pathogenesis, Immunity and Control)

Medical Microbiology: A Guide to Microbial Infections (Pathogenesis, Immunity and Control)

Editor: Queenie Mayes

AMERICAN
MEDICAL PUBLISHERS
www.americanmedicalpublishers.com

AMERICAN
MEDICAL PUBLISHERS
www.americanmedicalpublishers.com

Cataloging-in-Publication Data

Medical microbiology : a guide to microbial infections (pathogenesis, immunity and control) / edited by Queenie Mayes.
p. cm.
Includes bibliographical references and index.
ISBN 979-8-88740-253-6
1. Medical microbiology. 2. Pathogenic microorganisms. 3. Communicable diseases--Pathogenesis.
4. Communicable diseases--Immunological aspects. 5. Communicable diseases--Prevention.
6. Clinical immunology. I. Mayes, Queenie.
QR46 .M433 2023
616.01--dc23

American Medical Publishers,
41 Flatbush Avenue,
1st Floor, New York,
NY 11217, USA

ISBN 979-8-88740-253-6 (Hardback)

Contents

Preface

Medical microbiology refers to a sub discipline of microbiology which is applied in biology. The major aim of medical microbiology is the diagnosis, treatment and prevention of infectious diseases, which can be caused by microorganisms like viruses, bacteria, parasites and fungi. It is also focused on the study of different clinical applications of microbes for improving the health. Epidemiology is a significant aspect of medical microbiology, which investigates the causes, effect and patterns of health and disease. However, the clinical aspect is concerned with the microbial infections affecting the humans, and various methods for the treatment of infectious diseases. A detailed diagnosis of infectious disease comprises various techniques, such as genotyping, microbial culture, biochemical tests and microscopy. This book explores all the important aspects of medical microbiology in the present day scenario. Also included herein is a detailed explanation of pathogenesis, immunity and control of microbial infections. This book will serve as a reference to a broad spectrum of readers.

The information contained in this book is the result of intensive hard work done by researchers in this field. All due efforts have been made to make this book serve as a complete guiding source for students and researchers. The topics in this book have been comprehensively explained to help readers understand the growing trends in the field.

I would like to thank the entire group of writers who made sincere efforts in this book and my family who supported me in my efforts of working on this book. I take this opportunity to thank all those who have been a guiding force throughout my life.

Editor

1

Conservation of the OmpC Porin Among Typhoidal and Non-Typhoidal *Salmonella* Serovars

Nuriban Valero-Pacheco[1,2,3†‡], Joshua Blight[3†‡], Gustavo Aldapa-Vega[1,2], Phillip Kemlo[3], Marisol Pérez-Toledo[1,2†], Isabel Wong-Baeza[2], Ayako Kurioka[4], Christian Perez-Shibayama[5], Cristina Gil-Cruz[5], Luvia E. Sánchez-Torres[2], Rodolfo Pastelin-Palacios[6], Armando Isibasi[1], Arturo Reyes-Sandoval[3], Paul Klenerman[4‡] and Constantino López-Macías[1,7,8*‡]*

[1] Unidad de Investigación Médica en Inmunoquímica, Hospital de Especialidades del Centro Médico Nacional Siglo XXI, Instituto Mexicano del Seguro Social, Mexico City, Mexico, [2] Departamento de Inmunología, Escuela Nacional de Ciencias Biológicas, Instituto Politécnico Nacional, Mexico City, Mexico, [3] Nuffield Department of Medicine, The Henry Wellcome Building for Molecular Physiology, The Jenner Institute, University of Oxford, Oxford, United Kingdom, [4] Peter Medawar Building for Pathogen Research, University of Oxford, Oxford, United Kingdom, [5] Institute of Immunobiology, Kantonsspital St. Gallen, St. Gallen, Switzerland, [6] Facultad de Química, Universidad Nacional Autónoma de México, Mexico City, Mexico, [7] Visiting Professor of Immunology, Nuffield Department of Medicine, University of Oxford, Oxford, United Kingdom, [8] Mexican Translational Immunology Research Group, FOCIS Centres of Excellence, Cuernavaca, Mexico

***Correspondence:**
Paul Klenerman
paul.klenerman@ndm.ox.ac.uk
Constantino López-Macías
constantino@sminmunologia.mx;
constantino.lopez@imss.gob.mx

†Present address:
Nuriban Valero-Pacheco, Center for Immunity and Inflammation and Department of Microbiology, Biochemistry, and Molecular Genetics, New Jersey Medical School, Rutgers Biomedical and Health Sciences, Rutgers-The State University of New Jersey, Newark, NJ, United States
Joshua Blight, Department of Life Sciences, Imperial College London, Sir Alexander Fleming Building, London, United Kingdom
Marisol Pérez-Toledo, MRC Centre for Immune Regulation, Institute of Immunology and Immunotherapy, College of Medical and Dental Sciences, University of Birmingham, Birmingham, United Kingdom

‡These authors have contributed equally to this work

Salmonella enterica infections remain a challenging health issue, causing significant morbidity and mortality worldwide. Current vaccines against typhoid fever display moderate efficacy whilst no licensed vaccines are available for paratyphoid fever or invasive non-typhoidal salmonellosis. Therefore, there is an urgent need to develop high efficacy broad-spectrum vaccines that can protect against typhoidal and non-typhoidal *Salmonella*. The *Salmonella* outer membrane porins OmpC and OmpF, have been shown to be highly immunogenic antigens, efficiently eliciting protective antibody, and cellular immunity. Furthermore, enterobacterial porins, particularly the OmpC, have a high degree of homology in terms of sequence and structure, thus making them a suitable vaccine candidate. However, the degree of the amino acid conservation of OmpC among typhoidal and non-typhoidal *Salmonella* serovars is currently unknown. Here we used a bioinformatical analysis to classify the typhoidal and non-typhoidal *Salmonella* OmpC amino acid sequences into different clades independently of their serological classification. Further, our analysis determined that the porin OmpC contains various amino acid sequences that are highly conserved among both typhoidal and non-typhoidal *Salmonella* serovars. Critically, some of these highly conserved sequences were located in the transmembrane β-sheet within the porin β-barrel and have immunogenic potential for binding to MHC-II molecules, making them suitable candidates for a broad-spectrum *Salmonella* vaccine. Collectively, these findings suggest that these highly conserved sequences may be used for the rational design of an effective broad-spectrum vaccine against *Salmonella*.

Keywords: *Salmonella*, OmpC, immunogenicity, non-typhoidal, porin, vaccine, typhoid, salmonellosis

INTRODUCTION

Salmonella enterica infections remain a significant worldwide health problem, accounting for more than 120 million cases and approximately 1 million deaths annually (1, 2). These high morbidity and mortality rates are caused mainly by enteric fevers (typhoid and paratyphoid) and by non-typhoidal *Salmonella* (NTS) gastroenteritis (1–3). Furthermore, invasive NTS bacteremia (iNTS) is a common complication observed in immunocompromised adults and in young children with severe malaria and malnutrition (4). The current available licensed vaccines against *Salmonella* are the oral live attenuated Ty21a, the Vi capsular polysaccharide (Vi CPS), and the Vi-tetanus toxoid conjugate (Vi-TT), which only target the Typhi serovar, and have shown variable efficacy; 50% (95% CI 35–61%) for Ty21a, 55% (95% CI 30–70%) for Vi-CPS, and 54.6% (95% CI 26.8–71.8%) for Vi-TT (5, 6), while no licensed vaccines against iNTS are currently available (7). Although cross-reactivity through vaccination with the Ty21a vaccine can be induced against Paratyphi A, B, and Enteritidis serovars (8, 9), cross-protection has been reported only against Paratyphi B (10). Therefore, there is an urgent need for the development of novel broad-spectrum vaccines against *Salmonella*, which must be based on shared key structural components that induce protective immune responses against typhoidal and NTS serovars.

Porins are one of the most abundant outer-membrane proteins (Omp) in Gram-negative bacteria, which play a crucial role in the diffusion of small hydrophilic compounds, and are essential for bacterial survival and pathogenicity (11, 12). Porins are β-barrel structures consisting of 16 β-sheets (β), with 8 internal periplasmic turns (T) and 8 extracellular loops (L) (13, 14). *Salmonella* and other Gram-negative bacteria express two major porins, OmpC and OmpF (15–17). We have previously shown that *S.* Typhi OmpC and OmpF porins efficiently elicit innate immune responses through the TLR-mediated activation of antigen-presenting cells (18), which induce long-lasting porin-specific bactericidal antibody and cell-mediated immune responses (19–22). However, the basis of antigen specificity of *Salmonella* porins is not well-understood. Previous studies have shown that the porin OmpC shows a high degree of homology in terms of sequence and structure among Enterobacteriaceae porins (11, 13, 15, 23, 24). Therefore, antibody and cell-mediated cross-reactivity among *Salmonella* serovar porins has been widely reported in mouse models (19, 24–28). However, the degree of amino acid conservation of the porin OmpC among typhoidal and NTS serovars remains unknown. Through bioinformatics, we found that the typhoidal and NTS OmpC amino acid sequences can be classified into eight different clades that are independent of serovar classification. In addition, we found that the porin OmpC contains three distinct amino acid sequences, which are highly conserved among typhoidal and NTS serovars. These highly conserved sequences are located along the transmembrane β-sheet domains within the porin β-barrel. Furthermore, we found that one of the highly conserved OmpC sequences is present exclusively in *Salmonella* and not in other Enterobacterial porins and has the potential of binding to MHC-II molecules. Collectively, our results show that the porin OmpC of *Salmonella* contains highly conserved amino acid sequences, which could be used for the rational design of an effective, broad-spectrum vaccine against *Salmonella*.

MATERIALS AND METHODS

Conservation Analysis

Full-length protein sequences for OmpC porin from typhoidal and NTS serovars (Typhi, Paratyphi A, B, C, Typhimurium, Enteritidis, Dublin, and Gallinarum) were collected from the NCBI Entrez protein database using Taxonomy IDs (Txid). Subsequently, sequences for OmpC from all serovars were each aligned using Clustal Omega standalone binary 1.2.1 (29) and used to create a neighbor-joining tree using the Jukes-Cantor model resampled with 100 bootstraps and samples separated into clades (8 clades). Porin conservation was assessed using in-house developed software, based on a sliding window approach. Amino acid conservation within each clade was assessed using a 15 amino acid window with a mean conservation value (between 0 and 1) given for each window, determined by amino acid similarity. Windows with a mean value less than the first quartile of all windows was classed as conserved (intra-clade). Zero (0) represents a fully conserved window. This was used to generate an intra-conservation plot representing the mean window conservation across the entire proteome. Subsequently, conservation across clades (inter-clade) was assessed by identifying windows at the same position across clades that were conserved within their respective clades (i.e., mean window value below the first quartile) and given an arbitrary value between 0 and 1000 to indicate the magnitude of inter-clade conservation given. A consensus was created from the clades with shared conservation.

Porin Visualization

Salmonella Typhi OmpC full-length amino acid sequence was obtained from UniProt (P0A264-OMPC SALTI) (30), and the secondary structure was visualized using PDBSum (31). The three-dimensional *S.* Typhi OmpC (32) porin structure was obtained from PDB (ID: 3UU2). Geneious version 8.1.7, created by Biomatters (33), was used for porin 3D visualization.

TABLE 1 | Number of full-length amino acid sequences retrieved from the NCBI Entrez Protein database for the selected *Salmonella* OmpC porin.

Serovar	Txid	Number of sequences
Typhi	90370	24
Paratyphi A	54388	57
Paratyphi B	57045	40
Paratyphi C	57046	6
Dublin	98360	19
Enteritidis	149539	426
Typhimurium	90371	186
Gallinarum	594	3
	Total	761

MHC-II Peptide-Binding Prediction

To evaluate the potential immunogenicity of the OmpC conserved sequences, the Immuno Epitope Database (IEDB, https://www.iedb.org) MHC-II binding prediction tool was used. The MHCII binding predictions were performed on Oct/18/2019 using the IEDB analysis resource Consensus tool (34, 35). The predicted output is given in units of IC_{50}nM for combinatorial library and SMM_align; hence, a lower number indicates a higher affinity. According to the IEDB, as a rough guideline, peptides with IC_{50} values <50 nM are considered high affinity, <500 nM intermediate affinity and <5,000 nM low affinity. Most known epitopes have high or intermediate affinity (36).

BLAST Analysis

The conserved sequences of *Salmonella* OmpC porin were compared against Non-Redundant (nr) GenBank database using the standard protein Basic Local Alignment Search Tool (BLAST), BLASTP 2.10.0+, using the default options (37). Fast minimum evolution pairwise alignment trees were constructed using the default options of BLASTP 2.10.0+ (max seq. difference 0.85, Grishin distance).

Statistical Analysis

Statistics were calculated using linear regression in GraphPad Prism 6.0. *P* values ≤ 0.05 were considered as significant.

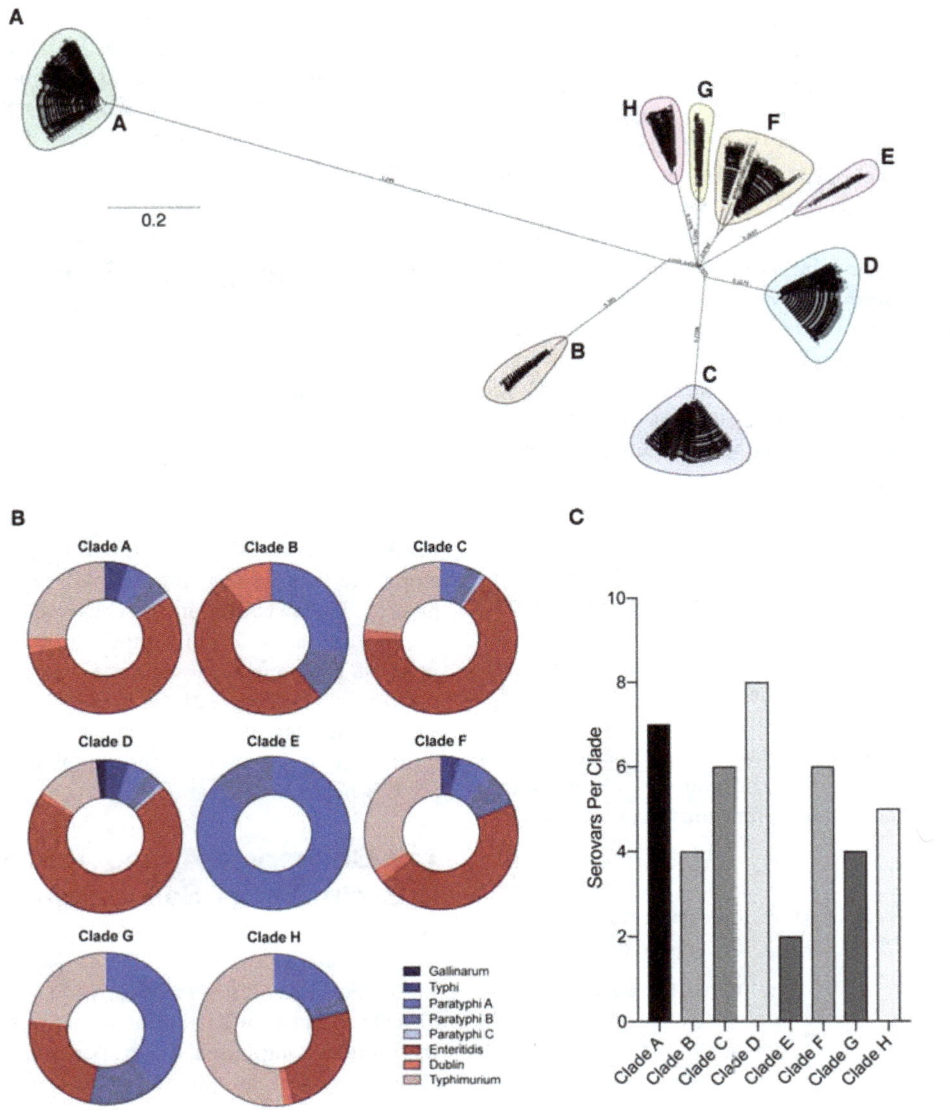

FIGURE 1 | Phylogeny of *Salmonella* OmpC protein. **(A)** Neighbor-joining tree of full-length *Salmonella* OmpC protein sequences. Full-length *Salmonella* OmpC protein sequences used to create a neighbor-joining tree using the Jukes-Cantor model with 100 bootstraps. Outgroups separated into 8 clades (A–H). **(B)** Prevalence of typhoidal and non-typhoidal *Salmonella* serovars among each OmpC clade. Full-length OmpC protein sequences were retrieved from NCBI and aligned using Clustal Omega, and intra-serovar OmpC conservation was assessed using in-house developed software utilizing a sliding window approach (for a detailed description see methods). The percentage of each *Salmonella* serovar OmpC amino acid sequence within *Salmonella* clades is shown. Typhoidal serovars are shown in blue while non-typhoidal serovars are shown in red. **(C)** Number of serovars per clade represented by a bar chart.

RESULTS

Identification of Conserved Amino Acid Sequences in the Porin OmpC Among Typhoidal and Non-Typhoidal *Salmonella* Serovars

To determine the degree of conservation among OmpC amino acid sequences from clinically relevant typhoidal (Typhi, Paratyphi A, B, and C) and non-typhoidal (Typhimurium, Enteritidis, Dublin, and Gallinarum) *Salmonella* serovars (38), we retrieved and aligned 761 *Salmonella* serovar OmpC amino acid sequences and assessed conservation within serovars using in-house developed software (see methods) (**Table 1**). However, sequences within serovars showed very poor identity, likely due to the serological classification of serovars (39). Therefore, OmpC sequences from these serovars were used to create a neighbor-joining tree and outgroups were classed into 8 separate clades (**Figure 1A**, **Table 2**). Each clade contained a mixture of serovars (**Figures 1B,C**). However, clades A, B, C, D, F, and H consisted of a majority of non-typhoidal serovars, while clades E and G were comprised of mostly typhoidal serovars, with clade E containing only sequences from Paratyphi A and B. As would be expected, the greater the number of sequences per clade the greater the number of serovars it contained ($R^2 = 0.7709$, $^{**}p = 0.00413$). We found that Clade D contained sequences from all 8 serovars analyzed, followed by clade A with 7 serovars, C and F with 6 serovars, clade H with 5 serovars, clades B and G with 4 serovars, and clade E with 2 serovars. In addition, we found that the most widely distributed serovars among the clades were Paratyphi A and B, which had sequences present in all of the clades. *Salmonella* Enteritidis was found in all but one of the clades analyzed (clade E), while Typhimurium and Dublin were found in 6 clades. Typhi and Paratyphi C serovars were only present in 3 clades, whereas Gallinarum was only found in one clade.

Next, we assessed the degree of conservation of full-length OmpC sequences within each clade (intra-clade; **Figure 2A**). Analysis showed a pattern of diversity and conservation across the protein unique to each clade, however some clades showed similar conservation fingerprints. For example, clades D and F showed a similar trend at the N-terminus, whereas clades F and G were more similar toward the C-terminus. There was no significant correlation between either the number of serovars per clade and the median conservation value for that clade ($R^2 = 0.09655$, $p = 0.6412$) and the number of sequences per clade and the median conservation value for that clade ($R^2 = 0.008383$, $p = 0.8293$).

TABLE 2 | Number of full-length amino acid sequences for each clade of *Salmonella* OmpC porin sequences.

Clade	Number of sequences
A	208
B	18
C	181
D	169
E	7
F	117
G	13
H	48
Total	761

Subsequently, conservation between clades was assessed (**Figure 2B**), which identified 5, 15, 23, 28, 16, 8, and 2% of the protein covered by regions conserved in all 8 or 7, 6, 5, 4, 3, and 2 clades respectively. Whereas, 3% of the protein sequence showed no conservation across clades, located centrally at position 236–246. Remarkably, when comparing more clades (>5) two regions of distinct cross clade conservation could be seen located at the 50–200 (X) and 320–430 (Y) amino acid positions, suggesting two regions of functional importance. Within these locations there were three regions (R1–R3) that showed a high degree of conservation among all of the *Salmonella* clades analyzed (**Table 3**). Collectively, these data show that the OmpC porin contains distinct amino acid sequences that are highly conserved among typhoidal and non-typhoidal *Salmonella* serovars.

The Conserved Amino Acid Sequences Are Located Along the β-Sheets of OmpC Porin

Next, we sought to identify the location of the conserved regions along the secondary structure of *S.* Typhi OmpC, the only available crystal structure of a *Salmonella* OmpC porin reported to date (**Figure 3A**) (32). Our results show that the sequence of the conserved region R1 (KGETQINDQLTGY) was located partially along the β3 β-sheet, the periplasmic turn T3, and part of the β4 β-sheet. The conserved region R2 (WTRLAFAGLKFA) was located along the β5 β-sheet. Finally, the conserved region R3 (GFANKTQNFEVVAQYQFDFGLRPSQAYLSKG) was located along the β13 β-sheet, the periplasmic turn T7, and the β14 β-sheet. The visualization the conserved amino acid sequences on the crystal *S.* Typhi OmpC porin structure showed that most of the conserved sequences were distributed along the porin β-barrel (**Figure 3B**). Collectively, our data show that the amino acid sequences conserved among *Salmonella* clades are located along the β-sheets and periplasmic turns of the OmpC porin β-barrel.

The Conserved Amino Acid Sequence R1 Is Exclusive for *Salmonella*

Because porins from Enterobacteriaceae show high-level sequence similarity (11, 13, 15, 24), we questioned whether the conserved sequences were exclusive to *Salmonella* porin OmpC. BLASTp analysis of R1 indicated that this amino acid sequence was found among several OmpC porins from *Salmonella enterica* serovars, as well as other *Salmonella* porins, such as OmpS2 and PhoE (E-value 3×10^{-4}, 100% identity). In addition, BLASTp results showed that the amino acid sequence from R1 (KGETQINDQLTGY) was also present in the OmpC and OmpF porins of the plant-associated genus *Pantoea* (40) (**Figure 4**). Conversely, the amino acid sequence of R2 (WTRLAFAGLKFA) was not exclusive to *Salmonella* serovars, since BLASTp results showed that this sequence was also found in the porins OmpC

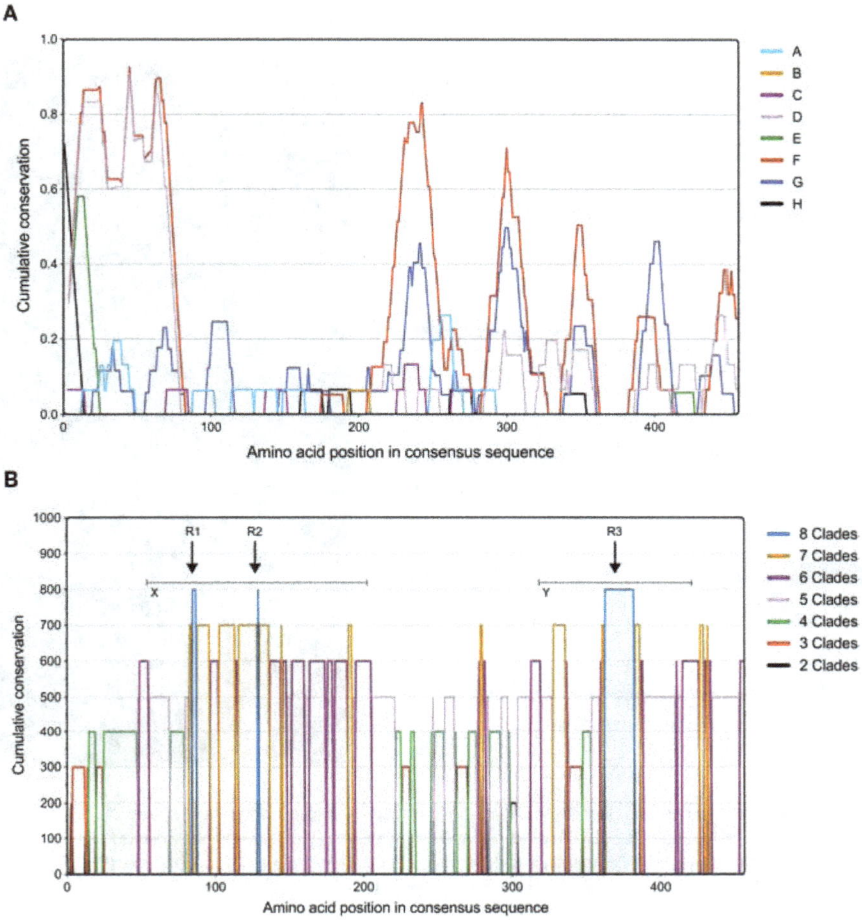

FIGURE 2 | Assessment of *Salmonella* OmpC clade conservation. **(A)** Intra-clade conservation of OmpC porin within typhoidal and non-typhoidal *Salmonella* serovars. Conservation of each *Salmonella* clade of the OmpC protein identified using a 15 amino acid sliding window approach (in-house software; for a detailed description see methods). The measure of OmpC amino acid conservation within *Salmonella* clades is shown in Y-axis (0–1), while X-axis shows the position in the aligned amino acid consensus sequence. A conservation value below the first quartile was classed as conserved for each clade. **(B)** Inter-clade conservation patterns in the protein sequence of OmpC porin among typhoidal and non-typhoidal *Salmonella* serovars. Full-length OmpC protein sequences were retrieved from NCBI and aligned using Clustal Omega, and inter-serovar conservation was assessed using in-house developed software. The measure of OmpC amino acid conservation between *Salmonella* clades is shown in Y-axis, while X-axis shows the position in the aligned amino acid consensus sequence. Colors indicate the number of clades that share conservation between each other. Arrows indicate the regions conserved among all *Salmonella* clades and gray bars indicate regions of distinct cross-clade conservation (see **Table 1**).

and OmpN of *Escherichia coli* and *Klebsiella sp.* (E-value 3×10^{-3}, 100% identity) (**Figure 5**). Finally, the amino acid sequence of R3 (GFANKTQNFEVVAQYQFDFGLRPSQAYLSKG) was found to be present in several *Salmonella enterica* serovar OmpC porins, however it was also present in other porins, such as PhoE, OmpC, and OmpF from other Enterobacteria, such as *E. coli*, *Enterobacter sp.*, *Citrobacter sp.*, *Klebsiella sp., and Rahnella sp.* (E-value 6×10^{-19}-4×10^{-18}, 90.62% identity) (**Figure 6**). Next, based on HLA allele frequencies and reference sets with maximal population coverage, we predicted the MHC-II alleles to which the conserved R1 seqeunce could bind (**Table 4**).

DISCUSSION

The development of novel tools for the detection of conserved sequences among vaccine candidates is particularly relevant to the discovery of shared antigenic determinants, which could be used for the rational design of broad-spectrum vaccines. In this study, we used in-house-developed software to evaluate the amino acid sequence conservation of the OmpC porin among typhoidal and NTS serovars. Although it has been reported that the porin OmpC has a high degree of homology in sequence and structure among Enterobacteriaceae porins, most of these

TABLE 3 | Conserved regions in the amino acid consensus sequences for the porin OmpC among the *Salmonella* serovars analyzed.

Conserved region	Amino acid sequence
R1	KGETQINDQLTGY
R2	WTRLAFAGLKFA
R3	GFANKTQNFEVVAQYQFDFGLRPSQAYLSKG

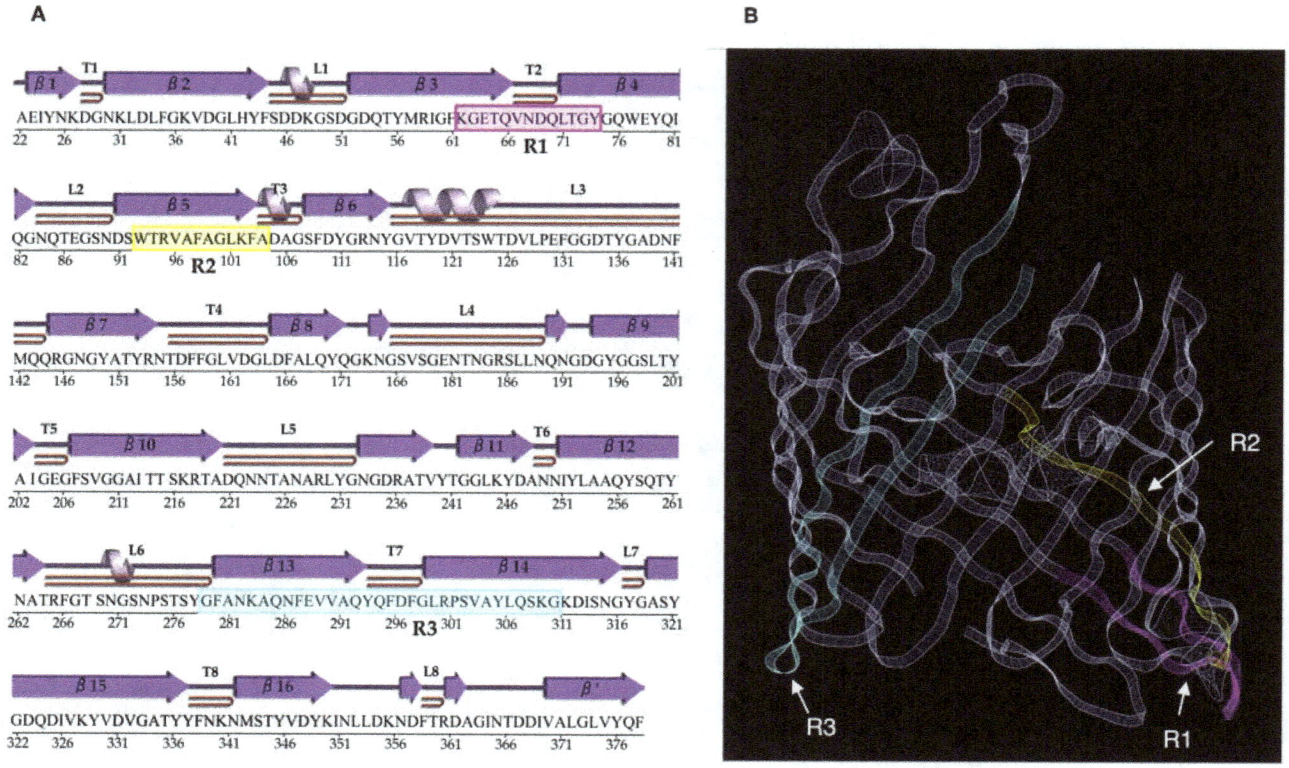

FIGURE 3 | The amino acid sequences conserved among *Salmonella* OmpC porin clades are located along the β-sheets of the β-barrel. **(A)** The secondary structure of the *S.* Typhi OmpC porin was modeled with PDBsum (ID: 3UU2). α-helices and β-sheets are numbered and shown in purple. The periplasmic turns are labeled T1–T8, and the extracellular loops are labeled L1–L8. The porin amino acid sequence is shown without the signal peptide. **(B)** Crystal structure of a *S.* Typhi OmpC monomer. **(A,B)** The conserved regions (R1–R3) among *Salmonella* clades are highlighted in colors, R1 (magenta), R2 (yellow), and R3 (cyan).

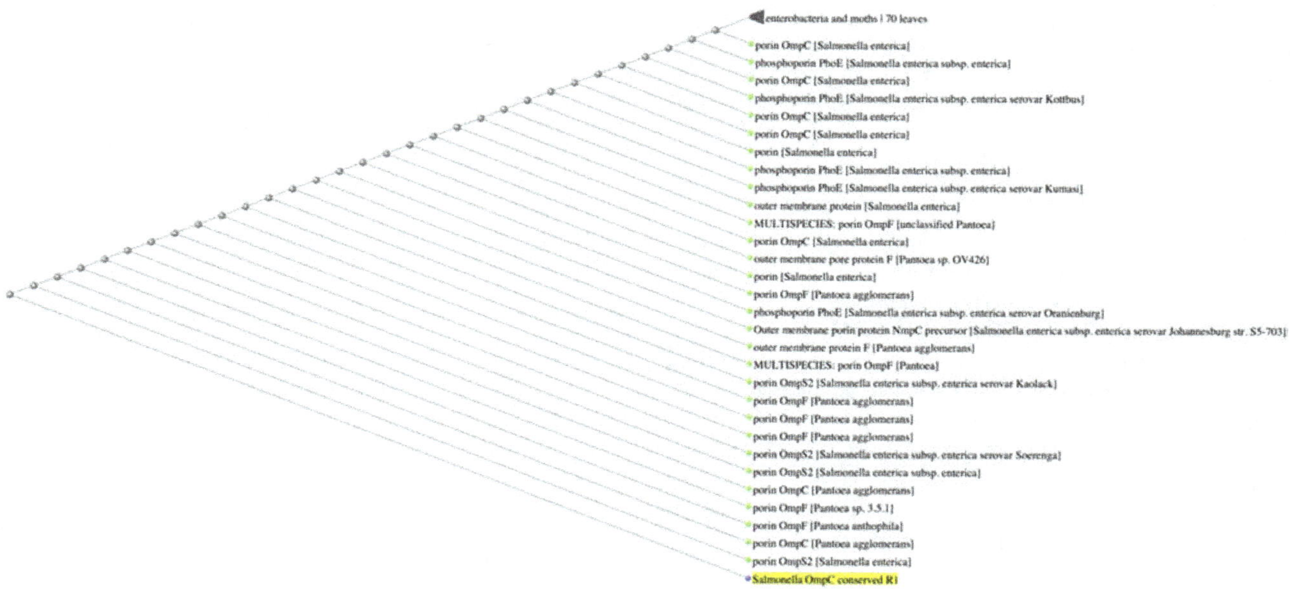

FIGURE 4 | The amino acid sequence of R1 is exclusive of *Salmonella* porins. Fast minimum evolution tree between the R1 sequence and the Non-Redundant (nr) GenBank database calculated by BLASTp.

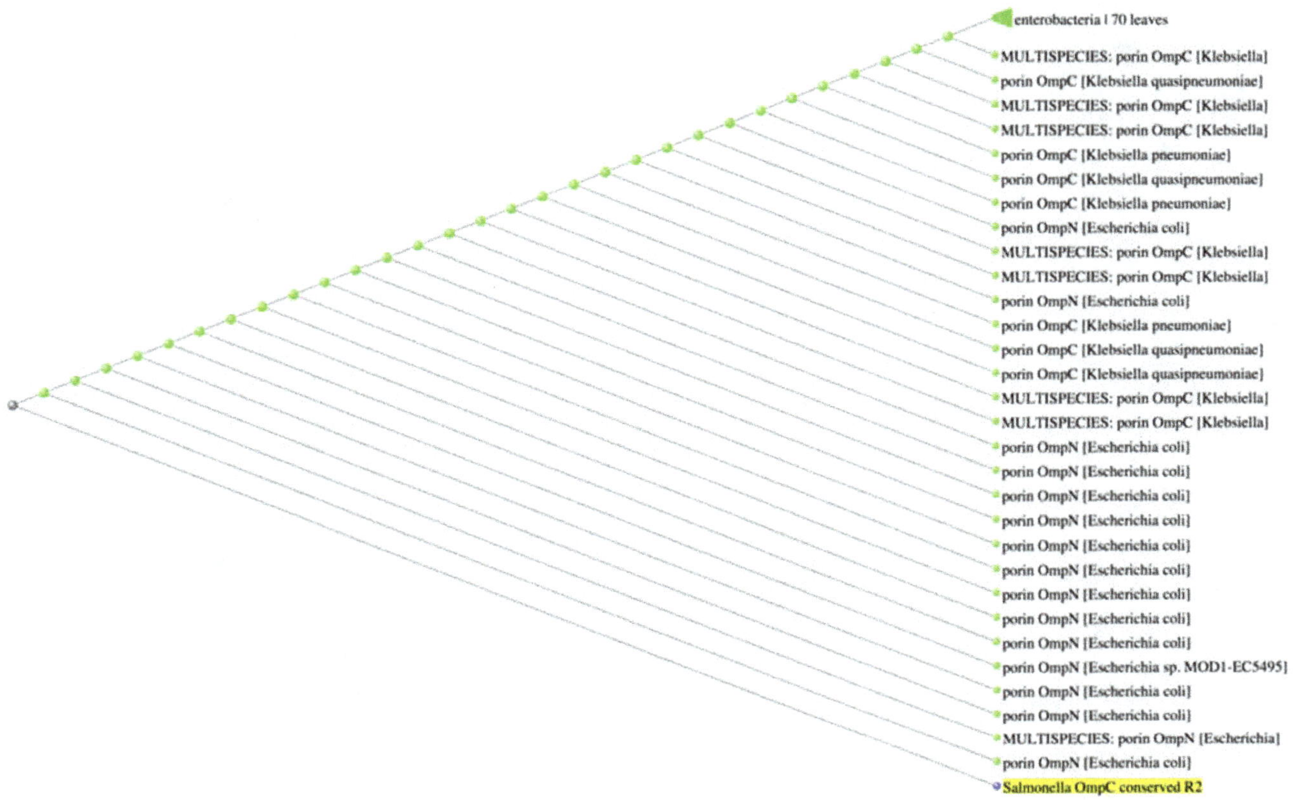

FIGURE 5 | The amino acid sequence of R2 is present in *Escherichia coli* and *Klebsiella sp.* porins. Fast minimum evolution tree between the R2 sequence and the Non-Redundant (nr) GenBank database calculated by BLASTp.

works have focused on defining the differences among amino acid sequences between the OmpC of *Salmonella* serovars and other Enterobacteria, but have not shown the degree of conservation of OmpC among serovars (11, 13, 15, 23, 24). To our knowledge, our work is the first to determine the degree of amino acid conservation of the OmpC porin among typhoidal and NTS serovars, and is the first work to define the conserved regions among *Salmonella* serovars OmpC porin.

Previous reports have shown that the OmpC transmembrane regions are homologous in sequence and structure among Enterobacteria (13, 41). Consequently, it was expected that most of the conserved sequences among *Salmonella* OmpC would be located along the transmembrane β-sheets of the porin β-barrel, as our results show. By contrast, none of the conserved amino acid regions were located along the surface-exposed loops; furthermore, we identified a region within the OmpC porin with no conservation across clades that corresponds to the external loop L4, which has been shown to be one of the regions with more antigenic variability within the OmpC (42–44). Our results show that the *Salmonella* OmpC conserved regions are located along the transmembrane β-sheets of the porin β-barrel, one explanation for this could be that some of the amino acid sequences contained in the conserved regions R1 and R3 of *Salmonella* OmpC are located in subunit contact regions, which are highly conserved among Enterobaceriaceae porins (24, 45). Likewise, it has been reported that the arginine residue (R-95) contained in the conserved region R2 is involved in pore formation (15, 46), which could explain the conservation of this region among *Salmonella* serovars.

The evidence that the conserved sequence in R1 was exclusively found in *Salmonella* porin sequences and not in other gut-associated Enterobacteria, suggests that the immune response that this sequence would induce should be *Salmonella*-specific. Conversely, the finding that the sequences contained in regions R2 and R3 were also found in porins of other commensal and pathogenic Enterobacteria, such as *E. coli, Klebsiella sp., Enterobacter sp., Citrobacter sp., Klebsiella sp., and Rahnella sp.*, suggests that the sequences of regions R2 and R3 are not exclusive of *Salmonella* porins. Our results show that the conserved OmpC sequences R1 can potentially bind to human MHC-II molecules. Similar results were found for human $CD4^+$ T cell epitopes conserved between meningococcal and gonococcal *Neisseria* porins (47, 48). Furthermore, it has been reported that Enterobacteriaceae porins have crucial antigenic epitopes corresponding to regions buried within the outer membrane, which are also highly conserved among Enterobacterial species (24). Some of the amino acid residues from the OmpC conserved region R1 (GFKGETQ) have also been shown to be highly conserved among Enterobacteriaceae porins because of their location in a crucial domain involved

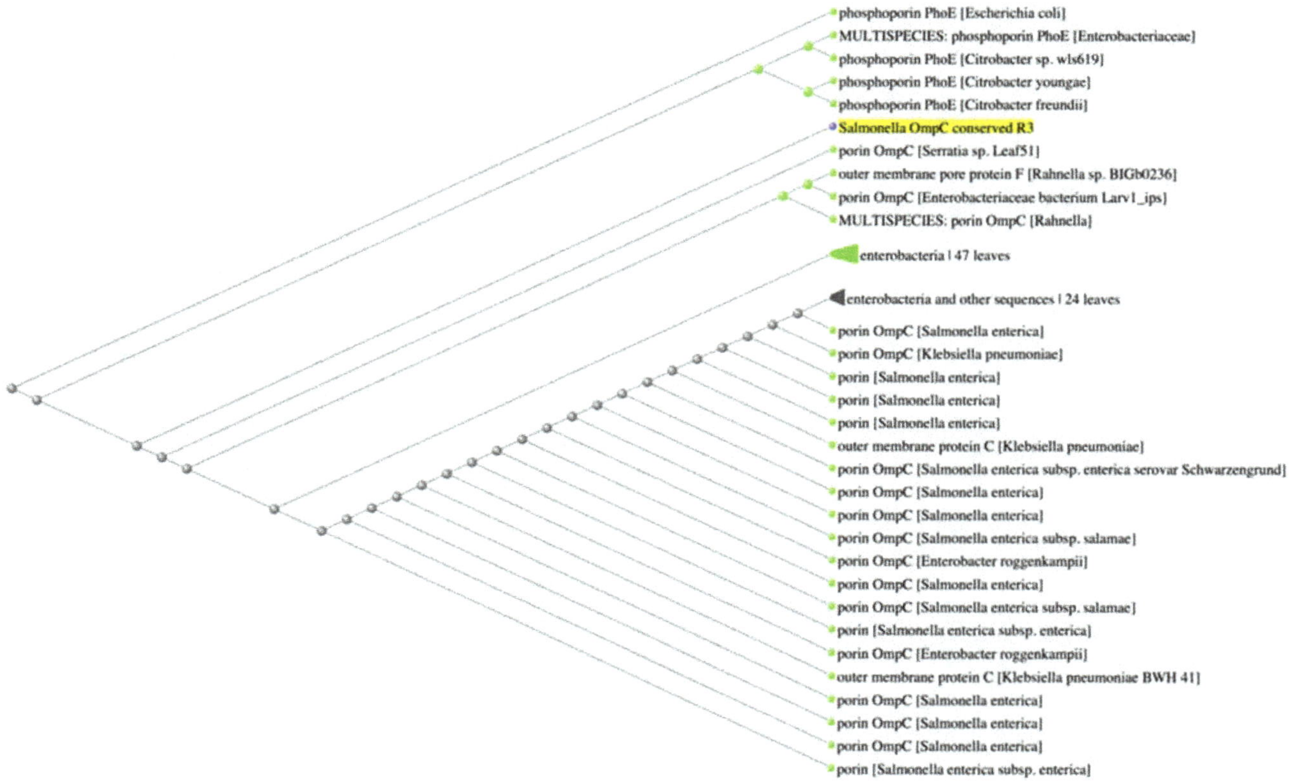

FIGURE 6 | The amino acid sequence of R3 can be found in *Salmonella* and other Enterobacerial porins. Fast minimum evolution tree between the R3 sequence and the Non-Redundant (nr) GenBank database calculated by BLASTp.

in porin subunit interactions (24, 45). In addition, some of the amino acid sequences conserved among *Salmonella* serovars (R1 and R3), have previously been reported as antibody targets or predicted as potential B cell epitopes (11, 24, 49); however, it remains unknown whether any of the conserved sequences can also be recognized by antibodies. In addition, further studies are needed to determine the contribution of MHC-restriction responses to the immunogenicity of the conserved OmpC peptides in T cells. Previous work identified two MHC-I-restricted epitopes in *Salmonella* OmpC porin (50), and strikingly, the amino acid sequence contained in one of the $CD8^+$ T cell-specific peptides contains identical or similar residues to the sequences contained in the conserved region R2 (TRVAFAGL). However, future work will need to focus on whether $CD8^+$ T cells from healthy donors or convalescent patients may also recognize some of the conserved OmpC sequences.

Although this work has shed some light regarding antigen specificity of the *Salmonella* OmpC porin among typhoidal and NTS serovars, there are still several questions left unanswered. For instance, it remains to be determined the cytokine profile produced by OmpC-specific $CD4^+$ T cells, as we have previously shown that vaccination of healthy volunteers with either the Ty21a vaccine or with *Salmonella* porins induces IFN-γ- and TNF-α-producing $CD4^+$ T cells (20, 22). Furthermore, it remains unknown whether the conserved OmpC peptide sequences can be also recognized by T cells from convalescent patients or healthy volunteers challenged with typhoidal and NTS *Salmonella* serovars. Because our current porin-based vaccine candidate is made of a mixture of OmpC and OmpF porins, it remains to be determined the degree of conservation of the porin OmpF among typhoidal and non-typhoidal *Salmonella* by means of the same methodology.

In conclusion, our work is the first to specifically establish the degree of conservation of the porin OmpC among typhoidal and non-typhoidal *Salmonella* serovars and to define the specific amino acid sequences with the highest degree of conservation among typhoidal and NTS serovars. Furthermore, we found that one of the highly conserved OmpC amino acid sequences is exclusive for *Salmonella* and has immunogenic potential for MHC-II binding. Considering that porins are highly immunogenic and protective vaccine candidates against *Salmonella* infections, our findings may lead to a better understanding of the basis of antigen specificity of *Salmonella* porins, which could be used to design tools for monitoring the porin-specific immune response after challenge or vaccination and could have direct implications for the rational design of a broad-spectrum vaccine against *Salmonella*.

TABLE 4 | MHC-II binding prediction for HLA allele frequencies and reference sets with maximal population coverage for the conserved amino acid sequence R1 among *Salmonella* OmpC porin.

HLA allele	Percentile rank	Adjusted rank
HLA-DRB3*01:01	18	28.07
HLA-DQA1*01:01/DQB1*05:01	39.5	61.59
HLA-DQA1*05:01/DQB1*02:01	50	77.97
HLA-DRB4*01:01	55	85.76
HLA-DQA1*03:01/DQB1*03:02	56	87.32
HLA-DQA1*01:02/DQB1*06:02	60.5	94.34
HLA-DRB1*12:01	61.5	95.9
HLA-DQA1*04:01/DQB1*04:02	64.5	100.58
HLA-DRB1*03:01	69	107.6
HLA-DPA1*01/DPB1*04:01	69.5	108.38
HLA-DPA1*01:03/DPB1*02:01	70	109.16
HLA-DPA1*02:01/DPB1*01:01	72	112.27
HLA-DPA1*03:01/DPB1*04:02	74.5	116.17
HLA-DRB3*02:02	75	116.95
HLA-DRB1*08:02	76	118.51
HLA-DRB1*13:02	76	118.51
HLA-DQA1*05:01/DQB1*03:01	82	127.87
HLA-DRB1*04:01	85	132.55
HLA-DRB1*11:01	85	132.55
HLA-DPA1*02:01/DPB1*05:01	85.5	133.33
HLA-DRB1*04:05	86	134.1
HLA-DRB1*01:01	87	135.66
HLA-DRB1*07:01	88	137.22
HLA-DRB1*09:01	92	143.46
HLA-DRB1*15:01	92	143.46
HLA-DRB5*01:01	95	148.14
HLA-DPA1*02:01/DPB1*14:01	96	149.7

AUTHOR CONTRIBUTIONS

NV-P and JB performed the experiments, analyzed the results, and wrote the paper. MP-T and GA-V analyzed the results and wrote the paper. PKe wrote the in-house computer program. AK, CP-S, and CG-C analyzed results and revised the manuscript. IW-B, LS-T, RP-P, and AI analyzed the results and revised the manuscript. AR-S, PKl, and CL-M designed the study, supervised the experiments, and revised the manuscript. All authors contributed to manuscript revision, read, and approved the submitted version.

FUNDING

This study received financial support from the Mexican National Research Council (CONACyT) projects: SEP-CONACYT CB-2015-256402, SRE-CONACYT 263683 and from Mexican Institute for Social Security (IMSS) Project Numbers: FIS/IMSS/PROT/G17/1682, and FIS/IMSS/PROT/MD17/1690 and by the Bacterial Vaccines (BactiVac) Network project BVNCP-07, funded by the GCRF Networks in Vaccines Research and Development which was co-funded by the MRC and BBSRC, all awarded to CL-M. SEP-CONACYT CB-2011-166946 awarded to RP-P. Association of Physicians of GB & Ireland Links with Developing Countries Scheme 2013/2014, from WT 091663MA awarded to PKl and CL-M. AR-S was a Jenner Investigator and a Wellcome Trust Career Development Fellow, supported by the WT 097395/Z/11/Z. NV-P, MP-T, and GA-V acknowledge Ph.D. scholarships received from IPN PIFI (Ref. 1924), IMSS (Ref. 99094890), and CONACyT (Refs. 339525 and 290749). NV-P also acknowledges financial support provided by IMSS through the Programa para el Desarrollo Profesional en Investigación Internacional de Estudiantes de Posgrado (PRODESI) program (Ref. R-2012-785-088). NV-P was an Academic Visitor at the Jenner Institute and at the Peter Medawar Building for Pathogen Research in the University of Oxford. CL-M acknowledges the support received from the IMSS-CIS Programa de Cooperación Internacional. JB acknowledges his D.Phil. scholarship from the Nuffield Department of Medicine, which was partly funded by an MRC research training and support grant (Ref. 1240480).

ACKNOWLEDGMENTS

The authors would like to thank Burkhard Ludewig for valuable comments and support to this project and Juan M. Inclan-Rico for critical reading and editing of the manuscript.

REFERENCES

1. MacLennan CA, Martin LB, Micoli F. Vaccines against invasive *Salmonella* disease: current status and future directions. *Hum Vaccin Immunother.* (2014) 10:1478–93. doi: 10.4161/hv.29054
2. Crump JA, Sjolund-Karlsson M, Gordon MA, Parry CM. Epidemiology, clinical presentation, laboratory diagnosis, antimicrobial resistance, and antimicrobial management of invasive *Salmonella* infections. *Clin Microbiol Rev.* (2015) 28:901–37. doi: 10.1128/CMR.00002-15
3. Buckle GC, Walker CL, Black RE. Typhoid fever and paratyphoid fever: Systematic review to estimate global morbidity and mortality for 2010. *J Glob Health.* (2012) 2:010401. doi: 10.7189/jogh.01.010401
4. Keestra-Gounder AM, Tsolis RM, Baumler AJ. Now you see me, now you don't: the interaction of *Salmonella* with innate immune receptors. *Nat Rev Microbiol.* (2015) 13:206–16. doi: 10.1038/nrmicro3428
5. Jin C, Gibani MM, Moore M, Juel HB, Jones E, Meiring J, et al. Efficacy and immunogenicity of a Vi-tetanus toxoid conjugate vaccine in the prevention of typhoid fever using a controlled human infection model of *Salmonella* Typhi: a randomised controlled, phase 2b trial. *Lancet.* (2017) 390:2472–80. doi: 10.1016/S0140-6736(17)32149-9
6. Milligan R, Paul M, Richardson M, Neuberger A. Vaccines for preventing typhoid fever. *Cochrane Database Syst Rev.* (2018) 5:CD001261. doi: 10.1002/14651858.CD001261.pub4
7. Tennant SM, MacLennan CA, Simon R, Martin LB, Khan MI. Nontyphoidal salmonella disease: current status of vaccine research and development. *Vaccine.* (2016) 34:2907–10. doi: 10.1016/j.vaccine.2016.03.072

8. Pakkanen SH, Kantele JM, Savolainen LE, Rombo L, Kantele A. Specific and cross-reactive immune response to oral *Salmonella* Typhi Ty21a and parenteral Vi capsular polysaccharide typhoid vaccines administered concomitantly. *Vaccine.* (2015) 33:451–8. doi: 10.1016/j.vaccine.2014.11.030
9. Wahid R, Fresnay S, Levine MM, Sztein MB. Cross-reactive multifunctional CD4+ T cell responses against *Salmonella* enterica serovars Typhi, Paratyphi A and Paratyphi B in humans following immunization with live oral typhoid vaccine Ty21a. *Clin Immunol.* (2016) 173:87–95. doi: 10.1016/j.clim.2016.09.006
10. Levine MM, Ferreccio C, Black RE, Lagos R, San Martin O, Blackwelder WC. Ty21a live oral typhoid vaccine and prevention of paratyphoid fever caused by Salmonella *enterica* Serovar Paratyphi B. *Clin Infect Dis.* (2007) 45(Suppl 1):S24–28. doi: 10.1086/518141
11. Arockiasamy A, Krishnaswamy S. Prediction of B-cell epitopes for *Salmonella* typhi OmpC. *J Biosci.* (1995) 20:235–43. doi: 10.1007/BF02703271
12. Nikaido H. Molecular basis of bacterial outer membrane permeability revisited. *Microbiol Mol Biol Rev.* (2003) 67:593–656. doi: 10.1128/MMBR.67.4.593-656.2003
13. Arockiasamy A, Krishnaswamy S. Homology model of surface antigen OmpC from *Salmonella* typhi and its functional implications. *J Biomol Struct Dyn.* (2000) 18:261–71. doi: 10.1080/07391102.2000.10506664
14. Balasubramaniam D, Arockiasamy A, Kumar PD, Sharma A, Krishnaswamy S. Asymmetric pore occupancy in crystal structure of OmpF porin from *Salmonella* typhi. *J Struct Biol.* (2012) 178:233–44. doi: 10.1016/j.jsb.2012.04.005
15. Puente JL, Juarez D, Bobadilla M, Arias CF, Calva E. The *Salmonella* ompC gene: structure and use as a carrier for heterologous sequences. *Gene.* (1995) 156:1–9. doi: 10.1016/0378-1119(94)00883-T
16. Santiviago CA, Toro CS, Bucarey SA, Mora GC. A chromosomal region surrounding the ompD porin gene marks a genetic difference between *Salmonella* typhi and the majority of *Salmonella* serovars. *Microbiology.* (2001) 147(Pt 7):1897–907. doi: 10.1099/00221287-147-7-1897
17. Tatavarthy A, Cannons A. Real-time PCR detection of *Salmonella* species using a novel target: the outer membrane porin F gene (ompF). *Lett Appl Microbiol.* (2010) 50:645–52. doi: 10.1111/j.1472-765X.2010.02848.x
18. Cervantes-Barragan L, Gil-Cruz C, Pastelin-Palacios R, Lang KS, Isibasi A, Ludewig B, et al. TLR2 and TLR4 signaling shapes specific antibody responses to *Salmonella* typhi antigens. *Eur J Immunol.* (2009) 39:126–35. doi: 10.1002/eji.200838185
19. Blanco F, Isibasi A, Raul Gonzalez C, Ortiz V, Paniagua J, Arreguin C, et al. Human cell mediated immunity to porins from *Salmonella* typhi. *Scand J Infect Dis.* (1993) 25:73–80. doi: 10.1080/00365549309169673
20. Salazar-Gonzalez RM, Maldonado-Bernal C, Ramirez-Cruz NE, Rios-Sarabia N, Beltran-Nava J, Castanon-Gonzalez J, et al. Induction of cellular immune response and anti-Salmonella *enterica* serovar typhi bactericidal antibodies in healthy volunteers by immunization with a vaccine candidate against typhoid fever. *Immunol Lett.* (2004) 93:115–22. doi: 10.1016/j.imlet.2004.01.010
21. Secundino I, Lopez-Macias C, Cervantes-Barragan L, Gil-Cruz C, Rios-Sarabia N, Pastelin-Palacios R, et al. *Salmonella* porins induce a sustained, lifelong specific bactericidal antibody memory response. *Immunology.* (2006) 117:59–70. doi: 10.1111/j.1365-2567.2005.02263.x
22. Carreno JM, Perez-Shibayama C, Gil-Cruz C, Lopez-Macias C, Vernazza P, Ludewig B, et al. Evolution of *Salmonella* Typhi outer membrane protein-specific T and B cell responses in humans following oral Ty21a vaccination: a randomized clinical trial. *PLoS ONE.* (2017) 12:e0178669. doi: 10.1371/journal.pone.0178669
23. Puente JL, Alvarez-Scherer V, Gosset G, Calva E. Comparative analysis of the *Salmonella* typhi and Escherichia coli ompC genes. *Gene.* (1989) 83:197–206. doi: 10.1016/0378-1119(89)90105-4
24. Simonet V, Mallea M, Fourel D, Bolla JM, Pages JM. Crucial domains are conserved in Enterobacteriaceae porins. *FEMS Microbiol Lett.* (1996) 136:91–7. doi: 10.1111/j.1574-6968.1996.tb08030.x
25. Isibasi A, Ortiz V, Vargas M, Paniagua J, Gonzalez C, Moreno J, et al. Protection against *Salmonella* typhi infection in mice after immunization with outer membrane proteins isolated from *Salmonella* typhi 9,12,d, Vi. *Infect Immun.* (1988) 56:2953–9.
26. Isibasi A, Ortiz-Navarrete V, Paniagua J, Pelayo R, Gonzalez CR, Garcia JA, et al. Active protection of mice against *Salmonella* typhi by immunization with strain-specific porins. *Vaccine.* (1992) 10:811–3. doi: 10.1016/0264-410X(92)90041-H
27. Gonzalez CR, Isibasi A, Ortiz-Navarrete V, Paniagua J, Garcia JA, Blanco F, et al. Lymphocytic proliferative response to outer-membrane proteins isolated from *Salmonella. Microbiol Immunol.* (1993) 37:793–9. doi: 10.1111/j.1348-0421.1993.tb01707.x
28. Toobak H, Rasooli I, Gargari SLM, Jahangiri A, Nadoushan MJ, Owlia P, et al. Characterization of the *Salmonella* typhi outer membrane protein C. *Korean J Microbiol Biotechnol.* (2013) 41:128–34. doi: 10.4014/kjmb.1207.07009
29. Sievers F, Wilm A, Dineen D, Gibson TJ, Karplus K, Li W, et al. Fast, scalable generation of high-quality protein multiple sequence alignments using Clustal Omega. *Mol Syst Biol.* (2011) 7:539. doi: 10.1038/msb.2011.75
30. UniProt C. UniProt: a hub for protein information. *Nucleic Acids Res.* (2015) 43(Database issue):D204–12. doi: 10.1093/nar/gku989
31. Laskowski RA, Hutchinson EG, Michie AD, Wallace AC, Jones ML, Thornton JM. PDBsum: a Web-based database of summaries and analyses of all PDB structures. *Trends Biochem Sci.* (1997) 22:488–90. doi: 10.1016/S0968-0004(97)01140-7
32. Prasanth P, Putcha BK, Arockiasamy A, Krishnaswamy S. *Crystal Structure of Outer Membrane Protein OmpC From* Salmonella *typhi* (2012). doi: 10.2210/pdb3UU2/pdb
33. Kearse M, Moir R, Wilson A, Stones-Havas S, Cheung M, Sturrock S, et al. Geneious Basic: an integrated and extendable desktop software platform for the organization and analysis of sequence data. *Bioinformatics.* (2012) 28:1647–9. doi: 10.1093/bioinformatics/bts199
34. Wang P, Sidney J, Dow C, Mothe B, Sette A, Peters B. A systematic assessment of MHC class II peptide binding predictions and evaluation of a consensus approach. *PLoS Comput Biol.* (2008) 4:e1000048. doi: 10.1371/journal.pcbi.1000048
35. Wang P, Sidney J, Kim Y, Sette A, Lund O, Nielsen M, et al. Peptide binding predictions for HLA DR, DP and DQ molecules. *BMC Bioinform.* (2010) 11:568. doi: 10.1186/1471-2105-11-568
36. Vita R, Mahajan S, Overton JA, Dhanda SK, Martini S, Cantrell JR, et al. The Immune Epitope Database (IEDB): 2018 update. *Nucleic Acids Res.* (2019) 47:D339–43. doi: 10.1093/nar/gky1006
37. Altschul SF, Madden TL, Schaffer AA, Zhang J, Zhang Z, Miller W, et al. Gapped BLAST and PSI-BLAST: a new generation of protein database search programs. *Nucleic Acids Res.* (1997) 25:3389–402. doi: 10.1093/nar/25.17.3389
38. Jones TF, Ingram LA, Cieslak PR, Vugia DJ, Tobin-D'Angelo M, Hurd S, et al. Salmonellosis outcomes differ substantially by serotype. *J Infect Dis.* (2008) 198:109–14. doi: 10.1086/588823
39. Wattiau P, Boland C, Bertrand S. Methodologies for *Salmonella* enterica subsp. enterica subtyping: gold standards and alternatives. *Appl Environ Microbiol.* (2011) 77:7877–85. doi: 10.1128/AEM.05527-11
40. Dutkiewicz J, Mackiewicz B, Kinga Lemieszek M, Golec M, Milanowski J. Pantoea agglomerans: a mysterious bacterium of evil and good. Part III Deleterious effects: infections of humans, animals and plants. *Ann Agric Environ Med.* (2016) 23:197–205. doi: 10.5604/12321966.1203878
41. Sujatha S, Arockiasamy A, Krishnaswamy S, Usha R. Molecular modelling of epitope presentation using membrane protein OmpC. *Indian J Biochem Biophys.* (2001) 38:294–7. Available online at: http://nopr.niscair.res.in/handle/123456789/15316
42. Paniagua-Solis JMO, Natalia Ortiz-Navarrete V, Ramirez G, Gonzalez C, Isibasi A. Predicted epitopes of *Salmonella* typhi OmpC porin are exposed on the bacterial surface. *Immunol Infect Dis.* (1995) 5:244–9.
43. Paniagua-Solis J, Sanchez J, Ortiz-Navarrete V, Gonzalez CR, Isibasi A. Construction of CTB fusion proteins for screening of monoclonal antibodies against *Salmonella* typhi OmpC peptide loops. *FEMS Microbiol Lett.* (1996) 141:31–6. doi: 10.1016/0378-1097(96)00200-5
44. Arockiasamy A, Murthy GS, Rukmini MR, Sundara Baalaji N, Katpally UC, Krishnaswamy S. Conformational epitope mapping of OmpC, a major cell surface antigen from *Salmonella* typhi. *J Struct Biol.* (2004) 148:22–33. doi: 10.1016/j.jsb.2004.03.011
45. Cowan SW, Schirmer T, Rummel G, Steiert M, Ghosh R, Pauptit RA, et al. Crystal structures explain functional properties of two *E. coli* porins. *Nature.* (1992) 358:727–33. doi: 10.1038/358727a0

46. Misra R, Benson SA. Genetic identification of the pore domain of the OmpC porin of *Escherichia coli* K-12. *J Bacteriol.* (1988) 170:3611–7. doi: 10.1128/jb.170.8.3611-3617.1988
47. Wiertz EJ, van Gaans-van den Brink JA, Schreuder GM, Termijtelen AA, Hoogerhout P, Poolman JT. T cell recognition of Neisseria meningitidis class 1 outer membrane proteins. Identification of T cell epitopes with selected synthetic peptides and determination of HLA restriction elements. *J Immunol.* (1991) 147:2012–8.
48. Wiertz EJ, van Gaans-van den Brink JA, Gausepohl H, Prochnicka-Chalufour A, Hoogerhout P, Poolman JT. Identification of T cell epitopes occurring in a meningococcal class 1 outer membrane protein using overlapping peptides assembled with simultaneous multiple peptide synthesis. *J Exp Med.* (1992) 176:79–88. doi: 10.1084/jem.176.1.79
49. Isibasi A, Paniagua J, Rojo MP, Martin N, Ramirez G, Gonzalez CR, et al. Role of porins from *Salmonella* typhi in the induction of protective immunity. *Ann N Y Acad Sci.* (1994) 730:350–2. doi: 10.1111/j.1749-6632.1994.tb44289.x
50. Diaz-Quinonez A, Martin-Orozco N, Isibasi A, Ortiz-Navarrete V. Two *Salmonella* OmpC K(b)-restricted epitopes for CD8+-T-cell recognition. *Infect Immun.* (2004) 72:3059–62. doi: 10.1128/IAI.72.5.3059-3062.2004

2

Bacterial RNA Contributes to the Down-Modulation of MHC-II Expression on Monocytes/Macrophages Diminishing CD4$^+$ T Cell Responses

M. Ayelén Milillo[1], Aldana Trotta[1], Agustina Serafino[1], José Luis Marin Franco[1], Fábio V. Marinho[2], Julieta Alcain[1], Melanie Genoula[1], Luciana Balboa[1], Sergio Costa Oliveira[2], Guillermo H. Giambartolomei[3†] and Paula Barrionuevo[1*†]

[1] Instituto de Medicina Experimental (CONICET-Academia Nacional de Medicina), Buenos Aires, Argentina, [2] Departamento de Bioquímica e Imunologia, Universidade Federal de Minas Gerais, Belo Horizonte, Brazil, [3] Instituto de Inmunología, Genética y Metabolismo, Hospital de Clínicas "José de San Martín" (CONICET-UBA), Buenos Aires, Argentina

***Correspondence:**
Paula Barrionuevo
pbarrion2004@yahoo.com.ar

† These authors have contributed equally to this work

Brucella abortus, the causative agent of brucellosis, displays many resources to evade T cell responses conducive to persist inside the host. Our laboratory has previously showed that infection of human monocytes with *B. abortus* down-modulates the IFN-γ-induced MHC-II expression. *Brucella* outer membrane lipoproteins are structural components involved in this phenomenon. Moreover, IL-6 is the soluble factor that mediated MHC-II down-regulation. Yet, the MHC-II down-regulation exerted by lipoproteins was less marked than the one observed as consequence of infection. This led us to postulate that there should be other components associated with viable bacteria that may act together with lipoproteins in order to diminish MHC-II. Our group has recently demonstrated that *B. abortus* RNA (PAMP related to pathogens' viability or *vita*-PAMP) is involved in MHC-I down-regulation. Therefore, in this study we investigated if *B. abortus* RNA could be contributing to the down-regulation of MHC-II. This PAMP significantly down-modulated the IFN-γ-induced MHC-II surface expression on THP-1 cells as well as in primary human monocytes and murine bone marrow macrophages. The expression of other molecules up-regulated by IFN-γ (such as co-stimulatory molecules) was stimulated on monocytes treated with *B. abortus* RNA. This result shows that this PAMP does not alter all IFN-γ-induced molecules globally. We also showed that other bacterial and parasitic RNAs caused MHC-II surface expression down-modulation indicating that this phenomenon is not restricted to *B. abortus*. Moreover, completely degraded RNA was also able to reproduce the phenomenon. MHC-II down-regulation on monocytes treated with RNA and L-Omp19 (a prototypical lipoprotein of *B. abortus*) was more pronounced than in monocytes stimulated with both components separately. We also demonstrated that *B. abortus* RNA along with its lipoproteins decrease MHC-II surface expression predominantly by a mechanism of inhibition of MHC-II expression. Regarding the signaling pathway, we demonstrated that IL-6 is a soluble factor implicated in *B. abortus* RNA and lipoproteins-triggered MHC-II surface down-regulation. Finally, CD4$^+$ T cells functionality was affected as macrophages treated with these components showed lower antigen presentation capacity. Therefore, *B. abortus* RNA and lipoproteins are two PAMPs that contribute to MHC-II down-regulation on monocytes/macrophages diminishing CD4$^+$ T cell responses.

Keywords: ***Brucella abortus*, bacterial RNA, monocytes/macrophages, MHC, antigen presentation/processing**

INTRODUCTION

For several years, the research in brucellosis was focused on understanding how *B. abortus* establishes a persistent infection inside its intracellular niche, the macrophage (1–5). Once inside the macrophage, *B. abortus* traffic through early and late endo/lysosomal compartments where a large percentage of bacteria are promptly eliminated (1, 2). But then, *Brucella* is able to form vacuoles derived from endoplasmic reticulum (ER) where the surviving bacteria begin to replicate dramatically (1, 3, 4). This particular ability of *Brucella* has been considered for years as the key mechanism to evade the immune response and establish a chronic infection. However, is *Brucella* really hidden from adaptive immunity? While *Brucella* is establishing its replicative niche, macrophages are able to present *Brucella*-derived peptides on MHC class I and class II molecules to T lymphocytes. Ratifying this phenomenon, CD4$^+$ and CD8$^+$ T cells have been found against *Brucella* in mouse, cattle, and human infections (6–9). Thus, a relevant question is how *B. abortus* persists in the presence of robust CD4$^+$ and CD8$^+$ T cell responses. Previous results from our laboratory demonstrated that *B. abortus* infection inhibits the IFN-γ-induced surface expression of MHC-II and MHC-I molecules on human monocytes/macrophages (10, 11). Consequently, macrophages infected with *B. abortus* exhibit decreased ability to present antigens to CD4$^+$ and CD8$^+$ T cells, respectively (10–12).

Regarding the MHC-II surface inhibition mediated by *B. abortus*, this phenomenon was also mimicked by HKBA (heat-killed *B. abortus*), suggesting the participation of a *Brucella* structural component (10). In line with this, a prototypical *B. abortus* lipoprotein [outer membrane protein 19 (Omp19)], decreased the surface expression of MHC-II molecules (10). Furthermore, all *Brucella* lipoproteins are capable of inhibiting MHC-II surface expression since Pam_3Cys (a synthetic lipohexapeptide that resemble the protein lipid moiety structure) also inhibited MHC-II expression (10). On the other hand, TLR (Toll-like receptor) 2 was the receptor involved in the MHC-II down-regulation mediated by HKBA or L-Omp19 (lipidated Omp19), and IL-6 was a soluble mediator implicated in this phenomenon (10). Recently we demonstrated that *B. abortus* lipoproteins inhibit MHC-II surface expression by decreasing the transcription of MHC-II genes (13). More specifically, *B. abortus* lipoproteins via IL-6 secretion inhibit the expression and activation of IFN-γ-induced IRF-1, decreasing the transcription of CIITA (the MHC-II master regulator) (13).

Despite the advances in the knowledge of MHC-II down-modulation by *B. abortus*, what specially caught our attention was that HKBA or *B. abortus* lipoproteins were less efficient at reducing IFN-γ-induced MHC-II surface expression than live bacteria (10, 13). Therefore, another component related to bacterial viability must be implicated in the down-modulation of MHC-II molecules. Recently, we have elucidated that the component of *B. abortus* responsible for the diminished MHC-I surface expression is its RNA, a pathogen-associated molecular pattern (PAMP) related to pathogens' viability or *vita*-PAMP (14). Interestingly, RNase-treated *B. abortus* RNA was also capable of inhibiting MHC-I expression to the same degree as native RNA (14). Both the intact molecules as well as the digested products of *B. abortus* RNA inhibit MHC-I surface expression by retaining these molecules within the Golgi apparatus (14). In addition, we demonstrated that *B. abortus* RNA down-modulates the IFN-γ-induced surface expression of MHC-I via TLR8 and by the EGFR signaling pathway (14, 15).

RNA, unlike conventional PAMPs (i.e., lipopolysaccharide, DNA and lipoproteins, among others), is found in viable bacteria but not in dead bacteria (14, 16, 17). Therefore, RNA could be another component involved in the MHC-II down-modulation in the context of *B. abortus* infection. The aim of this study was to investigate whether *B. abortus* RNA is able to modulate the IFN-γ-induced expression of MHC-II on monocytes/macrophages. Once this phenomenon was corroborated, we investigated the mechanisms and soluble mediators whereby *B. abortus* RNA alone or in combination with its lipoproteins was able to generate the inhibition of MHC-II surface expression. Finally, we evaluated if MHC-II down-modulation had biological relevance as we analyzed the antigen presentation of *B. abortus* RNA and lipoproteins-treated macrophages to CD4$^+$ T cells.

MATERIALS AND METHODS

Ethics Statement

In this study, human monocytes from adult blood donors in healthy state were utilized in agreement with the guidelines of the Ethical Committee of IMEX. Donors gave their informed consent before the study. With regard to animals, female mice from C57BL/6 strain were maintained under SPF conditions as previously described (14). All animal procedures were executed according to the rules for the use of laboratory animals of the National Institutes of Health and were authorized by the Animal Care and Use Committee of IMEX.

Bacteria Strains and *Trypanosoma cruzi*

B. abortus S2308, *Escherichia coli* 11105, *Staphylococcus aureus* 25923, and *Klebsiella pneumoniae* 700603 strains were cultivated in tryptose-soy agar in which yeast extract was added (Merck). The amount of bacteria on stationary-phase cultures was determined by the comparison of the OD at 600 nm with a standard curve. The experiments that involved infection of cells with live *Brucella abortus* were performed in biosafety level 3 (BSL-3) facilities, located at the ANLIS-Malbrán (Administración Nacional de Laboratorios e Institutos de Salud, Dr. Carlos G. Malbrán) (Buenos Aires, Argentina). With regard to *T. cruzi*, trypomastigotes from the Brazil strain were cultured overnight in Dulbecco's modified Eagle medium (Mediatech; pH 5.0), to transform trypomastigotes to amastigotes, as previously described (18).

Expression and Purification of *B. abortus* Recombinant Lipidated Omp19 (L-Omp19)

Lipoproteins were expressed in *E. coli* BL21 and purified as it was previously described (19). The final preparations contained <0.25 LPS U/μg of protein, determined by Limulus Amebocyte Lysate assay (Lonza). The purified proteins were kept at −80°C until use.

Cell Cultures

All the experiments were carried out in an incubator at 37°C and in an atmosphere with 5% CO_2. The standard medium used was composed of RPMI 1640 supplemented with 25 mM Hepes, 2 mM L-glutamine, 10% heat-inactivated fetal bovine serum (Gibco), 100 U of penicillin.ml^{-1} and 100 μg of streptomycin.ml^{-1}. Cells from the monocytic line THP-1, were purchased from the American Type Culture Collection (ATCC, Manassas, VA) and cultured as it was formerly described (19). In order to induce differentiation to monocytes, THP-1 cells at 5×10^5.ml^{-1} were cultured in 0.05 μM 1,25-dihydroxyvitamin D3 (EMD Millipore) for 72 h. In the experiments with primary human monocytes, peripheral blood mononuclear cells (PBMCs) were isolated by Ficoll-Hypaque gradient (GE Healthcare) centrifugation. Monocytes were purified from PBMCs by Percoll gradient (GE Healthcare) as previously described (10). To induce monocyte-derived DCs, monocytes were cultured at 2×10^6 cell/ml under a humidified atmosphere of 5% CO_2 at 37°C in standard medium supplemented with 50 ng/ml recombinant granulocyte-monocyte colony stimulating factor (GM-CSF) (Peprotech) and 10 ng/ml recombinant IL-4 (Prepotech) as described elsewhere (20). Bone marrow progenitors from C57BL/6 female mice were differentiated to mouse bone marrow-derived macrophages (BMDM) with recombinant monocyte colony stimulating factor (M-CSF) (PeproTech). These cells were then cultured as previously described (21).

Viability Assay

In order to determine cellular apoptosis, 5×10^5.ml^{-1} THP-1 cells were treated with *B. abortus* RNA, RNase-I-treated *B. abortus* RNA, L-Omp19 or their combination plus IFN-γ (Endogen) for 48 h. Cells treated with 2% paraformaldehyde (PFA) were included as a positive control of the technique. After 48 h, cells were washed and stained with 7-Amino-Actinomycin D (7-AAD; BD Biosciences) for 10 min at 0°C in darkness. Immediately after, cells were analyzed on a FACSCalibur® flow cytometer (BD Biosciences) or Sysmex Partec Cytometer (Sysmex Partec GmbH, Germany) and data were processed using FlowJo® 7.6 software.

RNA Preparation

5×10^8 CFU, 1×10^7 amastigotes or $5–10 \times 10^6$ PBMCs were suspended in 1 ml of Trizol Reagent (Invitrogen) and total RNA was isolated with *Quick*-RNA™ MiniPrep (Zymo Research) according to the manufacturer's instructions. RNA was quantified with OD at 260. The purity of the preparation was determined using a DeNovix DS-11 Spectrophotometer (DeNovix Inc.) with a ratio of absorbance 260/280 >2.0 and a ratio of absorbance 260/230 > 1.8. To exclude the potential effect of *B. abortus* DNA, some RNA preparations were incubated with DNase I (1 U/μg of RNA; Promega Corporation) in a buffer containing 400 mM Tris-HCl (pH 8.0), 100 mM $MgSO_4$, and 10 mM $CaCl_2$ for 30 min at 37°C and the reaction was stopped by addition of 20 mM EGTA and incubation for 10 min at 65°C. Additionally, to rule out the effect of *B. abortus* proteins in the effects mediated by *B. abortus* RNA, our preparations were treated with Proteinase K (200 μg/mL, Promega Corporation) for 60 min at 37°C, and the digestion was stopped by incubation at 96°C for 10 min.

In vitro Stimulation

Cells at 5×10^5.ml^{-1} were treated with *B. abortus* RNA, other prokaryotic or eukaryotic RNAs, *E. coli* RNase I (Life Technologies)-treated *B. abortus* RNA or *B. abortus* lipoproteins in the presence of 150 U.ml^{-1} IFN-γ for 48 h as it was formerly described (14). MHC-II, MHC-I, CD40, CD86, or CD80 expressions were assessed by flow cytometry. In the experiments that involved murine macrophages, BMDM were treated with different doses of *B. abortus* RNA in presence of 10 ng.ml^{-1} recombinant murine IFN-γ (PeproTech) for 48 h. Murine MHC-II expression was assessed by flow cytometry.

Cells Infection With *B. abortus*

5×10^5.ml^{-1} THP-1 were infected with a multiplicity of infection (MOI) of 100 *B. abortus* S2308 per cell in round-bottom polypropylene tubes (Falcon). This procedure was performed with 150 U.ml^{-1} IFN-γ for 2 h in standard medium without antibiotics. Afterwards, cells were extensively washed in order to remove uninternalized bacteria. Infected cells were maintained in culture in presence of IFN-γ, 100 μg.ml^{-1} gentamicin, and 50 μg.ml^{-1} streptomycin for other 48 h.

Influence of IL-6 on MHC-II Expression

In another set of experiments, 5×10^5.ml^{-1} THP-1 were incubated in presence of 150 U.ml^{-1} IFN-γ, *B. abortus* RNA (10 μg.ml^{-1}) and *B. abortus* L-Omp19 (1 μg.ml^{-1}) in the presence of neutralizing mAb for IL-6 (clone MQ2-13A5; eBioscience) or the isotype control at a concentration of 20 ng.ml^{-1}. After this, MHC-II expression was assessed by flow cytometry.

Flow Cytometry

Once *B. abortus* infection or stimulation of cells were performed, monocytes were stained with PE-labeled anti-human HLA-DR (clone L243, BD Pharmingen), FITC-labeled anti-human HLA-ABC (clone G46-2.6; BD Pharmingen) or isotype-matched control mAbs. To evaluate MHC-II expression, MHC-II bar graphs were performed on the MHC-II positive cells. In order to evaluate murine MHC-II surface expression, BMDMs were stained with PE-labeled anti-mouse MHC-II (I-A/I-E) (clone M5/114.15.2; e-Bioscience). To determine CD40, CD86, and CD80 surface expressions, in another set of experiments cells were stained with PE-labeled anti-human CD40 (clone 5C3; Biolegend), PE-labeled anti-human CD86 (clone IT2.2; BD) or FITC-labeled anti-human CD80 (clone 2D10; Biolegend). In all cases, monocytes were stained with 7-AAD for 10 min at 0°C in darkness. After that, all markers studied were analyzed on a FACSCalibur® flow cytometer (BD Biosciences) or Sysmex Partec Cytometer (Sysmex Partec GmbH, Germany), gating on viable cells (7-AAD negative cells). Data were processed using FlowJo® 7.6 software.

Confocal Microscopy Experiments

Confocal micrographs were performed as previously described (11). Briefly, 2 × 10^5 THP-1 cells/well were incubated in chamber-slides (Nunc) with 10 ng/ml PMA (Sigma-Aldrich) for 24 h to promote adherence. Then, cells were stimulated with *B. abortus* RNA (10 $\mu g.ml^{-1}$), RNase I-treated *B. abortus* RNA, *B. abortus* L-Omp19 (1 $\mu g.ml^{-1}$) or their combination with IFN-γ for 48 h. Afterwards, cells were treated with 2% PFA, permeabilized with 0.1% saponin and incubated with anti-HLA-DR mAb L243 (purified from murine hybridoma culture supernatants) and Alexa 546-labeled secondary Ab (Invitrogen). In order to detect Golgi apparatus, cells were labeled with a mAb specific for GM130 (BD Biosciences) followed by Alexa 488-labeled secondary Ab (Invitrogen). Then, slides were mounted and analyzed with a FV-1000 confocal microscope, as it was previously described (14).

Ag Presentation Assay

MHC class II-restricted response to OVA was assessed using the T cell hybridoma BO97.10, specific for OVA323-339 peptide on I-Ab on macrophages. BMDMs were stimulated with the different components in presence of murine IFN-γ for 48 h. Afterwards, these cells were exposed to OVA (100 μg/ml) for 3 h at 37°C. After washing, cells were suspended in complete medium at pH 7.3 and BO97.10 cells were added for 20 h. The production of IL-2 by BO97.10 was measured by ELISA (RD) as described previously (22).

Reagents

Neutralizing monoclonal antibody for human IL-6 (clone MQ2-13A5) was acquired from eBioscience.

Measurement of IL-6 Secretion

Human IL-6 was measured in culture supernatants by sandwich ELISA, as it was formerly described (19).

Statistical Analysis

Results were analyzed with one-way ANOVA followed by *post hoc* Tukey test or two-way ANOVA followed by *post hoc* Bonferroni test with GraphPad Prism software.

RESULTS

B. abortus RNA Participates in the Down-Modulation of IFN-γ-Induced MHC-II Surface Expression by Preventing the Up-Regulation of These Molecules

We evaluated if *B. abortus* RNA was a *vita*-PAMP involved in MHC-II down-regulation. For this purpose, cells from the human monocytic cell line THP-1 were stimulated with *B. abortus* RNA at several doses and in presence of human IFN-γ for 48 h. Then, the surface expression of MHC-II molecules was assessed by flow cytometry. This PAMP was able to diminish the IFN-γ-up-regulated MHC-II surface expression (**Figures 1A,B**), as it was previously seen in *B. abortus*-infected monocytes (10, 13). Moreover, we distinguished cells expressing MHC-II (MHC-II positive cells) or not (MHC-II null cells) (**Figure 1A**). We observed that *B. abortus* RNA decreases the MFI of MHC-II molecules within the MHC-II-expressing population (**Figures 1A,B**) and slightly increases the non-expressing population in a dose-dependent manner (**Figure 1C**). Since some phenol remains could still appear in RNA preparations, we performed a mock RNA extraction (i.e., in the absence of bacteria), and used it as a control. MHC-II expression was not altered due to the Trizol products (**Figure 1A**). We also performed experiments digesting our RNA preparations with DNase and Proteinase K. Then, we evaluated the effect of these preparations on MHC-II expression. Our results demonstrated that the preparations of DNase- and Proteinase K-digested RNA were able to inhibit MHC-II expression in the same way as intact RNA, indicating that potential contaminating DNA and proteins do not mediate the phenomenon of MHC-II inhibition (**Figures S1A,B** in Supplementary Material). In accordance with our published results (14), MHC-I was down-modulated by *B. abortus* RNA as well (**Figure 1D**). In order to rule out that MHC-II down-modulation was not due to cell apoptosis, we performed all the experiments gating on viable cells (7-AAD negative cells). Moreover, we confirmed that *B. abortus* RNA treatment did not change the percentage of viable cells (**Figure S2**). On the contrary, when cells were treated with paraformaldehyde (PFA), high percentages of non-viable cells were found (**Figure S2**). Next, we performed two sets of experiments to understand the exact mechanism by which *B. abortus* RNA down-regulates the IFN-γ-induced expression of MHC-II molecules, i.e., whether *B. abortus* RNA prevents the induction of MHC-II molecules by IFN-γ or it is able to modulate the MHC-II molecules once they are already induced by IFN-γ. We evaluate whether *B. abortus* RNA delayed the kinetic of MHC-II induction by IFN-γ and we evaluate if *B. abortus* RNA is able to down-regulate the MHC-II expression already induced by IFN-γ. For this, THP-1 cells were incubated with *B. abortus* RNA and IFN-γ for 48, 72, and 96 h. In addition, THP-1 cells were pre-incubated with IFN-γ for 24 h to induce MHC-II expression and then were stimulated with *B. abortus* RNA for additional 24 h. *B. abortus* RNA neither delays the kinetic of IFN-γ induction of MHC-II molecules (**Figure S3A**) nor it modifies the expression of MHC-II

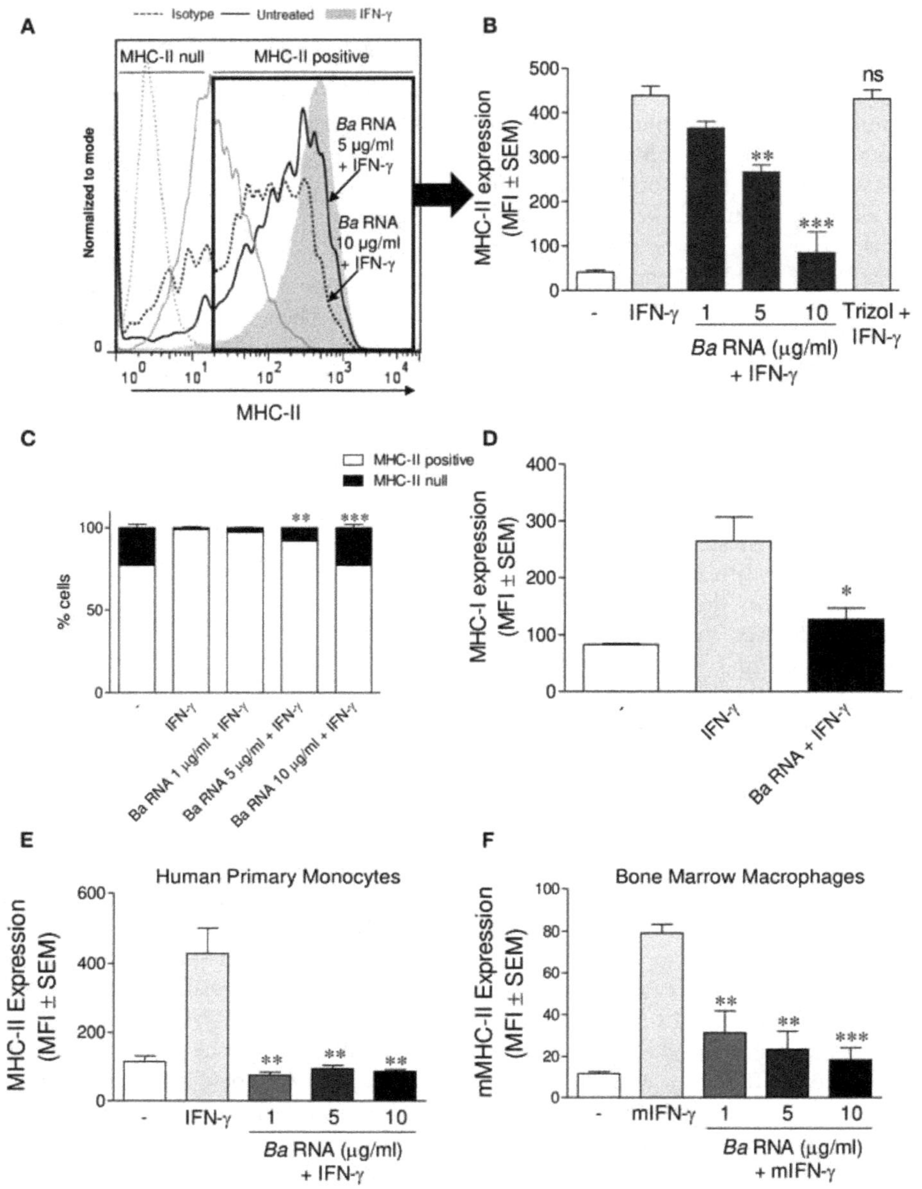

FIGURE 1 | *B. abortus* RNA down-modulates MHC-II on monocytes/macrophages. **(A,B)** THP-1 cells were treated with different doses of *B. abortus* RNA in the presence of IFN-γ for 48 h. MHC-II expression was evaluated by flow cytometry. **(A)** Flow cytometry histograms (showing MHC-II positive and null cells) representative of bars showed in **(B)**. **(B)** Bars represent the arithmetic means ± SEM of MHC-II positive cells corresponding to five independent experiments. Trizol extracted products in the absence of bacteria were used as a control. **(C)** Quantification of cells expressing MHC-II (MHC-II positive cells) or not (MHC-II null). Data is expressed as the percentage of cells ± SEM of three independent experiments. **(D)** THP-1 cells were treated with *B. abortus* RNA (10 μg/ml) in the presence of IFN-γ for 48 h. MHC-I expression was evaluated by flow cytometry. **(E,F)** Peripheral blood-purified monocytes **(E)** and bone marrow macrophages **(F)** were stimulated with different doses of *B. abortus* RNA in the presence of IFN-γ for 48 h. MHC-II expression was assessed by flow cytometry. Bars represent the arithmetic means ± SEM of five independent experiments. MFI, mean fluorescence intensity; mIFN-γ, murine IFN-γ. ns, non-significant. $^{*}P < 0.05$; $^{**}P < 0.01$; $^{***}P < 0.001$ vs. IFN-γ-treated cells.

molecules already induced by IFN-γ (**Figure S3B**). Moreover, to evaluate the effects of RNA on the basal expression of MHC-II, THP-1 cells were stimulated with *B. abortus* RNA in the absence of IFN-γ. *B. abortus* RNA was not able to down-modulate the basal expression of MHC-II (**Figure S3C**). Altogether, these results demonstrate that *B. abortus* RNA prevents the correct induction of MHC-II molecules by IFN-γ. Then, we searched if the MHC-II down-modulation could be reproduced in primary cultures of monocytes/macrophages. To achieve this, peripheral blood-isolated human monocytes or murine bone marrow-derived macrophages (BMDM) were stimulated with *B. abortus* RNA at several doses. Afterwards, MHC-II surface expression was evaluated by flow cytometry. *B. abortus* RNA was able to significantly down-modulate the IFN-γ-induced MHC-II expression on both primary cell cultures (**Figures 1E,F**). Thus, *B. abortus* RNA-mediated MHC-II down-modulation could be

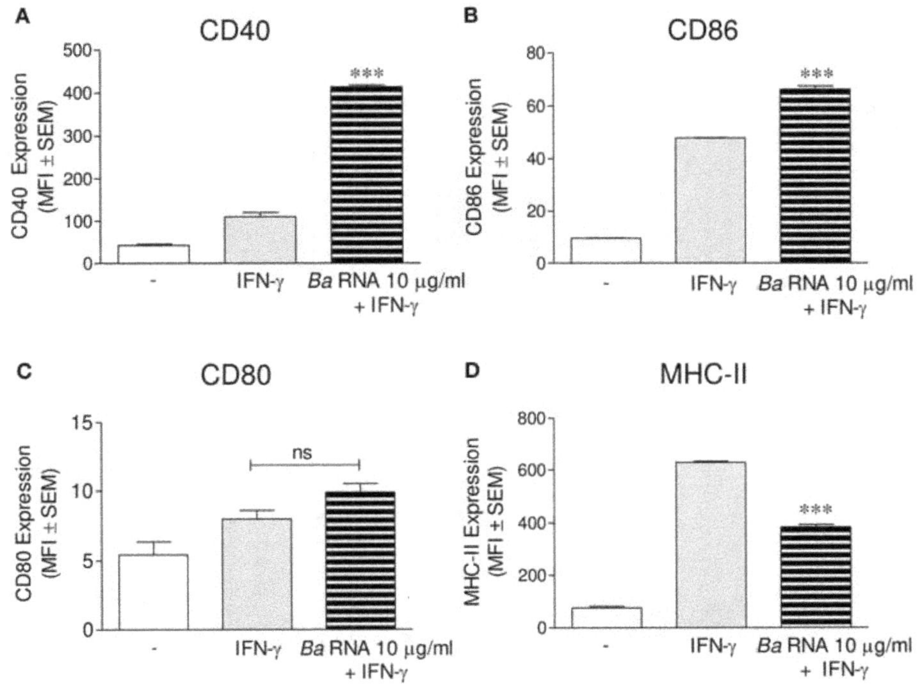

FIGURE 2 | *B. abortus* RNA does not down-modulate co-stimulatory molecules. **(A–D)** THP-1 cells were treated with *B. abortus* RNA (10 μg/ml) in the presence of IFN-γ for 48 h. CD40 **(A)**, CD86 **(B)**, and CD80 **(C)** expressions were assessed by flow cytometry. MHC-II expression was determined as a control **(D)**. Bars represent the arithmetic means ± SEM of five independent experiments. MFI, mean fluorescence intensity; ns, non-significant. $^{***}P < 0.001$ vs. IFN-γ-treated cells.

reproduced in different monocytes/macrophages cell cultures. Finally, we evaluated whether the down-modulation of IFN-γ-induced MHC-II and MHC-I surface expression mediated by *B. abortus* RNA was an exclusive phenomenon on MHC molecules or could be extended to other IFN-γ-induced molecules. To do this, THP-1 cells were treated with *B. abortus* RNA as we previously described. Then, the expression of the co-stimulatory molecules CD40, CD86, and CD80 was evaluated by flow cytometry. The expression of CD40 and CD86 was significantly increased in *B. abortus* RNA-treated monocytes (**Figures 2A,B**), while it did not affect the expression of CD80 compared to the cells treated only with IFN-γ (**Figure 2C**). The expression of MHC-II was evaluated in parallel as a control (**Figure 2D**). These results demonstrate that *B. abortus* RNA-mediated MHC inhibition is specific for these molecules, since this PAMP does not alter all IFN-γ-induced molecules globally. In conclusion, these results indicate that *B. abortus* RNA is a PAMP related to bacterial viability, which is implicated in the down-modulation of IFN-γ-induced MHC-II surface expression on monocytes/macrophages observed during *B. abortus* infection.

MHC-II Down-Modulation Could Be Extended to RNAs From Other Microorganisms

We next investigated whether the ability of *B. abortus* RNA to diminish the expression of MHC-II was an exclusive characteristic of the RNA of this bacterium or if it could be extended to RNAs of other microorganisms. To elucidate this, we purified RNA from *Klebsiella pneumoniae*, *Staphylococcus aureus*, and *Escherichia coli*. THP-1 cells were stimulated with these RNAs plus IFN-γ for 48 h. Afterwards, MHC-II surface expression was assessed by flow cytometry. All prokaryotic RNAs evaluated were able to inhibit MHC-II surface expression (**Figure 3A**). Furthermore, RNA purified from a parasite (*Trypanosoma cruzi*) was also able to decrease the surface expression of MHC-II (**Figure 3A**). However, even the maximum dose of peripheral blood mononuclear cells (PBMCs) RNA was incapable of down-modulating MHC-II surface expression (**Figure 3B**). Taken together, these results show that MHC-II surface expression inhibition is not restricted to *B. abortus* RNA. Nevertheless, human RNA does not affect MHC-II expression.

Completely Digested RNA Was Also Able to Down-Modulate MHC-II Expression

We next investigated if *B. abortus* RNA degradation products could also be implicated in MHC-II down-regulation, as they participate in MHC-I down modulation as well (14). For this, *B. abortus* RNA was treated with *E.coli* RNase I prior to stimulation of THP-1 cells in the presence of IFN-γ as we formerly described. As previously showed, the integrity of RNase-digested RNA is completely lost (14). Moreover, this digested RNA was able to down-modulate the IFN-γ-induced MHC-II surface expression to the same degree as non-digested RNA (**Figure 4**). As shown before, down-regulation of MHC-II was not the effect of the loss of live cells in RNase I-digested RNA stimulated cells, since this treatment did not change the percentage of viable

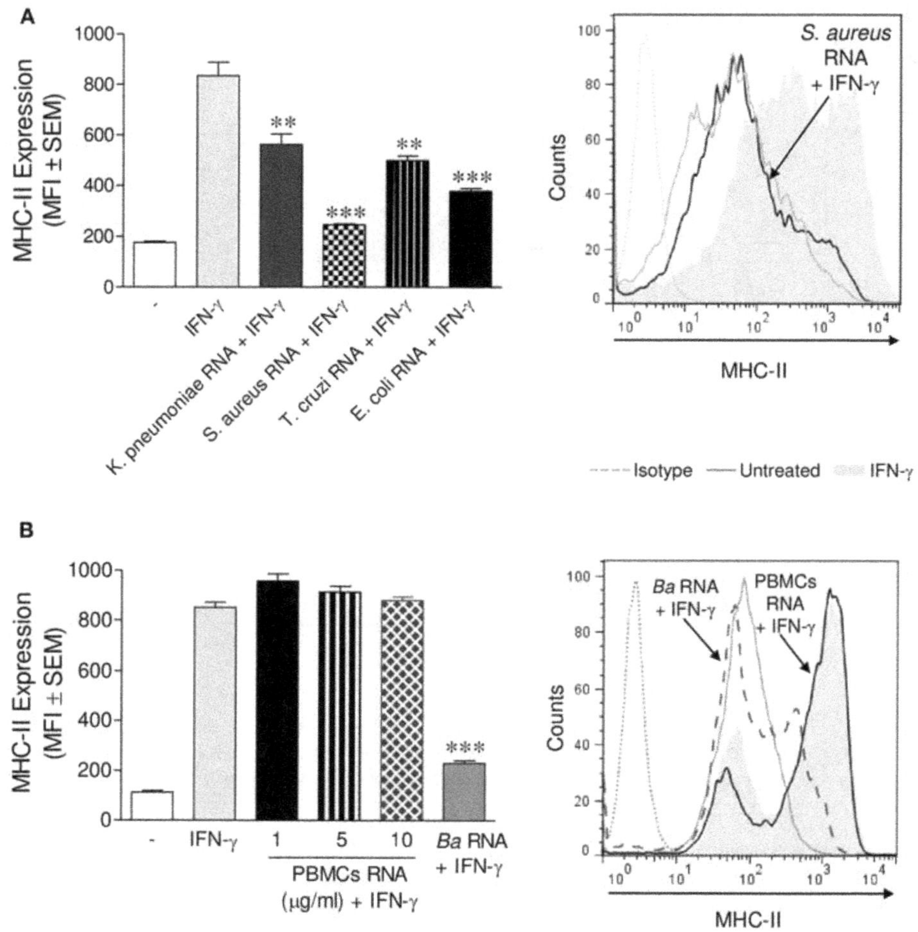

FIGURE 3 | MHC-II down-modulation could be extended to RNAs from different microorganisms. **(A)** THP-1 cells were treated with RNAs from *K. pneumoniae*, *S. aureus*, *E. coli*, and *T. cruzi* (10 μg/ml) in the presence of IFN-γ for 48 h. **(B)** THP-1 cells were treated with different doses of PBMCs RNA in the presence of IFN-γ for 48 h. *B. abortus* RNA (10 μg/ml)-treated cells were used as a control. MHC-II expression was assessed by flow cytometry. Bars represent the arithmetic means ± SEM of five independent experiments. MFI, mean fluorescence intensity. $^{**}P < 0.01$; $^{***}P < 0.001$ vs. IFN-γ-treated cells.

cells (**Figure S2**). In addition, THP-1 cells treated with RNase I had not changes in MHC-II expression compared to IFN-γ-only-treated cells (**Figure 4**). Globally, these results show that *B. abortus* RNA as well as its degradation products contribute to the MHC-II down-modulation mediated by *B. abortus*.

B. abortus RNA Along With Its Lipoproteins Mediate the MHC-II Down-Modulation Observed in *B. abortus* Infection

Taking into account that *B. abortus* lipoproteins (10, 13) and its RNA are components involved in the decrease of MHC-II surface expression, we wondered whether these components had a synergistic effect on MHC-II expression. For this, THP-1 cells were stimulated with *B. abortus* RNA, digested *B. abortus* RNA, the prototypical *B. abortus* lipoprotein L-Omp19 or the combination of each component in presence of IFN-γ for 48 h. MHC-II expression was assessed by flow cytometry. Again, MHC-II down-modulation was not due to the loss of viability in cells stimulated with L-Omp19 or with the combination of each component, since the percentage of viable cells did not change when compared to untreated cells (**Figure S2**). As it has been shown in **Figure 4**, *B. abortus* RNA and digested RNA were able to down-modulate MHC-II surface expression at similar levels (**Figure 5A**). L-Omp19 could also decrease the MHC-II expression induced by IFN-γ to the values of *B. abortus* RNA or its degradation products (**Figure 5A**). Furthermore, the combination of RNA and L-Omp19 induced a higher MHC-II down-modulation than merely RNA or L-Omp19 (**Figure 5A**). A similar effect was observed with the combination of digested *B. abortus* RNA and L-Omp19 (**Figure 5A**). Moreover, the combination of *B. abortus* RNA and L-Omp19 as well as digested *B. abortus* RNA and L-Omp19 showed MHC-II expression values similar to those obtained with THP-1 cells infected with *B. abortus* (**Figure 5A**). Taking into account that TLR8 is able to sense not only intact RNA but also RNA degradation products (23); and that we have previously demonstrated, that the down-modulation of MHC-I surface expression by intact and digested RNA is mediated by this receptor, we wanted to evaluate the participation of

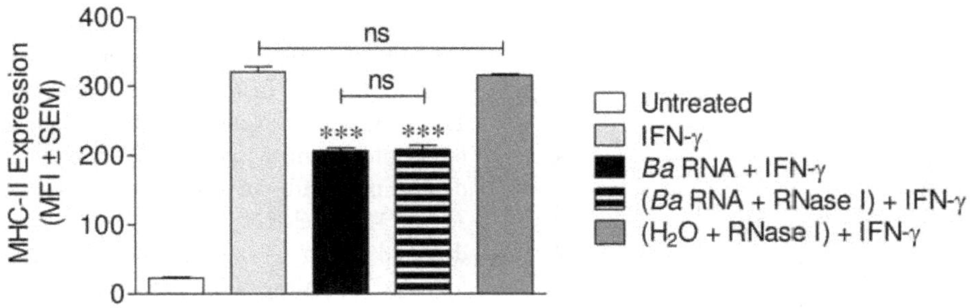

FIGURE 4 | Digested-*B. abortus* RNA is also able to down-modulate MHC-II. THP-1 cells were treated with *B. abortus* RNA (10 μg/ml) or RNase I-treated *B. abortus* RNA in the presence of IFN-γ for 48 h. Cells treated with RNase I were used as a control. MHC-II expression was assessed by flow cytometry. Bars represent the arithmetic means ± SEM of five independent experiments. MFI, mean fluorescence intensity; ns, non-significant. $^{***}P < 0.001$ vs. IFN-γ-treated cells.

TLR8 in *B. abortus* RNA and L-Omp19-mediated MHC-II down-modulation. Other researchers have demonstrated that in THP-1 cells, the pre-exposure to TLR8 ligands augments the response to a posterior stimulation with TLR2 ligands (24, 25). So, to evaluate the TLR8 involvement in *B. abortus* RNA and L-Omp19-mediated MHC-II down-modulation, THP-1 cells were pre-exposed to *B. abortus* RNA and then stimulated with L-Omp19 in the presence of IFN-γ. These results were compared to those obtained with simultaneous incubation with *B. abortus* RNA and L-Omp19 in the presence of IFN-γ. We observed a greater MHC-II down-regulation in cells pre-exposed to *B. abortus* RNA and then stimulated with L-Omp19 compared to cells that received both ligands simultaneously (**Figure 5B**). These results demonstrated that monocytes pre-exposed to TLR8 ligands are more responsive to TLR2 ligands. Overall, these results indicate that *B. abortus* RNA (viability-associated component) and *B. abortus* lipoproteins (structural components) constitute both *Brucella* virulence factors which contribute to MHC-II down-modulation in the context of the infection.

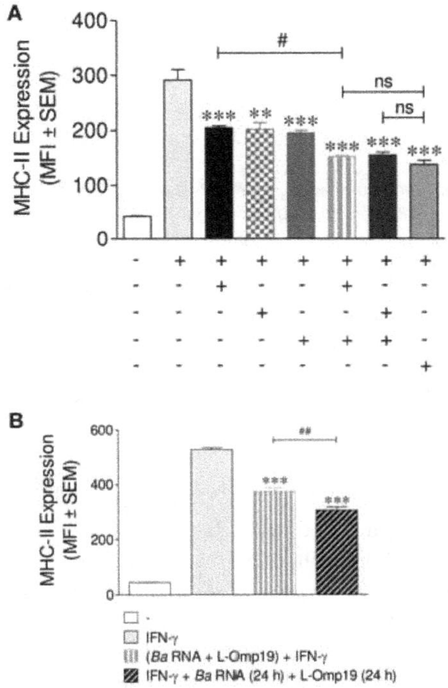

FIGURE 5 | *B. abortus* RNA and *B. abortus* L-Omp19 act synergistically in MHC-II inhibition. **(A)** THP-1 cells were infected with *B. abortus* (MOI 100:1) or treated with *B. abortus* RNA (10 μg/ml), digested *B. abortus* RNA, L-Omp19 (1 μg/ml) or their combination in the presence of IFN-γ for 48 h. **(B)** THP-1 cells were treated with IFN-γ and *B. abortus* RNA (5 μg/ml) for 24 h. Afterwards, L-Omp19 (1 μg/ml) was added for other 24 h. THP-1 cells treated with both stimuli simultaneously were used as control. MHC-II expression was assessed by flow cytometry. Bars represent the arithmetic means ± SEM of five independent experiments. MFI, mean fluorescence intensity; ns, non-significant. $^{**}P < 0.05$; $^{***}P < 0.001$ vs. IFN-γ-treated cells; $^{\#}P < 0.05$ vs. *Ba* RNA + IFN-γ; $^{\#\#}P < 0.01$ vs. (*Ba* RNA + L-Omp19) + IFN-γ.

IFN-γ-Induced MHC-II Surface Down-Regulation Mediated by *B. abortus* RNA and Its Lipoproteins Occurs at Late Time Points During Infection

Next, we wanted to evaluate the mechanism by which *B. abortus* RNA alone or together with lipoproteins was down-modulating MHC-II expression. Therefore, at first, we evaluated MHC-II down-regulation kinetics. In order to perform this, THP-1 cells were stimulated as previously described, with *B. abortus* RNA, RNase I-treated *B. abortus* RNA, the *B. abortus* lipoprotein L-Omp19 or the combination of each component in the presence of IFN-γ. At 6, 24, and 48 h, the surface expression of MHC-II was evaluated by flow cytometry. At 6 h, there is neither up-regulation of MHC-II on IFN-γ-treated cells nor MHC-II modulation with the different stimuli. However, at 24 h MHC-II expression on IFN-γ-treated cells is induced, being even accentuated at 48 h. At 24 h, L-Omp19 (but not *B. abortus* RNA and digested *B. abortus* RNA) significantly down-regulated MHC-II surface expression. Meanwhile at 48 h, *B. abortus* RNA, digested *B. abortus* RNA and L-Omp19 were able to significantly inhibit the MHC-II surface expression (**Figure 6**). Furthermore, at both times, as shown in **Figure 5A**, the combination of RNA (or digested *B. abortus* RNA) plus L-Omp19 induced a higher MHC-II down-modulation than merely RNA, digested RNA or L-Omp19 (**Figure 6**). We also demonstrate that *B. abortus* RNA

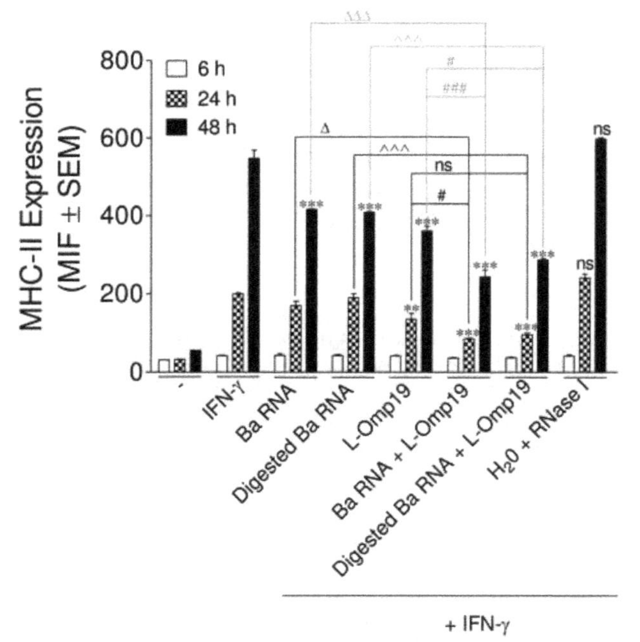

FIGURE 6 | MHC-II down-modulation begins after 24 h post-stimuli. THP-1 cells were treated with *B. abortus* RNA (10 μg/ml), digested *B. abortus* RNA, L-Omp19 (1 μg/ml) or their combination in the presence of IFN-γ for 6, 24, and 48 h. Cells treated with RNase I were used as a control. MHC-II expression was assessed by flow cytometry. Bars represent the arithmetic means ± SEM of five independent experiments. MFI, mean fluorescence intensity; ns, non-significant. $^{**}P < 0.01$; $^{***}P < 0.001$ vs. IFN-γ-treated cells; $^{\Delta}P < 0.05$; $^{\Delta\Delta\Delta}P < 0.001$ vs. *Ba* RNA; $^{\wedge\wedge\wedge}P < 0.001$ vs. Digested *Ba* RNA; $^{\#}P < 0.05$; $^{\#\#\#}P < 0.001$ vs. L-Omp19.

induced the expression of MHC-II on DCs (**Figure S4A**) and down-regulated the LPS-induced MHC-II expression on human monocytes (**Figure S4B**). Overall, these results demonstrate that *B. abortus* RNA, digested *B. abortus* RNA, and L-Omp19 alone or together decrease MHC-II only when these molecules are induced by a MHC-II up-regulator, such as IFN-γ. In turn, they show that when the induction of MHC-II mediated by IFN-γ is the highest (which is observed after 48 h post stimulation) the greater the degree of MHC-II surface inhibition generated by the components.

B. abortus RNA Along With Its Lipoproteins Decrease MHC-II Surface Expression Predominantly by a Mechanism of Inhibition of MHC-II Expression

Once the kinetics of MHC-II down modulation has been established, we then wondered the mechanism of this phenomenon. We have previously shown that lipoproteins of *B. abortus* decreased MHC-II expression by inhibiting MHC-II genes transcription (13). More recently, we demonstrated that *B. abortus* RNA down-modulates MHC-I by retaining them inside the Golgi apparatus rather than by transcriptional inhibition as occurred with MHC-II (14). So, we wanted to understand why *B. abortus* RNA alone or together with lipoproteins is able to down-modulate MHC-II. To do this, THP-1 cells were stimulated with *B. abortus* RNA, RNase I-treated *B. abortus* RNA, L-Omp19 or the combination of each component in the presence of IFN-γ for 6, 24, and 48 h. Then, MHC-II expression and localization were evaluated by confocal microscopy. The expression of MHC-II was determined with an anti-human MHC-II mAb followed by Alexa 546-labeled secondary antibody. Golgi apparatus was detected using a monoclonal antibody specific for GM130 followed by Alexa 488-labeled secondary Ab. In accordance with the kinetics results, at 6 h almost no MHC-II expression is observed under any condition (data not shown). At 24 h, IFN-γ-treated cells showed up-regulation of MHC-II surface expression. However, there was not a significant reduction on MHC-II expression mediated by *B. abortus* RNA, digested *B. abortus* RNA, L-Omp19 or their combination (data not shown). At 48 h, two populations were observed: cells with MHC-II expression confined to the cellular surface (named MHC-II-positive cells) and cells with no MHC-II expression on the cellular surface (named MHC-II null cells). As expected, the majority of the cells were MHC-II positive in IFN-γ-treated cells (**Figures 7A,B** and **Figure S5**). When cells were treated with *B. abortus* RNA and digested RNA, there was an increase in the number of MHC-II null cells. The same phenomenon was observed with L-Omp19. In addition, when the components were combined, the percentage of MHC-II null cells was even higher. As expected, the cells treated with IFN-γ and merely RNase I behaved similarly to those treated only with IFN-γ (**Figures 7A,B**).

Given the fact that MHC-II null cells are responsible for the down-modulation in MHC-II surface expression that we previously observed in the flow cytometry experiments, we wondered what mechanisms were causing this absence of MHC-II surface expression. Consequently, inside the MHC-II null population, we calculated the percentage of cells with MHC-II retained within the Golgi apparatus and the percentage of cells with no expression of MHC-II inside the cell at all. Cells treated with *B. abortus* RNA and digested RNA showed mainly a reduction in MHC-II intracellular expression although 17% of cells had MHC-II retained in Golgi apparatus (**Figures 7A,C** and **Figure S5**). However, when *B. abortus* RNA or digested RNA were combined with L-Omp19, the percentage of Golgi apparatus retention decreases to the values obtained for L-Omp19 alone (**Figures 7A,C**).

Taken together, these results demonstrate that there are two possible mechanisms involved in the down-modulation of MHC-II surface expression on monocytes/macrophages. However, the inhibition of MHC-II expression is the prevalent mechanism when cells are treated with *B. abortus* RNA together with lipoproteins.

IL-6 Is Involved in MHC-II Down-Modulation Mediated by *B. abortus* RNA and Its Lipoproteins

B. abortus lipoproteins mediate the down-regulation of MHC-II genes transcription, at least in part, via IL-6, as we previously

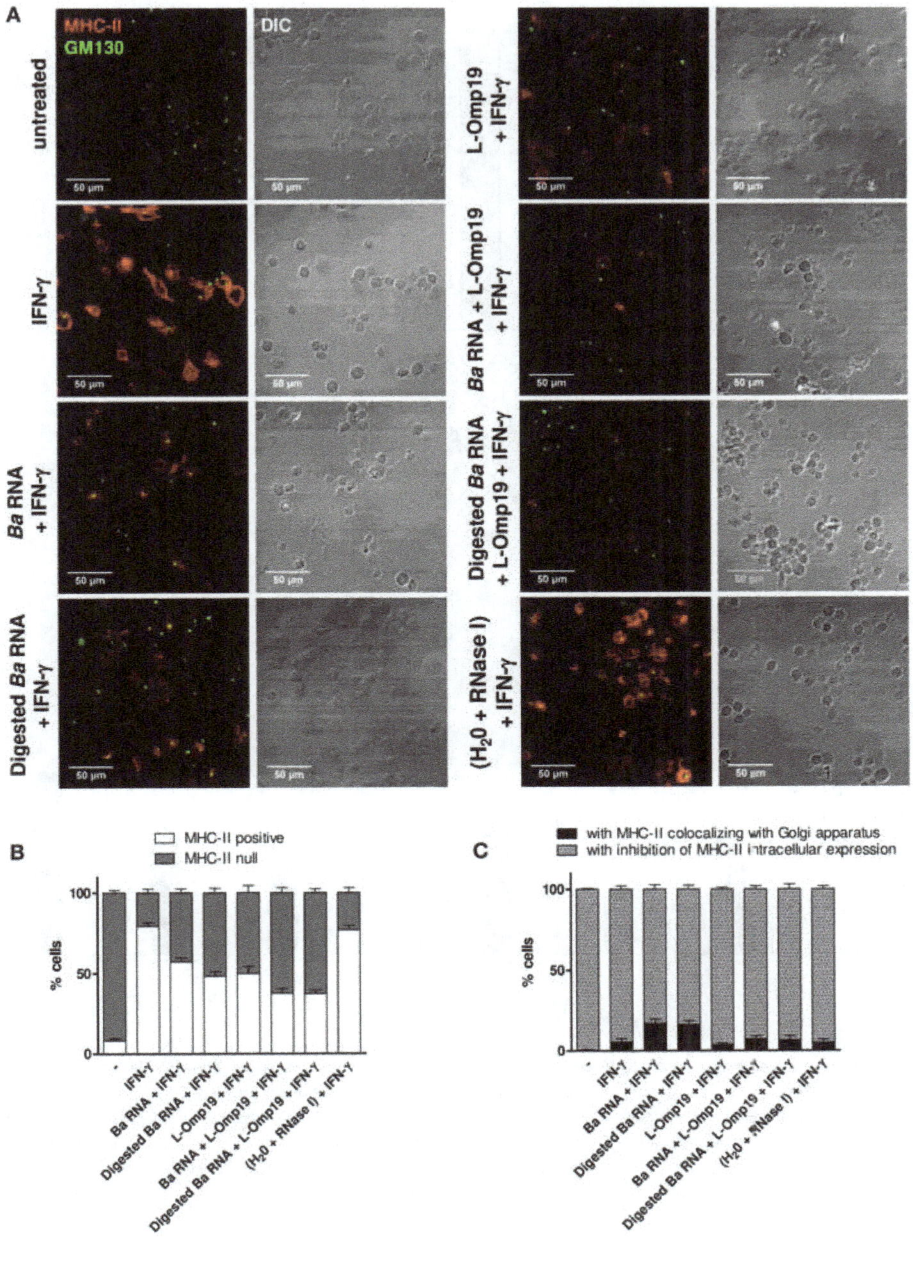

FIGURE 7 | *B. abortus* RNA and digested *B. abortus* RNA inhibit MHC-II expression on and inside the cells. **(A)** Confocal micrographs of THP-1 cells treated with *B. abortus* RNA (10 μg/ml), digested *B. abortus* RNA, L-Omp19 (1 μg/ml) or their combination in the presence of IFN-γ for 48 h. Cells treated with RNase I were used as a control. MHC-II was detected with a primary anti-human MHC-II Ab (L243) followed by Alexa 546-labeled secondary Ab (red). Golgi apparatus was detected using a mAb specific for GM130 followed by Alexa 488-labeled secondary Ab (green). Results are representative of three independent experiments. **(B)** Quantification of cells expressing MHC-II (MHC-II positive cells) or not (MHC-II null). Data is expressed as the percentage of cells ± SEM of three independent experiments. **(C)** Quantification of null cells with MHC-II colocalizing with Golgi apparatus or with inhibition of intracellular MHC-II expression. Data is expressed as the percentage of cells ± SEM of three independent experiments. The number of cells counted per experimental group was 200. DIC, differential interference contrast.

reported (13). As consequence, and given the fact that the main mechanism by which *B. abortus* RNA (alone or together with lipoproteins) down-modulates MHC-II surface expression is the inhibition of MHC-II inside the cell, we tested whether IL-6 could be a possible mediator in this phenomenon. In order to perform this, THP-1 monocytes were stimulated with *B. abortus* RNA, RNase I-treated *B. abortus* RNA, L-Omp19 or a combination of each component in the presence of IFN-γ for 48 h. Afterwards, secreted IL-6 was measured in the supernatants by ELISA sandwich. As previously demonstrated, L-Omp19 stimulates the secretion of IL-6 (**Figure 8A**). This cytokine was induced by *B. abortus* RNA and digested *B. abortus*

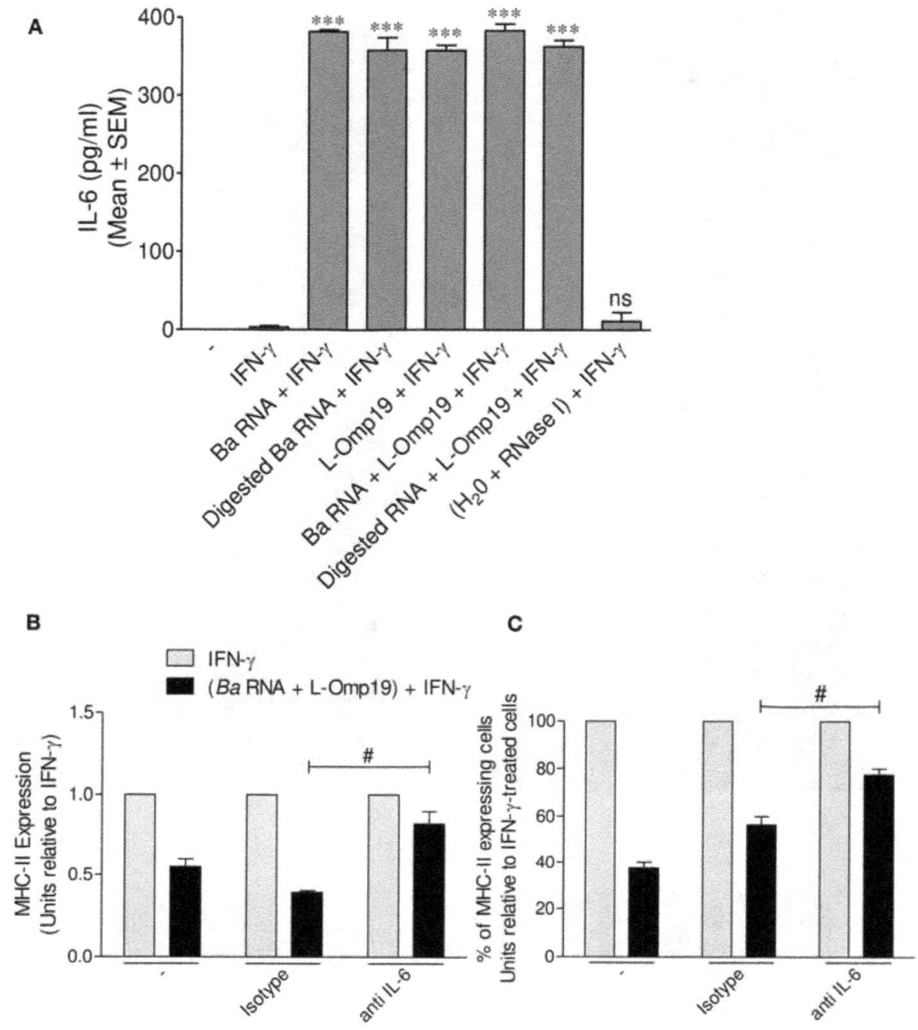

FIGURE 8 | IL-6 is a soluble mediator involved in *B. abortus* RNA and L-Omp19-mediated MHC-II down-modulation. **(A)** THP-1 cells were treated with *B. abortus* RNA (10 μg/ml), digested *B. abortus* RNA, L-Omp19 (1 μg/ml) or their combination in the presence of IFN-γ for 48 h. Then, supernatants were harvested and IL-6 secretion was quantified by ELISA sandwich. **(B,C)** THP-1 cells were treated with *B. abortus* RNA (10 μg/ml) and L-Omp19 (1 μg/ml) in the presence of IFN-γ and in the presence of neutralizing anti-IL-6 or its isotype control for 48 h. MHC-II expression was assessed by flow cytometry. **(B)** Bars represent the arithmetic means ± SEM of MHC-II positive cells corresponding to three independent experiments. **(C)** Quantification of cells expressing MHC-II (MHC-II positive cells). Data is expressed as the percentage of cells relative to IFN-γ ± SEM of three independent experiments. MFI, mean fluorescence intensity; ns, non-significant. ***$P < 0.001$ vs. IFN-γ-treated cells; #$P < 0.05$ vs. isotype control.

RNA as well (**Figure 8A**). Additionally, we stimulated THP-1 monocytes with the combination of *B. abortus* RNA, L-Omp19, and IFN-γ for 48 h in presence of an IL-6 neutralizing antibody or the isotype control. There was a partial recovery of the inhibition of IFN-γ-induced MHC-II expression when IL-6 was neutralized (**Figure 8B**). We also observed that the treatment with *B. abortus* RNA plus IFN-γ in the presence of anti-IL-6 not only increases the MFI of MHC-II molecules within the MHC-II-expressing cell population but also slightly increases the percentage of cells expressing MHC-II (**Figure 8C**). Therefore, this cytokine is one of the soluble mediators implicated in MHC-II down-modulation by *B. abortus* RNA and lipoproteins.

MHC-II Surface Inhibition Mediated by *B. abortus* RNA Alone or Together With Its Lipoproteins Correlates With Reduced Antigen Presentation to CD4+ T Cells

At last, we evaluate whether the down-regulation of MHC-II surface expression triggered by *B. abortus* RNA alone or together with lipoproteins had a functional correlation. For this purpose, we performed an antigen presentation assayusing a I-Ab-restricted T cell hybridoma specific for OVA 323-339 peptide (BO97.10). Murine BMDM were stimulated with *B. abortus* RNA, digested *B. abortus* RNA, L-Omp19 or the combination of each component in the presence of mIFN-γ (murine IFN-γ). After 48 h, BMDM were incubated with

OVA peptide and the T cell hybridoma BO97.10. As shown in **Figure 9**, the treatment with mIFN-γ induced the presentation of OVA peptide at 20 h, as supported by the capacity of BMDM to induce the secretion of IL-2 by BO97.10 cells. However, BMDM treated with *B. abortus* RNA, digested *B. abortus* RNA, L-Omp19 or the combination of each component plus mIFN-γ showed a significantly reduced capacity of OVA peptide presentation, as evidenced by decreased response of BO97.10 cells, related to BMDM treated only with mIFN-γ (**Figure 9**). As expected, BMDM treated with mIFN-γ and merely RNase I behaved similarly to those treated only with mIFN-γ (**Figure 9**). Overall, these results demonstrated that MHC-II down-regulation mediated by *B. abortus* RNA alone or together with lipoproteins is biologically relevant as it directly correlates with reduced antigen presentation to MHC-II-restricted $CD4^+$ T cells.

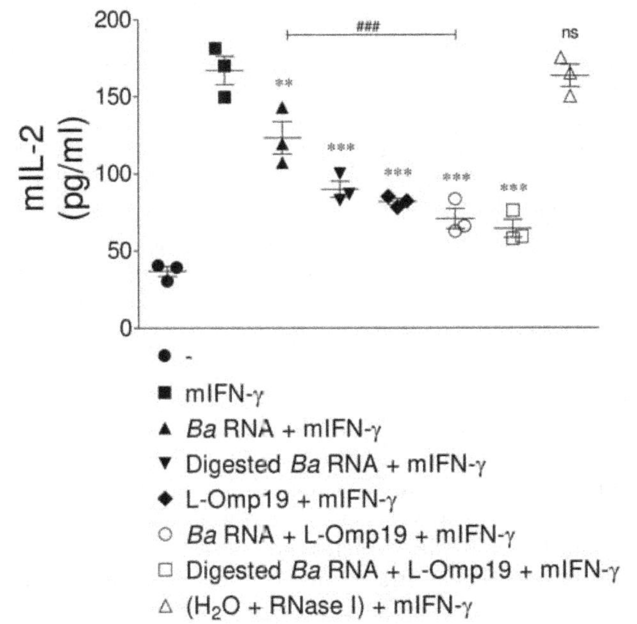

FIGURE 9 | MHC-II down-modulation correlates with diminished antigen presentation to $CD4^+$ T cells. BMM were treated with *B. abortus* RNA (10 μg/ml), digested *B. abortus* RNA, L-Omp19 (1 μg/ml) or their combination in the presence of mIFN-γ for 48 h. Then, cells were washed and incubated with 100 μg/ml of OVA peptide for 3 h at 37°C. Afterwards, cells were washed and co-cultured for 20 h at 37°C with BO97.10 cells, a T cell hybridoma specific for OVA peptide. T cell activation was measured by quantifying mIL-2 secretion in culture supernatants. $^{**}P < 0.01$; $^{***}P < 0.001$ vs. mIFN-γ-treated cells; ns, non-significant; $^{\#\#\#}P < 0.001$ vs. *Ba* RNA.

DISCUSSION

$CD4^+$ T cells are central to host resistance to *Brucella* infection (6–9). The secretion of IFN-γ by these cells enhances the bactericidal activity of *Brucella*-infected macrophages. Also, IFN-γ has an important role in activating macrophages. It enhances MHC-II expression on their surfaces, which results in increased antigen presentation to $CD4^+$ T cells (26–28). MHC-II genetic deficiency altering $CD4^+$ T lymphocytes completely impairs *Brucella* control in lungs, liver and spleen (29), highlighting the crucial role of these cells in the development of a protective response against infection. However, when bacteria are not fully eliminated, they are able to hide inside macrophages evading their eradication by the host immune system. One mechanism that would explain how *Brucella* is able to persist in the host chronically is the inhibition of MHC-II-restricted antigen presentation on *Brucella*-infected macrophages. We previously demonstrated that *B. abortus* infection down-regulates IFN-γ-induced MHC-II surface expression on monocytes/macrophages (10). Moreover, this down-modulation is caused by *B. abortus* lipoproteins (10, 13). However, these bacterial structural components were less efficient at reducing MHC-II surface expression than live bacteria, suggesting that another component related to bacterial viability must be involved in this phenomenon. In this study we demonstrated that *B. abortus* RNA, a component associated with viable bacteria, participates in the down-regulation of IFN-γ-induced expression of MHC-II molecules on monocytes/macrophages. The MHC-II surface inhibition was not the result of a detrimental effect of the RNA on monocytes (i.e., apoptosis or necrosis). Our results also demonstrate that *B. abortus* RNA neither delays the kinetic of IFN-γ induction of MHC-II molecules nor it modifies the expression of MHC-II molecules already induced by IFN-γ. On the contrary, *B. abortus* RNA prevents the correct induction of MHC-II molecules by IFN-γ. Moreover, MHC-II down-regulation was observed on cells of the monocytic line THP-1, on peripheral blood-purified human monocytes, and murine bone marrow-derived macrophages.

We have previously demonstrated that *B. abortus* RNA is also a component involved in *B. abortus*-mediated MHC-I surface inhibition (14). However, the inhibition of MHC molecules surface expression is not due to a global effect on IFN-γ-induced molecules. On the contrary, *B. abortus* RNA up-regulated the IFN-γ-induced expression of the co-stimulatory molecules CD40 and CD86, while it did not modify the expression of CD80. We also observed that MHC-II surface inhibition is not exclusive for *B. abortus* as it could be extrapolated to RNAs of other bacteria. Moreover, the phenomenon was observed with the RNA of the parasite *T. cruzi*. These results suggest that this singular immune regulation could happen in the context of other infectious processes.

Some years ago, it was demonstrated that the immune system is able to sense RNA degradation products through TLR8 (23). The fact that TLR8 recognizes degradation products nurtures the concept that bacterial or human phosphatases or nucleases might act before the activation of this receptor, as it has been previously proposed (30), phenomenon which could be compared to the prerequisite of the action of DNAse II in order to activate TLR9 (31, 32). In agreement with this idea, our results showed that *E.coli* RNase I-treated *B. abortus* RNA diminished MHC-II expression to the same extent as non-digested RNA. Therefore, our evidences suggest that the down-modulation of MHC-II by RNA and its degradation products is mediated by TLR8. In line with this, we recently published that the down-modulation of MHC-I surface expression by intact and digested RNA is mediated by hTLR8/mTLR7 as was demonstrated using BMDM from TLR7 [the TLR that acts as TLR8 in mice (33–35)] KO mice (14).

As we have previously demonstrated, HKBA was also capable of inhibiting MHC-II surface expression (10). Furthermore, *B. abortus* lipoproteins (structural components present in HKBA) were able to mimic the MHC-II down-modulation mediated by HKBA (10, 13). However, HKBA or *B. abortus* lipoproteins generated lower MHC-II reduction than live bacteria. Based on the evidences found in this study, we can now understand the differences in MHC-II down-modulation. Taking into account that RNA is rapidly eliminated when the bacteria lose their viability (14, 16, 17), in our previous experiments with HKBA, the MHC-II surface down-modulation was only mediated by lipoproteins. On the other hand, in the context of the infection, MHC-II surface down-modulation was not only mediated by lipoproteins but also by RNA. In line with this, we demonstrated that the combination of RNA and L-Omp19 induced higher MHC-II down-modulation than RNA or L-Omp19 alone. The synergism between RNA and lipoproteins can be understood in terms of cross-talk between TLRs. Immune responses to viral and bacterial pathogens depend on activation of intricate TLR-TLR interactions (36, 37). Stimulation of TLR8 alongside with TLR3 or TLR4 ligands on macrophages or DCs provoke a synergistic effect on activation of NF-kB and IFN regulatory factor (IRF), as it has been recently shown (36, 38). Bearing in mind this idea, Cervantes et al. showed that in human monocytes after TLR8 activation, the expression of TLR2 is induced (24). Other researchers have demonstrated that in THP-1 cells, the pre-exposure to 3M-002 (TLR8 ligand) augments the response to a posterior stimulation with TLR2 ligands (25). Another interesting finding is that CD14 is up regulated in monocytes that are differentiating to DCs when they are exposed to R848 (TLR7/8 ligand) (39). It has been described that CD14 facilitates the signaling through TLR2 mediated by bacterial lipoproteins (40–42). Our experiments of pre-exposure of THP-1 cells with *B. abortus* RNA before L-Omp19 (TLR2 ligand) corroborate in a functional way the involvement of TLR8 in MHC-II down-modulation.

Our kinetic studies demonstrated that MHC-II down-modulation by *B. abortus* RNA alone or in combination with *B. abortus* lipoproteins begins after 24 h post-stimuli, when MHC-II expression was induced by effect of IFN-γ. However, the maximum MHC-II surface down-modulation was observed at 48 h, in the moment of highest induction by IFN-γ. In turn, in agreement with previously published results (13, 43), *B. abortus* RNA alone or in combination with *B. abortus* lipoproteins is incapable of modulating MHC-II basal expression on monocytes. Our results also demonstrate that *B. abortus* RNA induced the expression of MHC-II on DCs. These results agree with our published results showing that *B. abortus* infection induces DCs maturation, as evidenced by the up-regulation of CD86, CD80, CCR7, CD83, MHC-II, MHC-I, and CD40 at 24 h post-infection (20). The apparent discrepancies between the MHC-II up-regulation in DCs and the down-regulation in monocytes/macrophages could be explain in terms of the kinetics of *Brucella* infection. One explanation is that activation of DCs with *B. abortus* is likely relevant at the onset of immune response, when Th1 and T CD8$^+$ responses are triggered. At later time points *Brucella* might be able to circumvent these responses to establish a chronic infection by means of different evasion mechanism such as down-modulation of MHC-II molecules in macrophages, where it dwells (12). Th1 cells and a high concentration of IFN-γ, a key cytokine in the induction of MHC-II expression, antigen processing and presentation by macrophages, integrate the immune response elicited against *Brucella*. However, in light of the obtained results, *B. abortus* might potentially inhibit the expression of MHC-II molecules regardless the triggering stimulus. In turn, our results suggest that the phenomenon could occur in the absence of an established production of IFN-γ, i.e., before the activation of the Th1 response, at early stages of *B. abortus* infection (with LPS as possible inducer of MHC-II). Nevertheless, MHC-II down-modulation is more pronounced in the moment of infection in which adaptive immunity begins to be relevant, i.e., when IFN-γ secreted by T lymphocytes is stimulating the presentation of *Brucella* antigens to MHC-II-restricted CD4$^+$ T cells.

One issue that merits discussion is the mechanism by which *B. abortus* RNA alone or in combination with lipoproteins is able to down-modulate MHC-II. We previously demonstrated that *B. abortus* lipoproteins down-regulate the IFN-γ-induced MHC-II surface expression by decreasing the transcription of MHC-II mRNA with the consequent inhibition of protein synthesis (13). Years later we demonstrated that *B. abortus* RNA decreases MHC-I surface expression by retaining these molecules within the Golgi apparatus (14). However, to our surprise, with *B. abortus* RNA we observed only a small percentage of cells with MHC-II molecules retained in the Golgi apparatus being the main mechanism the inhibition of the intracellular expression of these molecules. Regarding *B. abortus* lipoproteins, as expected, only intracellular inhibition of MHC-II expression was observed. On the other hand, when *B. abortus* RNA was combined with lipoproteins, the Golgi apparatus retention observed with merely RNA decreased, constituting MHC-II intracellular inhibition the principal mechanism. The confocal micrographs of *B. abortus* RNA plus lipoproteins allow us to evoke and understand what we previously observed in *B. abortus*-infected monocytes: a drastic reduction of MHC-II expression either in the surface or within the cell (11). Taken together, our results show that even for the treatment with *B. abortus* RNA alone, the predominant mechanism is the one previously described for lipoproteins. This mechanism is consistent with our kinetic experiments in which we observed a more pronounced inhibition at 48 h post-stimulation.

Another relevant question addressed in this study was the possible soluble mediators involved in the down-regulation of IFN-γ-induced MHC-II surface expression. We have demonstrated that IL-6 contributes to the inhibition of MHC-II expression mediated by *B. abortus* infection and their lipoproteins (10). Furthermore, we could discard the participation of IL-10 in this phenomenon (10). More recently, we demonstrated that *B. abortus* lipoproteins decrease the transcription of MHC-II and CIITA mRNA, and IRF-1 (regulatory transcriptional factor for CIITA) expression, trough IL-6 (13). On the other hand, we have recently demonstrated that *B. abortus* and its RNA induce the retention of MHC-I molecules within Golgi apparatus through EGFR signaling pathway (14, 15). Given that we demonstrated that the predominant mechanism of MHC-II surface down-modulation is the inhibition of expression of these molecules, we focus our attention on IL-6. Our results demonstrated that IL-6 is one soluble factor that participates in MHC-II down-regulation mediated by the combination of *B. abortus* RNA and lipoproteins. However, given the partial reversion of MHC-II surface down-modulation mediated by neutralizing Ab to IL-6, these results do not rule out that the EGFR pathway may also be involved. This pathway would explain the Golgi apparatus retention observed in a small percentage of cells.

Although we demonstrated that *B. abortus* RNA decreases MHC-II surface expression, it increases the expression of co-stimulatory molecules (CD40 and CD80). However, the global effect is the reduction of antigen presentation of *B. abortus* RNA stimulated-macrophages to $CD4^+$ T cells, which is an important functional correlation to our study. Moreover, *B. abortus* RNA in combination with lipoproteins leads to a lower antigen presentation.

Finally, we have elucidated that *B. abortus* RNA is a component associated to bacterial viability that along with lipoproteins participates in MHC-II surface down-modulation. Accordingly, through this phenomenon, the bacteria could prevent the $CD4^+$ T cell recognition in order to evade host immune response.

AUTHOR CONTRIBUTIONS

The experiments were designed and conceived by MM, GG, and PB. The experiments were performed by MM, AT, AS, JM, FM, JA, MG, and LB. Data was analyzed by MM. Materials, reagents were facilitated by SO and GG. They provided key suggestions to this work as well. All experiments were supervised by PB. The interpretation of data and the preparation of the manuscript were performed by MM and PB. The manuscript was reviewed by all authors.

ACKNOWLEDGMENTS

We thank the staff of the UOCCB (Unidad Operativa Centro de Contención Biológica), ANLIS-Malbrán (Administración Nacional de Laboratorios e Institutos de Salud Dr. Carlos G. Malbrán) (Buenos Aires, Argentina) for facilitating us the use of the BSL-3 laboratory. We are very grateful with Dr. Federico Fuentes for technical support with the analysis of confocal microscopies.

SUPPLEMENTARY MATERIAL

Figure S1 | Potential RNA contaminants are not involved in MHC-II down-modulation. **(A,B)** THP-1 cells were stimulated with DNase **(A)** or PK **(B)**-treated *B. abortus* RNA in the presence of IFN-γ for 48 h. Cells treated with DNase or PK alone were used as negative controls. Cells treated with *B. abortus* RNA were used as positive controls. MHC-II expression was assessed by flow cytometry. Bars represent the arithmetic means ± SEM of three independent experiments. MFI, mean fluorescence intensity; $^*P < 0.05$; $^{**}P < 0.01$; $^{***}P < 0.001$ vs. IFN-γ-treated cells; $^{\#\#\#}P < 0.001$ vs. negative controls.

Figure S2 | MHC-II down-modulation is not due to a loss of cell viability. THP-1 cells were treated with *B. abortus* RNA (10 μg/ml), L-Omp19 (1 μg/ml), RNase I-treated *B. abortus* RNA, or a combination of each component in the presence of IFN-γ for 48 h. Then the percentage of $7AAD^+$ cells were evaluated. Cells treated with Paraformaldehyde (PFA) were used as a positive control of the technique. $^{\#\#\#}P < 0.001$ vs. untreated cells.

Figure S3 | *B. abortus* RNA prevents the induction by IFN-γ of MHC-II. **(A)** THP-1 cells were treated with *B. abortus* RNA (5 μg/ml) in the presence of IFN-γ for 48, 72, or 96 h. **(B)** THP-1 cells were treated with IFN-γ for 24 h and then *B. abortus* RNA was added for other 24 h. **(C)** THP-1 cells were treated with *B. abortus* RNA for 48 h. MHC-II expression was assessed by flow cytometry. Bars represent the arithmetic means ± SEM of three independent experiments. MFI, mean fluorescence intensity; ns, non-significant; $^*P < 0.05$; $^{**}P < 0.01$; $^{***}P < 0.001$ vs. IFN-γ-treated cells; $^{\#\#\#}P < 0.001$ vs. (*Ba* RNA + IFN-γ).

Figure S4 | *B. abortus* RNA induced MHC-II expression on DCs while it inhibits the LPS-induced MHC-II on human monocytes. **(A)** DCs were treated with *B. abortus* RNA (1–10 μg/ml) or *E. coli* LPS (10 ng/ml) as a positive control of MHC-II induction for 24 h. **(B)** THP-1 cells were treated with *B. abortus* RNA (5 μg/ml) in the presence of *E coli* LPS (10 ng/ml) for 48 h. MHC-II expression was assessed by flow cytometry. Bars represent the arithmetic means ± SEM of three independent experiments. MFI, mean fluorescence intensity; $^{\#}P < 0.05$; $^{\#\#}P < 0.01$; $^{\#\#\#}P < 0.001$ vs. untreated cells; $^*P < 0.05$ vs. LPS-treated cells.

Figure S5 | *B. abortus* RNA and lipoproteins down-modulate MHC-II mainly by MHC-II inhibition inside the cells. Zooms of confocal micrographs of THP-1 cells treated with *B. abortus* RNA (10 μg/ml) or *B. abortus* RNA (10 μg/ml) plus L-Omp19 (1 μg/ml) in the presence of IFN-γ, as representative figures of MHC-II down-modulation mechanisms (retention in Golgi apparatus and MHC-II inhibition). MHC-II was detected with a primary anti-human MHC-II Ab (L243) followed by Alexa 546-labeled secondary Ab (red). Golgi apparatus was detected using a mAb specific for GM130 followed by Alexa 488-labeled secondary Ab (green). DIC, differential interference contrast.

REFERENCES

1. Celli J, de Chastellier C, Franchini DM, Pizarro-Cerda J, Moreno E, Gorvel JP. Brucella evades macrophage killing via VirB-dependent sustained interactions with the endoplasmic reticulum. *J Exp Med.* (2003) 198:545–56. doi: 10.1084/jem.20030088
2. Starr T, Ng TW, Wehrly TD, Knodler LA, Celli J. Brucella intracellular replication requires trafficking through the late endosomal/lysosomal compartment. *Traffic.* (2008) 9:678–94. doi: 10.1111/j.1600-0854.2008.00718.x
3. Gorvel JP, Moreno E. Brucella intracellular life: from invasion to intracellular replication. *Vet Microbiol.* (2002) 90:281–97. doi: 10.1016/S0378-1135(02)00214-6
4. Roop RM II, Bellaire BH, Valderas MW, Cardelli JA. Adaptation of the brucellae to their intracellular niche. *Mol Microbiol.* (2004) 52:621–30. doi: 10.1111/j.1365-2958.2004.04017.x
5. Starr T, Child R, Wehrly TD, Hansen B, Hwang S, Lopez-Otin C, et al. Selective subversion of autophagy complexes facilitates completion of the Brucella intracellular cycle. *Cell Host Microbe.* (2012) 11:33–45. doi: 10.1016/j.chom.2011.12.002
6. Moreno-Lafont MC, Lopez-Santiago R, Zumaran-Cuellar E, Paredes-Cervantes V, Lopez-Merino A, Estrada-Aguilera A, et al. Antigen-specific activation and proliferation of CD4+ and CD8+ T lymphocytes from brucellosis patients. *Trans R Soc Trop Med Hyg.* (2002) 96:340–7. doi: 10.1016/S0035-9203(02)90119-7

7. Moreno-Lafont MC, Lopez-Santiago R, Paredes-Cervantes V, Estrada-Aguilera A, Santos-Argumedo L. Activation and proliferation of T lymphocyte subpopulations in patients with brucellosis. *Arch Med Res.* (2003) 34:184–93. doi: 10.1016/S0188-4409(03)00020-1
8. Baldwin CL, Goenka R. Host immune responses to the intracellular bacteria Brucella: does the bacteria instruct the host to facilitate chronic infection? *Crit Rev Immunol.* (2006) 26:407–42. doi: 10.1615/CritRevImmunol.v26.i5.30
9. Skendros P, Pappas G, Boura P. Cell-mediated immunity in human brucellosis. *Microbes Infect.* (2011) 13:134–42. doi: 10.1016/j.micinf.2010.10.015
10. Barrionuevo P, Cassataro J, Delpino MV, Zwerdling A, Pasquevich KA, Garcia Samartino C, et al. Brucella abortus inhibits major histocompatibility complex class II expression and antigen processing through interleukin-6 secretion via Toll-like receptor 2. *Infect Immun.* (2008) 76:250–62. doi: 10.1128/IAI.00949-07
11. Barrionuevo P, Delpino MV, Pozner RG, Velasquez LN, Cassataro J, Giambartolomei GH. Brucella abortus induces intracellular retention of MHC-I molecules in human macrophages down-modulating cytotoxic CD8(+) T cell responses. *Cell Microbiol.* (2013) 15:487–502. doi: 10.1111/cmi.12058
12. Barrionuevo P, Giambartolomei GH. Inhibition of antigen presentation by Brucella: many more than many ways. *Microbes Infect.* (2019). doi: 10.1016/j.micinf.2018.12.004. [Epub ahead of print].
13. Velasquez LN, Milillo MA, Delpino MV, Trotta A, Fernandez P, Pozner RG, et al. Brucella abortus down-regulates MHC class II by the IL-6-dependent inhibition of CIITA through the downmodulation of IFN regulatory factor-1 (IRF-1). *J Leukoc Biol.* (2017) 101:759–73. doi: 10.1189/jlb.4A0416-196R
14. Milillo MA, Velasquez LN, Trotta A, Delpino MV, Marinho FV, Balboa L, et al. B. abortus RNA is the component involved in the down-modulation of MHC-I expression on human monocytes via TLR8 and the EGFR pathway. *PLoS Pathog.* (2017) 13:e1006527. doi: 10.1371/journal.ppat.1006527
15. Velasquez LN, Milillo MA, Delpino MV, Trotta A, Mercogliano MF, Pozner RG, et al. Inhibition of MHC-I by Brucella abortus is an early event during infection and involves EGFR pathway. *Immunol Cell Biol.* (2017) 95:388–98. doi: 10.1038/icb.2016.111
16. Sander LE, Davis MJ, Boekschoten MV, Amsen D, Dascher CC, Ryffel B, et al. Detection of prokaryotic mRNA signifies microbial viability and promotes immunity. *Nature.* (2011) 474:385–9. doi: 10.1038/nature10072
17. Mourao-Sa D, Roy S, Blander JM. Vita-PAMPs: signatures of microbial viability. *Adv Exp Med Biol.* (2013) 785:1–8. doi: 10.1007/978-1-4614-6217-0_1
18. Natale MA, Cesar G, Alvarez MG, Castro Eiro MD, Lococo B, Bertocchi G, et al. Correction: *Trypanosoma cruzi*-specific IFN-gamma-producing cells in chronic Chagas disease associate with a functional IL-7/IL-7R axis. *PLoS Negl Trop Dis.* (2019) 13:e0007168. doi: 10.1371/journal.pntd.0007168
19. Giambartolomei GH, Zwerdling A, Cassataro J, Bruno L, Fossati CA, Philipp MT. Lipoproteins, not lipopolysaccharide, are the key mediators of the proinflammatory response elicited by heat-killed *Brucella abortus*. *J Immunol.* (2004) 173:4635–42. doi: 10.4049/jimmunol.173.7.4635
20. Zwerdling A, Delpino MV, Barrionuevo P, Cassataro J, Pasquevich KA, Garcia Samartino C, et al. Brucella lipoproteins mimic dendritic cell maturation induced by *Brucella abortus*. *Microbes Infect.* (2008) 10:1346–54. doi: 10.1016/j.micinf.2008.07.035
21. Coria LM, Ibanez AE, Tkach M, Sabbione F, Bruno L, Carabajal MV, et al. A *Brucella* spp. Protease inhibitor limits antigen lysosomal proteolysis, increases cross-presentation, and enhances CD8+ T cell responses. *J Immunol.* (2016) 196:4014–29. doi: 10.4049/jimmunol.1501188
22. Regnault A, Lankar D, Lacabanne V, Rodriguez A, Thery C, Rescigno M, et al. Fcgamma receptor-mediated induction of dendritic cell maturation and major histocompatibility complex class I-restricted antigen presentation after immune complex internalization. *J Exp Med.* (1999) 189:371–80. doi: 10.1084/jem.189.2.371
23. Tanji H, Ohto U, Shibata T, Taoka M, Yamauchi Y, Isobe T, et al. Toll-like receptor 8 senses degradation products of single-stranded RNA. *Nat Struct Mol Biol.* (2015) 22:109–15. doi: 10.1038/nsmb.2943
24. Cervantes JL, La Vake CJ, Weinerman B, Luu S, O'Connell C, Verardi PH, et al. Human TLR8 is activated upon recognition of Borrelia burgdorferi RNA in the phagosome of human monocytes. *J Leukoc Biol.* (2013) 94:1231–41. doi: 10.1189/jlb.0413206
25. Mureith MW, Chang JJ, Lifson JD, Ndung'u T, Altfeld M. Exposure to HIV-1-encoded Toll-like receptor 8 ligands enhances monocyte response to microbial encoded Toll-like receptor 2/4 ligands. *AIDS.* (2010) 24:1841–8. doi: 10.1097/QAD.0b013e32833ad89a
26. Vitry MA, De Trez C, Goriely S, Dumoutier L, Akira S, Ryffel B, et al. Crucial role of gamma interferon-producing CD4+ Th1 cells but dispensable function of CD8+ T cell, B cell, Th2, and Th17 responses in the control of *Brucella melitensis* infection in mice. *Infect Immun.* (2012) 80:4271–80. doi: 10.1128/IAI.00761-12
27. Copin R, Vitry MA, Hanot Mambres D, Machelart A, De Trez C, Vanderwinden JM, et al. *In situ* microscopy analysis reveals local innate immune response developed around Brucella infected cells in resistant and susceptible mice. *PLoS Pathog.* (2012) 8:e1002575. doi: 10.1371/journal.ppat.1002575
28. Zhan Y, Cheers C. Endogenous gamma interferon mediates resistance to *Brucella abortus* infection. *Infect Immun.* (1993) 61:4899–901.
29. Hanot Mambres D, Machelart A, Potemberg G, De Trez C, Ryffel B, Letesson JJ, et al. Identification of immune effectors essential to the control of primary and secondary intranasal infection with *Brucella melitensis* in mice. *J Immunol.* (2016) 196:3780–93. doi: 10.4049/jimmunol.1502265
30. Geyer M, Pelka K, Latz E. Synergistic activation of Toll-like receptor 8 by two RNA degradation products. *Nat Struct Mol Biol.* (2015) 22:99–101. doi: 10.1038/nsmb.2967
31. Chan MP, Onji M, Fukui R, Kawane K, Shibata T, Saitoh S, et al. DNase II-dependent DNA digestion is required for DNA sensing by TLR9. *Nat Commun.* (2015) 6:5853. doi: 10.1038/ncomms6853
32. Pawaria S, Moody K, Busto P, Nundel K, Choi CH, Ghayur T, et al. Cutting edge: DNase II deficiency prevents activation of autoreactive B cells by double-stranded DNA endogenous ligands. *J Immunol.* (2015) 194:1403–7. doi: 10.4049/jimmunol.1402893
33. Pelka K, Shibata T, Miyake K, Latz E. Nucleic acid-sensing TLRs and autoimmunity: novel insights from structural and cell biology. *Immunol Rev.* (2016) 269:60–75. doi: 10.1111/imr.12375
34. Heil F, Hemmi H, Hochrein H, Ampenberger F, Kirschning C, Akira S, et al. Species-specific recognition of single-stranded RNA via toll-like receptor 7 and 8. *Science.* (2004) 303:1526–9. doi: 10.1126/science.1093620
35. Gorden KB, Gorski KS, Gibson SJ, Kedl RM, Kieper WC, Qiu X, et al. Synthetic TLR agonists reveal functional differences between human TLR7 and TLR8. *J Immunol.* (2005) 174:1259–68. doi: 10.4049/jimmunol.174.3.1259
36. Ghosh TK, Mickelson DJ, Solberg JC, Lipson KE, Inglefield JR, Alkan SS. TLR-TLR cross talk in human PBMC resulting in synergistic and antagonistic regulation of type-1 and 2 interferons, IL-12 and TNF-alpha. *Int Immunopharmacol.* (2007) 7:1111–21. doi: 10.1016/j.intimp.2007.04.006
37. Napolitani G, Rinaldi A, Bertoni F, Sallusto F, Lanzavecchia A. Selected toll-like receptor agonist combinations synergistically trigger a T helper type 1-polarizing program in dendritic cells. *Nat Immunol.* (2005) 6:769–76. doi: 10.1038/ni1223
38. Makela SM, Strengell M, Pietila TE, Osterlund P, Julkunen I. Multiple signaling pathways contribute to synergistic TLR ligand-dependent cytokine gene expression in human monocyte-derived macrophages and dendritic cells. *J Leukoc Biol.* (2009) 85:664–72. doi: 10.1189/jlb.0808503
39. Hackstein H, Knoche A, Nockher A, Poeling J, Kubin T, Jurk M, et al. The TLR7/8 ligand resiquimod targets monocyte-derived dendritic cell differentiation via TLR8 and augments functional dendritic cell generation. *Cell Immunol.* (2011) 271:401–12. doi: 10.1016/j.cellimm.2011.08.008
40. Sellati TJ, Bouis DA, Caimano MJ, Feulner JA, Ayers C, Lien E, et al. Activation of human monocytic cells by *Borrelia burgdorferi* and *Treponema pallidum* is facilitated by CD14 and correlates with surface exposure of spirochetal lipoproteins. *J Immunol.* (1999) 163:2049–56.
41. Aliprantis AO, Yang RB, Mark MR, Suggett S, Devaux B, Radolf JD, et al. Cell activation and apoptosis by bacterial lipoproteins through toll-like receptor-2. *Science.* (1999) 285:736–9. doi: 10.1126/science.285.5428.736
42. Hirschfeld M, Kirschning CJ, Schwandner R, Wesche H, Weis JH, Wooten RM, et al. Cutting edge: inflammatory signaling by *Borrelia burgdorferi* lipoproteins is mediated by toll-like receptor 2. *J Immunol.* (1999) 163:2382–6.

3

Differential Tick Salivary Protein Profiles and Human Immune Responses to Lone Star Ticks (*Amblyomma americanum*) from the Wild vs. a Laboratory Colony

L. Paulina Maldonado-Ruiz[1†], Lidia Montenegro-Cadena[2†], Brittany Blattner[2], Sapna Menghwar[2], Ludek Zurek[3] and Berlin Londono-Renteria[2]*

[1] Medical/Veterinary Entomology Laboratory, Department of Entomology, Kansas State University, Manhattan, KS, United States, [2] Vector Biology Laboratory, Department of Entomology, Kansas State University, Manhattan, KS, United States, [3] Department of Pathology and Parasitology, CEITEC Center for Zoonoses, University of Veterinary and Pharmaceutical Sciences, Brno, Czechia

***Correspondence:**
Berlin Londono-Renteria
blondono@ksu.edu

†These authors have contributed equally to this work

Ticks are a growing concern to human and animal health worldwide and they are leading vectors of arthropod-borne pathogens in the United States. Ticks are pool blood feeders that can attach to the host skin for days to weeks using their saliva to counteract the host defenses. Tick saliva, as in other hematophagous arthropods, contains pharmacological and immunological active compounds, which modulate local and systemic immune responses and induce antibody production. In the present study, we explore differences in the salivary gland extract (SGE) protein content of *Amblyomma americanum* ticks raised in a laboratory colony (CT) vs. those collected in the field (FT). First, we measured the IgG antibody levels against SGE in healthy volunteers residing in Kansas. ELISA test showed higher IgG antibody levels when using the SGE from CT as antigen. Interestingly, antibody levels against both, CT-SGE and FT-SGE, were high in the warm months (May–June) and decreased in the cold months (September–November). Immunoblot testing revealed a set of different immunogenic bands for each group of ticks and mass spectrometry data revealed differences in at 19 proteins specifically identified in the CT-SGE group and 20 from the FT-SGE group. Our results suggest that differences in the salivary proteins between CT-SGE and FT-SGE may explain the differential immune responses observed in this study.

Keywords: *Amblyomma americanum*, lone star tick, salivary proteins, human immune response, antibodies, seasonal response

INTRODUCTION

Ticks are obligate blood-feeding ectoparasites of a wide range of vertebrates and are important vectors of human and animal pathogens (1). Hard ticks (Ixodidae) feed once in each developmental stage for a prolonged period by deeply penetrating the epidermis, forming a pool of blood, and causing great damage to the host skin that could last from several days to weeks (2, 3). The saliva composition of the tick and other hematophagous arthropods is complex and includes vasodilators, anti-coagulation compounds, and platelet aggregation inhibitors (2, 4). In ticks, saliva composition changes at different time points (5, 6). Arthropods use saliva to counteract the response against injury caused during the process of blood feeding (piercing and tearing) that trigger host defense mechanisms as well as to facilitate the process of obtaining the blood. Evidence suggests that pathogens may take advantage of the immunomodulatory properties of the arthropod saliva to establish infection (7–9). Arthropod saliva modulates the transmission of pathogens either directly by enhancing pathogen invasion (10, 11) or indirectly by modulating host immune responses (12, 13).

Also, salivary proteins may induce potent antibody responses that can be associated with the intensity of exposure to arthropod saliva and can be used as a proxy to measure the degree of vector-host interaction (14, 15). The presence of anti-tick saliva antibodies in human serum can be measured by enzyme-linked immunosorbent assay (ELISA) as a biologic marker of tick exposure with epidemiologic applications. For instance, in the state of California, Lane et al. found a significant correlation between the antibodies to *Ixodes pacificus* and *Borrelia burgdorferi* (16). Previous studies also suggest that the vertebrate immune system exert immunological pressure on the arthropod (2). Specifically, studies report that arthropods may display differences in the composition of their saliva when exposed to different hosts (17, 18). The development of immunity against specific salivary proteins may impair feeding (11, 19, 20), thus it is expected that arthropods try to induce lower antibody levels against proteins that are special for blood feeding. Although the development of strong immunity against salivary proteins is rarely seen in nature (21), this characteristic is being exploited to develop anti-tick vaccines (22).

The lone star tick, *Amblyomma americanum*, is widely distributed across the Southeast and Midwest of the USA and have begun to spread to the central plains of the USA and to Canada (23, 24). This species is an important vector of *Francisella tularensis*, *Ehrlichia sp.*, and other pathogens (25, 26) and has been associated with triggering red meat allergy (27). Previous studies suggest a great diversity among *A. americanum* specimens collected in different states across the US. Also, among ticks raised in colony vs. the ones found in the wild (28). In this study, we tested the hypothesis that field collected *A. americanum* ticks have greater diversity in their salivary protein content than those raised in a colony for several generations, thus inducing different immune responses in the vertebrate hosts when feeding. Our preliminary approach was to explore the differences between ticks raised in a laboratory colony compared to those collected from the field by characterizing (a) the salivary gland extract protein content, (b) antibody levels against the salivary glands extract, and (c) the *in vitro* effect of tick salivary gland content on human cells using specific markers for inflammation and/or cell damage. Our aim was to identify important proteins subject to immunological pressure in the field and to detect specific salivary proteins that could be used to evaluate arthropod host interaction. Our preliminary results revealed important differences in the salivary content of ticks from the field that could potentially have an impact in pathogen transmission.

MATERIALS AND METHODS

Tick Specimens

Laboratory-reared colony non-fed *A. americanum* female adult ticks (CT) were obtained in 2017 from the Department of Entomology and Plant Pathology tick rearing facility at Oklahoma State University (Stillwater, OK). This tick colony was started in 1976 with engorged females collected in Oklahoma. Engorged females are introduced every 2 years in approximately equal numbers to mated colony females. All adult females are reared on sheep and kept at 94–96% humidity, and on a 12:12-hr light:dark cycle. All CT requested for this study were more than 2 months old (based on molting time). Field non-fed-questing *A. americanum* female adult ticks (FT) (unknown molting date) were collected from northeastern Kansas (Konza Prairie Biological Research Station) during summer in 2017 and 2018 using the cloth flagging method. Flags were made by attaching a 95 cm by 70 cm flannel cloth to a wooden utility handle (120 cm). Flagging was carried out by dragging the cloth over the grass area on the edge of the forest for 3–4 m. Ticks were removed from the cloth and placed in glass containers stored in a cooler with high humidity (>90% RH) until arrival to the laboratory. *A. americanum* females were identified by distinct morphological characteristics of ticks found in the state of Kansas (29). Main morphological features included; long palps and ornate scutum typical of genus *Amblyomma* and the distinct white spot located on the edge of scutum; characteristic of the *A. americanum* female (30). All ticks were stored at 4°C in 100% R.H (relative humidity) until used for the experiments.

Salivary Gland Extraction and Antigen Preparation

Ticks were surface sterilized using 0.5% sodium hypochlorite, 70% ethanol, and washed with sterile water before dissections. Ticks were immobilized on sterile dental wax and sterile phosphate buffer saline (PBS) was added. Tick dorsal integument was removed by a surgical scalpel and salivary glands were extracted. Dissections were performed initiating from anterior part of ticks to minimize the risk of contamination by avoiding midgut in posterior end. Salivary glands were removed and rinsed with PBS prior pooling based on the origin (FT and CT). Salivary gland extract (SGE) was obtained through freeze-thaw cycles (−80°C and 27°C/3 cycles). Protein concentration was measured using a NanoDropTM 2000 spectrophotometer (Thermo Fisher Scientific). Twenty ticks (10 FT and 10 CT) were selected for salivary gland dissections.

Human Blood Sampling

The protocols followed in the study were reviewed and approved by IRB #1206 from Kansas State University. Blood samples were obtained from 36 adult volunteers residing in Manhattan, Kansas thought finger prick. Blood samples were collected in filter papers (Whatman 903). Samples were collected in the summer 2018 (May–June), and only 27 of those could be followed in the fall (September–November). Blood was collected by the finger prick method as reported elsewhere (31) and blood drops were placed in. Dried blood spots in filter paper were eluted in PBS for further testing. At enrollment, tested individuals were provided with a questionnaire to gather information about age, gender, use of repellant, travel, and outdoor activities.

ELISA Antibody Levels Testing

Antibody levels were determined by an indirect ELISA following our previous published methodology (15). Total SGE from CT and FT were used as an antigen in the ELISA-based test conducted in 96-well ELISA plates (Nunc-Maxisorp, Nalgene Nunc International, Rochester, NY, USA). Plates were coated with 50 μl/well of tick SGE at a final concentration of 1 μg/ml prepared in 1X PBS and incubated overnight at 4°C. Blood from filter paper was eluted as follows, the fourth part of every dry blood spot (DBS) circle was eluted in 500 μl of PBS 1X overnight at 4°C. Plates were rinsed twice with washing buffer (1X PBS-0,05 % tween 20) and treated with blocking buffer (non-fat dry milk 2%, Tween 20 0.05%, 1X PBS) for 1.5 h at 37°C. Plates were then rinsed twice with washing buffer, and 50 μl/well of the eluted blood (1:50 diluted in blocking buffer) was incubated for 1.5 h at 37°C. After three washes, plates were incubated with horseradish peroxidase-conjugated goat anti-human IgG (Abcam, Ab81202) in a 1:1,000 dilution in blocking buffer. The colorimetric development was obtained using tetra-methyl-benzidine (TMB) (Gene-Script, Piscataway, NJ, USA). The reaction was stopped with 2N sulfuric acid and absorbance was measured at 450 nm. Two controls were included on each plate: (1) negative control: two wells with antigen and without sample as control for non-specific induction of color, caused by any of the reagents used in the test (2) positive control: 1 control per plate (same sample) to test plate variation and normalize OD (optical density) values as described elsewhere (15, 32). IgG antibody levels are reported as ΔOD = Average patient OD value (duplicate) minus the negative/blank control OD.

Tick SGE Protein Electrophoresis and Immunoblotting

For protein separation, the same amount (10 μg) of FT-SGE and CT-SGE were seeded in two miniprotean TGX gels (Bio-Rad) by duplicate. Precision Plus Protein™ 10–250 kDa Kaleidoscope™ (Thermo Fisher) was used as molecular weight marker and the gel was exposed to 150 V for 45 min. One gel was then washed with PBS and the proteins were visualized using the Pierce Silver Stain kit (Thermo Scientific) according to the manufacturer's instructions. A second gel was used for transferring proteins into a PVDF blotting membrane, trans-blot turbo (Bio-Rad). PVDF membrane with the tick salivary proteins was incubated overnight at 4°C with a 1:100 dilution of a pool of eluted blood samples (n = 10) from filter paper (as described above) using ELISA blocking buffer. After three washes with ELISA washing buffer, the membrane was incubated 2 h at room temperature with horseradish peroxidase-conjugated goat anti-human IgG (Abcam, Ab81202) in a 1:1,000 dilution in blocking buffer. The membrane was then washed three times with 1X PBS and incubated with TMB for membranes (Thermo Fisher) and the reaction was stopped with deionized water until the desired color was reached. Reactive proteins were measured using; My Image analysis software using the immunoblot picture as described elsewhere (15). Bands were identified and cut from the stained gel (sizes of ~10 and 20 kDa) and sent in duplicates for sequencing by UPLC-MS/MS.

Gel bands corresponding to immunogenic bands observed in the immunoblotting were sent for sequencing. Briefly, two independent samples for every band were obtained and analyzed. Every protein name was searched in the UNIPROT database and a blast search was performed. Gene ontology was also analyzed using UNIPROT. Features like protein weigh, identity with *A. americanum* and cell localization were recorded for all proteins. From the top 100 identified proteins using mass spectrometry (MS), 39 proteins were selected in total according to the occurrence probability >1.066 and expected weight.

Cell Lines

The Monocyte-like U937 (ATCC), endothelial HUVEC and neuroblastoma SH-SY5Y (Sigma-Aldrich) cell lines were used in this study to assess inflammation and cell damage. To evaluate the effect of SGE on immune on phagocytic cells (33) we used the mononuclear derived U937 cells were cultured in RPMI 1640 medium supplemented with 10% Fetal Bovine Serum (FBS) and penicillin/streptomycin 1%. Also, to evaluate the effect of endothelial tissue (34), we used HUVEC cells (Millipore-Sigma) cultured in endothelial cell growth medium following sellers' instructions. Since a significant number of viruses transmitted by ticks are neurotropic and arthropod salivary protein may disrupt the nerve-blood barrier, we used the SH-SY5Y neuroblastoma cells to evaluate the effect of SGE on neuronal physiology as described previously (35, 36). SH-SY5Y cells were cultured in DMEM medium supplemented with 15% heat-inactivated FBS and 1% Penicillin/streptomycin.

Cytokine Induction by Tick SGE

Cells were seeded in 24-well plates, 24 previous to the experiment. Cells were exposed to 1 μg/ml of SGE from either FT or CT an incubated for 24 h at 37°C and 5% of CO_2. After incubation, the cell pellet was collected and lysed using the RNA lysis buffer (Zymo Kit, cat R1055). Total RNA was extracted using Quick-RNA Kits (Zymo Research) and following manufacturer's instructions. RNA was used to produce cDNA using the RT2 First strand synthesis kit (Qiagen) and kept at −20°C until used.

In HUVEC cells, we measured the gene expression of fibronectin 1 (*FN1*) and thrombospondin (*TSP1*) (37, 38). For the SH-SY5Y cell line, we tested the *CASPASE 3*, *enolase 2*, Toll-interacting protein (*TOLLIP*), and myeloid differentiation factor-88 adaptor protein (*MyD88*) genes previously associated with injury/damage and immunity in these cells (39–42) (**Supplementary Table S1**). In addition, cytokine gene expression in the U937 cell line (macrophages) was evaluated using the Applied Biosystems® TaqMan® Array Human Cytokine Network 96-well Plate (Thermo Fisher) following the manufacturer's instructions. Afterward, genes that were found up-regulated were tested further to confirm the results. For this, we used a set of previously published primers: Interleukine (IL) IL8, IL-18, IL12a, IL1B and Tumor Necrosis Factor alfa (TNFα) (43–45), C-C Motif Chemokine Ligand 5 (CCL5), IL-10

(46), and Interferon gamma (IFNγ) (47). These reactions were performed using the PowerUp™ SYBR™ Green Master Mix (Thermo-fisher) in the Quantstudio 3 (Applied Biosystem) PCR thermocycler following manufacturer's instructions.

Data Analysis

The difference between two independent groups (i.e., antibody levels between males vs. females, fall vs. summer) was determined using the Mann-Whitney test with a $p < 0.05$. Correlation between to independent parameters was done using Spearman correlation method. Paired analysis (i.e., IgG antibodies in the summer vs. fall) we used Wilcoxon-matched pair test. Fold gene expression was calculated by the relative quantification $2^{-\Delta\Delta ct}$ method using the β2 macroglobulin as the housekeeping gene and cells without treatment as control. To test for statically significant differences ($p < 0.05$) between the independent groups Statistical analysis was performed using GraphPad Prism, version 8.1 (GraphPad Software Inc., La Jolla, CA).

RESULTS

Antibody Responses Against Whole SGE Proteins

To evaluate human immune responses against tick saliva, we collected blood samples from 36 volunteers living in Manhattan, KS, who reported no current illness at the time of sampling. The study sample was composed of 20 women and 16 men, with an age average of 39 years old (from 22 to 69 years) (**Table 1**). We collected samples from all 36 individuals in summer 2018, however, only 27 participants volunteered for a second sample in the Fall. Only 3 individuals tested (2 females, 1 male) reported to have traveled outside the US during summer, however, all volunteers reported to participate in outdoor activities during this time of the year and only 11 participants reported not using repellent during these activities.

Comparison of the IgG antibody levels against each SGE type (FT vs. CT) showed significantly higher antibody levels against the CT-SGE than against the FT-SGE (Mann-Whitney test, $p = 0.0094$). In addition, antibody levels against both SGE antigens were significantly higher in the summer months than in the Fall (Mann-Whitney test, $p < 0.05$), but no significant differences were observed when comparing antibody levels between males and females, or after comparing people using repellent or not (Mann-Whitney test, $p > 0.05$) (**Figures 2A–D**).

TABLE 1 | Summary of healthy volunteers participating in our study (individuals with outdoor activity associated with tick habitat).

	Males*	Females*	Total
Summer	16 (7)	20 (9)	36
Fall	12 (5)	15 (6)	27

*Outdoor activities included hiking, gardening, camping and yard work. *Individuals who traveled outside the US during summer (2 females, 1 male). Only 1 male and 1 female were tested again for fall.*

Salivary Profiles and Immunogenic Proteins in SGE From CT and FT

The SDS-PAGE analysis showed discrete differences in the SGE protein content from the CT-SGE and FT-SGE (**Figure 1A**). In general, higher protein content was observed in the CT-SGE in spite that equal amount of protein was loaded on each lane. However, the immunoblot testing the reactivity of human samples against both SGE revealed a significant strong reactivity with a band around ~25 kDa in the FT- SGE and a band around ~ 22 kDa for CT-SGE (**Figure 1B**). In addition, we observed a ~ 10-kDa band in both, CT and FT, although the band showed stronger reactivity in FT-SGE (**Figure 1C; Supplementary Figure S1**). Mass spectrometry of the 10 kDa band revealed a total of 19 proteins. Specifically, eight proteins were unique to the CT-SGE, seven unique to the FT-SGE, and four were shared between both groups (**Figure 1D**). In the case of the ~25–22 kDa portion, a total of 30 proteins were identified, 11 proteins specific to CT-SGE, 13 in the FT-SGE and six were shared by both groups. The list of proteins can be found in **Table 2**.

Since we used SGE and not saliva, we found both secreted and non-secreted proteins. Gene ontology revealed the function of 17 proteins, among those we could identify some with binding activity ($n = 9$), catalytic activity ($n = 6$), structural constituent of ribosome ($n = 3$), and lipid transporter activity ($n = 1$). From those proteins with an enzymatic activity we could identify hydrolases ($n = 4$), peptidases ($n = 3$), ferroxidase ($n = 1$), and kinases ($n = 1$). In addition, categorization by the biological process, we found proteins involved in cellular processes ($n = 10$), metabolic processes ($n = 6$), response to stimulus ($n = 2$) biological regulation ($n = 2$) and iron transport ($n = 1$). The only protein family found uniquely expressed as well as shared was the group of lipocalins, these proteins are found in the saliva of several arthropods and are abundant in tick saliva (48, 49). Our sequencing data revealed three lipocalins, one shared between tick groups and two individual lipocalins. BLAST analysis showed a 72% identity between a human lipocalin 2 protein (LCN2) (50) and the A0A0C9SE12 found in FT-SGE, while a 63% identity was found when comparing A0A0C9SAU2 from CT and only a 33% when comparing the shared A0A0C9SFF5. No other groups were found distributed among all categories analyzed (i.e., CT, FT, and shared.).

Cytokine Gene Expression

We tested the *in vitro* effect of CT-SGE and FT-SGE on human cells with the potential for interacting with the arthropod saliva during or after the blood feeding. Previous studies have shown the effect or arthropod saliva in the physiology of macrophages, endothelial cells and neurons (51). So, we explored the possibility that SGE from arthropods raised under different conditions may have a differential effect on host immunity. For this, we used a cytokine expression array and qRT-PCR to measure cytokine levels in the macrophage-like cell line U937 and exposed them to either CT-SGE or FT-SGE. Our results showed a slight upregulation (>1.0 fold) of IL-8, IL-10, and TNFα upon treatment with FT SGE (**Figure 3A**). Interestingly, the difference

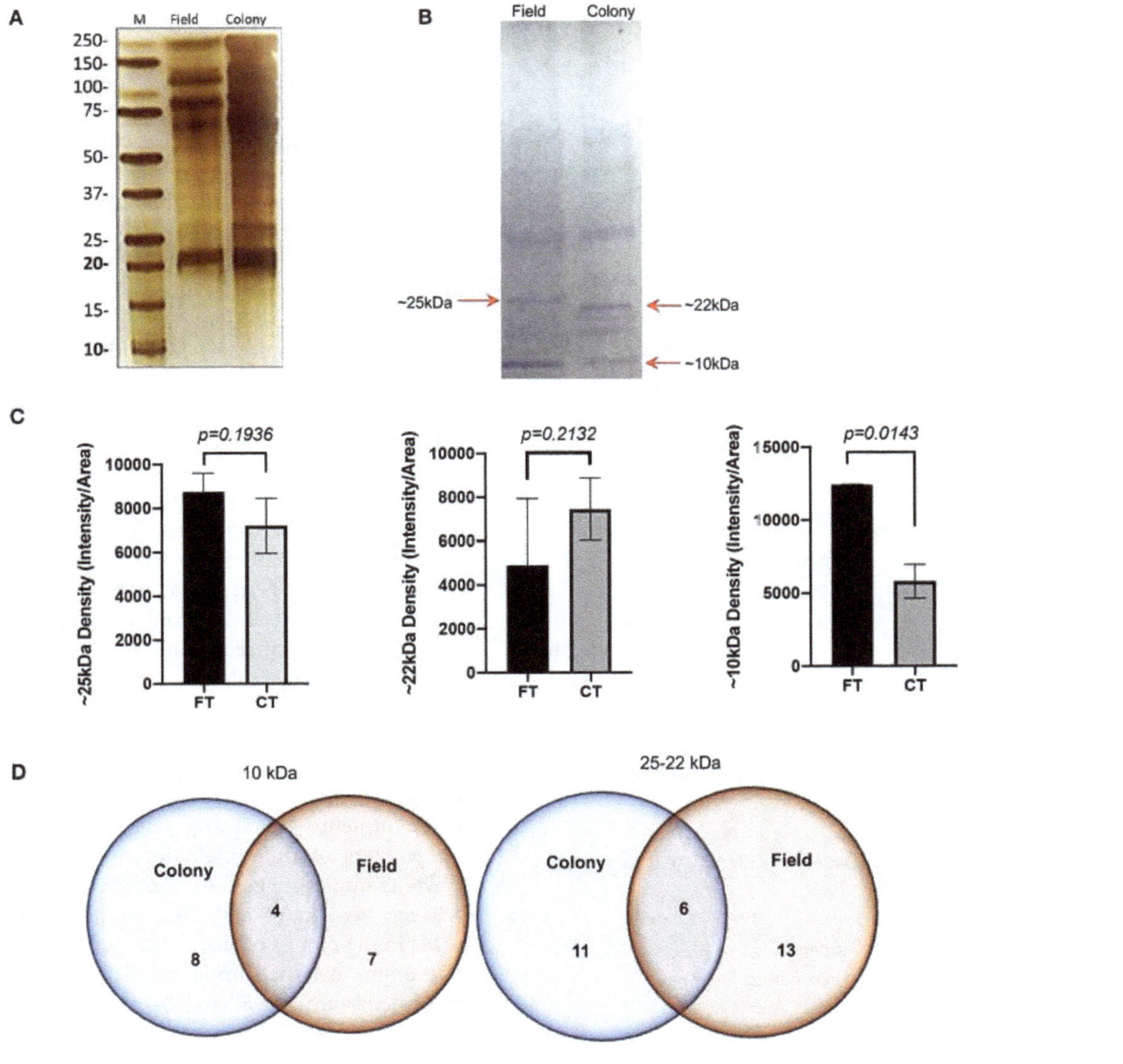

FIGURE 1 | SGE protein analysis Colony and Field. **(A)** Protein SDS-PAGE (silver stain). **(B)** Immunoblot using human samples from healthy volunteers. **(C)** Intensity comparison of immunogenic bands from the immunoblot, and **(D)** Schematic representation of proteins identified by mass spectrometry. Figure displaying the median with interquartile range. Significance evaluated by the Mann-Whitney test with a $p < 0.05$.

between SGE's was only significant in the TNFα levels (Mann-Whitney test, $p = 0.0159$) (**Figure 3B**). We did not find any significant differences in the expression of Fibronectin 1 and Thrombospondin 1 genes HUVEC cells (**Figure 3C**) or any of the genes tested in SH-SY5Y cells exposed to both groups of SGE, However, all these genes were upregulated in the SH-SY5Y upon incubation with the tick SGE (**Figure 3D**).

DISCUSSION

Arthropod saliva has recaptured attention in public health because of its involvement in the transmission of human pathogens. The use of antibodies against arthropod saliva as markers for bite exposure has been implemented to evaluate the risk of malaria and other mosquito-borne viruses with high reliability. In our study, we observed a significant reduction of anti-tick SGE antibodies from summer to fall suggesting a higher exposure to arthropod bites during the warmer months as observed previously. These results are in concordance to previous studies showing that antibodies against salivary proteins may be short-lived (52, 53). An unexpected finding was the higher antibody levels against the CT-SGE instead of the FT-SGE. Usually, colony arthropods are fed from the blood of one animal species for several generations. In this case, the colony ticks have been maintained in sheep for several years. Since several studies suggest that vertebrate host exert immunological pressure on salivary proteins, we speculate that the significantly higher concentration of salivary gland protein in the CT-SGE content may explain the observed results. Although the same concentration of SGE was used for all ELISAs, it is possible that the concentration of specific immunogenic proteins is higher in the CT-SGE than in the FT as revealed

TABLE 2 | List of proteins found by mass spectrometry in the ~25–22 and 10 kDa gel area corresponding to the immunogenic bands in the immunoblot.

Protein name	ID	MW
Only Field		
10 kDa Band		
Putative m13 family peptidase[1]	A0A0C9RVU2	11,956
Putative ribosomal protein s18c	A0A0C9RZJ8	17798
Putative myosin regulatory light chain ef-hand protein	A0A0C9SCS4	19,957
22–25 kDa Band		
Putative lipocalin-5[1]	A0A0C9SE12	25,502
Putative polynucleotide kinase 3' phosphatase	A0A0C9RUF1	29,836
Putative endoplasmic reticulum glucose-regulated protein grp94/endoplasmin hsp90 family	A0A0C9SDH1	27,206
Serine protease inhibitor[2]	A0A0E9Y1R8	24,603
Putative cell cycle-associated protein	A0A0C9S1G1	22,560
40S ribosomal protein S3a	A0A0C9S283	30,205
Putative phosphoserine phosphatase	A0A0C9SBN8	26,146
Only colony		
10 kDa Band		
Putative vitellogenin	A0A0C9RSG8	15,853
Histone H4	A0A0C9QYX1	11,667
Putative calmodulin	A0A0C9QZX5	16,811
Putative lipocalin-3 1 lipocalin	A0A0C9SAU2	17,939
22–25 kDa Band		
Signal peptidase complex subunit 3	A0A0C9RR64	20,224
Spectrin alpha chain-like protein	B5M765	26,729
Putative chaperonin subunit	A0A0C9R1F3	23,782
Putative 26s protease regulatory subunit 4-like protein	A0A0C9SBM8	25,824
Putative secreted protein 94[1]	A0A0C9S5A9	23,779
Shared		
10 kDa band		
Ferritin	Q6WNX6	19,853
Putative 40s ribosomal protein s27a	A0A0C9SCH5	17,949
Putative a-macroglobulin receptor[2]	A0A0C9SC71	15,655
Alpha-2-macroglobulin[2]	B5M727	19,026
22–25 kDa Band		
Putative heme lipoprotein	A0A0C9RTH2	23,282
Putative vitellogenin-2	A0A0C9S1B0	20,974
Putative lipocal-1 14 lipocalin	A0A0C9SFF5	23,504
Actin	B5M764	21,136
Putative polyubiquitin	A0A0C9S1S7	25,821
Putative laminin g domain protein	A0A0C9S253	28,976

[1]Signal peptide. [2]Secreted protein.

by our immunoblot. Our results suggest that the FT-SGE may have adapted to produce less concentration of highly immunogenic protein to induce fewer antibodies production and allow for longer feeding time. Importantly, immunogenic salivary proteins involved in blood feeding capable of inducing "good" antibody levels may be used as anti-arthropod vaccines (20, 22, 54).

A recent sialo-proteome study has reported up to 2,153 secreted proteins in *A. americanum* saliva and most of the proteins found in our study have been previously reported (20, 55). We found ten proteins only in FT-SGE, nine in CT-SGE only, and ten were shared between the two strains. Since we worked with SGE we found secreted and structural proteins. In the case of the FT SGE, three secreted proteins were uniquely found, a putative m13 family peptidase, a putative lipocalin-5 and a serine protease inhibitor. Another interesting protein found uniquely in the FT was a serine protease inhibitor (A0A0E9Y1R8). Among a wide range of functions, serine protease inhibitors are directly involved in the regulation of inflammation, blood clotting, wound healing, vasoconstriction. Also, several tick serine protease inhibitors are promising candidates for anti-tick vaccines (22, 56). In the case of the CT-SGE, we found an uncharacterized putative secreted protein 94 (A0A0C9S5A9) and a putative calmodulin (A0A0C9QZX5) among the proteins uniquely found in this tick group. Calmodulins are involved in calcium binding and previous studies describe a calmodulin involved in cellular signal transduction in *Haemaphysalis flava* (57).

Several proteins were found shared between the FT-SGE and the CT-SGE. Ferritin has previously found immunogenic in *A. americanum* salivary content (20). Ferritin has also been reported in salivary secretions from other ticks species where it plays important roles not only on iron metabolism and immunity but also as an anti-oxidant (58, 59). What may explain why it is important for both tick groups included in this study. Another important group of proteins found shared between tick groups were the α2-macroglobulin (α2M). These proteins are closely related to the C3, C4, and C5 components of the vertebrate complement system (60) and previous studies suggest a potential crosstalk of these molecules between vertebrates and invertebrates (61). The presence of α2Ms in the groups of shared proteins highlight the importance of immune defense during blood feedings since these groups of proteins are considered as early-acting innate immunity components, similar to opsonin (60). Also, a putative heme lipoprotein (A0A0C9RTH2) was found shared between CT and FT. A hem lipoprotein (HeLP) has been reported in the hemolymph of *Boophilus microplus*. This protein is able to bind up to 8 heme molecules and transports iron from the hemolymph to the tissues (62).

In this study, we explored for first the time the effect of tick saliva from different origin on neurons and endothelial cells *in vitro*. With this preliminary study, although no significant gene expression difference between strains was observed, our preliminary data suggest that both tick strains saliva could have an important impact in neuronal physiology, and further studies in this field are urgently needed. Although most of the cytokines measured were not significantly upregulated in concordance with previous studies suggesting an anti-inflammatory effect of tick saliva (63, 64), we observed a significantly higher expression of the pro-inflammatory cytokine TNFα (6-fold) in U937 cells when exposed to FT-SGE. Our hypothesis is that the presence of Lipocalin 5 in the FT-SGE may explain the discrepancies. In humans, a positive correlation of lipocalin-2 serum levels with serum TNFα levels was observed. There is a 72% identity between Lipocalin 2 and the putative Lipocalin

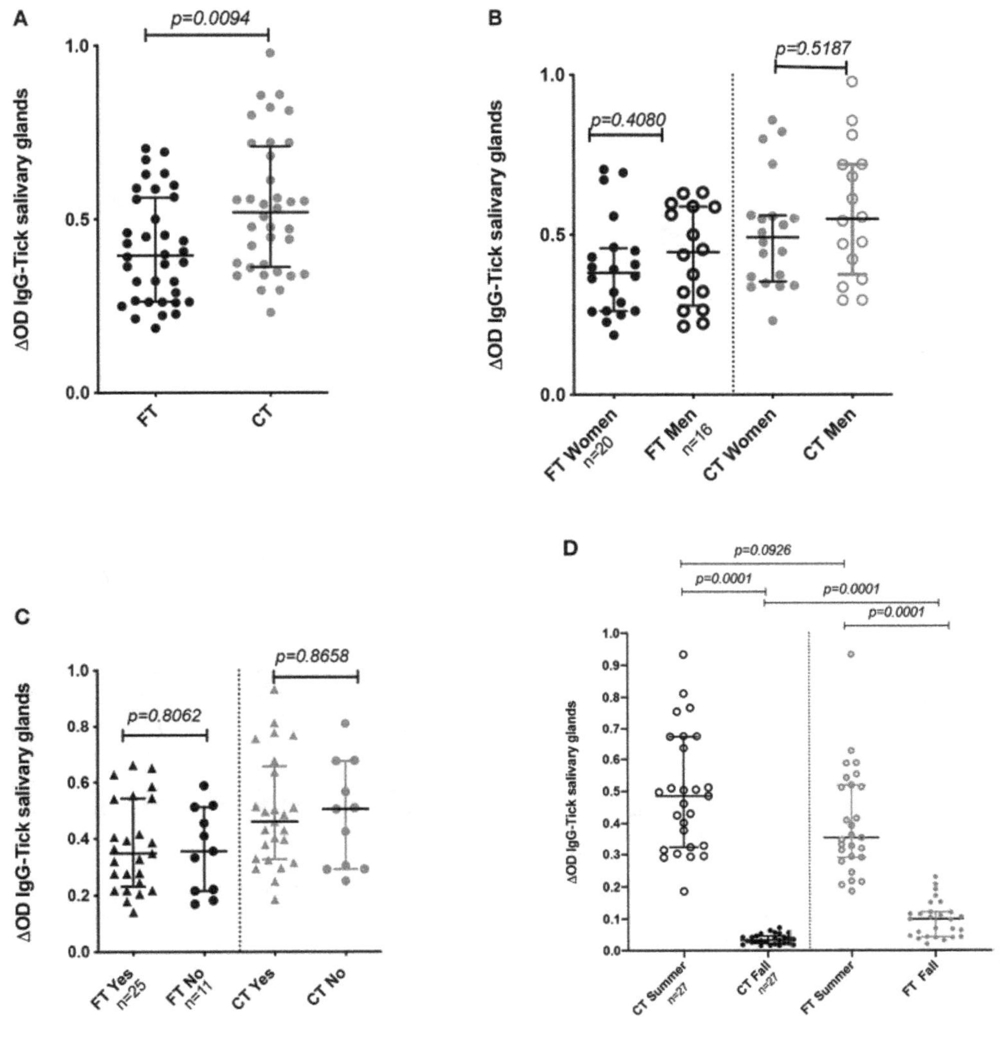

FIGURE 2 | IgG Antibody levels in human samples tested by ELISA. **(A)** Total IgG antibody levels against FT-SGE and CT-SGE. **(B)** Comparison of anti SGE antibodies levels in women and men enrolled in summer 2018. **(C)** Comparison of IgG antibodies levels by use of repellent. **(D)** Comparison of antibody levels in Summer and Fall of 2018. Figure displaying the median with interquartile range.Significance evaluated by the Mann-Whitney test with a $p < 0.05$.

5 found that may explain why we observed higher TNF in macrophages exposed to this SGE. While the other two lipocalins, Lipocalin 3 found uniquely in SGE from CT and lipocalin 1 revealing only 63 and 33%, respectively. Lipocalins are abundant proteins in the saliva of both soft and hard ticks. Also, a lipocalin from *Ixodes ricinus* (LIR) was associated with modulation of inflammation (65). These lipocalins are associated regulating skin immune responses through scavenging bio-amines decreasing the sensation of pain during the blood-feeding process and have been associated with toxicosis, a toxic reaction against tick and mite bites (66). In addition, higher levels of TNFα, downregulate B cell responses and is associated with lower immunoglobulin production (67, 68) which might explain lower antibody levels after exposure to field tick saliva.

Increasing evidence suggesting a close interaction between the immune and the nervous system in control of pain sensation. During feeding, arthropods should modulate pain sensation to guarantee their repletion. MyD88 mediates the majority of the Toll-Like Receptors (TLR) signaling and modulating the production of inflammatory cytokines (69). TLRs members are also expressed in nervous cells including microglia and astrocytes which modulate pain and itch conditions. Our study showed more than 4-fold upregulation of these genes in cells treated with FT-SGE. Interestingly, Tollip was also found upregulated. Previous studies suggest that Tollip promotes neuronal apoptosis and inflammation (70). Its upregulation similar to the MyD88 may suggest a proinflammatory effect of SGE on SH-SY5Y. In addition, our results showed an upregulation in enolase 2 and caspase 3. Enolase 2 is induced upon inflammatory signaling and it associated with degradation of the extracellular matrix, and caspase 3 is associated with cell apoptosis (71), suggesting a proinflammatory response in the central nervous system. This is of importance since tick bites can also be associated with Tick

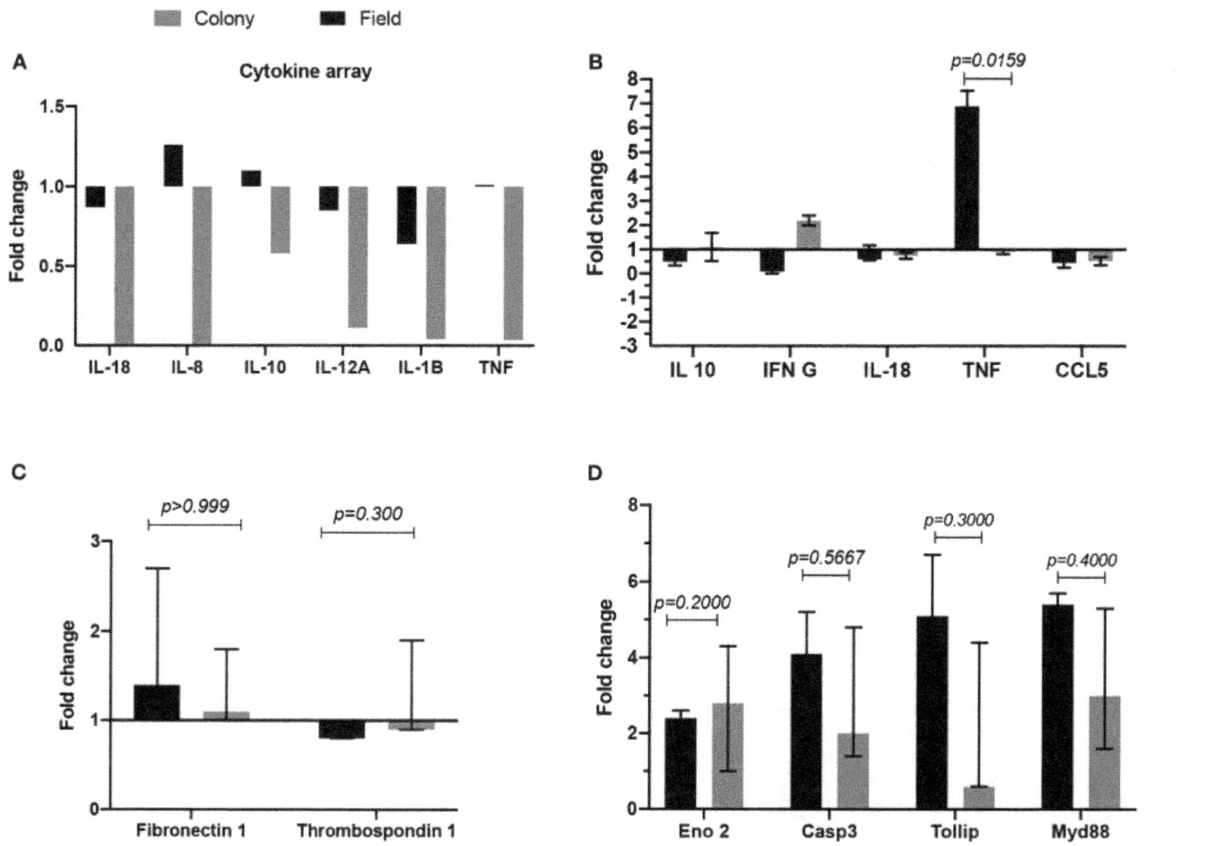

FIGURE 3 | Comparison of fold change gene expression between cells treated with either FT-SGE or CT-SGE. **(A)** Cytokine array values in U937 cells. **(B)** qRT-PCR results U937 cells cytokine testing. **(C)** Fold change gene expression in endothelial cells, and **(D)** gene expression in neurons. Figure displaying the median with interquartile range. Significance was tested by the Mann-Whitney test with a $p < 0.05$.

paralysis, a non-infectious disease caused by specific protein in tick saliva that demonstrates the effect of salivary proteins on the vertebrate nervous system (72, 73). However, It is important to disclose that we used immature/undifferentiated SH-SY5Y and the effect of tick saliva on mature neurons may be different (74).

These preliminary findings could also suggest that different cells types are affected by tick saliva during bites and that these cells have a specific response, which requires more attention to better elucidate their role during inflammation and pathogenesis of neuronal tick-borne infectious diseases. Indeed, our results showing overall differences in the response against CT-SGE and FT-SGE could be due to the underlying genetic difference between tick strains. Previous studies suggest that genetic variation of *A. americanum* is highly affected by their abundance in the environment as well as their aggressiveness as ectoparasite feeding in multiple hosts and can be significant in ticks collected from different geographical locations (23, 75). They also suggest that the lack of specificity in host preference of *A. americanum* may be responsible for the significant genetic variation among tick populations (75, 76). Age-related differences in the tick salivary component may also explain the differences observed between the two tick groups included in this study (2, 58). Specifically, ticks from the colony have a specific age-matched by the time of molting. However, ticks collected in the field may have different age (in days) and represent a more heterogeneous mixture of individuals. Nonetheless, our results highlight the importance of conducting this type of studies with field collected ticks and not laboratory reared ticks as they more closely resemble the expected responses when in contact with a human host.

Although interesting, our study has several limitations. Working with SGE instead of pure saliva introduces more components that could cause an interaction during the measurement of antibody responses. We aim to deepen our findings using pure saliva extract from both, colony and field ticks. Also, the number of volunteers was limited and information about their travel history was not recorded, these factors may have an impact in the observed response arthropod saliva since previous or chronic exposure to salivary proteins may impact antibody profiles (77). We anticipate enrolling at least 200 participants in a larger study to confirm the results to the current study using whole tick saliva as the antigen instead of SGE. However, we consider that the results provided in this preliminary study may lead to important conclusions and future directions.

CONCLUSION

This study shows that tick salivary gland protein content varies depending on the tick origin, indirectly showing that environmental conditions and probably host feeding preferences may have an impact on salivary gland content and immunogenicity. Also, our results suggest that salivary proteins from a tick can be used to measure the intensity of exposure to arthropod bites. However, not all salivary proteins are immunogenic, and this study reveals potential candidates to develop specific salivary biomarkers for *A. americanum* exposure.

ETHICS STATEMENT

The protocols followed in the study were reviewed and approved by IRB #1206 from Kansas State University. Blood samples were only collected from individuals agree to participate in the study and that had signed an informed consent. Dried blood spots in filter paper Whatman 903 were obtained from 36 healthy donors in the summer (May–June), and only 27 of those could be followed in the fall (September–November). Blood samples were obtained from adult volunteers residing in Manhattan, Kansas. At enrollment, tested individuals were provided with a questionnaire for an information about age, gender, use of repellant and outdoor activities.

AUTHOR CONTRIBUTIONS

LM-R: study design, sample collection, sample processing, analysis, writing, and reviewing. LM-C: study design, human cells *in vitro* testing, analysis, writing, and reviewing. BB: study design, sample collection, sample processing, analysis, writing, and reviewing. SM: writing and reviewing. LZ: analysis, writing, and reviewing. BL-R: study design, sample collection, analysis, writing, and reviewing.

ACKNOWLEDGMENTS

We thank the Kansas State University staff and students that participated in the study providing their blood samples. We would also like to acknowledge Yoonseong Park for his contribution on the reviewing process. Publication of this article was funded in part by the Kansas State University Open Access Publishing Fund.

REFERENCES

1. Brites-Neto J, Duarte KM, Martins TF. Tick-borne infections in human and animal population worldwide. *Vet World.* (2015) 8:301–15. doi: 10.14202/vetworld.2015.301-315
2. Simo L, Kazimirova M, Richardson J, Bonnet SI. The essential role of tick salivary glands and saliva in tick feeding and pathogen transmission. *Front Cell Infect Microbiol.* (2017) 7:281. doi: 10.3389/fcimb.2017.00281
3. Nuttall PA. Wonders of tick saliva. *Ticks Tick Borne Dis.* (2019) 10:470–81. doi: 10.1016/j.ttbdis.2018.11.005
4. Titus RG, Bishop JV, Mejia JS. The immunomodulatory factors of arthropod saliva and the potential for these factors to serve as vaccine targets to prevent pathogen transmission. *Parasite Immunol.* (2006) 28:131–41. doi: 10.1111/j.1365-3024.2006.00807.x
5. Kotal J, Langhansova H, Lieskovska J, Andersen JF, Francischetti IM, Chavakis T, et al. Modulation of host immunity by tick saliva. *J Proteomics.* (2015) 128:58–68. doi: 10.1016/j.jprot.2015.07.005
6. Perner J, Kropackova S, Kopacek P, Ribeiro JMC. Sialome diversity of ticks revealed by RNAseq of single tick salivary glands. *PLoS Negl Trop Dis.* (2018) 12:e0006410. doi: 10.1371/journal.pntd.0006410
7. Kazimirova M, Thangamani S, Bartikova P, Hermance M, Holikova V, Stibraniova I, et al. Tick-borne viruses and biological processes at the tick-host-virus interface. *Front Cell Infect Microbiol.* (2017) 7:339. doi: 10.3389/fcimb.2017.00339
8. Hermance ME, Thangamani S. Tick saliva enhances powassan virus transmission to the host, influencing its dissemination and the course of disease. *J Virol.* (2015) 89:7852–60. doi: 10.1128/JVI.01056-15
9. Nuttall PA. Tick saliva and its role in pathogen transmission. *Wien Klin Wochenschr.* (2019) 10:1–12. doi: 10.1007/s00508-019-1500-y
10. Schuijt TJ, Hovius JW, van Burgel ND, Ramamoorthi N, Fikrig E, van Dam AP. The tick salivary protein Salp15 inhibits the killing of serum-sensitive Borrelia burgdorferi sensu lato isolates. *Infect Immun.* (2008) 76:2888–94. doi: 10.1128/IAI.00232-08
11. Andrade BB, Teixeira CR, Barral A, Barral-Netto M. Haematophagous arthropod saliva and host defense system: a tale of tear and blood. *An Acad Bras Cienc.* (2005) 77:665–93. doi: 10.1590/S0001-37652005000400008
12. Scholl DC, Embers ME, Caskey JR, Kaushal D, Mather TN, Buck WR, et al. Immunomodulatory effects of tick saliva on dermal cells exposed to Borrelia burgdorferi, the agent of Lyme disease. *Parasit Vectors.* (2016) 9:394. doi: 10.1186/s13071-016-1638-7
13. Wikel S. Ticks and tick-borne pathogens at the cutaneous interface: host defenses, tick countermeasures, a suitable environment for pathogen establishment. *Front Microbiol.* (2013) 4:337. doi: 10.3389/fmicb.2013.00337
14. Londono-Renteria B, Cardenas JC, Giovanni JE, Cardenas L, Villamizar P, Rolon J, et al. *Aedes aegypti* anti-salivary gland antibody concentration and dengue virus exposure history in healthy individuals living in an endemic area in Colombia. *Biomedica.* (2015) 35:572–81. doi: 10.7705/biomedica.v35i4.2530
15. Londono-Renteria B, Patel JC, Vaughn M, Funkhauser S, Ponnusamy L, Grippin C, et al. Long-lasting permethrin-impregnated clothing protects against mosquito bites in outdoor workers. *Am J Trop Med Hyg.* (2015) 93:869–74. doi: 10.4269/ajtmh.15-0130
16. Lane RS, Moss RB, Hsu YP, Wei T, Mesirow ML, Kuo MM. Anti-arthropod saliva antibodies among residents of a community at high risk for Lyme disease in California. *Am J Trop Med Hyg.* (1999) 61:850–9. doi: 10.4269/ajtmh.1999.61.850
17. Huang YS, Higgs S, Vanlandingham DL. Arbovirus-mosquito vector-host interactions and the impact on transmission and disease pathogenesis of arboviruses. *Front Microbiol.* (2019) 10:22. doi: 10.3389/fmicb.2019.00022
18. Nuttall PA, Labuda M. Tick-host interactions: saliva-activated transmission. *Parasitology.* (2004) 129 (Suppl. 1):S177–89. doi: 10.1017/S0031182004005633
19. Ferreira BR, Szabo MJ, Cavassani KA, Bechara GH, Silva JS. Antigens from Rhipicephalus sanguineus ticks elicit potent cell-mediated immune responses in resistant but not in susceptible animals. *Vet Parasitol.* (2003) 115:35–48. doi: 10.1016/S0304-4017(03)00190-0
20. Radulovic ZM, Kim TK, Porter LM, Sze SH, Lewis L, Mulenga A. A 24–48 h fed Amblyomma americanum tick saliva immuno-proteome. *BMC Genomics.* (2014) 15:518. doi: 10.1186/1471-2164-15-518
21. Ribeiro JM. How ticks make a living. *Parasitol Today.* (1995) 11:91–3. doi: 10.1016/0169-4758(95)80162-6

22. Sprong H, Trentelman J, Seemann I, Grubhoffer L, Rego RO, Hajdusek O, et al. ANTIDotE: anti-tick vaccines to prevent tick-borne diseases in Europe. *Parasit Vectors.* (2014) 7:77. doi: 10.1186/1756-3305-7-77
23. Childs JE, Paddock CD. The ascendancy of Amblyomma americanum as a vector of pathogens affecting humans in the United States. *Annu Rev Entomol.* (2003) 48:307–37. doi: 10.1146/annurev.ento.48.091801.112728
24. Barrett AW, Noden BH, Gruntmeir JM, Holland T, Mitcham JR, Martin JE, et al. County scale distribution of *Amblyomma americanum* (Ixodida: Ixodidae) in Oklahoma: addressing local deficits in tick maps based on passive reporting. *J Med Entomol.* (2015) 52:269–73. doi: 10.1093/jme/tju026
25. Raghavan RK, Peterson AT, Cobos ME, Ganta R, Foley D. Current and future distribution of the Lone Star Tick, *Amblyomma americanum* (L.) (Acari: Ixodidae) in North America. *PLoS ONE.* (2019) 14:e0209082. doi: 10.1371/journal.pone.0209082
26. Mani RJ, Metcalf JA, Clinkenbeard KD. *Amblyomma americanum* as a bridging vector for human infection with *Francisella tularensis*. *PLoS ONE.* (2015) 10:e0130513. doi: 10.1371/journal.pone.0130513
27. Crispell G, Commins SP, Archer-Hartman SA, Choudhary S, Dharmarajan G, Azadi P, et al. Discovery of alpha-gal-containing antigens in north american tick species believed to induce red meat allergy. *Front Immunol.* (2019) 10:1056. doi: 10.3389/fimmu.2019.01056
28. Monzon JD, Atkinson EG, Henn BM, Benach JL. Population and evolutionary genomics of *Amblyomma americanum*, an expanding arthropod disease vector. *Genome Biol Evol.* (2016) 8:1351–60. doi: 10.1093/gbe/evw080
29. Centers for Disease Control and Prevention. *Tickborne diseases of the United States.* (2019). Available online at: https://www.cdc.gov/ticks/tickbornediseases/tickID.html
30. Sonenshine DE, Nicholson, WL. Ticks (Ixodida). In: Mullen GR, Durden LA, editors. *Medical and Veterinary Entomology*. Statesboro, GA: Academic Press (2002). p. 517–58.
31. Londono-Renteria BL, Eisele TP, Keating J, James MA, Wesson DM. Antibody response against *Anopheles albimanus* (Diptera: Culicidae) salivary protein as a measure of mosquito bite exposure in Haiti. *J Med Entomol.* (2010) 47:1156–63. doi: 10.1603/ME09240
32. Londono-Renteria B, Drame PM, Weitzel T, Rosas R, Gripping C, Cardenas JC, et al. *An. gambiae* gSG6-P1 evaluation as a proxy for human-vector contact in the Americas: a pilot study. *Parasit Vectors.* (2015) 8:533. doi: 10.1186/s13071-015-1160-3
33. Conway MJ, Londono-Renteria B, Troupin A, Watson AM, Klimstra WB, Fikrig E, et al. *Aedes aegypti* D7 saliva protein inhibits dengue virus infection. *PLoS Negl Trop Dis.* (2016) 10:e0004941. doi: 10.1371/journal.pntd.0004941
34. Vogt MB, Lahon A, Arya RP, Kneubehl AR, Spencer Clinton JL, Paust S, et al. Mosquito saliva alone has profound effects on the human immune system. *PLoS Negl Trop Dis.* (2018) 12:e0006439. doi: 10.1371/journal.pntd.0006439
35. T.Nascimento GD, Vieira PS, Cogo SC, Dias-Netipanyj MF, Franca Junior N, Camara DAD, et al. Antitumoral effects of *Amblyomma sculptum* Berlese saliva in neuroblastoma cell lines involve cytoskeletal deconstruction and cell cycle arrest. *Rev Bras Parasitol Vet.* (2019) 28:126–33. doi: 10.1590/s1984-296120180098
36. Shipley MM, Mangold CA, Kuny CV, Szpara ML. Differentiated human SH-SY5Y cells provide a reductionist model of herpes simplex virus 1 neurotropism. *J Virol.* (2017) 91:e00958-17. doi: 10.1128/JVI.00958-17
37. Gokyu M, Kobayashi H, Nanbara H, Sudo T, Ikeda Y, Suda T, et al. Thrombospondin-1 production is enhanced by Porphyromonas gingivalis lipopolysaccharide in THP-1 cells. *PLoS ONE.* (2014) 9:e115107. doi: 10.1371/journal.pone.0115107
38. Tabata S, Ikeda R, Yamamoto M, Shimaoka S, Mukaida N, Takeda Y, et al. Thymidine phosphorylase activates NFkappaB and stimulates the expression of angiogenic and metastatic factors in human cancer cells. *Oncotarget.* (2014) 5:10473–85. doi: 10.18632/oncotarget.2242
39. Pimentel-Nunes P, Goncalves N, Boal-Carvalho I, Afonso L, Lopes P, Roncon-Albuquerque R Jr, et al. Decreased Toll-interacting protein and peroxisome proliferator-activated receptor gamma are associated with increased expression of Toll-like receptors in colon carcinogenesis. *J Clin Pathol.* (2012) 65:302–8. doi: 10.1136/jclinpath-2011-200567
40. Gu H, Jiao Y, Yu X, Li X, Wang W, Ding L, et al. Resveratrol inhibits the IL-1beta-induced expression of MMP-13 and IL-6 in human articular chondrocytes via TLR4/MyD88-dependent and -independent signaling cascades. *Int J Mol Med.* (2017) 39:734–40. doi: 10.3892/ijmm.2017.2885
41. Du M, Wang X, Tan X, Li X, Huang D, Huang K, et al. Nkx2-5 is expressed in atherosclerotic plaques and attenuates development of atherosclerosis in apolipoprotein E-deficient mice. *J Am Heart Assoc.* (2016) 5:e004440. doi: 10.1161/JAHA.116.004440
42. Li Y, Chen R, Bowden M, Mo F, Lin YY, Gleave M, et al. Establishment of a neuroendocrine prostate cancer model driven by the RNA splicing factor SRRM4. *Oncotarget.* (2017) 8:66878–88. doi: 10.18632/oncotarget.19916
43. Feng M, Kang M, He F, Xiao Z, Liu Z, Yao H, et al. Plasma interleukin-37 is increased and inhibits the production of inflammatory cytokines in peripheral blood mononuclear cells in systemic juvenile idiopathic arthritis patients. *J Transl Med.* (2018) 16:277. doi: 10.1186/s12967-018-1655-8
44. Wang B, Wei G, Liu B, Zhou X, Xiao H, Dong N, et al. The role of high mobility group box 1 protein in interleukin-18-induced myofibroblastic transition of valvular interstitial cells. *Cardiology.* (2016) 135:168–78. doi: 10.1159/000447483
45. Kawka E, Witowski J, Fouqet N, Tayama H, Bender TO, Catar R, et al. Regulation of chemokine CCL5 synthesis in human peritoneal fibroblasts: a key role of IFN-gamma. *Mediators Inflamm.* (2014) 2014:590654. doi: 10.1155/2014/590654
46. Plotnikova MA, Klotchenko SA, Vasin AV. Development of a multiplex quantitative PCR assay for the analysis of human cytokine gene expression in influenza A virus-infected cells. *J Immunol Methods.* (2016) 430:51–5. doi: 10.1016/j.jim.2016.01.005
47. Kim S, Kim YK, Lee H, Cho JE, Kim HY, Uh Y, et al. Interferon gamma mRNA quantitative real-time polymerase chain reaction for the diagnosis of latent tuberculosis: a novel interferon gamma release assay. *Diagn Microbiol Infect Dis.* (2013) 75:68–72. doi: 10.1016/j.diagmicrobio.2012.09.015
48. Sanchez D, Ganfornina MD, Gutierrez G, Marin A. Exon-intron structure and evolution of the Lipocalin gene family. *Mol Biol Evol.* (2003) 20:775–83. doi: 10.1093/molbev/msg079
49. Paesen GC, Adams PL, Nuttall PA, Stuart DL. Tick histamine-binding proteins: lipocalins with a second binding cavity. *Biochim Biophys Acta.* (2000) 1482:92–101. doi: 10.1016/S0167-4838(00)00168-0
50. Wolk K, Wenzel J, Tsaousi A, Witte-Handel E, Babel N, Zelenak C, et al. Lipocalin-2 is expressed by activated granulocytes and keratinocytes in affected skin and reflects disease activity in acne inversa/hidradenitis suppurativa. *Br J Dermatol.* (2017) 177:1385–93. doi: 10.1111/bjd.15424
51. Fontaine A, Diouf I, Bakkali N, Misse D, Pages F, Fusai T, et al. Implication of haematophagous arthropod salivary proteins in host-vector interactions. *Parasit Vectors.* (2011) 4:187. doi: 10.1186/1756-3305-4-187
52. Londono-Renteria B, Cardenas JC, Cardenas LD, Christofferson RC, Chisenhall DM, Wesson DM, et al. Use of anti-Aedes aegypti salivary extract antibody concentration to correlate risk of vector exposure and dengue transmission risk in Colombia. *PLoS ONE.* (2013) 8:e81211. doi: 10.1371/journal.pone.0081211
53. Fontaine A, Pascual A, Orlandi-Pradines E, Diouf I, Remoue F, Pages F, et al. Relationship between exposure to vector bites and antibody responses to mosquito salivary gland extracts. *PLoS ONE.* (2011) 6:e29107. doi: 10.1371/journal.pone.0029107
54. Rego ROM, Trentelman JJA, Anguita J, Nijhof AM, Sprong H, Klempa B, et al. Counterattacking the tick bite: towards a rational design of anti-tick vaccines targeting pathogen transmission. *Parasit Vectors.* (2019) 12:229. doi: 10.1186/s13071-019-3468-x
55. Karim S, Ribeiro JM. An insight into the sialome of the lone star tick, *Amblyomma americanum*, with a glimpse on its time dependent gene expression. *PLoS ONE.* (2015) 10:e0131292. doi: 10.1371/journal.pone.0131292
56. Sugino M, Imamura S, Mulenga A, Nakajima M, Tsuda A, Ohashi K, et al. A serine proteinase inhibitor (serpin) from ixodid tick Haemaphysalis longicornis; cloning and preliminary assessment of its suitability as a candidate for a tick vaccine. *Vaccine.* (2003) 21:2844–51. doi: 10.1016/S0264-410X(03)00167-1
57. Liu L, Cheng TY, He XM. Proteomic profiling of the midgut contents of *Haemaphysalis flava*. *Ticks Tick Borne Dis.* (2018) 9:490–5. doi: 10.1016/j.ttbdis.2018.01.008

58. Tirloni L, Reck J, Terra RM, Martins JR, Mulenga A, Sherman NE, et al. Proteomic analysis of cattle tick Rhipicephalus (Boophilus) microplus saliva: a comparison between partially and fully engorged females. *PLoS ONE.* (2014) 9:e94831. doi: 10.1371/journal.pone.0094831
59. Lewis LA, Radulovic ZM, Kim TK, Porter LM, Mulenga A. Identification of 24h ixodes scapularis immunogenic tick saliva proteins. *Ticks Tick Borne Dis.* (2015) 6:424–34. doi: 10.1016/j.ttbdis.2015.03.012
60. Sottrup-Jensen L, Stepanik TM, Kristensen T, Lonblad PB, Jones CM, Wierzbicki DM, et al. Common evolutionary origin of alpha 2-macroglobulin and complement components C3 and C4. *Proc Natl Acad Sci USA.* (1985) 82:9–13. doi: 10.1073/pnas.82.1.9
61. Londono-Renteria B, Grippin C, Cardenas JC, Troupin A, Colpitts TM. Human C5a protein participates in the mosquito immune response against dengue virus. *J Med Entomol.* (2016) 53:505–12. doi: 10.1093/jme/tjw003
62. Maya-Monteiro CM, Daffre S, Logullo C, Lara FA, Alves EW, Capurro ML, et al. HeLp, a heme lipoprotein from the hemolymph of the cattle tick, *Boophilus microplus*. *J Biol Chem.* (2000) 275:36584–9. doi: 10.1074/jbc.M007344200
63. Tian Y, Chen W, Mo G, Chen R, Fang M, Yedid G, et al. An immunosuppressant peptide from the hard tick *Amblyomma variegatum*. *Toxins.* (2016) 8:E133. doi: 10.3390/toxins8050133
64. Ramachandra RN, Wikel SK. Modulation of host-immune responses by ticks (Acari: Ixodidae): effect of salivary gland extracts on host macrophages and lymphocyte cytokine production. *J Med Entomol.* (1992) 29:818–26. doi: 10.1093/jmedent/29.5.818
65. Beaufays J, Adam B, Decrem Y, Prevot PP, Santini S, Brasseur R, et al. Ixodes ricinus tick lipocalins: identification, cloning, phylogenetic analysis and biochemical characterization. *PLoS ONE.* (2008) 3:e3941. doi: 10.1371/journal.pone.0003941
66. Mans BJ, Louw AI, Neitz AW. The major tick salivary gland proteins and toxins from the soft tick, *Ornithodoros savignyi*, are part of the tick Lipocalin family: implications for the origins of tick toxicoses. *Mol Biol Evol.* (2003) 20:1158–67. doi: 10.1093/molbev/msg126
67. Frasca D, Romero M, Diaz A, Alter-Wolf S, Ratliff M, Landin AM, et al. A molecular mechanism for TNF-alpha-mediated downregulation of B cell responses. *J Immunol.* (2012) 188:279–86. doi: 10.4049/jimmunol.1003964
68. Rieckmann P, Tuscano JM, Kehrl JH. Tumor necrosis factor-alpha (TNF-alpha) and interleukin-6 (IL-6) in B-lymphocyte function. *Methods.* (1997) 11:128–32. doi: 10.1006/meth.1996.0396
69. Liu XJ, Liu T, Chen G, Wang B, Yu XL, Yin C, et al. TLR signaling adaptor protein MyD88 in primary sensory neurons contributes to persistent inflammatory and neuropathic pain and neuroinflammation. *Sci Rep.* (2016) 6:28188. doi: 10.1038/srep28188
70. Li M, Feng B, Wang L, Guo S, Zhang P, Gong J, et al. Tollip is a critical mediator of cerebral ischaemia-reperfusion injury. *J Pathol.* (2015) 237:249–62. doi: 10.1002/path.4565
71. Haque A, Ray SK, Cox A, Banik NL. Neuron specific enolase: a promising therapeutic target in acute spinal cord injury. *Metab Brain Dis.* (2016) 31:487–95. doi: 10.1007/s11011-016-9801-6
72. Borawski K, Pancewicz S, Czupryna P, Zajkowska J, Moniuszko-Malinowska A. Tick paralysis. *Przegl Epidemiol.* (2018) 72:17–24.
73. Pienaar R, Neitz AWH, Mans BJ. Tick paralysis: solving an enigma. *Vet Sci.* (2018) 5:E53. doi: 10.3390/vetsci5020053
74. Shipley MM, Mangold CA, Szpara ML. Differentiation of the SH-SY5Y human neuroblastoma cell line. *J Vis Exp.* (2016) 53193. doi: 10.3791/53193
75. Trout RT, Steelman CD, Szalanski AL. Population genetics of *Amblyomma americanum* (Acari: Ixodidae) collected from Arkansas. *J Med Entomol.* (2010) 47:152–61. doi: 10.1093/jmedent/47.2.152
76. Barrett LG, Thrall PH, Burdon JJ, Linde CC. Life history determines genetic structure and evolutionary potential of host-parasite interactions. *Trends Ecol Evol.* (2008) 23:678–85. doi: 10.1016/j.tree.2008.06.017
77. Cardenas JC, Drame PM, Luque-Burgos KA, Berrio JD, Entrena-Mutis E, Gonzalez MU, et al. IgG1 and IgG4 antibodies against *Aedes aegypti* salivary proteins and risk for dengue infections. *PLoS ONE.* (2019) 14:e0208455. doi: 10.1371/journal.pone.0208455

4

Immune Response Modulation by Caliciviruses

Yoatzin Peñaflor-Téllez, Adrian Trujillo-Uscanga, Jesús Alejandro Escobar-Almazán and Ana Lorena Gutiérrez-Escolano*

Departamento de Infectómica y Patogénesis Molecular, Centro de Investigación y de Estudios Avanzados, IPN, Mexico City, Mexico

***Correspondence:**
Ana Lorena Gutiérrez-Escolano
alonso@cinvestav.mx

Noroviruses and Sapoviruses, classified in the *Caliciviridae* family, are small positive-stranded RNA viruses, considered nowadays the leading cause of acute gastroenteritis globally in both children and adults. Although most noroviruses have been associated with gastrointestinal disease in humans, almost 50 years after its discovery, there is still a lack of comprehensive evidence regarding its biology and pathogenesis mainly because they can be neither conveniently grown in cultured cells nor propagated in animal models. However, other members of this family such as Feline calicivirus (FCV), Murine norovirus (MNV), Rabbit hemorrhagic disease virus (RHDV), and Porcine sapovirus (PS), from which there are accessible propagation systems, have been useful to study the calicivirus replication strategies. Using cell cultures and animal models, many of the functions of the viral proteins in the viral replication cycles have been well-characterized. Moreover, evidence of the role of viral proteins from different members of the family in the establishment of infection has been generated and the mechanism of their immunopathogenesis begins to be understood. In this review, we discuss different aspects of how caliciviruses are implicated in membrane rearrangements, apoptosis, and evasion of the immune responses, highlighting some of the pathogenic mechanisms triggered by different members of the *Caliciviridae* family.

Keywords: calicivirus, apoptosis, immunopathogenesis, replicative complexes, HuNoV, FCV, RHDV, MNV

INTRODUCTION

Human caliciviruses (HuCVs), comprised by human noroviruses (HuNoV) and sapoviruses (HuSaV), are the leading cause of acute gastroenteritis globally (1), affecting millions of people each year (1, 2). They are considered the most common cause of acute diarrhea in both children and adults in industrialized countries; however, almost 50 years after its discovery, there is still a lack of comprehensive epidemiological evidence of the role of noroviruses in developing countries (3). Although most noroviruses have been associated with gastrointestinal disease in humans, knowledge regarding its biology and pathogenesis have been hampered because they cannot be conveniently grown in cell culture or propagated in animal models (4, 5). As a result, much of our knowledge on the basic mechanisms of norovirus biology has been largely inferred from studies on other animal caliciviruses that can be successfully propagated *in vitro* as well as in live models (5).

The *Caliciviridae* family is composed of small non-enveloped viruses of ~27–35 nm in diameter, with a single-stranded RNA of positive polarity genome of ~7.6–8.6 kilobases (kb) in length. This family currently comprises five genera: *Norovirus, Sapovirus, Lagovirus, Vesivirus, and Nebovirus* that are ubiquitous in the environment. Moreover, other six new genera*: Recovirus, Valovirus, Nacovirus, Bavovirus, Minovirus, and Salovirus* have been proposed (6–12).

Caliciviruses have a broad host range and cause a wide spectrum of diseases in their hosts, including digestive tract infections, vesicular lesions and reproductive failure, stomatitis, upper respiratory tract and systemic diseases, and hemorrhagic disease (6).

Replicative Cycle

Calicivirus Attachment, Entry, and RNA Uncoating

Caliciviruses require attachment to their target cells through the interaction with oligosaccharides present in the cell surface. Many noroviruses, neboviruses, and lagoviruses require saccharides in histo-blood group antigens (HBGAs) [reviewed in (13) and (14), whereas vesiviruses and murine norovirus (MNV) use sialic acid (15, 16)]. Bile salts and divalent cations are also key mediators of norovirus entry (17). Like many other viruses, the members of the *Caliciviridae* family enter their host cell by receptor-mediated endocytosis. Protein receptors of three caliciviruses have been identified; the Junctional Adhesion Molecule 1 (JAM-1) for FCV (18, 19) and for Hom-1 calicivirus on human cells (20), and the CD300lf and CD300ld molecules for MNV (21, 22). Moreover, Annexin A2 has been implicated in the attachment and entry of the Rabbit vesivirus (RaV) (23). Although no more proteinaceous receptors have been described for other caliciviruses, it is known that RHDV interaction with HBGAs triggers the entry to its target cells (13); moreover, occludin is required as a coreceptor for porcine sapovirus (PSaV) entry to epithelial cells from porcine kidney LLC-PK cells with dissociated tight junctions (24).

Caliciviruses enter their host cells by triggering different endocytosis pathways following receptor engagement (24–27). The acidification of late endosomes is an essential step in the viral entry process (28, 29); however, the ways by which the virus escapes the endosome degradation and delivers the genome into the cytosol are poorly understood. New insights into calicivirus uncoating process come from a recent finding that demonstrates the formation of a portal on the capsid of FCV after JAM-1 engagement that allows the opening of the capsid shell for the release of the genomic RNA into the cytoplasm passing through the endosomal membrane (30).

CALICIVIRUS GENOME TRANSLATION AND REPLICATION

Calicivirus genome translation occurs immediately after the viral genome is released into the cytoplasm. Its genome is single-stranded of positive polarity RNA that is covalently bound to the viral protein genome-linked (VPg) at its 5′ end, and is polyadenylated; it is flanked by two short non-translated regions (NTR) that contain important regulatory elements for viral translation, replication, and morphogenesis (**Figure 1**). VPg linked to the 5′ end of the calicivirus genome serves as a proteinaceous cap that interacts with translation initiation factors, including the canonic cap-binding proteins; eIF4F, eIF4E, eIF4A, and eIF3 (31–38).

Calicivirus genomes are of ~7.5–8.6 Kb in length and contain from two to four open reading frames (ORF). The non-structural (NS) proteins are encoded in the ORF1, expressed as a polyprotein that is cleaved by the action of its own protease into 6 or 7 individual proteins designated non structural (NS) 1 through 7: NS1/2 or N-term, NS3 or helicase, NS4, NS5 or VPg, NS6 or protease, and NS7 or RNA dependent RNA polymerase (RdRp). The structural proteins VP1 and VP2 are encoded in the ORF2 and 3 from the subgenomic RNA as in noroviruses and vesiviruses; other caliciviruses encoded VP1 in the ORF1 [reviewed in (39, 40)]. MNV contain a fourth ORF that encodes the virulence factor (VF) 1, involved in evasion of innate immunity (41). In FCV, VP1 is encoded as a precursor that is cleaved by the viral protease-polymerase NS6/7 to produce the mature VP1 and a small protein of 124 amino acids known as the leader of the capsid protein (LC) (42) which has recently been shown to be involved in triggering apoptosis (43). The NS proteins, enhance translation rounds of the viral genome and lead the cell to the establishment of a pathogenic phenotype, inducing membrane proliferation that will induce the formation of the replication complexes (RCs), or viral factories and alter the vesicular secretory pathway to evade both the innate and acquired antiviral immune response and trigger apoptosis.

Calicivirus genome replication occurs in the RCs and involves the production of a negative-sense RNA template through the action of the NS7 protein, from which the genomic and subgenomic RNAs are produced (4, 39). Both VP1 and VP2 translation also takes place near the RC at late stages of infection.

Maturation and Exit

Calicivirus exit has been associated with the induction of apoptosis as a mechanism to facilitate the dissemination of viral progeny in the host. Moreover, Santiana et al. have reported a non-lytically release of norovirus particles inside exosomes into stool that contribute to the fecal-oral transmission of multiple viral particles collectively to the next host (44). The role of apoptosis will be described in more detail below since it is essential for the establishment of the calicivirus immunopathogenic phenotype.

CYTOPATHIC EFFECT AND MEMBRANE REARRANGEMENTS IN CALICIVIRUS INFECTED CELLS

All positive-stranded RNA viruses replicate in association with cytoplasmic membranes from the host cell where membrane compartments, known as RCs or viral factories are induced by viral NS proteins in coordination with host factors to facilitate productive RNA replication. Packaging of the viral genome also occurs in these compartments, providing an environment protected from host cell immunity. The membrane rearrangements induced by these viruses can be derived from a variety of organelles including the endoplasmic reticulum (ER) and Golgi apparatus, lipid droplets, endosomes, lysosomes,

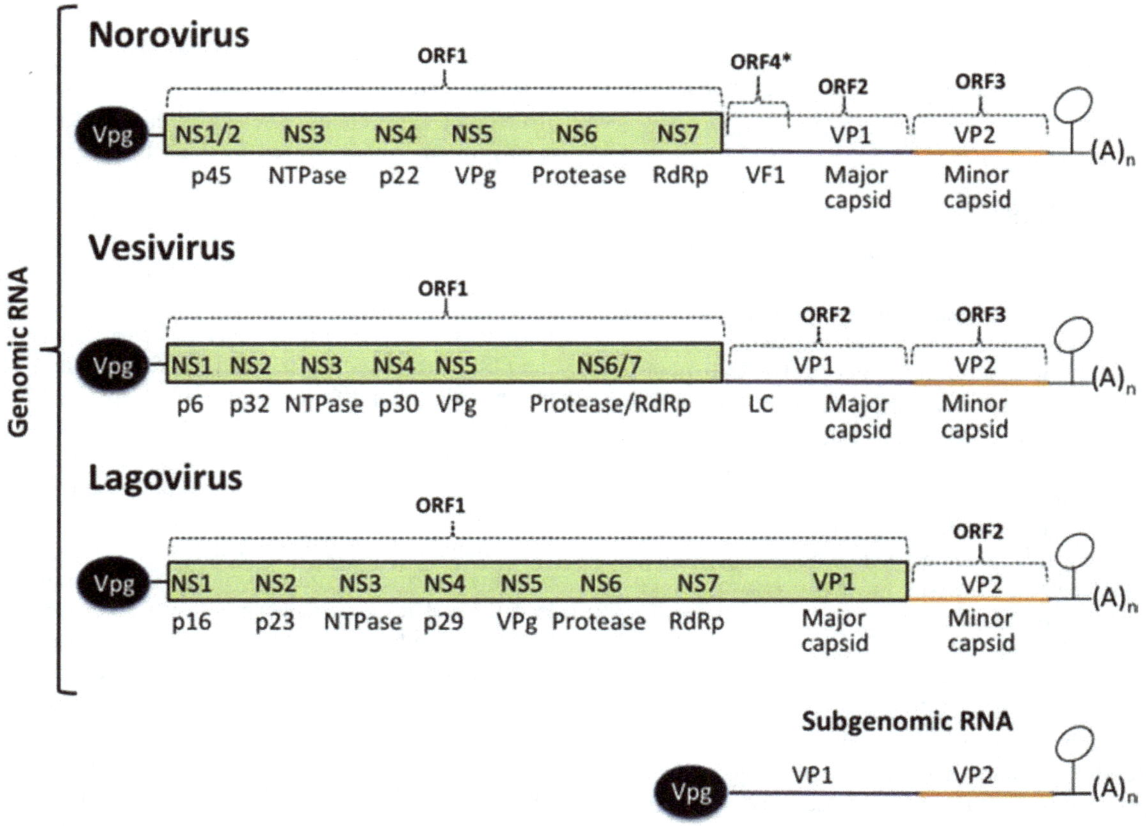

FIGURE 1 | Calicivirus genome organization. All calicivirus genomes are 5′ Vpg-linked and polyadenylated at their 3′ ends. They contain an ORF 1 that encodes for the non-structural proteins NS1–NS7. The structural proteins VP1 and VP2 are encoded form the ORF 2 and 3 (*Noroviruses* and *Vesiviruses*) or form the ORF 1 and 2 (*Lagoviruses, Neboviruses, Becoviruses,* and *Sapoviruses*) are translated form the subgenomic RNA. The MNV Virulence Factor 1 (VF1) encoded from the ORF 4, the FCV Leader of the capsid (LC), and HuSaPV ORF-3 protein are unique among caliciviruses. Stem-loop structures present in the 3′ UTRs form the genomic and the subgenomic RNAs are indicated.

peroxisomes, chloroplasts, and mitochondria [reviewed in (45, 46)].

The first reports regarding the alteration of intracellular membranes caused by a calicivirus infection were published since the early 70s (47–49). In FCV, proteins p32 (NS2), p39 (NS3), and p30 (NS4) proteins were found to cause ER-derived origin membranous vesicles (50). Thus, as suggested by Bailey et al. the initiation step of RC formation may take place on the ER, but other components of the secretory pathway may be involved as this structure matures (50).

The expression of the RHDV viral protein p23, which is equivalent to the MNV NS1/2 and homolog of the FCV p32, has been shown to localize in the ER, as well as the helicase p29 (51). Interestingly, expression of the recombinant RdRp alone or in the context of the entire polyprotein from both RHDV and RCV cause a striking redistribution of Golgi but not ER membranes (51–53).

The expression of the N-terminal (NS1/2) non-structural protein from NV, was found to colocalize with the Golgi apparatus and induce intracellular membrane rearrangements (54), in contrast to the ER localization patterns of the homologous proteins from RHDV, MNV, and FCV (51, 55). A phenotypically abnormal Golgi was also shown as the result of both NV replication and the expression of the NS protein p22 (NS4) that was also involved in the inhibition of the cellular protein secretion pathway (ER to Golgi trafficking; 57). The antagonism of the secretory pathway produced by NV NS4 has been proposed to facilitate viral pathogenesis, probably as an interferon (IFN) and/or cytokine signaling deactivator (56). More recently, the expression of norovirus GII.4 ORF1 polyprotein was shown to produce the accumulation of single, double, and multi membrane vesicles likely built from the ER, that resemble those reported during MNV infection (57). Moreover, the expression of single proteins revealed different membrane alterations: NS1/2 induced proliferation of smooth ER membranes, NS3 was found associated with ER membranes around lipid droplets, and NS4 caused an even more pronounced effect than NS3 and was the only protein capable of inducing both single and double-membrane vesicles when expressed alone (57).

The differences in the intracellular localization of the NS proteins from several members of the *Caliciviridae* family, in both transfected and infected environments, indicate a high level of variation in the intracellular replication mechanisms; however, as with many other positive RNA viruses, membranes of the secretory pathway participate in the RC formation. Therefore, besides its role in viral replication, membrane rearrangement, and fragmentation of the Golgi network may also result in the alteration of the intracellular transport and secretion of host cell proteins involved in the evasion of host immune responses.

APOPTOSIS IN CALICIVIRUS INFECTED CELLS

During calicivirus infection, intrinsic apoptosis occurs to facilitate the dissemination of viral progeny in the host (58–63). Recent evidence suggests that apoptosis is used by noroviruses as a mechanism to suppress the translation of induced interferon-stimulated genes (ISG) in order to diminish the host innate immune response to infection (64).

The first reports of apoptosis induced by a calicivirus were observed in experimentally infected rabbits with RHDV that undergo liver cell death due to apoptosis (59, 65). Moreover, all cell types supporting viral replication in experimentally infected rabbits present apoptosis upon infection, such as lung macrophages, intravascular monocytes, endothelial cells (59), granulocytes, and lymphocytes (66). The RHDV VP2 (VP10) was the first viral protein associated with the induction of apoptosis in transfected cells (67). More recently, the ectopic expression of the viral trypsin-like cysteine-protease NS6 was found to cause the activation of caspase−3,−8, and−9 in rabbit (RK13), as well as in human (HepG2 and HeLa) cells (68), suggesting that apoptosis plays a central role in the pathogenesis of this virus.

Intrinsic apoptosis in FCV infection has been well-characterized and several reports have evidenced both morphological (chromatin condensation, DNA fragmentation, plasma membrane blebbing, and cell shrinkage) as well as molecular changes (Bax translocation to the mitochondria, cytochrome C and the Second Mitochondria-derived Activator of Caspases, and Direct IAP-Binding protein with Low PI, Smac/DIABLO release to the cytosol, and caspase−9 and−3 activation) (43, 58, 61–63). The FCV protein LC, which is unique among the *Caliciviridae* members, is responsible for the cytopathic effect characterized in infected CrFK cells by cell rounding and caspases activation and induction of the intrinsic apoptotic pathway (43, 69).

MNV infection is known to cause the induction of mitochondrial apoptosis via activation of caspase−3,−7, and−9 as well as induction of cathepsin B activity (60, 70). Even though, no single MNV-1 protein has been associated with the downregulation of survivin or induction of apoptosis (60), the expression of the MNV ORF1 polyprotein induces apoptosis in a virus-free cell model characterized by caspase-9 activation and survivin downregulation (71), indicating that one or more NS proteins are pro-apoptotic in the absence of viral replication. Furthermore, caspase-mediated cleavage of MNV-CR6 strain NS1/2 protein potentiates apoptosis through further caspase activation (72).

Replication of HuNoV causes apoptosis in the epithelial cells of small intestinal tissue sections (duodenum) of pig enterocytes characterized by nuclear displacement, chromatin condensation, and reduced number of organelles (73). The same morphological changes as well as caspase-3 activation were observed in infected human epithelial cells (74), particularly in enterocytes and sub-epithelial macrophages from intestinal transplant recipients with calicivirus enteritis (75–77). The increased apoptosis shown in crypt enterocytes in these immunosuppressed patients is generally considered to be the cause of intestinal allograft rejection and enteritis, while increased apoptosis of villus enterocytes and sub-epithelial macrophages is associated with enteritis (75, 76).

In vitro studies regarding the viral molecules implicated in the induction of apoptosis have identified two different NS proteins form HuNoV GII namely NS4 protein (p20) from norovirus GII.4 variant 2002, and the helicase NS3 or NTPase (P41) from the norovirus GII.4/YJB1/2009/Chiayi. This pro-apoptotic activity was enhanced by the co-expression with N-term or p22 (78). However, no protein encoded by NV, a GI.I strain, has been implicated in the induction of apoptosis.

THE IMMUNE RESPONSE TO CALICIVIRUS INFECTION

Calicivirus infection is generally acute, although it can also be persistent, lasting weeks or even months after the appearance of the first symptoms. Depending on the virus, the infection can be limited to certain organs or can be systemic. The immune response of calicivirus involves both the innate and acquired components; here, we want to briefly outline some general aspects of calicivirus immunity to better understand the strategies that these viruses have developed to evade the immune response.

Innate Immune Response

The innate immune response triggered by calicivirus is mediated by the interferon (IFN) pathway, as has been reported in several virus families. During norovirus infection, potent antiviral activities induced by different types of IFNs have been documented. MNV infected cells increase the expression of IFN and IFN related genes (IRG) through the dsRNA PAMP receptor MDA-5 that recognizes the viral genome (79, 80). MDA5 activates the interferon response factors (IRF) 3 and 7 and the NF-κB pathways through the mitochondrial antiviral signaling (MAVS) protein, leading to the expression of the interferon stimulated genes (ISGs) and pro-inflammatory cytokines. HuNoV RNA replication is also sensitive to several types of interferon, and various ISGs such as RTP4, HPSE, RIG-I, and MDA5 were identified as anti-norovirus effectors; particularly, the dsRNA sensors MDA-5 and RIG-I are potent inhibitors of HuNoV (81). IRF activation also occurs during RHDV infection of rabbit peripheral blood cells, and the potential role of leukocytes and their cytokines in infection has also been studied (82, 83). Regarding FCV infection, the 2,280 strain activates the IFN-β promoter and expression

(84), as well as other ISGs like IRF-1 that hinder viral replication (85).

Adaptative Immune Response

The adaptive or acquired immune response in calicivirus infection involves both humoral and cellular elements that help to control and eradicate the infection. Specific antibodies have been detected in several animals and humans after being exposed to caliciviruses. Induction of a humoral response has been documented with an attenuated strain of FCV in housecats (86), and with a wild type strain of RHDV in young rabbits (87), although different levels of protection against reinfection are achieved; moreover, it is also known that humoral response is required to completely clear MNV infection (88). A high prevalence of serum antibodies to HuNoV has been widely documented in children and adults; however, the protective role in the infection clearance is still a subject of discussion (89). The production and characterization of monoclonal antibodies (mAbs) that recognize specific sequences or structural regions of the epitopes of HuNoVs viral-like particles (VLPs) have helped to identify and characterize the antigens in distinct strains of HuNoVs, as well as its prevalence in distinct HuNoVs genotypes and the capacity of the virus to overcome its blockage. Two extensive and complete reviews about the characterization of the antigen epitopes of the HuNoV genotype GII.4 and its use in providing a road map for the design of candidate vaccines to cover distinct strains with major prevalence around the world as well as in the antigenic diversity of noroviruses have been recently published (90, 91).

Being the intestinal mucosa the main niche of the norovirus infection, it is natural that an important element of the host's humoral response is the production of immunoglobulin A (IgA). It has been proposed that IgA confers certain degree of protection, since HuNoV-exposed patients that already had higher saliva-HuNoV specific IgA did not show gastroenteritis symptoms (92). Moreover, a higher preexisting fecal HuNoV-specific IgA inverse-correlated with both peak of virus levels in stool and time of virus shedding, suggesting that IgA not only confers protection, but can control and produce a quicker clearance of infection (92). Specific IgA sera from HuNoV GI.1-infected patients has the ability to neutralize GI.1 VLPs binding and other GI VLPs such as GI.3 and GI.4 to carbohydrate ligands, reinforcing the idea of some level of cross-reacting protection, at least in the same genogroup (93). Moreover, it seems like IgA is more effective than IgG in blocking the virion binding to HBGA (94).

Although not extensively known, a specific cellular immune response occurs during MNV [reviewed in (95)] and FCV infection, where both monocytes and monocyte-derived dendritic cells (DC) presenting FCV peptides are capable of activating T $CD8^+$ and $CD8^-$ in an *in vitro* model; moreover, FCV-specific CD4+ T cells are present in the spleen of vaccinated cats (95–97). Although more information regarding the role of T cells in controlling HuNoV infection is required, some information has been discussed previously (98, 99).

EVASION OF THE IMMUNE RESPONSE

Upon a viral infection, the host cells activate a complex immune response to eliminate the invading pathogens; however, viruses have developed different strategies to escape such immune control mechanisms and to complete an effective replication and spread to a new host [reviewed in (100–102)]. Caliciviruses, as positive-sense single-stranded RNA viruses that replicate in the cytoplasm, have developed different strategies to prevent recognition of its components.

Evasion of Type I IFN Immune Response

IFN plays a role in controlling calicivirus infection, as expected these viruses have adopted mechanisms for evading IFN signaling. STAT-1 and IFNs type I and II have essential roles in the clearance of MNV infections since they limit the viral replication in the intestine and viral dissemination to peripheral tissues and prevent apoptosis in intestinal cells (103–105). However, infection with the persistent MNV strain S99 caused a poor STAT-1 activation and IFN-β production, suggesting that the establishment of persistent infection in mice is possibly the result of a hampered innate immune response.

Infection with the FCV strains F9, Bolin, HRB-SS failed to induce an IFN-β response (84). To this regard, Yumiketa et al. (106) reported that the expression of the FCV NS protein 39 (NS3) suppresses IFN-β and ISG15 mRNA production and IRF-3 phosphorylation and dimerization induced by dsRNA, suggesting that this viral protein hampers type 1 IFN production by preventing IRF-3 activation (106). The identification of the viral molecules and the mechanisms followed by these viruses to control the IFN response is an area of active research and the proteins involved in inhibiting the cellular protein secretion pathway are targets for investigation. One example is the HuNoV NS protein 22 that antagonizes the secretory pathway; thus, it is probably a key factor in deactivating IFN and cytokine signaling (56).

Role of Type III IFN in Calicivirus Infection Tropism, Persistence, and Transmission

IFN pathway impairment may play a role in calicivirus persistence, as both IFN-β and IFN-λ levels are not augmented in mice infected with the MNV-CR6 persistent strain, in comparison to the non-persistent strain MNV-CW3 (107). Moreover, IFN-λ treatment in mice confers protection against MNV-CR6 persistent strain for up to 2 weeks, and mice receiving this treatment 25 days post infection with this strain, showed a reduction in viral shedding at 2 days of treatment and total virus clearance within 1 week (107), suggesting that the main site of action of IFN-λ is in the intestine, reducing viral dissemination. Another possible role of IFN-λ against MNV infection is protection from contagion; blood and intestinal overexpression of IFN-λ and its stimulated genes in IFN-α/β and IFN-γ knockout mice generated protection against MNV when exposed to seeders and infected mice shedding virus through their stool (108). The relationship between the gut microbiome and IFN-λ in calicivirus infection has been briefly studied using antibiotic-treated mice, where persistent infection and replication in the intestine is only prevented in treated mice that have a functional IFN-λ pathway. This review showed that the commensal microbiome in mice gut fosters MNV infection by downregulating the IFN-λ pathway (109).

Interactions of Caliciviruses With the Microbiota

Many caliciviruses access their hosts through mucosal surfaces that contain a diversity of commensal pathogens; thus, in these sites they interact with hundreds of differential commensal bacteria, which are part of the host immune defense [reviewed in (109–111)]. Particularly, pathogens infecting the intestine, such as HuNoVs and MNVs encounter these microbes with a harmful of beneficial result to the host. On one hand, it has been reported that the *Lactobacillus* genus can inhibit MNV replication *in vitro* by the up-regulation of IFN-β and IFN-γ expression (112), indicating its protective role from this viral infection and suggesting that commensal bacteria in mucosal sites are part of the antiviral response against pathogenic viruses (110).

On the other hand, and contrary to this benefit of the gut microbiota, enteric bacteria are a stimulatory factor for norovirus infection; both HuNoVs and MNV require the presence of HBGA-expressing enteric bacteria to infect B cells *in vitro* and likely *in vivo* (113). More recently, the ability of different HuNoV strains to bind to naturally occurring bacteria strains isolated from human stool as well as to selected reference strains was reported (114). In this same work, a selective binding of Tulane virus, a calicivirus that infects the gastrointestinal tract of rhesus monkeys to some of these bacteria was also observed (114). Binding of caliciviruses to bacteria may facilitate the entry into their target cells and the development of infection; thus, microbiota could be a mechanism of calicivirus evasion.

NS1 From Persistent MNV CR6 Strain Impairs IFN-λ Response

It has been reported that the NS1/2 gene of the persistent MNV-CR6 strain is responsible for the virus tropism and persistence, since a chimeric acute CW3 strain expressing the NS1/2 from CR6 becomes persistent, changing its tropism to the proximal colon of infected mice (72); however, only the NS1 region is responsible for this tropism and persistence. It was recently demonstrated that NS1 protein from MNV-CR6 persistent strain is a product of caspase 3 cleavage, and secreted by a non-classical secretion pathway, downregulating the IFN-λ response in the intestine of infected mice (115). Moreover, mice immunized with MNV-CR6 NS1 gained protection against infection and achieved a better prophylaxis than the one obtained by immunization with VLPs or VP1 protein alone. This phenomenon may be conserved between noroviruses, as the secretion of NS1 from HuNoV GI.1 has also been demonstrated. Thus, NS1 protein from MNV (and possibly from other caliciviruses) is an immune response modulator, particularly affecting the IFN III pathway and influencing virus tropism and host persistence.

Calicivirus Infection and Translational Control

Viruses rely absolutely on the protein synthesis machinery of the host cells; thus, they have developed remarkable strategies to inhibit cellular protein synthesis to prevent competition of ribosome recruitment by host mRNAs. Moreover, inhibition of *de novo* cellular protein synthesis may also contribute to neutralize the stress responses and host innate defenses to infection (116).

Caliciviruses can alter the global translational control of the host by: (1) directly or indirectly targeting cellular translation factors and (2) by altering host ribonucleoprotein (mRNP) compartmentalization, particularly disrupting the assembly of cytoplasmic stress granules (SGs).

1) Targeting cellular translation factors. VPg from the FCV and MNV interact with eukaryotic initiation factors such as eIF3, eIF4E, eIF4A, and eIF4G to promote its own translation; thus hijacking the host protein machinery (31–34, 36). Moreover, infection with FCV alters the global host translation by targeting two eukaryotic initiation factors: eIF4G and the poly A binding protein (PABP) by the action of the viral protease-polymerase NS6/7 (117, 118). MNV infection causes phosphorylation of eIF4E through the MAPK pathway, contributing to changes in the translational state of specific host mRNAs (119). To this regard, a fraction of PABP is also cleaved during MNV infection by the action of the protease NS6 and as a consequence, a reduction in the translation of induced ISGs takes place (64).

Besides the direct targeting of cellular translation factors by viral proteins, induction of apoptosis by viral infections results in the activation of caspases, cellular proteases that also mediates the cleavage of cellular translation initiation factors (120). During MNV infection, cleavage of eIF4GI and eIF4GII occur as a consequence of caspase 3 activation; thus, apoptosis also contributes to the global inhibition of cell translation and evasion of the immune response (64). Caspases also causes the cleavage of nucleoporins (Nups), the principal components of the nuclear pore complex that mediate protein and RNA traficking between the nucleus and the cytoplasm (121). We have observed that during MNV and FCV infection, Nup270 (Tpr) and Nup153 are targets of caspases (unpublished data), suggesting that alterations in the nucleo-cytoplasmic transport may contribute to avert the innate immune response.

Thus, modification of translation initiation factors by calicivirus infection (summarized in **Table 1**), not only favors viral protein synthesis but also hinders the translation of genes induced by the innate immune response (64, 103).

2) Compartmentalization. Upon infection, inhibition of bulk host protein synthesis can also be regulated by the induction of stress granules (SGs) that are important components of the host antiviral defense. SGs are non-membranous, transiently assembled ribonucleoprotein (RNPs) complexes were cell translation can be stalled by sorting non-essential

TABLE 1 | Calicivirus proteins involved in translational control.

Virus	Viral proteins	Cellular protein targets	Mechanisms	References
FCV MNV	VPg	eIF3, eIF4F	Interacting with cellular factors and usurp the host protein synthesis machinery	(31, 33, 34, 36)
FCV	NS6/7 protease/polymerase	eIF4G	Processing translation factors and inhibiting global cellular protein synthesis	(118)
FCV MNV	NS6/7 and NS6 proteases	PABP	Reduction in the translation of induced interferon stimulated genes (ISGs)	(64, 117)
MNV		eIF4E phosphorylation	Affecting translational state of specific host mRNAs	(119)
FCV	NS6/7 protease/polymerase	G3BP1 and G3BP2	Impairs formation of stress granules	(122)
MNV		G3BP1	Impairs formation of stress granules	(123)

mRNA away in response to stress [reviewed in (124–126)]. However, as gene expression of heterologous viral RNAs can also be regulated in these structures, inhibition of SG formation can occur by viraly-encoded factors to confront this antiviral response and maximize virus replication efficiency. FCV infection impairs the assembly of SGs through the cleavage of the SG-nucleating proteins (G3BP1 and G3BP2) by the viral protease-polymerase NS6/7 (122), while MNV infection restricts SG nucleation and formation by recruiting G3BP1 protein to its replication sites, with the equally consequence to prevent SG formation and enhance replication (123) (**Figure 2**).

High Mutational Rates, Genetic Diversity, and Evasion of the Immune Response

RNA viral populations consist on a spectrum of different genomes that result of the high mutational rates derived form the characteristically low fidelity of viral RdRp, as well as molecular recombination and gene segment reassortment. These viruses with extremely high mutation rates exhibit a faster replication, that results in the establishment of the infection in the cell before the immune response can hamper it, and present significant genetic diversity that allow them to evolve, and thus, avoid the cell antiviral systems (127).

One of the first studies on calicivirus mutation rate and evolution showed that isolates collected during a year from a single immunosuppressed patient with chronic diarrhea and viral shedding of HuNoV, presented few changes in the ORF1, but accumulated changes in the P domain of the capsid protein VP1, that were subject to immune pressure (128). Similar changes have been observed in the SaV VP1 codifying region (129). Mutations in the viral capsid protein are one of the immunity-driven mechanisms, to evade a humoral response of the host; particularly information encoded in the P2 subdomain could direct different mechanisms to escape immunological memory [reviewed in (130)].

Analysis of the fidelity of the replicase from HuNoVs involved in gastroenteritis outbreaks have shown that the RdRp from the HuNoV GII.4 strain, responsible for the majority of outbreaks worldwide, has the highest evolution rate compared with other less frequently detected strains, suggesting that the high prevalence of certain strains around the world is a consequence of the genetic diversity of their genomes, which result in a greater capacity to response to new environments. Interestingly, comparison of the evolution properties of several pandemic GII.4 strains to non-pandemic strains found that GII.4 viruses undergo evolution at a much higher rate than the non-pandemic strains (131). Moreover, the presence of non-synonymous mutations in all the HuNoV genotypes analyzed were localized to common structural residues in the capsid, which indicates that these sites are most probably under immune selection (131).

High mutation rate in calicivirus and its importance to achieve efficient viral replication can be observed when a strain with a detrimental phenotype is repeatedly passed through cellular culture until it reaches wild type characteristics. Examples of this has been documented, as the reversion of the LC mutants in FCV (69) and VF1 mutants in MNV (41). Studies in the evolution of an hypervariable region of the FCV capsid protein known to contain neutralization epitopes has shown that the altered viral antigenic profile produced in persistently infected cats generate sequences not detected by the host, that may also result in an evasion of the immune response (132).

MNV VF1 Factor Antagonizes the Innate Immune Response

A rather unique characteristic in MNV's genome is the presence of a fourth ORF that encodes for the protein VF1 in the subgenomic RNA. The protein VF1 locates to the mitochondria and has been suggested to participate in the control of the virus-induced apoptosis and an anti-innate immune activity through the downregulation of the interferon immune response. The protein VF1 interferes with the expression of antiviral genes including IFN-β, the IFN-stimulated gene ISG54, and CXCL10 (41, 133, 134). A similar ORF that overlaps the VP1 coding region is present in genogroup I sapoviruses, although the production of a protein from this ORF has not been demonstrated (135); yet, its conservation in both MNV and sapoviruses suggests that the product of this ORF plays a critical role in virus pathogenesis.

Prostaglandins and Nitric Oxide Production in Calicivirus Infection

Prostaglandins (PG) are IFN antagonists that modulate the production of the innate immunity effector nitric oxide (NO), involved in the control of many infections. It has

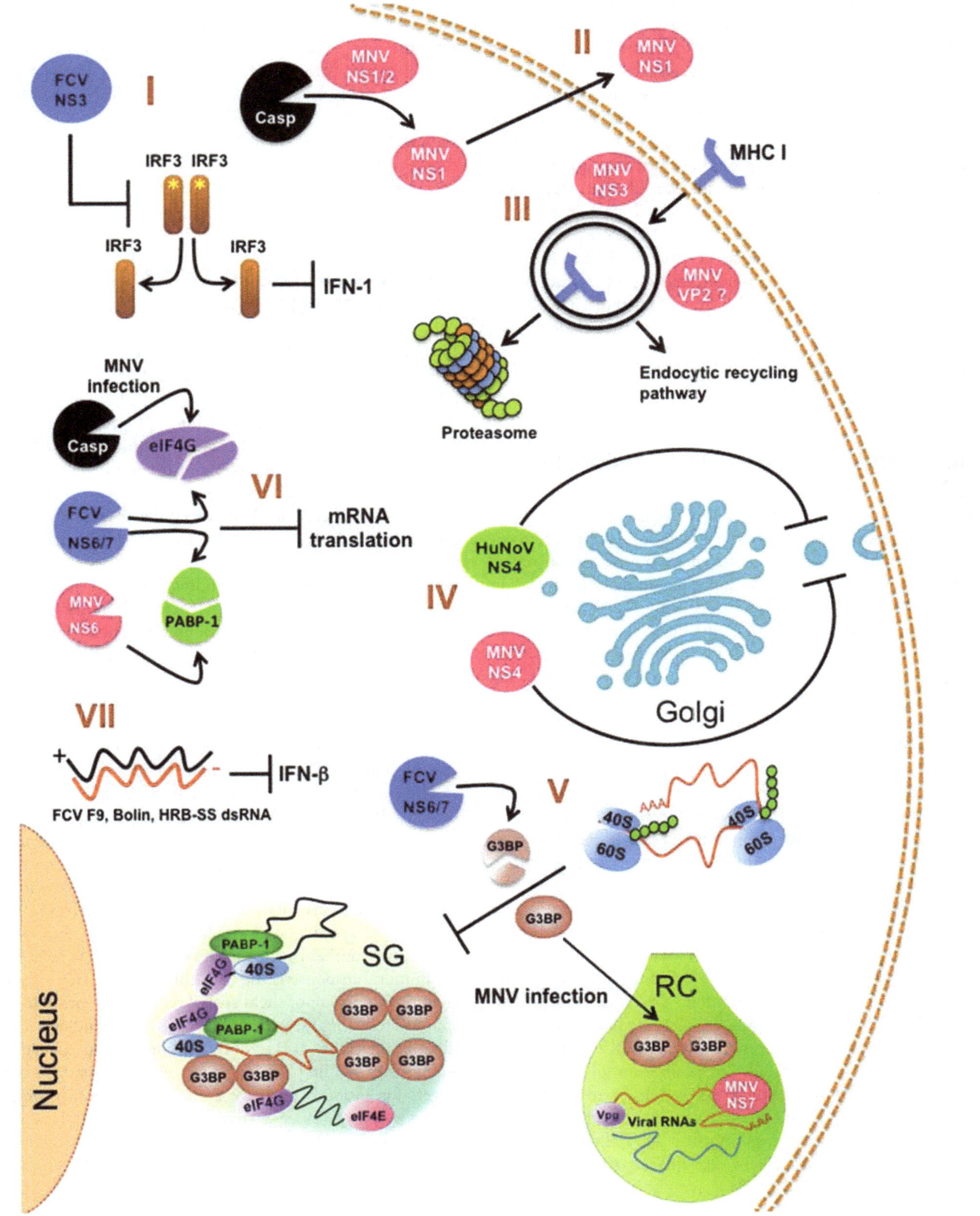

FIGURE 2 | Innate immune pathways inhibition by calicivirus infection. (I) FCV NS3 prevents IRF-3 activation and hampers type 1 IFN production. (II) Caspase-mediate cleavage of MNV NS1/2 for persistent infection of intestinal epithelial cells. (III) Internalization and degradation of MHC I by the action of MNV NS3 protein. (IV) Inhibition of the cellular protein secretion pathway (ER to Golgi trafficking) by HuNoV NS4 (p22) and MNV NS4 (p18). (V) Stress granules (SG) impairment by FCV and MNV infection. (VI) Inhibition of the global cell translation by MNV and FCV infection. (VII) Impairment of INF-β response by FCV strains F9, Bolin, HRB-SS. RC (replicative complex) is indicated. *Indicates phosphorylation.

been reported that levels of NO increase in the digestive tract of patients suffering from acute gastroenteritis caused by noroviruses (136). During PSaV infection, there is an increased activation of the cyclooxygenase-2/Prostaglandin E_2 (COX-2/PGE_2) and an inhibition of the NO production. The inhibition of the COX/PGE_2 pathway caused an increase of NO production and a reduction of the viral replication, indicating that PSaV hampers the antiviral response to provide an environment appropriate for efficient replication. The increase of both COX-2 mRNA and protein levels is produced during the infection and by the expression of the viral proteins VPg and protease-polymerase NS6/7 (137). A similar activation is also observed during FCV and MNV infection, suggesting a crucial role for the COX2/PGE_2 signaling pathway in the replication of the *Caliciviridae*; however, the viral factors that modulate the evasion of the immune response in these particular viruses remain to be determined (138).

Impairment of Antigen Presentation by MNV

As previously discussed above, the mechanisms underlying norovirus persistence or clearance are not well-understood; however, studies of MNV persistence strains and its effect on lymphocyte TCD8+ activation suggest that the infection of macrophages and dendritic cells with MNV impairs the antigen presentation pathway by reducing the surface expression of MHC class I proteins early during infection (111). This reduction is the consequence of the MHC class I internalization via the endocytic recycling pathway and proteasome-dependent degradation. This phenotype is likely to be caused by the NS3 protein, the NTPase involved in viral genome replication (**Figure 2**). This reduction of MHC class I levels hinders the presentation of viral peptides, the activation of $CD8^+$ T cells, and the initiation of the cellular immune response (111). This evasion of antigen presentation most certainly has a role in the clearance of the virus from the host, because it is known that the CD8+ T lymphocytes of mice infected with the persistent MNV-CR6 strain have a differential gene expression than those of the acute strain CW3-infected mice; this distinct gene expression alters the TCD8+ cells localization in the mouse organism, as well as its capacity to respond to activation by proliferation. The results suggest that there are at least two ways of how calicivirus dampers TCD8+ mediated immunity: (1) the reduction in the presentation of MNV antigens by enteric infected cells through internalization of the MHC-I proteins and (2) the distinct expression of differentiation clusters in TCD8+ activated cells presented with the MNV persistent strain antigens, resulting in a suboptimal activation and relocalization of these cells, creating an special niche in the intestine, with fewer TCD8+ lymphocytes where MNV replication can be efficiently achieved (139, 140). The role of the NS1/2 protein of the MNV persistent strain CR6 in the TCD8+ cell response modulation has not been thoroughly studied, but it is known that a MNV CR6 strain lacking a functional NS1/2 (CR6D121/131G) cannot efficiently replicate in wild type nor in $Rag^{-/-}$ mice lacking B and T cell immune response; suggesting that NS1 does not affect acquired immune response and, therefore the TCD8+ differential activation by the persistent strain has to be through another unknown mechanism (115).

Another protein that is involved in the modulation of the immune response is the MNV minor capsid protein VP2 that can regulate antigen presentation (133, 134). Some calicivirus proteins involved in the modulation of the immune response are shown in **Table 2**.

EVASION OF THE HUMORAL RESPONSE BY CALICIVIRUSES

It is well-known that calicivirus infection triggers a humoral response with an impact in the control of the infection, virus propagation or spread through the host. The calicivirus capsids are composed of 180 copies of the VP1 protein that contains 2 principal domains: (1) The amino terminal S (shell) domain proximal to the viral genome, and (2) the carboxi-terminal P (protruding) domain, that dimerizes to form protrusions on the capsid surface. The P domain, the most common target for antibodies in the host is divided in 2 subdomains, P1 that interacts with the S domain and P2 that is the protruding region of P that contain the binding sites for cellular receptors and neutralizing antibodies (141). Multiple efforts for a vaccine development that generates humoral protection against HuNoV have been made; however, the high mutation rate in amino acids from the distinct capsid epitopes combined with selective pressure from the host, damper cross reaction, and longlasting protection both after vaccination and infection; constant changes in genomic populations thorough the world every 5 years are another major problem in vaccine development (142).

The D epitope, adjacent to the P domain in the HuNoV VP1, responsible for the binding with the glycans from the HBGAs, can experience variations in its sequence that result in both a change in affinity for a specific HBGA group as well as an escape from the blockade antibodies. The plasticity of this region has an impact in the tropism of a particular HuNoV genotype as well as in the herd immunity of a population exposed to a particular strain (98, 143).

Another mechanisms of HuNoVs involved in the evasion of the humoral response is the "breathing" of the viral capsid; this phenomenon result of slight spatial rearrangements of the virion epitopes reducing their exposure to hosts antibodies without an effect in infectivity (141). Moreover, amino acid changes in the regions surrounding the conserved epitopes that are constant targets for antibody blockage are also a mechanism of evasion of this response, since a steric effect can result in a reduced antibody binding to the epitope. Posttranslational modifications of amino acids in the viral capsid have also an effect in the virion binding to its HBGA co-receptor (144); however, its effect in the antibodies binding to the viral capsid remains to be determined.

The structure of HuNoV, MNV, RHDV, and FCV virions determined by cryo-electron microscopy studies have shown differences in the size of the P-S linker domains that result in

TABLE 2 | Calicivirus factors involved in the modulation of the immune response.

Genes	Virus	Viral factors	Immune regulatory functions	References
Norovirus	MNV	Virulence factor 1	Downregulation of the IFN immune response	(41)
		NS3	Reduction of the MHC-I protein in the cell surface Decrease in viral antigen presentation Altered CD8+ T cells response	(111)
		Unknown	NO reduction by COX_2/PGE2 pathway activation	(138)
		NS1/2	Impairment of IFN III pathway	(115)
		VP2	Regulation of antigen presentation	(133, 134)
	HuNoV MNV	NS4(p22) NS4 (p18)	Impairment of INF and cytokine signaling	(56)
Vesivirus	FCV	dsRNA	Induction of IFN-b promoter by FCV strain 2280 Lack of IFN-b induction by FCV strains F9, Bolin ad HRB-SS	(84)
		NS3 (p39)	Downregulation of Interferon 1 pathway by preventing IRF-3 activation	(106)
		NS6/7	Sgs assembly disruption by G3BP-1 and G3BP-2 cleavage	(122)
		Unknown	NO reduction by COX_2/PGE2 pathway activation	(138)
Sapovirus	PSaV	VPg and NS6/7	NO reduction by COX_2/PGE2 pathway activation	(137)

distinct dominant epitopes and antibody binding sites [reviewed in (141)]. Particularly in MNV there is a greater flexibility between these P-S domains that could help the virus evade the humoral immune response through diverse mechanisms, like the P-S linker rupture by hosts proteases that results in the release of the P domains as decoys to avoid antibody interaction with the virion; however, since these conformational states seems to be not conserved among all calicivirus, they may not be a common strategy for a successful virus replication and thrive. To this regard, cryo-electron microscopy studies have shown that FCV binding to its receptor occurs in its compressed state (145).

Conformational changes in the P epitope have effects on the neutralizing capability of antibodies to successfully bind to the virion, as a closed or open state in the P dimer expose or hide distinct regions of the epitopes that result in a less efficient virion neutralization response. All these mechanisms regarding changes in the structure of the virion as a way to avoid the humoral immune response have been recently described in more detail in the excellent review by Smith et al. (141).

CONCLUSIONS

All viruses encode for viral factors that are key elements in the regulation of the viral replicative cycle, and as a consequence, in the establishment of infection. During calicivirus infection, several cellular pathways are altered to achieve a successful viral production and viral spread, as well as an effective evasion of the immune response. Infections produced by the members of the *Caliciviridae* family depend on similar pathways; however, the viral factors involved in its regulation are not always the same, which may lead to the diversity of viral tropism and immunopathogenesis. Moreover, the corresponding proteins have multiple functions, not all of which are currently well-understood; thus, knowing the multiple roles of these viral factors will impact on the development of new strategies for the control of calicivirus infection both in humans and animals.

AUTHOR CONTRIBUTIONS

YP-T, AT-U, JE-A, and AG-E collaborated equally in the bibliographical research and writing. AG-E coordinated and edited the manuscript.

ACKNOWLEDGMENTS

We would like to acknowledge Juan E. Ludert for critical comments on the manuscript.

REFERENCES

1. Pires SM, Fischer-Walker CL, Lanata CF, Devleesschauwer B, Hall AJ, Kirk MD, et al. Aetiology-specific estimates of the global and regional incidence and mortality of diarrhoeal diseases commonly transmitted through food. *PLoS ONE.* (2015) 10:e0142927. doi: 10.1371/journal.pone.0142927
2. Ahmed SM, Hall AJ, Robinson AE, Verhoef L, Premkumar P, Parashar UD, et al. Global prevalence of norovirus in cases of gastroenteritis: a systematic review and meta-analysis. *Lancet Infect Dis.* (2014) 14:725–30. doi: 10.1016/S1473-3099(14)70767-4
3. Ayukekbong JA, Mesumbe HN, Oyero OG, Lindh M, Bergstrom T. Role of noroviruses as aetiological agents of diarrhoea in developing countries. *J Gen Virol.* (2015) 96:1983–99. doi: 10.1099/vir.0.000194
4. Thorne LG, Goodfellow IG. Norovirus gene expression and replication. *J Gen Virol.* (2013) 95(Pt 2):278–91.doi: 10.1099/vir.0.059634-0

5. Vashist S, Bailey D, Putics A, Goodfellow I. Model systems for the study of human norovirus biology. *Future Virol.* (2009) 4:353–67. doi: 10.2217/fvl.09.18
6. Desselberger U. Caliciviridae other than noroviruses. *Viruses.* (2019) 11:286. doi: 10.3390/v11030286
7. Farkas T, Sestak K, Wei C, Jiang X. Characterization of a rhesus monkey calicivirus representing a new genus of Calicivitidae. *J Virol.* (2008) 82:5408–16. doi: 10.1128/JVI.00070-08
8. L'Homme Y, Sansregret R, Plante-Fortier E, Lamontagne AM, Ouardani M, Lacroix G, et al. Genomic characterization of swine caliciviruses representing a new genus of Caliciviridae. *Virus Genes.* (2009) 39:66–75. doi: 10.1007/s11262-009-0360-3
9. Liao Q, Wang X, Wang D, Zhang D. Complete genome sequence of a novel calicivirus from a goose. *Arch Virol.* (2014) 159:2529–31. doi: 10.1007/s00705-014-2083-6
10. Mikalsen AB, Nilsen P, Froystad-Saugen M, Lindmo K, Eliassen TM, Rode M, et al. Characterization of a novel calicivirus causing systemic infection in atlantic salmon (*Salmo salar* L.): proposal for a new genus of caliciviridae. *PLoS ONE.* (2014) 9:e107132. doi: 10.1371/journal.pone.0107132
11. Mor SK, Phelps NBD, Ng TFF, Subramaniam K, Primus A, Armien AG, et al. Genomic characterization of a novel calicivirus, FHMCV-2012, from baitfish in the USA. *Arch Virol.* (2017) 162:3619–27. doi: 10.1007/s00705-017-3519-6
12. Wolf S, Reetz J, Otto P. Genetic characterization of a novel calicivirus from a chicken. *Arch Virol.* (2011) 156:1143–50. doi: 10.1007/s00705-011-0964-5
13. Ruvoen-Clouet N, Ganiere JP, Andre-Fontaine G, Blanchard D, Le Pendu J. Binding of rabbit hemorrhagic disease virus to antigens of the ABH histo-blood group family. *J Virol.* (2000) 74:11950–4. doi: 10.1128/JVI.74.24.11950-11954.2000
14. Tan M, Jiang X. Norovirus-host interaction: multi-selections by human histo-blood group antigens. *Trends Microbiol.* (2011) 19:382–8. doi: 10.1016/j.tim.2011.05.007
15. Stuart AD, Brown TDK. α2,6-linked sialic acid acts as a receptor for *Feline calicivirus. J Gen Virol.* (2007) 88:177–86. doi: 10.1099/vir.0.82158-0
16. Taube S, Perry JW, Yetming K, Patel SP, Auble H, Shu LM, et al. Ganglioside-linked terminal sialic acid moieties on murine macrophages function as attachment receptors for murine noroviruses. *J Virol.* (2009) 83:4092–101. doi: 10.1128/JVI.02245-08
17. Graziano VR, Wei J, Wilen CB. Norovirus attachment and entry. *Viruses.* (2019) 11:495. doi: 10.3390/v11060495
18. Makino A, Shimojima M, Miyazawa T, Kato K, Tohya Y, Akashi H. Junctional adhesion molecule 1 is a functional receptor for feline calicivirus. *J Virol.* (2006) 80:4482–90. doi: 10.1128/JVI.80.9.4482-4490.2006
19. Pesavento PA, Stokol T, Liu H, van der List DA, Gaffney PM, Parker JS. Distribution of the feline calicivirus receptor junctional adhesion molecule a in feline tissues. *Vet Pathol.* (2011) 48:361–8. doi: 10.1177/0300985810375245
20. Sosnovtsev SV, Sandoval-Jaime C, Parra GI, Tin CM, Jones RW, Soden J, et al. Identification of human junctional adhesion molecule 1 as a functional receptor for the Hom-1 calicivirus on human cells. *MBio.* (2017) 8:e00031-17. doi: 10.1128/mBio.00031-17
21. Haga K, Fujimoto A, Takai-Todaka R, Miki M, Doan YH, Murakami K, et al. Functional receptor molecules CD300lf and CD300ld within the CD300 family enable murine noroviruses to infect cells. *Proc Natl Acad Sci USA.* (2016) 113:E6248–55. doi: 10.1073/pnas.16055 75113
22. Orchard RC, Wilen CB, Doench JG, Baldridge MT, McCune BT, Lee YC, et al. Discovery of a proteinaceous cellular receptor for a norovirus. *Science.* (2016) 353:933–6. doi: 10.1126/science.aaf1220
23. Gonzalez-Reyes S, Garcia-Manso A, del Barrio G, Dalton KP, Gonzalez-Molleda L, Arrojo-Fernandez J, et al. Role of annexin A2 in cellular entry of rabbit vesivirus. *J Gen Virol.* (2009) 90(Pt 11):2724–30. doi: 10.1099/vir.0.013276-0
24. Alfajaro MM, Cho EH, Kim DS, Kim JY, Park JG, Soliman M, et al. Early porcine sapovirus infection disrupts tight junctions and uses occludin as a coreceptor. *J Virol.* (2019) 93:e01773-18. doi: 10.1128/JVI.01 773-18
25. Kreutz LC, Seal BS. The pathway of feline calicivirus entry. *Virus Res.* (1995) 35:63–70. doi: 10.1016/0168-1702(94)00077-P
26. Stuart AD, Brown TD. Entry of feline calicivirus is dependent on clathrin-mediated endocytosis and acidification in endosomes. *J Virol.* (2006) 80:7500–9. doi: 10.1128/JVI.02452-05
27. Gerondopoulos A, Jackson T, Monaghan P, Doyle N, Roberts LO. Murine norovirus-1 cell entry is mediated through a non-clathrin-, non-caveolae-, dynamin- and cholesterol-dependent pathway. *J Gen Virol.* (2010) 91(Pt 6):1428–38. doi: 10.1099/vir.0.016717-0
28. Shivanna V, Kim Y, Chang KO. The crucial role of bile acids in the entry of porcine enteric calicivirus. *Virology.* (2014) 456–7:268–78. doi: 10.1016/j.virol.2014.04.002
29. Soliman M, Kim DS, Park JG, Kim JY, Alfajaro MM, Baek YB, et al. Phosphatidylinositol 3-Kinase/Akt and MEK/ERK signaling pathways facilitate sapovirus trafficking and late endosomal acidification for viral uncoating in LLC-PK cells. *J Virol.* (2018) 92:e01674-18. doi: 10.1128/JVI.01674-18
30. Conley MJ, McElwee M, Azmi L, Gabrielsen M, Byron O, Goodfellow IG, et al. Calicivirus VP2 forms a portal-like assembly following receptor engagement. *Nature.* (2019) 565:377–81. doi: 10.1038/s41586-018-0852-1
31. Chaudhry Y, Nayak A, Bordeleau ME, Tanaka J, Pelletier J, Belsham GJ, et al. Caliciviruses differ in their functional requirements for eIF4F components. *J Biol Chem.* (2006) 281:25315–25. doi: 10.1074/jbc.M602230200
32. Chung L, Bailey D, Leen EN, Emmott EP, Chaudhry Y, Roberts LO, et al. Norovirus translation requires an interaction between the C Terminus of the genome-linked viral protein VPg and eukaryotic translation initiation factor 4G. *J Biol Chem.* (2014) 289:21738–50. doi: 10.1074/jbc.M114.550657
33. Daughenbaugh KF, Fraser CS, Hershey JWB, Hardy ME. The genome-linked protein VPg of the Norwalk virus binds eIF3, suggesting its role in translation initiation complex recruitment. *EMBO J.* (2003) 22:2852–9. doi: 10.1093/emboj/cdg251
34. Daughenbaugh KF, Wobus CE, Hardy ME. VPg of murine norovirus binds translation initiation factors in infected cells. *Virol J.* (2006) 3:33. doi: 10.1186/1743-422X-3-33
35. Goodfellow I. The genome-linked protein VPg of vertebrate viruses - a multifaceted protein. *Curr Opin Virol.* (2011) 1:355–62. doi: 10.1016/j.coviro.2011.09.003
36. Goodfellow I, Chaudhry Y, Gioldasi I, Gerondopoulos A, Natoni A, Labrie L, et al. Calicivirus translation initiation requires an interaction between VPg and eIF4E. *EMBO Rep.* (2005) 6:968–72. doi: 10.1038/sj.embor.7400510
37. Herbert TP, Brierley I, Brown TDK. Identification of a protein linked to the genomic and subgenomic mRNAs of feline calicivirus and its role in translation. *J Gen Virol.* (1997) 78:1033–40. doi: 10.1099/0022-1317-78-5-1033
38. Hosmillo M, Chaudhry Y, Kim DS, Goodfellow I, Cho KO. Sapovirus translation requires an interaction between VPg and the cap binding protein eIF4E. *J Virol.* (2014) 88:12213–21. doi: 10.1128/JVI.01650-14
39. Alhatlani B, Vashist S, Goodfellow I. Functions of the 5' and 3' ends of calicivirus genomes. *Virus Res.* (2015) 206:134–43. doi: 10.1016/j.virusres.2015.02.002
40. Gutierrez-Escolano AL. Host-cell factors involved in the calicivirus replicative cycle. *Future Virol.* (2014) 9:147–60. doi: 10.2217/fvl.13.125
41. McFadden N, Bailey D, Carrara G, Benson A, Chaudhry Y, Shortland A, et al. Norovirus regulation of the innate immune response and apoptosis occurs via the product of the alternative open reading frame 4. *PLoS Pathog.* (2011) 7:e1002413. doi: 10.1371/journal.ppat.1002413
42. Sosnovtsev SV, Sosnovtseva SA, Green KY. Cleavage of the feline calicivirus capsid precursor is mediated by a virus-encoded proteinase. *J Virol.* (1998) 72:3051–9.
43. Barrera-Vazquez OS, Cancio-Lonches C, Hernandez-Gonzalez O, Chavez-Munguia B, Villegas-Sepulveda N, Gutierrez-Escolano AL. The feline calicivirus leader of the capsid protein causes survivin and XIAP downregulation and apoptosis. *Virology.* (2019) 527:146–58. doi: 10.1016/j.virol.2018.11.017
44. Santiana M, Ghosh S, Ho BA, Rajasekaran V, Du WL, Mutsafi Y, et al. Vesicle-cloaked virus clusters are optimal units for inter-organismal viral transmission. *Cell Host Microbe.* (2018) 24:208–20.e208. doi: 10.1016/j.chom.2018.07.006
45. Denison MR. Seeking membranes: positive-strand RNA virus replication complexes. *PLoS Biol.* (2008) 6:e270. doi: 10.1371/journal.pbio.0060270

46. Harak C, Lohmann V. Ultrastructure of the replication sites of positive-strand RNA viruses. *Virology.* (2015) 479–80:418–33. doi: 10.1016/j.virol.2015.02.029
47. Green KY, Mory A, Fogg MH, Weisberg A, Belliot G, Wagner M, et al. Isolation of enzymatically active replication complexes from feline calicivirus-infected cells. *J Virol.* (2002) 76:8582–95. doi: 10.1128/JVI.76.17.8582-8595.2002
48. Love DN, Sabine M. Electron microscopic observation of feline kidney cells infected with a feline calicivirus. *Arch Virol.* (1995) 48:16. doi: 10.1007/BF01317964
49. Peterson JE, Studdent MJ. Feline picornavirus. Structure of the virus and electron microscopic observations on infected cell cultures. *Archiv Gesamte Virusforoschung.* (1970) 32:12. doi: 10.1007/BF01249961
50. Bailey D, Kaiser WJ, Hollinshead M, Moffat K, Chaudhry Y, Wileman T, et al. Feline calicivirus p32, p39 and p30 proteins localize to the endoplasmic reticulum to initiate replication complex formation. *J Gen Virol.* (2010) 91(Pt 3):739–49. doi: 10.1099/vir.0.016279-0
51. Urakova N, Frese M, Hall RN, Liu J, Matthaei M, Strive T. Expression and partial characterisation of rabbit haemorrhagic disease virus non-structural proteins. *Virology.* (2015) 484:69–79. doi: 10.1016/j.virol.2015.05.004
52. Urakova N, Strive T, Frese M. RNA-dependent RNA polymerases of both virulent and benign rabbit caliciviruses induce striking rearrangement of golgi membranes. *PLoS ONE.* (2017) 12:e0169913. doi: 10.1371/journal.pone.0169913
53. Urakova N, Warden AC, White PA, Strive T, Frese M. A motif in the F homomorph of rabbit haemorrhagic disease virus polymerase is important for the subcellular localisation of the protein and its ability to induce redistribution of golgi membranes. *Viruses.* (2017) 9:E202. doi: 10.3390/v9080202
54. Fernandez-Vega V, Sosnovtsev SV, Belliot G, King AD, Mitra T, Gorbalenya A, et al. Norwalk virus N-terminal nonstructural protein is associated with disassembly of the Golgi complex in transfected cells. *J Virol.* (2004) 78:4827–37. doi: 10.1128/JVI.78.9.4827-4837.2004
55. Hyde JL, Mackenzie JM. Subcellular localization of the MNV-1 ORF1 proteins and their potential roles in the formation of the MNV-1 replication complex. *Virology.* (2010) 406:138–48. doi: 10.1016/j.virol.2010.06.047
56. Sharp TM, Guix S, Katayama K, Crawford SE, Estes MK. Inhibition of cellular protein secretion by norwalk virus nonstructural protein p22 requires a mimic of an endoplasmic reticulum export signal. *PLoS ONE.* (2010) 5:e13130. doi: 10.1371/journal.pone.0013130
57. Doerflinger SY, Cortese M, Romero-Brey I, Menne Z, Tubiana T, Schenk C, et al. Membrane alterations induced by nonstructural proteins of human norovirus. *PLoS Pathog.* (2017) 13:e1006705. doi: 10.1371/journal.ppat.1006705
58. Al-Molawi N, Beardmore VA, Carter MJ, Kass GEN, Roberts LO. Caspase-mediated cleavage of the feline calicivirus capsid protein. *J Gen Virol.* (2003) 84:1237–44. doi: 10.1099/vir.0.18840-0
59. Alonso C, Oviedo JM, Martin-Alonso JM, Diaz E, Boga JA, Parra F. Programmed cell death in the pathogenesis of rabbit hemorrhagic disease. *Arch Virol.* (1998) 143:321–32. doi: 10.1007/s007050050289
60. Bok K, Prikhodko VG, Green KY, Sosnovtsev SV. Apoptosis in murine norovirus-infected RAW264.7 cells is associated with downregulation of survivin. *J Virol.* (2009) 83:3647–56. doi: 10.1128/JVI.02028-08
61. Natoni A, Kass GEN, Carter MJ, Roberts LO. The mitochondrial pathway of apoptosis is triggered during feline calicivirus infection. *J Gen Virol.* (2006) 87:357–61. doi: 10.1099/vir.0.81399-0
62. Roberts LO, Al-Molawi N, Carter MJ, Kass GEN. *Apoptosis* in cultured cells infected with feline calicivirus. *Apoptosis.* (2003) 1010:587–90. doi: 10.1196/annals.1299.110
63. Sosnovtsev SV, Prikhod'ko EA, Belliot G, Cohen JI, Green KY. Feline calicivirus replication induces apoptosis in cultured cells. *Virus Res.* (2003) 94:1–10. doi: 10.1016/S0168-1702(03)00115-1
64. Emmott E, Sorgeloos F, Caddy SL, Vashist S, Sosnovtsev S, Lloyd R, et al. Norovirus-mediated modification of the translational landscape via virus and host-induced cleavage of translation initiation factors. *Mol Cell Proteomics.* (2017) 16(4 Suppl. 1):S215–29. doi: 10.1074/mcp.M116.062448
65. Jung JY, Lee BJ, Tai JH, Park JH, Lee YS. Apoptosis in rabbit haemorrhagic disease. *J Comp Pathol.* (2000) 123:135–40. doi: 10.1053/jcpa.2000.0403
66. Niedzwiedzka-Rystwej P, Hukowska-Szematowicz B, Tokarz-Deptula B, Trzeciak-Ryczek A, Dzialo J, Deptula W. Apoptosis of peripheral blood leucocytes in rabbits infected with different strains of rabbit haemorrhagic disease virus. *Acta Biochim Pol.* (2013) 60:65–9. doi: 10.18388/abp.2013_1952
67. Liu G, Ni Z, Yun T, Yu B, Chen L, Zhao W, et al. A DNA-launched reverse genetics system for rabbit hemorrhagic disease virus reveals that the VP2 protein is not essential for virus infectivity. *J Gen Virol.* (2008) 89(Pt 12):3080–5. doi: 10.1099/vir.0.2008/003525-0
68. Chen M, Liu X, Hu B, Fan Z, Song Y, Wei H, et al. Rabbit hemorrhagic disease virus non-structural protein 6 induces apoptosis in rabbit kidney cells. *Front Microbiol.* (2018) 9:3308. doi: 10.3389/fmicb.2018.03308
69. Abente EJ, Sosnovtsev SV, Sandoval-Jaime C, Parra GI, Bok K, Green KY. The feline calicivirus leader of the capsid protein is associated with cytopathic effect. *J Virol.* (2013) 87:3003–17. doi: 10.1128/JVI.02480-12
70. Furman LM, Maaty WS, Petersen LK, Ettayebi K, Hardy ME, Bothner B. Cysteine protease activation and apoptosis in Murine norovirus infection. *Virol J.* (2009) 6:139. doi: 10.1186/1743-422X-6-139
71. Herod MR, Salim O, Skilton RJ, Prince CA, Ward VK, Lambden PR, et al. Expression of the murine norovirus (MNV) ORF1 polyprotein is sufficient to induce apoptosis in a virus-free cell model. *PLoS ONE.* (2014) 9:e90679. doi: 10.1371/journal.pone.0090679
72. Robinson BA, Van Winkle JA, McCune BT, Peters AM, Nice TJ. Caspase-mediated cleavage of murine norovirus NS1/2 potentiates apoptosis and is required for persistent infection of intestinal epithelial cells. *PLoS Pathog.* (2019) 15:e1007940. doi: 10.1371/journal.ppat.1007940
73. Cheetham S, Souza M, Meulia T, Grimes S, Han MG, Saif LJ. Pathogenesis of a genogroup II human norovirus in gnotobiotic pigs. *J Virol.* (2006) 80:10372–81. doi: 10.1128/JVI.00809-06
74. Troeger H, Loddenkemper C, Schneider T, Schreier E, Epple HJ, Zeitz M, et al. Structural and functional changes of the duodenum in human norovirus infection. *Gut.* (2009) 58:1070–7. doi: 10.1136/gut.2008.160150
75. Kaufman SS, Chatterjee NK, Fuschino ME, Magid MS, Gordon RE, Morse DL, et al. Calicivirus enteritis in an intestinal transplant recipient. *Am J Transpl.* (2003) 3:764–8. doi: 10.1034/j.1600-6143.2003.00112.x
76. Kaufman SS, Chatterjee NK, Fuschino ME, Morse DL, Morotti RA, Magid MS, et al. Characteristics of human calicivirus enteritis in intestinal transplant recipients. *J Pediatr Gastroenterol Nutr.* (2005) 40:328–33. doi: 10.1097/01.MPG.0000155182.54001.48
77. Morotti RA, Kaufman SS, Fishbein TM, Chatterjee NK, Fuschino ME, Morse DL, et al. Calicivirus infection in pediatric small intestine transplant recipients: pathological considerations. *Hum Pathol.* (2004) 35:1236–40. doi: 10.1016/j.humpath.2004.06.013
78. Yen JB, Wei LH, Chen LW, Chen LY, Hung CH, Wang SS, et al. Subcellular localization and functional characterization of GII.4 norovirus-encoded NTPase. *J Virol.* (2018) 92:e01824-17. doi: 10.1128/JVI.01824-17
79. Enosi Tuipulotu D, Netzler NE, Lun JH, Mackenzie JM, White PA. TLR7 agonists display potent antiviral effects against norovirus infection via innate stimulation. *Antimicrob Agents Chemother.* (2018) 62:e02417-17. doi: 10.1128/AAC.02417-17
80. McCartney SA, Thackray LB, Gitlin L, Gilfillan S, Virgin HW, Colonna M. MDA-5 recognition of a murine norovirus. *PLoS Pathog.* (2008) 4:e1000108. doi: 10.1371/annotation/3ce83911-9ccf-4452-a690-2816d0e94c10
81. Dang W, Xu L, Yin Y, Chen S, Wang W, Hakim MS, et al. IRF-1, RIG-I and MDA5 display potent antiviral activities against norovirus coordinately induced by different types of interferons. *Antiviral Res.* (2018) 155:48–59. doi: 10.1016/j.antiviral.2018.05.004
82. Trzeciak-Ryczek A, Tokarz-Deptula B, Deptula W. Expression of IL-1β, IL-2, IL-10, TNF-β and GM-CSF in peripheral blood leukocytes of rabbits experimentally infected with rabbit haemorrhagic disease virus. *Vet Microbiol.* (2016) 186:71–81. doi: 10.1016/j.vetmic.2016.02.021
83. Trzeciak-Ryczek A, Tokarz-Deptula B, Deptula W. Expression of IL-1Ra, IL-6, IL-8, IL-18, TNF-α and IFN-γ genes in peripheral blood leukocytes of rabbits infected with RHDV (Rabbit Haemorrhagic Disease Virus). *Dev Comp Immunol.* (2017) 76:310–5. doi: 10.1016/j.dci.2017.07.005
84. Tian J, Zhang X, Wu H, Liu C, Liu J, Hu X, et al. Assessment of the IFN-βresponse to four feline caliciviruses: infection in CRFK cells. *Infect Genet Evol.* (2015) 34:352–60. doi: 10.1016/j.meegid.2015.06.003

85. Liu Y, Liu X, Kang H, Hu X, Liu J, Tian J, et al. Identification of feline interferon regulatory factor 1 as an efficient antiviral factor against the replication of feline calicivirus and other feline viruses. *Biomed Res Int.* (2018) 2018:2739830. doi: 10.1155/2018/2739830
86. Wensman JJ, Samman A, Lindhe A, Thibault JC, Berndtsson LT, Hosie MJ. Ability of vaccine strain induced antibodies to neutralize field isolates of caliciviruses from Swedish cats. *Acta Vet Scand.* (2015) 57:86. doi: 10.1186/s13028-015-0178-z
87. Ferreira PG, Dinis M, Costa E, Silva A, Aguas AP. Adult rabbits acquire resistance to lethal calicivirus infection by adoptive transfer of sera from infected young rabbits. *Vet Immunol Immunopathol.* (2008) 121:364–9. doi: 10.1016/j.vetimm.2007.09.005
88. Chachu KA, Strong DW, LoBue AD, Wobus CE, Baric RS, Virgin HW. Antibody is critical for the clearance of murine norovirus infection. *J Virol.* (2008) 82:6610–7. doi: 10.1128/JVI.00141-08
89. Lindesmith LC, McDaniel JR, Changela A, Verardi R, Kerr SA, Costantini V, et al. Sera antibody repertoire analyses reveal mechanisms of broad and pandemic strain neutralizing responses after human norovirus vaccination. *Immunity.* (2019) 50:1530–41.e1538. doi: 10.1016/j.immuni.2019.05.007
90. Mallory ML, Lindesmith LC, Graham RL, Baric RS. GII.4 human norovirus: surveying the antigenic landscape. *Viruses.* (2019) 11:177. doi: 10.3390/v11020177
91. van Loben Sels JM, Green KY. The antigenic topology of norovirus as defined by B and T cell epitope mapping: implications for universal vaccines and therapeutics. *Viruses.* (2019) 11:E432. doi: 10.3390/v11050432
92. Ramani S, Neill FH, Opekun AR, Gilger MA, Graham DY, Estes MK, et al. Mucosal and cellular immune responses to norwalk virus. *J Infect Dis.* (2015) 212:397–405. doi: 10.1093/infdis/jiv053
93. Lindesmith LC, Beltramello M, Swanstrom J, Jones TA, Corti D, Lanzavecchia A, et al. Serum immunoglobulin a cross-strain blockade of human noroviruses. *Open Forum Infect Dis.* (2015) 2:ofv084. doi: 10.1093/ofid/ofv084
94. Sapparapu G, Czako R, Alvarado G, Shanker S, Prasad BV, Atmar RL, et al. Frequent use of the IgA isotype in human B cells encoding potent norovirus-specific monoclonal antibodies that block HBGA binding. *PLoS Pathog.* (2016) 12:e1005719. doi: 10.1371/journal.ppat.1005719
95. Newman KL, Leon JS. Norovirus immunology: of mice and mechanisms. *Eur J Immunol.* (2015) 45:2742–57. doi: 10.1002/eji.201545512
96. de Groot-Mijnes JD, van der Most RG, van Dun JM, te Lintelo EG, Schuurman NM, Egberink HF, et al. Three-color flow cytometry detection of virus-specific CD4+ and CD8+ T cells in the cat. *J Immunol Methods.* (2004) 285:41–54. doi: 10.1016/j.jim.2003.10.019
97. Vermeulen BL, Gleich SE, Dedeurwaerder A, Olyslaegers DA, Desmarets LM, Dewerchin HL, et al. *In vitro* assessment of the feline cell-mediated immune response against feline panleukopeniavirus, calicivirus and felid herpesvirus 1 using 5-bromo-2'-deoxyuridine labeling. *Vet Immunol Immunopathol.* (2012) 146:177–84. doi: 10.1016/j.vetimm.2012.03.004
98. Debbink K, Lindesmith LC, Donaldson EF, Baric RS. Norovirus immunity and the great escape. *PLoS Pathog.* (2012) 8:e1002921. doi: 10.1371/journal.ppat.1002921
99. Malm M, Hyoty H, Knip M, Vesikari T, Blazevic V. Development of T cell immunity to norovirus and rotavirus in children under five years of age. *Sci Rep.* (2019) 9:3199. doi: 10.1038/s41598-019-39840-9
100. Alcami A, Koszinowski UH. Viral mechanisms of immune evasion. *Trends Microbiol.* (2000) 8:410–8. doi: 10.1016/S0966-842X(00)01830-8
101. Beachboard DC, Horner SM. Innate immune evasion strategies of DNA and RNA viruses. *Curr Opin Microbiol.* (2016) 32:113–9. doi: 10.1016/j.mib.2016.05.015
102. Moreno-Altamirano MMB, Kolstoe SE, Sánchez-García FJ. Virus control of cell metabolism for replication and evasion of host immune responses. *Front Cell Infect Microbiol.* (2019) 9:15. doi: 10.3389/fcimb.2019.00095
103. Karst SM, Wobus CE, Lay M, Davidson J, Virgin HW. STAT1-dependent innate immunity to a Norwalk-like virus. *Science.* (2003) 299:1575–8. doi: 10.1126/science.1077905
104. Mumphrey SM, Changotra H, Moore TN, Heimann-Nichols ER, Wobus CE, Reilly MJ, et al. Murine norovirus 1 infection is associated with histopathological changes in immunocompetent hosts, but clinical disease is prevented by STAT1-dependent interferon responses. *J Virol.* (2007) 81:3251–63. doi: 10.1128/JVI.02096-06
105. Niendorf S, Klemm U, Mas Marques A, Bock CT, Hohne M. Infection with the persistent murine norovirus strain MNV-S99 suppresses IFN-β release and activation of Stat1 *in vitro*. *PLoS ONE.* (2016) 11:e0156898. doi: 10.1371/journal.pone.0156898
106. Yumiketa Y, Narita T, Inoue Y, Sato G, Kamitani W, Oka T, et al. Nonstructural protein p39 of feline calicivirus suppresses host innate immune response by preventing IRF-3 activation. *Vet Microbiol.* (2016) 185:62–7. doi: 10.1016/j.vetmic.2016.02.005
107. Nice TJ, Baldridge MT, McCune BT, Norman JM, Lazear HM, Artyomov M, et al. Interferon-lambda cures persistent murine norovirus infection in the absence of adaptive immunity. *Science.* (2015) 347:269–73. doi: 10.1126/science.1258100
108. Rocha-Pereira J, Jacobs S, Noppen S, Verbeken E, Michiels T, Neyts J. Interferon lambda (IFN-lambda) efficiently blocks norovirus transmission in a mouse model. *Antiviral Res.* (2018) 149:7–15. doi: 10.1016/j.antiviral.2017.10.017
109. Baldridge MT, Turula H, Wobus CE. Norovirus regulation by host and microbe. *Trends Mol Med.* (2016) 22:1047–59. doi: 10.1016/j.molmed.2016.10.003
110. Domínguez-Díaz C, García-Orozco A, Riera-Leal A, Padilla-Arellano JR, Fafutis-Morris M. Microbiota and its role on viral evasion: is it with us or against us? *Front Cell Infect Microbiol.* (2019) 9:7. doi: 10.3389/fcimb.2019.00256
111. Fritzlar S, Jegaskanda S, Aktepe TE, Prier JE, Holz LE, White PA, et al. Mouse norovirus infection reduces the surface expression of major histocompatibility complex class I proteins and inhibits CD8(+) T cell recognition and activation. *J Virol.* (2018) 92:e00286-18. doi: 10.1128/JVI.00286-18
112. Lee H, Ko G. Antiviral effect of vitamin A on norovirus infection via modulation of the gut microbiome. *Sci Rep.* (2016) 6:25835. doi: 10.1038/srep25835
113. Jones MK, Watanabe M, Zhu S, Graves CL, Keyes LR, Grau KR, et al. Enteric bacteria promote human and mouse norovirus infection of B cells. *Science.* (2014) 346:755–9. doi: 10.1126/science.1257147
114. Almand EA, Moore MD, Outlaw J, Jaykus LA. Human norovirus binding to select bacteria representative of the human gut microbiota. *PLoS ONE.* (2017) 12:e0173124. doi: 10.1371/journal.pone.0173124
115. Lee S, Liu H, Wilen CB, Sychev ZE, Desai C, Hykes BL, et al. A secreted viral nonstructural protein determines intestinal norovirus pathogenesis. *Cell Host Microbe.* (2019) 25:845–857.e845. doi: 10.1016/j.chom.2019.04.005
116. Walsh D, Mathews MB, Mohr I. Tinkering with translation: protein synthesis in virus-infected cells. *Cold Spring Harb Perspect Biol.* (2013) 5:a012351. doi: 10.1101/cshperspect.a012351
117. Kuyumcu-Martinez M, Belliot G, Sosnovtsev SV, Chang KO, Green KY, Lloyd RE. Calicivirus 3C-like proteinase inhibits cellular translation by cleavage of poly(A)-binding protein. *J Virol.* (2004) 78:8172–82. doi: 10.1128/JVI.78.15.8172-8182.2004
118. Willcocks MM, Carter MJ, Roberts LO. Cleavage of eukaryotic initiation factor eIF4G and inhibition of host-cell protein synthesis during feline calicivirus infection. *J Gen Virol.* (2004) 85(Pt 5):1125–30. doi: 10.1099/vir.0.19564-0
119. Royall E, Doyle N, Abdul-Wahab A, Emmott E, Morley SJ, Goodfellow I, et al. Murine norovirus 1 (MNV1) replication induces translational control of the host by regulating eIF4E activity during infection. *J Biol Chem.* (2015) 290:4748–58. doi: 10.1074/jbc.M114.602649
120. Marissen WE, Gradi A, Sonenberg N, Lloyd RE. Cleavage of eukaryotic translation initiation factor 4GII correlates with translation inhibition during apoptosis. *Cell Death Differ.* (2000) 7:1234–43. doi: 10.1038/sj.cdd.4400750
121. Ferrando-May E, Cordes V, Biller-Ckovric I, Mirkovic J, Gorlich D, Nicotera P. Caspases mediate nucleoporin cleavage, but not early redistribution of nuclear transport factors and modulation of nuclear permeability in apoptosis. *Cell Death Differ.* (2001) 8:495–505. doi: 10.1038/sj.cdd.4400837
122. Humoud MN, Doyle N, Royall E, Willcocks MM, Sorgeloos F, van Kuppeveld F, et al. Feline calicivirus infection disrupts assembly of cytoplasmic stress granules and induces G3BP1 cleavage. *J Virol.* (2016) 90:6489–501. doi: 10.1128/JVI.00647-16

123. Fritzlar S, Aktepe TE, Chao YW, Kenney ND, McAllaster MR, Wilen CB, et al. Mouse norovirus infection arrests host cell translation uncoupled from the stress granule-PKR-eIF2α axis. *MBio.* (2019) 10:e00960-19. doi: 10.1128/mBio.00960-19
124. Lloyd RE. How do viruses interact with stress-associated RNA granules? *PLoS Pathog.* (2012) 8:e1002741. doi: 10.1371/journal.ppat.1002741
125. Reineke LC, Lloyd RE. Diversion of stress granules and P-bodies during viral infection. *Virology.* (2013) 436:255–67. doi: 10.1016/j.virol.2012.11.017
126. Zhang Q, Sharma NR, Zheng ZM, Chen M. Viral regulation of RNA granules in infected cells. *Virol Sin.* (2019) 34:175–91. doi: 10.1007/s12250-019-00122-3
127. Regoes RR, Hamblin S, Tanaka MM. Viral mutation rates: modelling the roles of within-host viral dynamics and the trade-off between replication fidelity and speed. *Proc Biol Sci.* (2013) 280:20122047. doi: 10.1098/rspb.2012.2047
128. Nilsson M, Hedlund KO, Thorhagen M, Larson G, Johansen K, Ekspong A, et al. Evolution of human calicivirus RNA *in vivo*: accumulation of mutations in the protruding P2 domain of the capsid leads to structural changes and possibly a new phenotype. *J Virol.* (2003) 77:13117–24. doi: 10.1128/JVI.77.24.13117-13124.2003
129. Iwakiri A, Ganmyo H, Yamamoto S, Otao K, Mikasa M, Kizoe S, et al. Quantitative analysis of fecal sapovirus shedding: identification of nucleotide substitutions in the capsid protein during prolonged excretion. *Arch Virol.* (2009) 154:689–93. doi: 10.1007/s00705-009-0358-0
130. Donaldson EF, Lindesmith LC, Lobue AD, Baric RS. Viral shape-shifting: norovirus evasion of the human immune system. *Nat Rev Microbiol.* (2010) 8:231–41. doi: 10.1038/nrmicro2296
131. Bull RA, Eden JS, Rawlinson WD, White PA. Rapid evolution of pandemic noroviruses of the GII.4 lineage. *PLoS Pathog.* (2010) 6:e1000831. doi: 10.1371/journal.ppat.1000831
132. Radford AD, Turner PC, Bennett M, McArdle F, Dawson S, Glenn MA, et al. Quasispecies evolution of a hypervariable region of the feline calicivirus capsid gene in cell culture and in persistently infected cats. *J Gen Virol.* (1998) 79(Pt 1):1–10. doi: 10.1099/0022-1317-79-1-1
133. Roth AN, Karst SM. Norovirus mechanisms of immune antagonism. *Curr Opin Virol.* (2016) 16:24–30. doi: 10.1016/j.coviro.2015.11.005
134. Zhu S, Regev D, Watanabe M, Hickman D, Moussatche N, Jesus DM, et al. Identification of immune and viral correlates of norovirus protective immunity through comparative study of intra-cluster norovirus strains. *PLoS Pathog.* (2013) 9:e1003592. doi: 10.1371/journal.ppat.1003592
135. Thackray LB, Wobus CE, Chachu KA, Liu B, Alegre ER, Henderson KS, et al. Murine noroviruses comprising a single genogroup exhibit biological diversity despite limited sequence divergence. *J Virol.* (2007) 81:10460–73. doi: 10.1128/JVI.00783-07
136. Sowmyanarayanan TV, Natarajan SK, Ramachandran A, Sarkar R, Moses PD, Simon A, et al. Nitric oxide production in acute gastroenteritis in Indian children. *Trans R Soc Trop Med Hyg.* (2009) 103:849–51. doi: 10.1016/j.trstmh.2009.05.003
137. Alfajaro MM, Choi JS, Kim DS, Seo JY, Kim JY, Park JG, et al. Activation of COX-2/PGE2 promotes sapovirus replication via the inhibition of nitric oxide production. *J Virol.* (2017) 91:e01656–16. doi: 10.1128/JVI.01 656-16
138. Alfajaro MM, Cho EH, Park JG, Kim JY, Soliman M, Baek YB, et al. Feline calicivirus- and murine norovirus-induced COX-2/PGE2 signaling pathway has proviral effects. *PLoS ONE.* (2018) 13:e0200726. doi: 10.1371/journal.pone.0200726
139. Tomov VT, Osborne LC, Dolfi DV, Sonnenberg GF, Monticelli LA, Mansfield K, et al. Persistent enteric murine norovirus infection is associated with functionally suboptimal virus-specific CD8 T cell responses. *J Virol.* (2013) 87:7015–31. doi: 10.1128/JVI.03 389-12
140. Tomov VT, Palko O, Lau CW, Pattekar A, Sun Y, Tacheva R, et al. Differentiation and protective capacity of virus-specific CD8(+) T cells suggest murine norovirus persistence in an immune-privileged enteric niche. *Immunity.* (2017) 47:723–38.e725. doi: 10.1016/j.immuni.2017.09.017
141. Smith HQ, Smith TJ. The dynamic capsid structures of the noroviruses. *Viruses.* (2019) 11:E235. doi: 10.3390/v11030235
142. Lindesmith LC, Donaldson EF, Lobue AD, Cannon JL, Zheng DP, Vinje J, et al. Mechanisms of GII.4 norovirus persistence in human populations. *PLoS Med.* (2008) 5:e31. doi: 10.1371/journal.pmed.0050031
143. Lindesmith LC, Brewer-Jensen PD, Mallory ML, Yount B, Collins MH, Debbink K, et al. Human norovirus epitope D plasticity allows escape from antibody immunity without loss of capacity for binding cellular ligands. *J Virol.* (2019) 93:e01813-18. doi: 10.1128/JVI.01813-18
144. Mallagaray A, Creutznacher R, Dulfer J, Mayer PHO, Grimm LL, Orduna JM, et al. A post-translational modification of human Norovirus capsid protein attenuates glycan binding. *Nat Commun.* (2019) 10:1320. doi: 10.1038/s41467-019-09251-5
145. Bhella D, Goodfellow IG. The cryo-electron microscopy structure of feline calicivirus bound to junctional adhesion molecule A at 9-angstrom resolution reveals receptor-induced flexibility and two distinct conformational changes in the capsid protein VP1. *J Virol.* (2011) 85:11381–90. doi: 10.1128/JVI.05621-11

5

Immune Response to Mucosal *Brucella* Infection

Rubén López-Santiago[1], Ana Beatriz Sánchez-Argáez[1], Liliana Gabriela De Alba-Núñez[1], Shantal Lizbeth Baltierra-Uribe[2] and Martha Cecilia Moreno-Lafont[1]*

[1] Departamento de Inmunología, Escuela Nacional de Ciencias Biológicas, Instituto Politécnico Nacional, Mexico City, Mexico, [2] Departamento de Microbiología, Escuela Nacional de Ciencias Biológicas, Instituto Politécnico Nacional, Mexico City, Mexico

***Correspondence:**
Martha Cecilia Moreno-Lafont
mmlafont@gmail.com;
mlafont@ipn.mx

Brucellosis is one of the most prevalent bacterial zoonosis of worldwide distribution. The disease is caused by *Brucella* spp., facultative intracellular pathogens. Brucellosis in animals results in abortion of fetuses, while in humans, it frequently manifests flu-like symptoms and a typical undulant fever, being osteoarthritis a common complication of the chronic infection. The two most common ways to acquire the infection in humans are through the ingestion of contaminated dairy products or by inhalation of contaminated aerosols. *Brucella* spp. enter the body mainly through the gastrointestinal and respiratory mucosa; however, most studies of immune response to *Brucella* spp. are performed analyzing models of systemic immunity. It is necessary to better understand the mucosal immune response induced by *Brucella* infection since this is the main entry site for the bacterium. In this review, some virulence factors and the mechanisms needed for pathogen invasion and persistence are discussed. Furthermore, some aspects of local immune responses induced during *Brucella* infection will be reviewed. With this knowledge, better vaccines can be designed focused on inducing protective mucosal immune response.

Keywords: brucellosis, gut immunity, *Brucella* vaccines, intracellular infection, respiratory tract immunity

INTRODUCTION

The discovery of brucellosis took place in Malta during the Crimean war in 1859. The British troops had been suffering high fever, so the Royal British medical staff was called in. David Bruce was the officer who investigated what he called Malta fever or Mediterranean fever. In 1887, he managed to isolate and cultivate the bacterium responsible for the disease (1).

Later, Themistocles Zammit found that people who lived in farms, reared goats, and drank milk from these animals showed the same symptoms as Mediterranean fever patients. Using this finding, Zammit reproduced the infection in healthy goats and successfully isolated the bacterium in blood and milk. He deduced that the British army contracted the infection by consuming milk from infected animals in the local region. Therefore, in 1906 a decision was made to ban goat's milk consumption as a preemptive measure to control the disease among the British army. However, Malta fever was not eradicated in the region and suspicions arose regarding the consumption of ice-cream, cheese, and fudge made from contaminated milk (1, 2).

Zammit's contribution proved that brucellosis is mostly transmitted orally. Later, other contagion routes were reported (respiratory, parenteral, or by contact) and considered occupational hazards.

Although it has been well-established that *Brucella* enters the organism orally, the bacterium has not been properly defined as enteropathogenic, which has caused certain controversy. The infection by *Brucella* spp. does not cause diarrhea, a characteristic symptom of enteropathogenic bacteria (3, 4). Diarrhea is caused by inflammation due to the recruitment of cells, as neutrophils, producing damage to the epithelium, and compromising the integrity of the mucosa, which triggers inflammatory diarrhea (5). Studies *in vivo* have demonstrated that mice intragastrically inoculated with *B. melitensis* do not recruit neutrophils in the small intestine, while histological sections do not show considerable inflammation (6). On the contrary, enteropathogens as *Salmonella, Vibrio cholera*, and *Escherichia coli* do cause the characteristic inflammatory reaction and trigger diarrhea (5). Additionally, *Brucella* seems to transit only the intestine and does not appear to invade it and create as replicative niche in it (3, 4).

Animal models in which *Brucella* spp. is orally or intragastrically inoculated show that the bacterium can be recovered from the small intestine, particularly from gut-associated lymphoid tissue (GALT) as Peyer's patches (PP) and mesenteric lymph nodes (MLN). The bacterium is located in these tissues from an early stage of the infection and up to 21 days afterwards, as demonstrated by plating homogenates from the organs. This suggests that *Brucella* remains at these sites to replicate (6). However, infection in these models is achieved using high bacterial doses, 10^8-10^{10} colony forming units (CFU), which might force gastrointestinal tract tissues to be colonized by the bacterium (3, 4).

Although *Brucella* spp. enters the body mainly through the mucous membranes of the gastrointestinal tract and the respiratory tract, most of the anti-*Brucella* immunity studies performed so far use experimental models of parenteral infection, mainly intraperitoneal, which gives easy and rapid access to the spleen and other organs of the reticuloendothelial system (**Figure 1**). In this review we will discuss the concepts of innate mucosal immunity involved in mucosal protection against *Brucella* infection. The mechanisms used by *Brucella* spp. to evade the elements of oral, intestinal, and repiratory mucosal immunity will also be analyzed. In addition, the recent concept of T-cell-mediated immunity operating in the intestinal mucosa, whose characteristics differ from the systemic immunity developing in the spleen, will be discussed. The understanding of Brucella's interactions with the elements of mucosal immunity and the possibilities of experimental models should allow this information to be used to explain why this infectious disease tends to be chronic, and what will be the best vaccination strategies through these pathways.

ORAL CAVITY, FIRST CONTACT SITE FOR *BRUCELLA* SPP.

The oral cavity is the first site of contact of *Brucella* spp. with the host and it is provided with an immune system mechanism belonging to mucosa-associated lymphoid tissue (MALT). Therefore, *Brucella* should initiate an immune recognition response in this tissue. The oral cavity is a highly hostile site: not only is it exposed to pathogens that enter by this route, as *Brucella*, *E. coli*, and *Samonella*, but it is also in constant contact with air antigens, food, or microbiota, and is subjected to mechanical damage by mastication. Consequently, the oral mucosa has defense mechanisms and tolerance similar to GALT (7, 8).

Initially, when *Brucella* enters the oral cavity, it encounters barriers such as saliva, which contains elements that eliminate or control microbial growth, such as lysozyme, lactoferrin, nystadine, peroxidases and immunoglobulins, mainly type A (IgA). Along with saliva, there is also the gingival crevicular fluid that covers the space between the teeth and the gingiva, known as the gingival sulcus. This fluid contains complement molecules, antibodies, neutrophils, and plasma cells. Therefore, the mixture of saliva and gingival crevicular fluid forms an initial strong barrier against pathogenic microorganisms (**Figure 1**). However, it is unknown whether *Brucella* is susceptible to this barrier or able to evade it (8).

In the mucosal tissue there are also phagocytic cells that recognize pathogens as *Brucella*. Phagocytic cells as dendritic cells and macrophages (antigen-presenting cells, APCs) able to capture antigens and migrate to the nearest regional lymph node, in this case the cervical lymph node, are distributed along the specialized tissue of the oral cavity. Once they have captured antigens from the oral mucosa, APCs migrate to the lymph node to present the antigen to the lymphocytes and send the appropriate activation signal (8, 9).

In spite of being the first contact *Brucella* has with the host, the response of the immune system against *Brucella* in this site has been poorly studied. Still, there are reports of brucellosis patients showing inflammation in the cervical lymph nodes who had apparently become infected by consuming products contaminated with *Brucella*. These findings led to the development of an animal model inducing infection with *B. melitensis* by three different routes of administration for subsequent comparison. The first one consisted of depositing the bacteria directly in the oral cavity of the mouse, the second one involved the administration of the bacteria with an oropharyngeal probe, while the third way of administration was performed intraperitoneally. It was found that, regardless of the administration route, *Brucella* infection induced inflammation of the cervical lymph node. The viable bacterium was also recovered from the first days after infection and *Brucella* was determined to persist in the GLN until 50 days after inoculation. Regardless of the administration route and because more bacteria were found in GLN than in other tissues, it is suspected that GLN may be a selective *Brucella* niche (10).

This suggests that from the first moment after ingesting food contaminated with *Brucella*, the bacterium is recognized and taken by some APCs belonging to the oral mucosa and later migrates to the cervical lymph node. Cell analysis of the inflamed cervical lymph node from the model described above indicates that there is an increase in CD68+ cells, a marker expressed by macrophages (10).

Knowledge of the passage of *Brucella* in the oral mucosa is practically unknown; for example, whether there is a participation of amygdales and/or adenoids, which are lymphoid

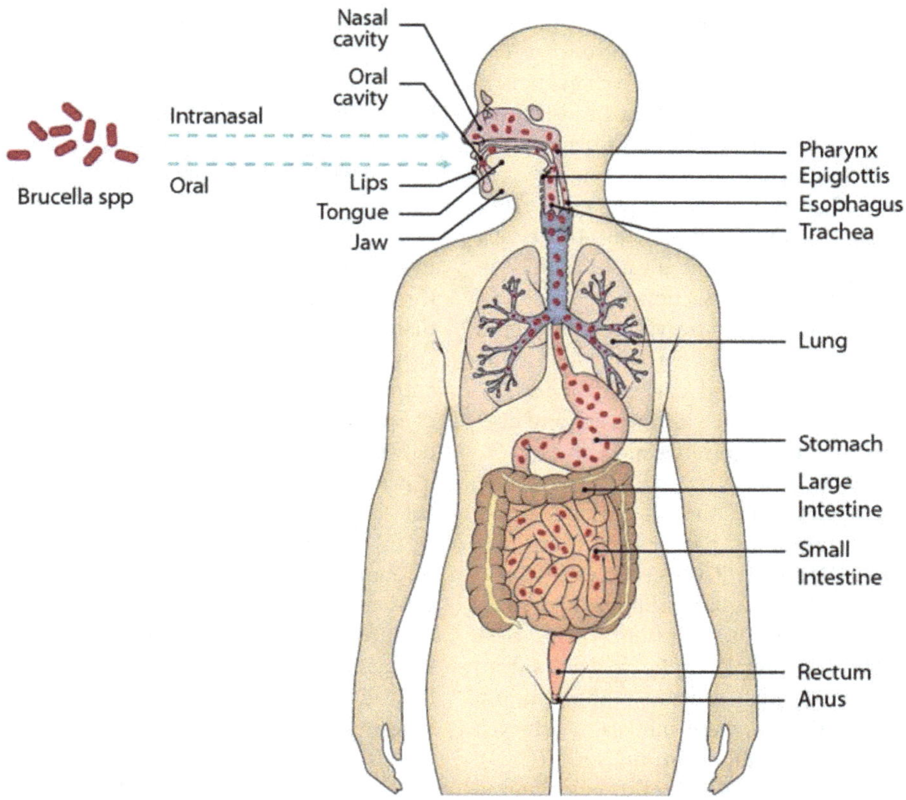

FIGURE 1 | Main mucous membranes affected by the entry of *Brucella* through the oral and intranasal routes. When ingesting food contaminated with *Brucella*, the oral cavity is the first site of contact of the bacteria with the host, although it is very little time that remains there, in the oral cavity there are elements of the immune system belonging to MALT that should recognize the presence of *Brucella* and eliminate it. After the oral cavity *Brucella* could enter the gastrointestinal tract along with the alimentary bolus through the esophagus up to the stomach. In the stomach *Brucella* is apparently able to resist the pH of gastric juices, then enters the small intestine, where it will face physical and chemical barriers, as well as different cell lines and lymphoid tissue belonging to GALT. Following this route is likely to reach the large intestine and even that the bacteria was eliminated by feces, however unknown.

tissue of the oral cavity. Similarly, it is unknown if the recognition of *Brucella* produces an inflammatory response in the epithelium of the oral cavity or if the response induced in the GLN extends to other sites of the host.

The oral cavity has been considered very little as the body's first point of contact with *Brucella* spp. Since the oral mucosa is the initial site of infection, more attention should be paid to the role of the lymph nodes draining to the head and neck. It is therefore possible that the oral route is a potential vaccination route.

INTERPLAY OF *BRUCELLA* THROUGH THE GASTROINTESTINAL TRACT

The gastrointestinal tract is daily exposed to a wide variety of innocuous antigens from foods and microbiota, and, eventually, pathogenic antigens (11–14). The integrity of the intestinal tissue depends on a local immune system consisting of physical barriers, molecules, several cell strains, and specialized lymphoid tissue associated to the intestine (**Figure 2**) (14, 15). The epithelium is covered with a mucus barrier that protects it against direct contact with most of the bacteria, both in the stomach and the intestine. This mucus contains a glycoprotein called mucin, which has viscous and glutinous properties to trap microorganisms that are then expelled with the aid of the peristaltic movement in the intestine (11, 15). Besides mucin, the intestinal mucosa contains proteins secreted by Paneth cells, including β-defensins, lysozyme, cathelicidins, and phospholipase A2, which act as antimicrobial agents.

On the other hand, bile salts released in the small intestine create conjugates with detergent action that damage the bacterial wall and prevent microbiota growth (11, 16). Finally, in the intestinal mucus are immunoglobulins with the capacity to neutralize antigens from intestinal lumen, mostly IgA. Cells from the intestinal epithelium are joined between them by a variety of molecules. Among these intercellular interactions are close conjunctions, whose molecules prevent antigens from entering the lamina propria via the lumen (17). The main effector site of the intestinal immune response is the lamina propria; there APCs (as CD68+ macrophages and dendritic cells, DC) are located and show an immature phenotype and high phagocytic activity. Also, polymorphonuclear cells (neutrophils, mastocytes, and eosinophils) are found in the lamina propria, especially when there is an inflammatory response. The lamina propria is

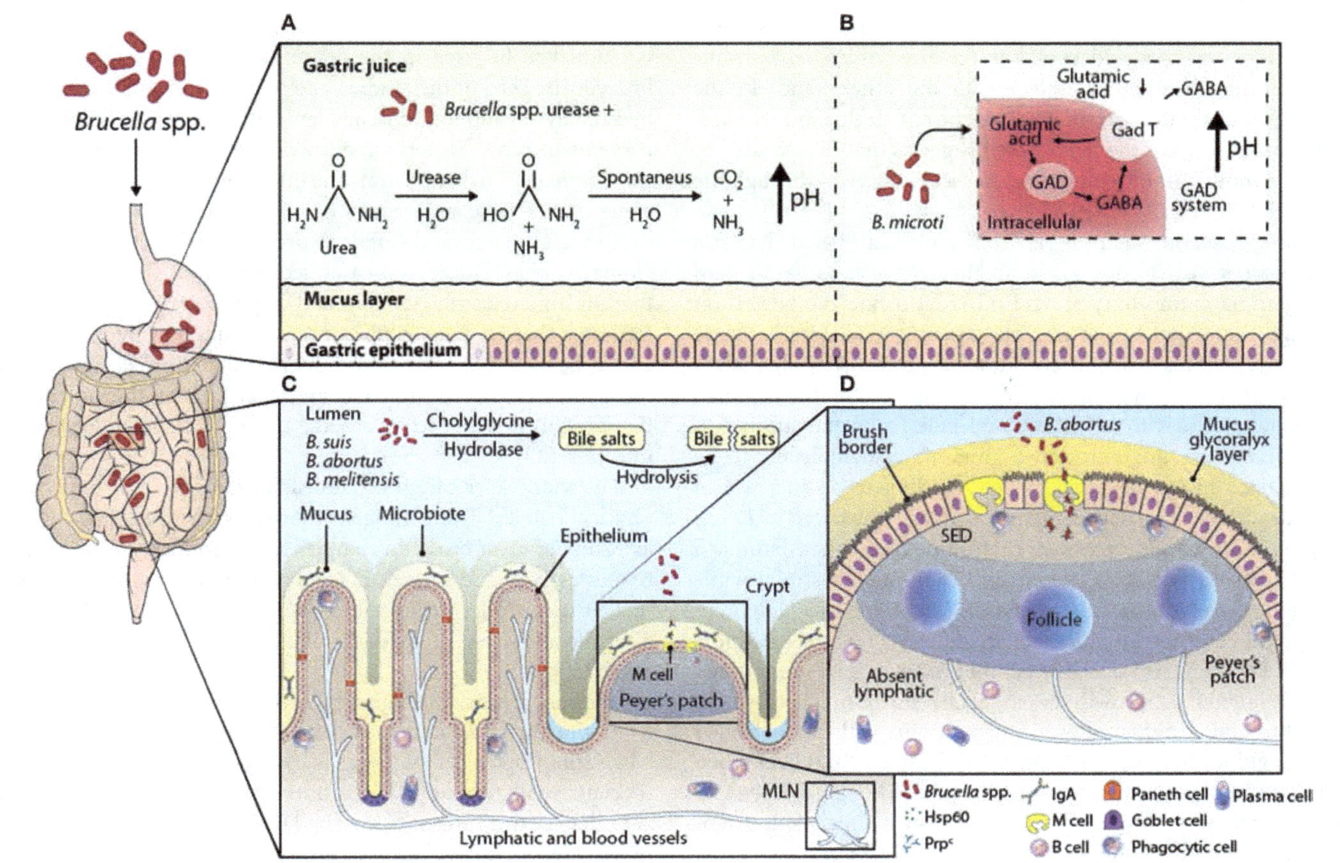

FIGURE 2 | Illustration of the proposed models of the interaction of *Brucella* strains with GALT. When *Brucella* reaches the stomach, it encounters the main chemical barrier, the pH of gastric juices. Some *Brucella* spp. possess the enzyme urease, which is able to catalyze the hydrolysis of urea into carbamate and ammonia; carbamate is degraded by spontaneous hydrolysis into ammonia and carbon dioxide, creating a basic environment in the environment by increasing the pH **(A)**. It has been described in *B. microti* the GAD system that consists of transporting glutamic acid into the bacterium and with the help of the enzyme glutamate decarboxylase (GAD) convert glutamic acid into gamma amino butyric acid (GABA), this reaction consumes a proton that alkalinizes the extracellular medium of the bacterium, which would help *B. microti* survive in an extremely acidic environment such as the pH of the stomach **(B)**. The bile salts in the small intestine have an antimicrobial role, because they are capable of damaging the membrane of some bacteria, the strains *B. suis, B. abortus*, and *B. melitensis* possess the enzyme cholylglycine hydrolase, an enzyme that catalyzes the hydrolysis of bile salts, inhibiting their microbicidal activity **(C)**. In addition to the chemical barriers present in the gastrointestinal tract, there is the most important physical barrier, the monolayer of epithelial cells of the intestine. It has not been fully clarified how *Brucella* crosses this barrier, however it has been proposed that it is through M cells, specialized enterocytes that are found above the sub-epithelial dome (SED), in the epithelium region associated with the follicle. The M cells on its apical side express highly the cellular prion protein (Prpc), this protein is a receptor and one of its ligands is the Hsp60 protein, secreted by *B. abortus* through its type IV secretion system, which suggests that the interaction of the receptor and its ligand promotes the entry of the bacteria into the intestine **(D)**.

also populated by T and B lymphocytes that migrate from their activation site in the lymphoid tissue to the intestine (9, 11).

The GALT is constituted by PP, isolated lymphoid follicles, and MLN. These are considered the main sites inducing the adaptive immune response since they are also the location of antigen presentation to T lymphocytes and activation of B lymphocytes, which create germinal centers (13, 17).

Given that the mouth is the natural entry for *Brucella* spp. the gastrointestinal tract is the most exposed tissue, which the bacterium uses to disseminate and start the infection, apparently, evading the local immune response. The pH of the stomach is useful to degrade proteins and is considered a chemical barrier that pathogens must confront during their transit (15). Some bacteria, as *Helicobacter pylori*, produce an enzyme with urease activity that is considered a virulence factor. This is because the enzyme hydrolyzes urea, ammonia, and carbamate, creating a basic environment in the medium. This alkaline condition promotes bacterial growth while urease byproducts provide a source of nitrogen. However, urease can compromise the integrity of the epithelial tissue (18). Urease activity could be a favorable factor to *Brucella* spp. persistence through the stomach. In the sequencing of *Brucella* spp. genome, two urease operons (*ure1* and *ure2*) were found in its chromosome 1 (19). The only *Brucella* species that does not produce urease is *B. ovis*, which is not transmitted orally but sexually in animals. This incapacity is likely to be caused by the absence of the enzyme.

The biological function of urease and its role in the pathogenesis have been evaluated in strains manipulated to eliminate operons *ure1* and *ure2*. The mutated strains were intragastrically inoculated to BALB/c mice. The researchers observed a lower colonization in the small intestine, as compared against the one observed in the wild strain *B. abortus 2308*. Still, there was no evidence that the urease-deficient strains colonize the liver or the spleen. On the other hand, in the intraperitoneal inoculation, urease-deficient strains did colonize both the spleen and the liver, which suggests that urease is a key factor, although not the only one, to secure survival through the stomach (**Figure 2A**) (6, 19–21).

Some bacteria such as *E. coli* and lactic acid bacteria (*Lactococcus lactis*) have a system that converts glutamic acid into gamma amino-butyric acid (GABA) inside the bacterium through the action of the enzyme glutamic acid decarboxylase (GAD) (22). This reaction consumes a proton that alkalinizes the intracellular environment of the bacterium. In addition, this system allows for a GABA molecule to be transported to the extracellular medium and a glutamic acid molecule to be internalized in the bacterial cytosol, leading to an increase in the extracellular pH. This system is primarily involved in *E. coli* resistance in extremely acidic environments, such as stomach pH. The GAD system is present in the *B. microti* strain, while the gene involved in this system is identified as *gadBC*. In the presence of a glutamic acid medium *B. microti* can grow at a pH of 2.5; however, when the *gadBC* gene is modified into *B microti* its growth in an acidic medium decrease. *In vivo*, the oral administration of these strains with the modified genes significantly decreases their CFU in spleen and liver when compared to the *B. microti* strain without the modified *gadBC* genes. Then, it is suggested that this system is a mechanism that *Brucella* can employ to resist the stomach pH (**Figure 2B**) (23).

The presence of *gadBC* genes has been identified with *in silico* analysis present in almost all species of *Brucella*; still, the functionality of the GAD system is not present in more pathogenic species such as *B. abortus, B. canis, B. melitensis, B. neotomae, and B. suis* (24).

Bile salts are secreted in the small intestine as conjugates with detergent properties that promote dispersion and enzymatic degradation of fats. This property also has an effect on the membrane of some bacteria; therefore, bile salts are considered to play an antimicrobial role (16). It has been described that *B. abortus, B. melitensis*, and *B. suis* synthesize an enzyme hydrolyzing bile salts, called cholyglycine hydrolase, coded by gene *chg*. This enzyme is also found in intestinal microbiota bacteria as *Lactobacillus* and *Bacteroidetes*, which suggests that microbiota bacteria require this enzyme to prevent the detergent action of bile salt conjugates (25).

The function of *Brucella* spp. cholyglycine hydrolase has been studied in strains in which gene *chg* has been previously eliminated. Studies prove the relevance of this enzyme during transit in the intestine when the knock-out strain is orally administered to mice. A decrease in the chg$^{-/-}$ bacteria disseminated to the spleen was observed in comparison with wild bacteria that were orally administered. This study demonstrated that the viability of *Brucella* spp. transit in the gut depends on the integrity of cholyglycine hydrolase. This finding suggests cholyglycine is relevant as a virulence factor, aiding the bacteria to avoid the microbicide activity of bile salt conjugates (**Figure 2C**) (26).

Unlipidated 19 kDa outer membrane protein, U-Omp19, is a *Brucella* protein without lipid fraction. This modified protein is studied to be used in the development of a vaccine against brucellosis. During the studies, the sequence of this protein has been analyzed and found to be identical to the protease inhibitor proteins of other bacteria, mainly of the Inh family of *Erwinia chrysanthemi*. To demonstrate the inhibitory function of U-Omp, experiments were performed *in vitro*: U-Omp was incubated in a casein system and different proteases characteristic of the stomach (pepsin) and proteases secreted from the pancreas to the intestine (elastase, trypsin, and α quymotrypsin). The study indicates that U-Omp inhibits protease function by preventing casein degradation. The results suggest that *Brucella* can evade the proteases of the stomach and intestine of the host with this protein in order to invade the mucosal tissue and establish infection (27).

The monolayer of epithelial cells in the gut is an important physical barrier. The pathogens that reach the intestinal lumen, as *Brucella*, must cross this barrier to disseminate toward other tissues as liver and spleen. Evidence in animal models suggests that *Brucella* goes from the intestinal lumen into the small intestine and, from there, disseminates to other organs as spleen and liver (6).

The mechanism through which *Brucella* spp. is translocated from the intestinal lumen to tissue remains unclear. Still, it has been proposed that *Brucella* is introduced by enterocytes specialized in trapping lumen antigens, called M cells, which later deliver the antigen to nearby DC (6, 28). M cells are found in a region of PP, called follicle-associated epithelium. PP are distributed along the small intestine and their anatomy, cell distribution, and functions are similar to those of a node, except PP do not have capsule nor afferent lymphatic vessels (13, 29).

Studies *in vitro* demonstrated that *B. melitensis* can cross a monolayer of human epithelial cells differentiated to M cells but does not go through a monolayer of non-differentiated enterocytes, suggesting that M cells promote the transit of *Brucella* through the epithelial monolayer (6). Studies *in vivo* on the association between *Brucella* and PP were done in ligated loops, closing the ends of an intestinal section containing at least one PP where the bacterium as inoculated. These studies allowed for the observation of *B. abortus*-GFP by confocal microscopy within the follicle-associated epithelium of the Peyer's patches, a region that is rich in M cells (28). A more thorough understanding of the role M cells play was achieved studying the cellular prion protein (PrP^{C}) highly expressed at the apical end of M cells. This protein is a receptor, one of its identified ligands is the heat-shock protein Hsp60, secreted by *B. abortus* through its type-IV secretion system. This suggests that the interaction between PrP^{C} and Hsp60 promotes infection by macrophages, so PrP^{C} could be a *Brucella* receptor (30). The observation that *B. abortus* inoculated in the ligated loop associated to PrP^{C} is related to the high efficiency with which the bacterium is internalized in PP. In PrP^{C}-deficient mice (prnp$^{-/-}$), a lower amount of internalized *B. abortus* internalized in the ligated PP loop was observed. However, when *Brucella* is inoculated orally in prnp$^{-/-}$ mice, no PP were detected (31). These observations confirm the role of PrP^{C} in the capture and internalization of the bacterium by M cells, which provide *Brucella* spp. An efficient penetration into the organism (**Figure 2D**).

It must be noted that strains of *B. abortus, B. melitensis, B. suis, B. canis,* and *B. abortus* RB51 adhere to epithelial cells CaCo-2 and HT29 inside which they can replicate. Infection of cell lines Caco-2 and HT29 with *Brucella* strains does not induce the secretion of pro-inflammatory cytokines as TNFα, IL-1β, MCP-1, IL-10, or TGF-β; however, they produce IL-8 and chemokine CCL-20 (32). The absence of inflammatory response to the infection by *Brucella* spp. has also been observed in histological sections of the small intestine from intragastrically inoculated mice. These sections do not show neutrophil infiltration, which would be favored by IL-8 and CCL-20 secretion (6).

Despite the mechanisms mentioned on the entry of *Brucella* spp. in the organism, it is still unclear how *Brucella* avoids each barrier of the intestinal immune system. Similarly, we have yet to clarify how and why *Brucella* remains in the gut and GALT (as PP and MLN) for so long. Submandibular maxillary lymph nodes (which drain oral cavity, eyes, and nasal mucosa) can be a niche or reservoir for *Brucella* to remain silent and for periods of up to 50 days (33). This proposal could also be considered for organs as PP or MLN in which viable *Brucella* has also been found to remain for extended periods. It is also important to elucidate how *Brucella* spp. virulence factors affect innate immune response and GALT adaptive response. Once this is understood, experts will be able to develop vaccines that protect the exposed tissue of the gastrointestinal mucosa.

Although *Brucella* cannot be considered as an enteropathogen, it passes through the intestine in a natural infection. Although this has long been known to be the pathway of entry for this pathogen, most studies of pathogenesis and the immune response against *Brucella* spp. have been conducted by inoculating the bacterium intraperitoneally. This route favors systemic infection in early post-infection times, with early and easy colonization of the bacteria in the spleen. However, as it is not the natural route of infection, it does not allow knowing the immunity mechanisms that could contain the infection before its systemic dissemination. It is possible that the intestine, an effective barrier to bacterial invaders, is a possible reservoir of *Brucella* spp. For this reason, it is essential to have a detailed knowledge of the mechanisms of innate and acquired immunity that develop in the intestinal mucous membrane toward the various components of *Brucella* spp. that allow its systemic dissemination.

MUCOSAL OF RESPIRATORY TRACT. OTHER PORTAL OF ENTRY OF *BRUCELLA* SPP.

Oral exposure is the major route of infection and aerosol exposure is the most common source of occupationally acquired brucellosis caused by the manipulation of contaminated secretions of ill animals or by contact with laboratory cultures and tissue samples (34, 35). *Brucella* spp. can be easily aerosolized, with the additional hazard of its low infectious dose. The human infection has a variety of presentations, mainly affecting the reticuloendothelial system and complications had been reported; pulmonary involvement is sporadic (36, 37). Because of its potential spread by aerosols, *Brucella* has been classified as a biological agent of threat (38).

On the arrival of bacteria to the nasopharynx, the first step in pathogenesis is the adhesion to target molecules through different microbial ligands, most of them unknown so far. It has been reported an adhesin of *B. abortus* with an immunoglobulin-like domain. Although this protein has been involved in the adhesion to epithelial cells (39) the colonization of these bacteria in the respiratory tract has not been reported as is the case with species such as *Bordetella pertussis*, which usually enters and resides into the upper respiratory tract (40). In humans and other species, the inhalation of aerosols contaminated with *Brucella* leads to colonization of organs such as the lymph nodes, spleen, and liver (41).

The inhalation of aerosol or the intranasal instillation in mice is considered the most natural pathway of entry of *Brucella,* since the bacteria must trespass the first defense mechanisms (42). Epithelial barriers, mucus, defensins, and lysozyme avoid the colonization and entry to respiratory tract. It has been described that *Brucella abortus* PliC is a lysozyme inhibitor and it could participate in the brucellosis pathogenesis (43). Epithelial cells produce defensins, cytokines and chemokines in response to *B. abortus.* β-defensin 2 has antimicrobial activity against several pathogens and *in vitro* model β-defensin 2 does not seem to be effective against *Brucella,* but it could participate in recruiting immune cells and increase the dissemination of the bacteria (44).

In the nasal mucosa, secretory IgA and to a lesser extent IgG are other defense mechanisms. However, some evidences suggest that humoral immune response mediated by IgA may not play a central role in restraint against *Brucella* so the pathogen can even penetrate the epithelial barrier (45).

Epithelial cells and phagocytic cells are the first cells to be contacted by inhaled microorganisms. Some pathogens find temporary refuge from host immunity by sliding between epithelial cells (46). Furthermore, *Brucella* invades lung epithelial cells and alveolar macrophages where it avoids its degradation by inhibiting and modulating the endocytic traffic. In this way, these infected cells could promote the extrapulmonary dissemination of the bacteria within host tissues (47, 48). There is evidence that following intratracheal inoculation of *Brucella* in animal models, the bacteria spread to the spleen, draining cervical lymph node, tracheobronchial lymph nodes and mediastinal lymph nodes (47, 49), Therefore, immune response in mediastinal and cells homing to lungs have to be analyzed with more detail to clarify the immune responses that could mediate immune protection against mucosal infection.

Cytokines IL-1, IL-6, and TNF-α are important mediators of systemic and local inflammatory responses, but in lungs this triad do not have a key role. It has been shown that IL-1 and IL-6 deficiencies do not impact on the course of *Brucella* infection in the lungs, liver, or spleen. However, TCR-δ, TAP1, IL-17RA, and IFN-γR deficiencies affect *Brucella* control in the lungs (50). Recently, it was reported that IL-1R, probably through IL-1β action, and the NLRP3 and AIM2 inflammasomes have a protective effect on respiratory *Brucella* infection (51).

The induction of cellular-mediated responses is important in the clearance of *Brucella* from the lung, liver, and spleen, and the protection should be optimal when immunization and challenge routes are identical (45, 52). The live vaccines have shown to be effective in protection against brucellosis and these studies in animals have allowed to define the systemic immunity, but most of these studies performed parenteral vaccination and there is limited information of the mucosal response induced by the natural route of entry of *Brucella* (53).

Although no immunization route has shown total protection against intranasal challenge it has been found a significant reduction of bacterial load compared to the unvaccinated animals. Generally, it has been observed that intranasal immunization of *Brucella* induces systemic and mucosal immune responses (45, 52).

RESPONSE OF T LYMPHOCYTES TO INFECTION BY *BRUCELLA*

Brucella is one of the non-commensal pathogenic microorganisms that enter the organism through the intestinal mucosa and destabilize the commensal biota. Other pathogens such as *Escherichia coli* (ETC, EPEC, EIEC, etc.), *Shigella, Salmonella,* and *Yersinia* (54) colonize the gut and lead to the synthesis of proinflammatory molecules as TNF-α and IL-18, which are produced by macrophages in response to the infection (55).

Brucella abortus is captured by macrophages, where it causes the inhibition of several intracellular processes, as phagosome-lysosome fusion and respiratory burst through components as lipopolysaccharide (LPS) and those of the type-IV secretion system, which are virulence factors (6, 56–58). The most relevant virulence mechanism of *Brucella* spp. is its ability of survival and replication within these phagocytic cells as well as its mechanisms to evade intracellular death. *Brucella* spp. can infect different cell strains as macrophages, monocytes, DC, epithelial cells, and B lymphocytes (3). This characteristic is shared by other bacterial species that behave as intracellular pathogens, as *Mycobacterium tuberculosis* and *Salmonella enterica serovar Typhi* (59, 60), so the mechanisms of induced immunity are partially similar.

During the severe stage of the disease, which lasts 2 weeks approximately, the bacteria multiply rapidly. In the chronic stage, lasting 5–6 weeks, the bacterial concentration stabilizes and then decreases slowly, although there are some remaining bacteria in the liver, spleen, and lymph nodes even after 5 months (57).

The lamina propria of the intestine is inhabited by a number of cell lines, including CD4+, CD8+, γδT, and activated B lymphocytes, plasmatic cells, macrophages, eosinophils, and several populations of DC that take part in the regulation of the mucosa immune response (61). Additionally, stimulated enterocytes do have the ability to produce proinflammatory cytokines IL-1, IL-6, IL-7, and IL-8 (17).

The natural invasion of the host by *Brucella* induces a specific immune response mediated by Th1 lymphocytes that protects against the development of the disease, similar to the one observed in infections caused by other intracellular pathogens as *Salmonella* and *Mycobacterium tuberculosis.* Th1 lymphocytes are characterized by the production of proinflammatory cytokines as IL-1β, IL-6, TNF-α, and more importantly, IFN-γ (59). These proinflammatory cytokines play a protective role since they activate macrophages to increase their bactericide capacity and cytotoxic T lymphocytes (CTL) that kill infected cells (62–65). It has been observed that IFN-γ and IL-12 production by macrophages is induced by IL-17 (66). Also, the differentiation to Th17 lymphocytes is induced by a combination of IL-1, IL-6, and the transforming growth factor β (TGF-β). The *in vivo* participation of IL-23 in this differentiation process is necessary to achieve a stable differentiation and proliferation of Th17 cells when activated (67).

IL-17-producing cells, found in the lamina propria, play an essential role against microorganisms infecting the gastrointestinal tract (68). IL-17 production has also been observed in the lung and oral cavity mucosa. The cells producing the cytokine migrate toward these sites due to CCR6 expression. It has been established that IL-17 response at these mucosal sites is mainly directed against extracellular bacteria and fungi (69). Its protective role in infections caused by intracellular pathogens was initially controversial. In infections caused by *Listeria monocytogenes*, IL-17 response is produced by γδT lymphocytes in the liver, which apparently leads to the arrival of neutrophils in the organ. Nevertheless, mice lacking IL-17 receptor (IL-17RA$^{-/-}$) survive infection by *L. monocytogenes* (70). Contrastingly, IL-17 is necessary to generate a protective immune response against *M. tuberculosis* induced by vaccination.

The role of IL-17 seems to be differentially relevant with respect to *Brucella* species, against which protection is created. In oral vaccination of BALB/c mice with *B. melitensis* strain from which gene *znuA* (involved in zinc transportation) or *B. abortus* RB51 strain induced a similar protection against the intranasal challenge with *B. melitensis* 16M. The mice that showed IFN-γ deficiency (IFN-γ$^{-/-}$) also exhibited a state of protection, albeit less significant than the one observed in BALB/c wild-type mice. The protection in both mice strains was parallel to IL-17 and IL-22 response. However, IL-17 and IL-22 production was higher in IFN-γ$^{-/-}$mice than in wild type BALB/c mice, which would suggest that IL-17 and IL-22 compensate for the absence of IFN-γ. The *in vivo* neutralization of IL-17 with specific antibodies only affected the protection conferred by strain RB51 but did not affect the one provided by mutant Δ*znuA* (71). This proved that IL-17 is relevant to induce the protection provided by strain RB51 when administered orally.

Other studies have demonstrated the role that IL-17 plays in the protection against brucellosis induced by vaccination in the intestinal mucosa (72). *B. abortus* inhibits the host's proteases through Omp19 and limits the antigenic proteolysis of cells from PP and MLN, increasing the bacterial concentration in the gut mucosa inside monocytes and DC. However, in mice immunized with ovalbumin together with *Brucella* U-Omp19 as adjuvant, the anti-ovalbumin response of Th1, Th17, and CD8+ T lymphocytes was increased in the gut mucosa and system, leading to a high production of IFN-γ and IL-17 (27).

Abkar et al. (73) orally immunized BALB/c mice with protein U-Omp19 incorporated into N-trimethyl chitosan (TMC/Omp19) nanoparticles. They compared the response with that observed in mice immunized with intraperitoneal TMC/Opm19 after being challenged with virulent *B. abortus* strains 544 and *B. melitensis* 16M. The results showed that vaccination with oral TMC/Opm19 generated a protection considerably higher than the one induced by intraperitoneal vaccination. In addition, the intraperitoneal vaccination induced Th1- and Th2-type responses while the oral vaccination induced Th1 and Th17 cell response. These results demonstrate that the oral presentation of *Brucella* spp. antigens induce a more efficient response in which IL-17 production is deeply involved.

Lymphoid aggregates (particularly $\gamma\delta$T lymphocytes, cryptopatches) have been identified in the lamina propria of mice. In these aggregates, T$\gamma\delta$ and CD8+$\alpha\alpha$ lymphocytes suffer extrathymic maturation (74). Only a few studies on the role of $\gamma\delta$T cells have been reported; however, it is well-known that they are relevant in the early stages of infection since TCR$\delta^{-/-}$ mice are more susceptible to infection by *B. abortus* than wild-type C57BL/6. During the first week post infection, there was an increase in $\gamma\delta$T cells, which abated after 2 weeks. On the other hand, IFN$\gamma^{-/-}$ mice, from which $\gamma\delta$T cells were eliminated, showed a considerable increase in susceptibility to the infection by *B. abortus* (75).

In contrast, CD4+CD25+ Tregs cells are involved in the early stages of infection by *Brucella*, reducing the capacity of response of CD4+ effector T cells. The elimination of CD4+CD25+ Tregs cells with anti CD25 antibodies triggered an enhanced protective response against *B. abortus* in BALB/c mice, along with an increase in IFN-γ production compared with the response of mice without anti CDC25 treatment. In persistent infection, CD4+CD25+ Tregs cells maintain their suppressor function (76).

At the beginning of the infection by *B. abortus*, the number of Tregs and effector T cells was increased (76, 77). In this early stage of the infection, Tregs can negatively regulate the function of effector T cells through the production of IL-10 (78). Splenocytes can also produce IL-10 after the stimulus by PrpA protein of *B. abortus* and thus promoting the persistence of the infection (79). This suggests a deleterious role of the anti-*Brucella* immune response mediated by Treg and IL-10 production.

It is remarkable that in other infectious processes, CD4+CD25+ Treg and IL-10 protect against the infection or the disease. This has been observed in the tuberculosis murine model (80), and in infections caused by *Helicobacter pylori* (81), *Pneumocystis carinnii* (82), or trypanosomiasis (83).

It is well-established that the development of Th1 cell-mediated immune response is important in protection against *Brucella* spp. Particular emphasis has been placed on the role of IFN-γ in protecting against infection caused by *Brucella* spp. This conclusion has been drawn from studies done on animals infected by parenteral pathways, in which a systemic infection develops directly. Protective immunity in the intestine continues to be dependent on T cells, but it has become clear that other subpopulations are involved. In addition, a delicate balance must be maintained in the gut between pro-inflammatory, classically anti-*Brucella*, and anti-inflammatory responses. This knowledge is required for the design of vaccines that must be applied through the digestive tract to generate local immunity in the intestinal mucosa.

ANTIGENIC COMPONENTS OF *BRUCELLA* AS VIRULENCE FACTORS

Brucella spp. is an intracellular pathogen that invades and proliferates within the host's cells. The virulence of this strain is associated to the intracellular replication capacity in phagocytic and non-phagocytic cells (84). *Brucella* spp. lacks the typical virulence factors as toxins, fimbria, pili, and plasmids (85). Contrastingly, this intracellular pathogen has different antigenic elements that provide it with virulence and allow it to establish in the host's cells.

Lipopolysaccharide

Brucella, as genus, has two colonial morphologies: smooth and rough. In general, *Brucella* strains of rough morphology are attenuated or show reduced virulence, with the exception of species *B. ovis* and *B. canis*, that are virulent and naturally rough. The LPS of *Brucella* is one of its main virulence factors and is considered non-conventional when compared against other Gram-negative LPS, as those from the *Enterobacteriaceae* family. Neither *B. abortus* LPS nor that of *B. melitensis* activate complement or macrophages while their endotoxic activity is extremely reduced (86, 87).

The LPS of *Brucella* spp. is constituted by three main components: lipid A, core, and O side chain, which is the immunodominant component. Lipid A is inserted in the external membrane and has a backbone of diaminoglucose; acyl groups are the longest chain, C18–C19 or C29 instead of C12 to C14 of conventional LPS. The core, to which acylated chains are bound, has a polysaccharide sequence conserved among *Brucella* species. The bond between the acylated chain and core is through an amide linkage instead of ester and amide linkages. The O side chain of smooth LPS from *Brucella* is a chain of repeating units of sugars with a variability that allows for the differentiation of the species (88).

LPS from *Brucella* exhibits low endotoxicity due to poor macrophage recognition by heterodimer TLR-2/MD2, considered the main LPS receptor in Gram-negative bacteria that also transduces activation signals within macrophages. In consequence *Brucella* LPS does not induce a response in macrophages or DC *in vivo* or *in vitro*. The stimulation of macrophages or DC with *Brucella* spp. LPS does not induce the expression of activation markers on the cell surface nor does it induce the production of proinflammatory cytokines. In contrast, *Brucella* spp. LPS seems to deregulate macrophages and DC according to their function of antigen presenting cells, so it does not allow for the activation or proliferation of T lymphocytes. This low induction in the immune response mediated by cells could be the way in which *Brucella* evades from the beginning of the infection. It allows *Brucella* to establish, triggering the chronicity of the infection (89).

It has been demonstrated that the core is a virulence factor, since wadC mannosyl transferase mutants increase interaction with MD2, leading to a higher production of cytokines. On the other hand, the loss of the O-chain creates attenuated strains that allow the infected cell to carry the vesicle containing *Brucella* to the lysosomal compartment, where the bacterium is eliminated. Smooth strains evade from this intracellular death pathway, suggesting that the O side chain of LPS is involved in the transportation of the vesicle containing *Brucella* to other non-lysosomal compartments, or avoidance of transport to such lysosomal compartment (90). *Brucella* spp. LPS also prevents the activation of the complement, with which it also avoids opsonization by subcomponent C3b, decreasing recognition by phagocytic cells through receptors for the complement. Additionally, it prevents the generation of anaphylatoxins C3a and C5a, hampering the consequent proinflammatory response (86, 87).

Cyclic β-1,2-Glucan

Cyclic glucans are intrinsic components of Gram-negative bacteria that have a high structural variability and are responsible for maintaining homeostasis against osmolarity changes (91). *Brucella* spp. cyclic glucans are accumulated in the periplasm and are constituted by a backbone of glucose units bound by b-1,2 links with a polymerization degree of 17–25 monomers (92). Mutants of the genes responsible for the synthesis and transport of glucan to the periplasm show decreased survival and multiplication of the bacterium in BALB/c mice spleen. The mutant strain of the gene *cgs* (cyclic glucan synthase), responsible for glucan synthesis induces a response that is almost exclusive of Thl lymphocytes (93). It has been demonstrated that the cyclic glucan of *Brucella* spp. acts upon the host cell membrane at the lipid rafts. Then, the bacterium controls the maturation of the vacuoles in which it is internalized, preventing lysosome fusion, and allowing to reach the replication niche (94). The cyclic β- 1,2-glucan of *Brucella* spp. promotes splenomegaly in mice as a consequence of monocyte, DC, and neutrophil recruitment by IL-12 and TNF-α induction (95). Studies *in vitro* have demonstrated that *Brucella* spp. induces DC activation via TLR4, MyD88 and TRIF, but not through CD14, increasing the antigen-specific response of CD8+ T lymphocytes (96).

Type IV Secretion System and BvrR/BvrS

Brucella spp. has a two-component system BvrR/BvrS. This system directly and indirectly controls the expression of operon virB, coding the type IV secretion system (T4SS) (97). The two-component BvrR/BvrS system of *Brucella* spp. is constituted by a histidine-kinase sensor located in the cytoplasmic membrane (BvrS) and a cytoplasmic regulator (BvrR). The mutant strains in the BvrR/BvrS system are avirulent in mice, show a lower capacity to invade macrophages and HeLa cells and are unable to replicate intracellularly (98).

The *Brucella* BvrR/BvrS two-component regulatory system is essential to detect changes in the phagosomal environment. In addition, it allows the bacterium to modify the lifestyle from extracellular to intracellular (99). The BvrR/BvrS system controls the conformation of the LPS structure and the expression of Omp (99–101). This system is also necessary to switch off extracellular survival genes and express the genes needed for invasion and intracellular survival (97).

The *Brucella* T4SS, constituted by 12 components, has been evaluated using *in vitro* and *in vivo* models. The *in vitro* infection of different cell lines demonstrated that the T4SS is essential to allow for the intracellular replication of the bacterium. In animal models it has been observed that T4SS is necessary for the onset of the infection (102). Recently it has been published that BvrR is a good candidate for a DNA vaccine in the murine brucellosis model, but many studies are missing (103).

Enzyme Superoxide Dismutase

The survival of *Brucella* within the macrophage has been associated to the synthesis of several proteins: antioxidant enzymes as KatE and Cu,Zn superoxide dismutase (Cu/Zn SOD). Superoxide dismutases (SODs) are metalloenzymes that catalyze the dismutation of superoxide ions, being an important mechanism of antioxidant defense (104). Periplasmic SODs are a key element of the defense mechanisms several pathogens must protect against the respiratory burst of the host's phagocytic cells. This is a previous survival step that allows for the later replication of the bacteria within phagocytes (105).

Brucella spp. Cu/Zn SOD is located in the periplasmic space of the cell wall. The bacterial count of *B. abortus* Cu/Zn SOD mutants recovered from BALB/c mice is much lower when compared to the amount recovered from wild *B. abortus* (106). This result demonstrated the key role that Cu/Zn SOD plays in the virulence of the bacterium.

Urease

This enzyme catabolizes the hydrolysis of urea in carbon and ammonic dioxide. Urease has been reported as a virulence factor for many pathogens, which induce direct toxicity in renal tissue and the formation of kidney stones. It allows for the transit of microorganisms as *Yersinia, Klebsiella*, and *Helicobacter pylori* to colonize the stomach and promotes the bacterium in an acid environment. Sangari et al. (21) evaluated urease operon mutants that were efficiently eliminated, evidencing that the presence of the enzyme promotes its survival and thus promotes infection.

VACCINES

The most effective strategy to prevent the spread of brucellosis in humans, besides the pasteurization of dairy products, has been the control of cattle through vaccination. Although there are effective vaccines to control brucellosis, the disease has not been eradicated from most of the countries around the world (107). The available vaccines present several disadvantages as the interference with the immune response induced by diagnosis methods; some cause abortions in pregnant animals while the immunity they generate does not protect the cattle vaccinated throughout their reproductive life (107, 108). To date, there is no vaccine for safe application in humans since it is considered that even those strains known for their stability can revert their attenuated state (they must be applied as live vaccine) and trigger the disease in the vaccinated population. Vaccination programs

TABLE 1 | Ideal *Brucella* vaccine (107).

1. Constituted by living bacteria able to generate a potent Th1-type response.
2. Not induce the production of antibodies that may interfere with diagnosis tests to detect infected animals.
3. An attenuated strain that does not cause disease nor persistent infection in animal.
4. Not be pathogenic for humans, preventing accidental contamination during the administration of the vaccine.
5. Induce long-term protection with only one dose, without causing abortions even when administered to pregnant females.
6. Not induce antibody response when applying boosters.
7. Stable and not revert to its virulent state *in vivo* or *in vitro*.
8. Affordable for its massive application and easy to produce and administer.

mostly focus on females because it has been suggested that some vaccines may damage the male reproductive system (109).

According to Ko and Splitter (84), Dorneles et al. (107), Nicoletti (110), and Schurig et al. (111) the ideal vaccine against brucellosis must have the following characteristics: (1) it must be constituted by living bacteria able to generate a potent Th1-type response; (2) it must not induce the production of antibodies that may interfere with diagnosis tests to detect infected animals, regardless of the route or dosage and age of animals; (3) it must be an attenuated strain that does not cause disease nor persistent infection in animals; (4) it must not be pathogenic for humans, preventing accidental contamination during the administration of the vaccine; (5) it must induce long-term protection with only one dose, without causing abortions even when administered to pregnant females; (6) it must not induce antibody response when applying boosters; (7) it must be stable and not revert to its virulent state *in vivo* or *in vitro*; and (8) it must be affordable for its massive application and easy to produce and administer (**Table 1**).

Most of the vaccines currently used aim to prevent the disease caused by *B. abortus* (strains 19, RB51, 45/20, and SR82) and *B. melitensis* (strain Rev. 1) (108, 112). Vaccine strains for *B. suis*, *B. ovis*, and *B. canis* have been developed experimentally without reaching massive application. **Table 2** summarize the classification of Brucella vaccines.

LIVE, ATTENUATED VACCINES

These vaccines are given parenterally and generate immunity against systemic infection. However, as previously discussed, local mucosal immunity can precisely prevent systemic spread. It should be studied whether the use of live vaccines could maintain long-lasting immunity in the gastrointestinal and/or respiratory mucosa. Developing and maintaining local immunity will be important, as some evidence suggests that mucous membranes are reservoirs of *Brucella* spp.

B. abortus S19

This strain was originally isolated from milk in 1923. It was accidentally attenuated after keeping it at room temperature for a year. Its use as vaccine in cattle started in 1941 (108, 111, 142). Strain S19 is indicated for its application in calves since it causes epididymitis in male adults and is associated to abortion in pregnant females (143). Animals vaccinated with *B. abortus* S19 develop antibodies against LPS because the strain is smooth. Therefore, it is not possible to differentiate between animals vaccinated with this strain and naturally infected animals (108, 144). Recently, it was noticed that immune response is different among breeds of cattle, as the Shawial breed responded less to the 19S vaccine than the crossbread animals (145).

B. abortus 45/20

This strain was derived from an isolated smooth strain obtained from an infected cow (called 45) in 1922. After passages through guinea pig, strain 45 was obtained and, after 20 passages, the rough phase was isolated; therefore, the strain was named 45/20. This strain had to be administered inactivated by heating along with an adjuvant. It can revert to its virulent smooth form, so it has to be inactivated before applying it as vaccine (108, 111). Unfortunately, the protection and antibody response assays showed high variability, which questioned the efficacy of the vaccine. Additionally, some animals exhibited hypersensitivity reactions on the injection site of the vaccine. These inconveniences led to the interruption in the use of this strain as vaccine (107).

B. abortus RB51

Smooth strains commonly show phase variation into rough strains. This change in phenotype is usually accompanied by a decrease in the strain's virulence. However, some species are naturally rough, as *B. ovis* and *B. canis*. These last are pathogenic for a natural host, but the number of animal species they infect is reduced when compared against the diversity of hosts where smooth strains can be isolated. Based on these observations and the experience creating strain 45/20, experts began looking for a notably attenuated rough mutant that could colonize the host for the time needed to induce a protective immune response (111).

The strain *B. abortus* RB51 was obtained after successive passages of the virulent smooth strain *B. abortus* 2308 in a culture medium with rifampicin or penicillin. Strain RB51 shows a rough phenotype and lacks the LPS polysaccharide O-chain. It is highly stable and does not revert to the virulent smooth phenotype (142). The absence of O-chain does not induce the formation of antibodies, which allows for the differentiation between vaccinated and naturally infected animals (107). In contrast, the strain induces a strong Th1-type cell response, which confers a high protective efficiency. This effectiveness is due to the induction of IFN-γ response, which leads to the activation of cytotoxic T lymphocytes, which eliminate the infected cells, and increase the bactericide activity of macrophages (143). In 1990, the use of strain RB51 as vaccine of choice in the USA was implemented to control bovine brucellosis and is currently applied in several Latin American countries (108). The fact that it was selected as rifampicin-resistant is a considerable disadvantage since it is the first-choice antibiotic against brucellosis when streptomycin cannot be administered (146).

TABLE 2 | Classification of *Brucella* vaccines.

Classification	Vaccine	Route of administration	Immunological parameter evaluated	References
Vaccines from recombinant strains	*RB51WboA* *RB51SOD* RB51SOD/WboA	Intraperitoneal in BALB/c mice	Concentration of IFN-γ in culture supernatants of splenocytes upon *in vitro* stimulation. Clearance of challenge infection with *B. abortus* 2308 and *B. melitensis* 16 M measure as CFU in spleen in mice previously vaccinated with mutant strains. Development of IgG2a: *RB51SOD,* developed antibodies to SOD *RB51WboA,* develop to the O-side chain RB51SOD/WboA, develop to SOD and the O-side chain.	(113–117)
	Mutants in genes *wbkA* and *per*	Intraperitoneal in BALB/c mouse	Clearance of challenge infection with *B. abortus* 2308 measure as CFU in spleen in mice previously vaccinated with mutant strains.	(118–120)
	S2308DATP	Intraperitoneal in BALB/c mouse	Clearance of challenge infection with *B. abortus* 2308 measure as CFU in spleen and blood in mice previously vaccinated with mutant strains. Evaluation in the expression of MCH I, MHC II and costimulatory molecules CD40, CD80 and CD86. IgG evaluation.	(121)
	B. abortus Δpgk	Intraperitoneal BALB/c, 129/Sv, C57BL/6, and IRF-1 KO mice	Clearance of challenge infection with *B. abortus* 2308 measure as CFU in spleen in BALB/c, 129/Sv, C57BL/6, and 129/Sv mice previously vaccinated with mutant strains, *B. abortus* S19, RB51. IFN-γ production by spleen cells of IRF-1 KO mice vaccinated with S19, RB51, or the Δpgk mutant strain.	(122)
	S19ΔvjbR	Vaccination intraperitoneally BALB/c mouse with a sustained-release vehicle to enhance vaccination efficacy was evaluated utilizing the live S19ΔvjbR::Kan in encapsulated alginate microspheres containing a non-immunogenic eggshell precursor protein of the parasite *Fasciola hepatica*	Clearance of challenge infection with *B. abortus* 2308 measure as CFU in spleen in mice previously vaccinated with S19 and mutant strains encapsulated and non-encapsulated.	(123, 124)
		IRF-1$^{-/-}$ mice were vaccinated intraperitoneally with *B. abortus* S19ΔvjbR	Clearance of challenge infection with *B. melitensis* 16M measure as CFU in spleen in mice previously vaccinated with S19ΔvjbR	(125)
	ΔznuA	Intraperitoneal in BALB/c mouse	Clearance of challenge infection with *B. abortus* 2308 measure as CFU in spleen in mice previously vaccinated with S19, RB51 and mutant strains.	(126, 127)
Probiotic vector	*Lactococcus lactis* expressing antigen L7/L12 of *B. abortus*	Intragastric gavage in BALB/c mouse	Evaluation of fecal anti-L7/L12 IgA and systemic IgG anti-L7/L12. The mutant strain was challenged by intraperitoneal injection with *B. abortus* 2308, and the clearance in the spleen was measure.	(128)
	Lactococcus lactis expressing Cu, Zn superoxide dismutase (SOD) of *B. abortus*	Oral in BALB/c mouse with *L. lactis* expressing Cu/Zn alone or in combination with *L. lactis* expressing IL-12	Evaluation of the presence IgG1, IgG2a, IgM, and sIgA from nasal and bronchoalveolar lavages. Lymphocyte proliferation assay after oral immunization. The mutant strain was challenged by intraperitoneal injection with *B. abortus* 2308, and the clearance in the spleen was measure.	(129)

(Continued)

TABLE 2 | Continued

Classification	Vaccine	Route of administration	Immunological parameter evaluated	References
Bacterial vector:	*Salmonella typhimurium* expressing BCSP31, Omp3b, and SOD proteins of *Brucella abortus*	Intraperitoneal and oral in BALB/c mouse	Evaluation of IgG, TNF-α, and IFN-γ. The mixture of mutant strains was challenged by intraperitoneal injection with *B. abortus* 544, and the clearance in the spleen was measure.	(130)
	Salmonella typhimurium expressing BLS, Omp19, prpA, and SOD proteins of *Brucella abortus*	Intraperitoneal in guinea pigs	Histopathological assessment in lungs, liver, spleen, and uterus. The mixture of mutant strains was challenged by intraperitoneal injection with *B. abortus* 544, and the clearance in the spleen and liver was measure.	(131)
		Intraperitoneal in pregnant guinea pigs	Histopathological assessment in lungs, liver, spleen, and uterus. The mixture of mutant strains was challenged by intraperitoneal injection with *B. abortus* 544, and the clearance in the spleen and liver was measure.	(132)
Attenuated strains	*B. neotomae*	Intraperitoneal in BALB/c mouse with *B. neotomae* and *B. neotomae* mutant strains	Levels in serum of total IgG, as well as IgG1, IgG2a, IgG2b, IgG3, and IgM. IL-2, GM-CSF, IFN-γ, TNF-α, IL-4, IL-5, IL-10, IL-12p70 cytokines were tested in the collected supernatants of splenocytes from vaccinated mice. Cells from spleens of vaccinated mice were stained, to determine the proportion of CD4+ and CD8+ T cells that secreted IFN-γ. *B. neotomae* and *B. neotomae* mutant strains were challenged by intraperitoneal injection with *B. melitensis* 16M, *B. abortus* 2308, or *B. suis* 1330, and the clearance in the spleen was measure.	(133)
		Oral in BALB/c mouse	Levels in serum of total IgG, as well as IgG1, IgG2a, IgG2b, IgG3, and IgM. Levels in intestinal secretions of total IgG, IgM, and IgA. Cells from spleens of vaccinated mice were stained, to determine the proportion of CD4+ and CD8+ T cells that secreted IFN-γ and TNF-α. *B. neotomae* was challenged by intraperitoneal injection with *B. abortus* 2308 and the clearance in the spleen, liver and lungs was measure.	(134)
	znuA B. melitensis	Oral in BALB/c mouse and IFN-$\gamma^{-/-}$ BALB/c mouse	Evaluation for colonization in spleens, Peyer's patches, and mesenteric lymph nodes (MLNs). Splenocyte production of IFN-γ, IL-17 and IL-22, was evaluated, pre and post challenge. Vaccination with *znuA B. melitensis* and *B. abortus* RB51, was nasally challenge with *B. melitensis* 16M. Clearance in the spleen and lungs was measure. Spleen grown was measure.	(71)
			Evaluation of Lc T CD4+ and CD8+.	(135)
	B. melitensis WR201	Oral in BALB/c mice	Vaccination with the mutant strain was nasally challenge with *B. melitensis* 16M, clearance in the spleen, liver and lungs was measure. Determination of IgG and IgM in serum and IgA in saliva. Splenocyte cytokine production of IL-2 and IFN-γ.	(136)
Viral vectors	Influenza virus vectors expressing proteins Omp16, Omp19, SOD, or L7/L12	Pregnant sheeps and goats Subcutaneous and conjunctival routes	Serum samples for determine antigen-specific humoral IgG, IgG2a, IgG1 antibodies, and whole blood for T cell stimulation index and IFN-γ production.	(137)

(Continued)

TABLE 2 | Continued

Classification	Vaccine	Route of administration	Immunological parameter evaluated	References
			Challenged with a virulent strain of *B. melitensis*16M, concentration of the bacteria in lymph nodes (submandibular, retropharyngeal, right subscapular, left subscapular, mediastinal, bronchial, portal, para-aortic, pelvic, mesenterican dudder), parenchymal organs (liver, kidney, spleen, and bone marrow) and placenta.	
Cell subunit vaccines	BLSOMP31	Conjuntival in lambs	Samples of serum, saliva, nasal, preputial and lacrimal secretions for detection of IgG. Samples of saliva, nasal, preputial and lacrimal secretions for detection of IgG and IgA anti-BLSOmp31 levels. IFN-γ in blood samples. Intradermal reaction to BLSOmp3.	(138)
Non-pathogenic alphaproteobacteria (NPAP) antigens	*Ochrobactrum anthropi, Sinorhizobium meliloti, Mesorhizobium loti, Agrobacterium tumefaciens*	Subcutaneous, intraperitoneal and Intragastric in BALB/c mouse	The subcutaneous and intraperitoneal vaccine administration was challenge intravenously with *B. melitensis* H38. Clearance in the spleen was measure. The intragastric vaccine administration was challenge with *B. abortus* 2308. Clearance in the spleen was measure. Serum IgG against *B. abortus* cytosolic antigens in mice immunized intraperitoneally with cytosolic fractions of NPAP. Serum IgG and IgA and fecal IgA against *B. abortus* cytosolic antigens in mice orally immunized.	(139)
Nanoparticles	Omp31-loaded N-trimethyl chitosan nanoparticles	Intraperitoneal and oral in BALB/c mouse	Determination of IgG1 and IgG2a and IgM in serum. Anti-Omp31 IgA was determined in fecal samples. Cytokine (IFN-γ, IL-12, IL-4, and IL-17) response in splenocytes. The vaccine was challenge with *B. melitensis* 16M, clearance in the spleen was measure.	(140)
Outer membrane vesicles (OMVS)	(OMVs) of *B. melitensis* 16M	Intramuscular in BALB/c mouse	Serum immunoglobulin IgG1 and IgG2a isotypes with specificity to OMVs. Cytokine response of Bone Marrow-Derived Dendritic Cells (BMDC) from Balb/c mouse, Th1 (IFN-γ, IL-2, IL-6, IL-12, and TNF-α), DC2-mediated Th2 (IL-4 and IL-10), and DC17-mediated Th17 (IL-17, IL-23, and TGF-β). Mice were challenge intraperitoneal with *B. melitensis* 16M, clearance in the spleen was measure.	(141)

B. abortus SR82

Strain SR82 was developed in the former Soviet Union and was first applied as vaccine for cattle in 1988. It is recognized by the R and S phase antisera. It is as efficient as vaccine S19 but does not induce false positives in serological diagnosis tests because the presence of antibodies against R phase can be evaluated (107, 147).

B. melitensis Rev1

Strain Rev1 is smooth, behaves as attenuated strain, and is applied to goats and sheep. It was derived from *B. melitensis* 16M and requires the addition of streptomycin to the medium for its growth. This requirement is a disadvantage since streptomycin is the first-option antibiotic for brucellosis treatment, usually administered together with tetracycline (109, 111, 146); its administration is preferably conjunctival. This strain also induces the production of antibodies that interfere with the diagnosis: vaccinated animals cannot be differentiated from those that are naturally infected (109).

Vaccination with live strains has proven to have a highly protective efficiency in cattle and wildlife animals. This is because the bacterium remains viable in the host for a certain time and replicates. This promotes an immune response mediated by T lymphocytes against components of the pathogen, guaranteeing its effectiveness as protection-inducing agent against brucellosis (84, 148).

MUCOSAL VACCINES

The mucus membranes, covering the intestinal and urogenital tracts, conjunctiva, auditory canal, and exocrine gland ducts, have a highly specialized mucosal immune system that protects these surfaces against external attacks (149, 150). The design of vaccines that activate immunity in the mucus membranes seem to be promising. However, for a vaccine to be successful, it must be absorbed by the intestinal epithelium and captured by antigen-presenting cells in the intestine. It must also induce local response of B and T lymphocytes but must not create tolerance (151). Vaccines that are applied in the mucosa, particularly those that are orally administered, face dilution by mucous secretion; they may be trapped in the mucus and excluded with it or degraded by mucosal enzymes (152).

PROBIOTIC VECTORS

Several authors have explored the use of lactobacilli as vectors to generate oral vaccines. This possibility has been explored since probiotics easily survive in the gastrointestinal tract without hurting it, maintaining a close association with the epithelium. In addition, some authors have studied their immunomodulatory properties (153, 154). Because of this last property they have been applied together with vaccines for intracellular organisms. For instance, *L. rhamnosus* is adjuvant for vaccination with polymorphic membrane protein C (N-Pmpc) administered in the conjunctiva and increases the humoral and specific cell immune responses (155).

The following experiences have been documented when probiotics are applied together with vaccines to prevent brucellosis.

Lactococcus Lactis Expressing Antigen L7/L12 of *B. abortus*

L7/L12 is a ribosomal protein inducing cell-type response. Ribeiro et al. (156) transformed *L. lactis* using gene L7/L12. The vaccine administered orally in BALB/c mice induced significant IgA levels in feces against L7/L12, but no specific antibodies were found in serum; therefore, a systemic response was not triggered. The intraperitoneal application of the probiotic created a better protection (128).

Lactococcus Lactis Expressing Cu, Zn Superoxide Dismutase (SOD) of *B. abortus*

Bermúdez-Humarán et al. (157) showed that when administered in C57BL/6 mice by nasal route, *L. lactis* transformed to produce IL-12 in conjunction with *L. lactis*, and E7 antigen of the human papillomavirus type 16 (human papillomavirus type 16 E7 antigen) presented a Th1-type response induced with significant secretion of IFN-γ in splenocytes. Based on this study two recombinant strains of *L. lactis*, one expressing Cu/Zn SOD and another expressing IL-12, were administered to BALB/c mice orally. The animals produced significant SOD-specific sIgA in nasal and bronchoalveolar lavage and T cell proliferation as a response to re-stimulation with SOD or crude *Brucella* protein extract. Protection against challenge with *B. abortus* 2308 was similar to the one observed in mice vaccinated with RB51 and it was better when administered together with the two recombinant *L. lactis* strains (129).

BACTERIAL VECTORS

Salmonella typhimurium Expressing BCSP31, Omp3b, and SOD Proteins of *Brucella abortus*

BALB/c mice were intraperitoneally and orally immunized with the mix of *S. typhimurium* recombinant strains. The concentration of IgG, TNF-α, and IFN-γ in serum of mice immunized in both routes (except the recombinant one expressing Omp3b, orally administered) was significantly higher when compared against the control inoculated with wild-type *S. typhimurium*. Protection against challenge with intraperitoneal *B. abortus* 544 was higher in mice vaccinated with the mix of recombinant bacteria administered orally (130).

Salmonella typhimurium Expressing BLS, Omp19, prpA, and SOD Proteins of *Brucella abortus*

A vaccine using an attenuated *S. typhimurium* strain was designed and proved to be well-tolerated when administered orally or subcutaneously; it induces low production of TNF-α and lower cytotoxicity (158). *S. typhimurium* transformed to express Cu/Zn SOD, lumazine synthase (BLS), Omp-19, and proline racemase protein A (prpA) (131, 158) induces a good level of protection against challenge with *B. abortus* 544 when orally administered. This protection correlated with Th1 and Th17 response (72).

In addition, researchers have conducted experiments in which the vaccine additioned with *B. abortus LPS* is intraperitoneally administered to guinea pigs. Protection against challenge with *B. abortus* 544 was acceptable and did not generate histopathological damage in lungs, liver, spleen, and uterus (132, 159).

ATTENUATED STRAINS

B. neotomae

One of the options evaluated in the creation of new vaccines against brucellosis is the use of *Brucella* strains that are non-pathogenic for humans or cattle. One of these naturally attenuated strains is *B. neotomae*, a smooth strain isolated from desert mice.

Moustafa et al. (133) designed four vaccine strains from *B. neotomae: B. neotomae* irradiated with gamma rays, which maintains the bacterium metabolically active but prevents its replication, *B. neotomae* SOD, and *B. neotomae* Bp26 (26 kDa). The strains were intraperitoneally administered to BALB/c mice that were challenged with *B. abortus* 2308, *B. melitensis* 16M, and *B. suis* 1330. The highest protection was provided by the irradiated strain, which also induced the production of IFN-γ, IL-12p70, IL-5, and IL-10. Based on this result, Dabral et al. (134) orally vaccinated BALB/c mice with the irradiated *B. neotomae* strain and *B. abortus* RB51 as reference. In both groups of mice, antigen-specific CD4+ and CD8+ T cells secreting IFN-γ and TNF-α were induced. The challenge with intraperitoneal and intranasal *B. abortus* demonstrated that protection induced by *B. neotomae* was better than the one by RB51.

znuA B. melitensis

Yang et al. (126) demonstrated that *B. abortus* strain znuA showed a deficiency while transporting zinc but generated a good protective response. They generated the same gene deletion in *B. melitensis* and orally vaccinated BALB/c mice that were later challenged nasally with *B. melitensis* 16M. The vaccine induced Th1 response in the spleen and respiratory lymph nodes, inducing 10-fold more CD8+ T lymphocytes producing IFN-γ than CD4+ T lymphocytes. Additionally, a systemic and mucosal Th-17 response was generated (71, 135). Two weeks after the administration, no colonies of the mutant strain were detected in spleen, PP or MLN. In contrast, mice immunized with RB51 and S19 still showed the bacterium in the organs after 2 weeks. This result indicates that *B. melitensis znuA* is less virulent (160, 161).

B. melitensis WR201

This is a purine-auxotrophic strain harboring operon *purEK* deletion. The orally administered bacteria are no longer isolated from spleen, lungs, and liver 8 weeks after immunization. It induces a good protection against nasal challenge with *B. melitensis* 16M (136).

VIRAL VECTORS

Influenza virus vectors expressing proteins Omp16, Omp19, SOD, or L7/L12 were administered subcutaneously and through the conjunctiva along with the adjuvant Montanide^{TM} Gel 01 in goats and sheep simultaneously. The vaccination induced 70% protection in pregnant animals against challenge with *B. melitensis* 16M (137).

CELL SUBUNIT VACCINES

BLSOMP31

Decameric *Brucella* lumazine synthase (BLS) has been proven to be a protein able to carry antigens without altering their conformation due to its physicochemical and immunogenic properties. In addition, it induces activation of CD8+ T lymphocyte response and IFN-γ production (162). Estein et al. (163) used BLS and added an exposed loop of Omp31 and proved that this combination induced protection against challenge with *B. ovis* administered parenterally to goats. The same antigen was administered at the conjunctiva to 5-month-old muttons, using a thermoresponsive and mucoadhesive gel and chitosan as carriers (BLSOmp31-P407-Ch). The antigen generated specific lgG- and lgA-specific response, increased IFN-γ in serum, and development of an intradermal reaction at 90 days post infection (138).

ALPHAPROTEOBACTERIA

Since it has been proven that there is a cross-reactivity between *Brucella* and non-pathogenic alphaproteobacteria (NPAP) antigens, Delpino et al. (26) vaccinated BALB/c mice with *Ochrobactrum anthropi, Sinorhizobium meliloti, Mesorhizobium loti, Agrobacterium tumefaciens*, or *Brucella melitensis* H38 as positive control. The best response to the intravenous challenge with *B. abortus* 2308 was found in mice vaccinated with *O. anthropi*, *M. loti*, and *B. melitensis* H38, compared against the response in mice administered PBS and that in mice vaccinated with cytosolic extracts.

Delpino et al. (26) also orally immunized using live NPAP and heat-killed *B. abortus* 2308, while they orally challenged using *B. abortus* 2308. The results showed that *O. anthropi* induced a strong lgA anti-*Brucella* response in serum and feces. Oral vaccination with NPAP induced high protection levels but reduced ones in mice vaccinated with heat-killed *B. abortus* 2308.

NANOPARTICLES

The oral administration with Omp31-loaded *N*-trimethyl chitosan nanoparticles in BALB/c mice induced a combination of Th1-Th17 responses, and a strong response of IFN-γ, IL-12, and IL-17. The mice challenged with *B. melitensis* 16M showed a significant level of protection in the spleen 4 weeks after vaccination (140).

OUTER MEMBRANE VESICLES

It has been observed that Gram-negative bacteria can secrete membrane vesicles, which carry molecular components associated to the virulence of the bacterium they are derived from Dorneles et al. (107). Vesicles of Gram-negative bacteria derive from the outer membrane. The proteomic analysis of the outer membrane vesicles (OMVs) of *B. melitensis* 16M proved that they contain, among others, Omp16, Omp19, Omp25, Omp31, Cu/Zn SOD, IalB, InvB GroES, and bp26 (141, 164). OMVs are recognized by membrane and cytoplasmic receptors as NOD receptors (nucleotide binding oligomerization domain-like receptors) in eukaryotic cells and induce immune response. OMVs obtained from strain VTRM1 induced IL-12, TNF-α, and IFN-γ response significantly higher than that induced by strain 16M in DC derived from bone marrow. OMVs obtained from *B. melitensis* 16M were intraperitoneally applied as vaccine to BALB/c mice and induced a slightly reduced protection level against challenge with 16M, when compared with the challenge with *B. melitensis* Rev1 (2.64 vs. 1.9 logarithmic units). Interestingly, OMVs obtained from mutant rough *B. melitensis* VTRM1 conferred a much higher protection level (3.08 logarithmic units) (141). These results are promising since they suggest the possibility of obtaining an acellular vaccine to be applied in humans. However, its efficacy must be proven orally as an edible vaccine to induce local immunity, which must stop infection at the entry site.

CONCLUDING REMARKS

The studies discussed in this review indicate current research on interactions between *Brucella* and its host mucosa. *Brucella* spp. is a pathogen that enters its host preferably through the mucosa of the gastrointestinal tract. Infection is eventually reported through the respiratory tract, either in the laboratory by inhalation of contaminated aerosols, or in the field by inhalation of dust particles including bacteria. Systemic immunity is well-known, since most experimental studies administer the bacteria intraperitoneally, where it establishes interactions with cellular populations different from those found in mucous membranes. As discussed, some studies suggest that in the intestine *Brucella* spp. interacts with dendritic cells, and that these represent a variety of populations with antagonistic functions. It has been observed that an important population of dendritic cells induces tolerogenic responses, so the role of dendritic cells with proinflammatory function should be studied.

In systemic infection the proinflammatory response is fundamental to establish the anti *Brucella* immunity, as it activates Th1 cells, which through the IFN-g stimulate the bactericidal activity of macrophages. In the mucosa a reaction must be subject to strong control as it can be deleterious. The role of cytotoxic T lymphocytes should be explored in more detail, as in systemic immunity studies they are essential to eliminate cells infected with *Brucella* spp. Preliminary results suggest their activation in the gut, but the role of Th17 cells in the gut as well as in the oral cavity and gut should be confirmed. It is possible that these cellular populations have a critical participation in these sites in view of the evidence suggesting that mucous membranes are reservoir sites for *Brucella* spp. which could be an important basis for the chronicity of *Brucella* infection. The study in some of these areas is growing exponentially and may translate into new vaccines and therapies. The new vaccines are involving the use of compounds derived from specific bacteria or bacteria as probiotics that protect mucosal surfaces and induce immunity.

New vaccines should increase protection against brucellosis, an intracellular bacterial infection that is difficult to treat. Much remains to be learned from the study of the interaction between *Brucella* and his host. The knowledge gained from these studies should also be translated into better therapeutic treatments to protect against this important chronic infectious disease.

AUTHOR CONTRIBUTIONS

RL-S contributed with the T-cell immunity and compilation of the paper's chapters. AS-A contributed with the chapter related to gut immunity. LD contributed with the chapter related to *Brucella* vaccines. SB-U contributed with the chapter related to respiratory tract immunity. MM-L contributed with the whole organization, the critical review and edition.

REFERENCES

1. Wyatt HV. Lessons from the history of brucellosis. *Rev Sci Tech.* (2013) 32:17–25. doi: 10.20506/rst.32.1.2181
2. Wyatt HV. How themistocles zammit found malta fever (brucellosis) to be transmitted by the milk of goats. *J R Soc Med.* (2005) 98:451–4. doi: 10.1177/014107680509801009
3. Gorvel JP, Moreno E. *Brucella* intracellular life: from invasion to intracellular replication. *Vet Microbiol.* (2002) 90:281–97. doi: 10.1016/S0378-1135(02)00214-6
4. Gorvel JP, Moreno E, Moriyó N. Is *Brucella* an enteric pathogen? *Nat Rev Microbiol.* (2009) 7:250. doi: 10.1038/nrmicro2012-c1
5. Tsolis RM, Young GM, Solnick JV, Baumler AJ. From bench to bedside: stealth of enteroinvasive pathogens. *Nat Rev Microbiol.* (2008) 6:883–92. doi: 10.1038/nrmicro2012
6. Paixao TA, Roux CM, den Hartigh AB, Sankaran-Walters S, Dandekar S, Santos RL, et al. Establishment of systemic *Brucella melitensis* infection through the digestive tract requires urease, the type IV secretion system, and lipopolysaccharide O antigen. *Infect Immun.* (2009) 77:4197–208. doi: 10.1128/IAI.00417-09
7. Feller L, Altini M, Khammissa RA, Chandran R, Bouckaert M, Lemmer J. Oral mucosal immunity. *Oral Surg Oral Med Oral Pathol Oral Radiol.* (2013) 116:576–83. doi: 10.1016/j.oooo.2013.07.013

8. Meyle J, Dommisch H, Groeger S, Giacaman RA, Costalonga M, Herzberg M. The innate host response in caries and periodontitis. *J Clin Periodontol.* (2017) 44:1215–25. doi: 10.1111/jcpe.12781
9. Walker DM. Oral mucosal immunology: an overview. *Ann Acad Med Singapore.* (2004) 33:27–30.
10. von Bargen K, Gagnaire A, Arce-Gorvel V, de Bovis B, Baudimont F, Chasson L, et al. Cervical lymph nodes as a selective niche for *Brucella* during oral infections. *PLoS ONE.* (2014) 10:e0121790. doi: 10.1371/journal.pone.0121790
11. Acheson D, Luccioli S. Microbial-gut interactions in health and disease. Mucosal immune responses. *Best Pract Res Clin Gastroenterol.* (2004) 18:387–404. doi: 10.1016/j.bpg.2003.11.002
12. Forchielli ML, Walker WA. The effect of protective nutrients on mucosal defense in the immature intestine. *Acta Paediatr Suppl.* (2005) 94:74–83. doi: 10.1080/08035320510043592
13. Forchielli M, Walker W. The role of gut-associated lymphoid tissues and mucosal defence. *Br J Nutr.* (2005) 93:S41–8. doi: 10.1079/BJN20041356
14. Jeon MK, Klaus C, Kaemmerer E, Gassler N. Intestinal barrier: molecular pathways and modifiers. *World J Gastrointest Pathophysiol.* (2013) 4:94–9. doi: 10.4291/wjgp.v4.i4.94
15. Schenk M, Mueller C. The mucosal immune system at the gastrointestinal barrier. *Best Pract Res Clin Gastroenterol.* (2008) 22:91–409. doi: 10.1016/j.bpg.2007.11.002
16. Hofmann AF, Eckman L. How bile acids confer gut mucosal protection against bacteria. *Proc Natl Acad Sci USA.* (2006) 103:4333–4. doi: 10.1073/pnas.0600780103
17. Mowat AM, Agace WW. Regional specialization within the intestinal immune system. *Nat Rev Immunol.* (2014) 14:667–85. doi: 10.1038/nri3738
18. Smoot DT, Mobley HLT, Chippendale GR, Lewison JF, Resau JH. *Helicobacter pylori* urease activity is toxic to human gastric epithelial cells. *Infect Immun.* (1990) 58:1992–4.
19. Sangari FJ, Seoane A, Cruz-Rodríguez M, Agüero J, García-Lobo JM. Characterization of the urease operon of *Brucella abortus* and assessment of its role in virulence of the bacterium. *Infect Immun.* (2007) 75:774–80. doi: 10.1128/IAI.01244-06
20. Bandara AB, Contreras A, Contreras-Rodríguez A, Martins AM, Dobrean V, Poff-Reichow S, et al. *Brucella suis* urease encoded by *ure1* but not *ure2* is necessary for intestinal infection of BALB/c mice. *BMC Microbiol.* (2007) 7:57. doi: 10.1186/1471-2180-7-57
21. Sangari FJ, Cayon AM, Seoane A, García-Lobo JM. *Brucella abortus ure2* region contains an acid-activated urea transporter and a nickel transport system. *BMC Microbiol.* (2010) 10:107. doi: 10.1186/1471-2180-10-107
22. De Biase D, Tramonti A, Bossa F, Visca P. The response to stationary-phase stress conditions in *Escherichia coli*: role and regulation of the glutamic acid decarboxylase system. *Mol Microbiol.* (1999) 32:1198–211.
23. Occhialini A, Jimenez de Bagues MP, Saadeh B, Bastianelli D, Hanna N, De Biase D, et al. The glutamic acid decarboxylase system of the new species *Brucella microti* contributes to its acid resistance and to oral infection of mice. *J Infect Dis.* (2012) 206:1424–32. doi: 10.1093/infdis/jis522
24. Damiano MA, Bastianelli D, Al Dahouk S, Kohler S, Cloeckaert A, De Biase D, et al. Glutamate decarboxylase-dependent acid resistance in *Brucella* spp.: distribution and contribution to fitness under extremely acidic conditions. *Appl Environ Microbiol.* (2015) 81:578–86. doi: 10.1128/AEM.029 28-14
25. Tanaka H, Hashiba H, Kok J, Mierau I. Bile salt hydrolase of *Bifidobacterium longum*—Biochemical and genetic characterization. *Appl Environ Microbiol.* (2000) 66:2502–12. doi: 10.1128/AEM.66.6.2502-2512.2000
26. Delpino MV, Marchesini MI, Estein SM, Comerci DJ, Cassataro J, Fossati CA, et al. A bile salt hydrolase of *Brucella abortus* contributes to the establishment of a successful infection through the oral route in mice. *Infect Immun.* (2007) 75:299–305. doi: 10.1128/IAI.00952-06
27. Ibañez AE, Coria LM, Carabajal MV, Delpino MV, Risso GS, González-Cobiello P, et al. A bacterial protease inhibitor protects antigens delivered in oral vaccines from digestion while triggering specific mucosal immune responses. *J Control Release.* (2015) 220:18–28. doi: 10.1016/j.jconrel.2015.10.011
28. Salcedo SP, Marchesini MI, Lelouard H, Fugier E, Jolly G, Balor S, et al. *Brucella* control of dendritic cells maturation is dependent on the TIR-containing protein Btp1. *PLoS Pathogen.* (2008) 4:e21. doi: 10.1371/journal.ppat.0040021
29. Man AL, Prieto-García ME, Nicoletti C. Improving M cell mediated transport across mucosal barriers: do certain bacteria hold the keys? *Immunology.* (2004) 113:15–22. doi: 10.1111/j.1365-2567.2004.01964.x
30. Watarai M, Kim S, Erdenebaatar J, Makino SI, Horiuchi M, Shirahata T, et al. Cellular prion protein promotes *Brucella* infection into macrophages. *J Exp Med.* (2003) 198:5–17. doi: 10.1084/jem.20021980
31. Nakato G, Hase K, Suzuki M, Kimura M, Ato M, Hanazato M, et al. Cutting edge: *Brucella abortus* exploits a cellular prion protein on intestinal M cells as an invasive receptor. *J Immunol.* (2012) 189:540–1544. doi: 10.4049/jimmunol.1103332
32. Ferrero MC, Fossati CA, Rumbo M, Baldi PC. *Brucella* invasion of human intestinal epithelial cells elicits a weak proinflammatory response but a significant CCL20 secretion. *FEMS Immunol Med Microbiol.* (2012) 66:45–57. doi: 10.1111/j.1574-695X.2012.00985.x
33. von Bargen K, Gorvel JP, Salcedo SP. Internal affairs: investigating the *Brucella* intracellular lifestyle. *FEMS Microbiol Rev.* (2012) 36:533–62. doi: 10.1111/j.1574-6976.2012.00334.x
34. Corbel, M. (2006). *Brucellosis in Humans and Animals.* Geneva: World Health Organization.
35. Traxler RM, Lehman MW, Bosserman EA, Guerra MA, Smith TL. A literature review of laboratory-acquired brucellosis. *J Clin Microbiol.* (2013) 51:3055–62. doi: 10.1128/JCM.00135-13
36. Solera J, Solís García del Pozo J. Treatment of pulmonary brucellosis: a systematic review. *Exp Rev Anti Infect Ther.* (2017) 15:33–42. doi: 10.1080/14787210.2017.1254042
37. Uluğ M, Can-Uluğ N. Pulmonary involvement in brucellosis. *Can J Infect Dis Med Microbiol.* (2012) 23:e13–5. doi: 10.1155/2012/164892
38. Pappas G, Panagopoulou P, Christou L, Akritidis N. *Brucella* as a biological weapon. *Cell Mol Life Sci.* (2006) 63:2229–36. doi: 10.1007/s00018-006-6311-4
39. Czibener C, Merwaiss F, Guaimas F, Del Giudice MG, Serantes DAR, Spera JM, et al. BigA is a novel adhesin of *Brucella* that mediates adhesion to epithelial cells. *Cell Microbiol.* (2016) 18:500–13. doi: 10.1111/cmi.1 2526
40. Massillo C, Gorgojo J, Lamberti Y, Rodriguez ME. *Bordetella pertussis* entry into respiratory epithelial cells and intracellular survival. *Path Dis.* (2013) 69:194–204. doi: 10.1111/2049-632X.12072
41. Henning LN, Gillum KT, Fisher DA, Barnewall RE, Krile RT, Anderson MS, et al. The pathophysiology of inhalational brucellosis in BALB/c mice. *Sci Rep.* (2012) 2:495–495. doi: 10.1038/srep00495
42. Smither SJ, Perkins SD, Davies C, Stagg AJ, Nelson M, Atkins HS. Development and characterization of mouse Models of infection with aerosolized *Brucella melitensis* and *Brucella suis. Clin Vaccine Immunol.* (2009) 16:779–83. doi: 10.1128/CVI.00029-09
43. Um SH, Kim JS, Kim K, Kim N, Cho HS, Ha NC. Structural basis for the inhibition of human Lysozyme by PliC from *Brucella abortus. Biochemistry.* (2013) 52:9385–93. doi: 10.1021/bi401241c
44. Hielpos MS, Ferrero MC, Fernández AG, Bonetto J, Giambartolomei GH, Fossati CA, et al. CCL20 and beta-Defensin 2 production by human lung epithelial cells and macrophages in response to *Brucella abortus* infection. *PLoS ONE.* (2015) 10:e0140408–e0140408. doi: 10.1371/journal.pone.0140408
45. Surendran N, Sriranganathan N, Lawler H, Boyle SM, Hiltbold EM, Heid B, et al. Efficacy of vaccination strategies against intranasal challenge with *Brucella abortus* in BALB/c mice. *Vaccine.* (2011) 29:2749–55. doi: 10.1016/j.vaccine.2011.01.090
46. Virji M. Bacterial adherence and tropism in the human respiratory tract. In: Nataro JP, Cohen PS, Mobley HLT, Weiser JN, editors. *Colonization of Mucosal Surfaces.* Washington, DC: ASM Press (2005) p. 97–116.
47. Archambaud C, Salcedo SP, Lelouard H, Devilard E, de Bovis B, Van Rooijen N, et al. Contrasting roles of macrophages and dendritic cells in controlling initial pulmonary Brucella infection. *Eur J Immunol.* (2010) 40:3458–71. doi: 10.1002/eji.201040497
48. Ferrero MC, Fossati CA, Baldi PC. Smooth *Brucella* strains invade and replicate in human lung epithelial cells without inducing cell death. *Microbes Infect.* (2009) 11:476–83. doi: 10.1016/j.micinf.2009.01.010

49. Hensel ME, Garcia-Gonzalez DG, Chaki SP, Samuel J, Arenas-Gamboa AM. Characterization of an intratracheal aerosol challenge model of *Brucella melitensis* in guinea pigs. *PLoS ONE.* (2019) 14:e0212457. doi: 10.1371/journal.pone.0212457
50. Hanot Mambres D, Machelart A, Potemberg G, De Trez C, Ryffel B, Letesson J-J, et al. Identification of immune effectors essential to the control of primary and secondary intranasal infection with *Brucella melitensis* in mice. *J Immunol.* (2016) 196:3780–93. doi: 10.4049/jimmunol.1502265
51. Hielpos MS, Fernández AG, Falivene J, Alonso Paiva IM, Muñoz González F, Ferrero MC, et al. IL-1R and inflammasomes mediate early pulmonary protective mechanisms in respiratory *Brucella abortus* infection. *Front Cell Infect Microbiol.* (2018) 8:391. doi: 10.3389/fcimb.2018.00391
52. Surendran N, Sriranganathan N, Boyle SM, Hiltbold EM, Tenpenny N, Walker M, et al. Protection to respiratory challenge of *Brucella abortus* strain 2308 in the lung. *Vaccine.* (2013) 31:4103–10. doi: 10.1016/j.vaccine.2013.06.078
53. Lalsiamthara J, Lee JH. Development and trial of vaccines against *Brucella. J Vet Sci.* (2017) 18:281–90. doi: 10.4142/jvs.2017.18.S1.281
54. Hooper LV. Bacterial contributions to mammalian gut development. *Trends Microbiol.* (2004) 12:129–34. doi: 10.1016/j.tim.2004.01.001
55. Sansonetti PJ. War and peace at mucosal surfaces. *Nat Rev Immunol.* (2004) 4:953–64. doi: 10.1038/nri1499
56. Billard E, Cazeivielle C, Dornand J, Gross A. High susceptibility of human dendritic cells to invasion by the intracellular pathogens *Brucella suis, B. abortus and B. melitensis. Infect. Immun.* (2005) 73:8418–24. doi: 10.1128/IAI.73.12.8418-8424.2005
57. Hong PC, Tsolis RM, Ficht TA. Identification of genes required for chronic persistence of *Brucella abortus* in mice. *Infect Immun.* (2000) 68:4102–7. doi: 10.1128/IAI.68.7.4102-4107.2000
58. Roux CM, Rolan HG, Santos RL, Beremand PD, Thomas TL, Adams LG, et al. *Brucella* requires a functional Type IV secretion system to elicit innate immune responses in mice. *Cell Microbiol.* (2007) 9:1851–69. doi: 10.1111/j.1462-5822.2007.00922.x
59. Byndloss MX, Tsolis RM. *Brucella* spp. virulence factors and immunity. *Annu Rev Anim Biosci.* (2016) 4:111–27. doi: 10.1146/annurev-animal-021815-111326
60. Byndloss MX, Rivera-Chavez F, Tsolis RM, Baumler AJ. How bacterial pathogens use type III and type IV secretion systems to facilitate their transmission. *Curr Op Microbiol.* (2017) 35:1–7. doi: 10.1016/j.mib.2016.08.007
61. Kato T, Owen RL. Absence of EGF receptors and of EGF uptake in Peyer's patch dome epithelium. *Adv Exp Med Biol.* (1994) 355:295–301. doi: 10.1007/978-1-4615-2492-2_50
62. Brandao AP, Oliveira FS, Carvalho NB, Vieira LQ, Azevedo V, Macedo GC, et al. Host susceptibility to *Brucella abortus* infection is more pronounced in IFN-γ knockout than IL-12/β2-microglobulin double deficient mice. *Clin Dev Immunol.* (2012) 2012:589494. doi: 10.1155/2012/589494
63. Murphy EA, Sathiyaseelan J, Parent MA, Zou B, Baldwin CL. Interferon gamma is crucial for surviving a *Brucella abortus* infection in both resistant C57BL/6 and susceptible BALB/ mice. *Immunology.* (2001) 103:511–8. doi: 10.1046/j.1365-2567.2001.01258.x
64. Zhan Y, Cheers C. Endogenous interleukin-12 is involved in resistance to *Brucella abortus* infection. *Infect Immun.* (1995) 63:1387–90.
65. Zhan Y, Cheers C. Control of IL-12 and IFN-gamma production in response to live or dead bacteria by TNF and other factors. *J Immunol.* (1998) 161:1447–53.
66. Onishi RM, Gaffen SL. Interleukin-17 and its target genes: mechanisms of interleukin-17 function in disease. *Immunology.* (2010) 129:311–21. doi: 10.1111/j.1365-2567.2009.03240.x
67. Korn T, Bettelli E, Oukka M, Kuchroo VK. IL-17 and Th17 cells. *Annu Rev Immunol.* (2009) 27:485–517. doi: 10.1146/annurev.immunol.021908.132710
68. Marks BR, Craft J. Barrier immunity and IL-17. *Semin Immunol.* (2009) 21:164–71. doi: 10.1016/j.smim.2009.03.001
69. O'Quinn DB, Palmer MT, Lee YK, Weaver CT. Emergence of the Th17 pathway and its role in host defense. *Adv Immunol.* (2008) 99:115–63. doi: 10.1016/S0065-2776(08)00605-6
70. Hamada S, Umemura M, Shiono T, Tanaka K, Yahagi A, Begum MD, et al. IL-17A produced by gamma delta T cells plays a critical role in innate immunity against *Listeria monocytogenes* infection in the liver. *J Immunol.* (2008) 181:3456–63. doi: 10.4049/jimmunol.181.5.3456
71. Clapp B, Skyberg JA, Yang X, Thornburg T, Walters N, Pascual DW. Protective live oral brucellosis vaccines stimulate Th1 and Th17 cell responses. *Infect Immun.* (2011) 79:4165–74. doi: 10.1128/IAI.05080-11
72. Pasquevich KA, Ibanez AE, Coria LM, Garcia-Samartino C, Estein S, Zwerdling M, et al. An oral vaccine based on U-Omp19 induces protection against *B. abortus* mucosal challenge by inducing an adaptive IL-17 immune response in mice. *PLoS ONE.* (2011) 6:e16203. doi: 10.1371/journal.pone.0016203
73. Abkar M, Lotfi AS, Amani J, Eskandari K, Ramandi MF, Salimian J, et al. Survey of Omp19 immunogenicity against *Brucella abortus* and *Brucella melitensis:* influence of nanoparticulation versus traditional immunization. *Vet Res Comm.* (2015) 39:217–28. doi: 10.1007/s11259-015-9645-2
74. Kanamori Y, Ishimaru K, Nanno M, Maki K, Ikuta K, Nariuchi H, et al. Identification of novel lymphoid tissues in murine intestinal mucosa where clusters of c-kit+IL-7R+Thy1+ lympho-hemopoietic progenitors develop. *J Exp Med.* (1996) 184:1449–59. doi: 10.1084/jem.184.4.1449
75. Skyberg JA, Thornburg T, Rollins M, Huarte E, Jutila MA, Pascual DW. Murine and bovine γδ T cells enhance innate immunity against *Brucella abortus* infections. *PLoS ONE.* (2011) 6:e21978. doi: 10.1371/journal.pone.0021978
76. Pasquali P, Thornton AM, Vendetti S, Pistoia C, Petrucci P, Tarantino M, et al. CD4+CD25+ T regulatory cells limit effector T cells and favor the progression of brucellosis in BALB/c mice. *Microbes Infect.* (2010) 12:3–10. doi: 10.1016/j.micinf.2009.09.005
77. Belkaid Y, Rouse BT. Natural regulatory T cells in infectious disease. *Nat Immunol.* (2005) 6:353–60. doi: 10.1038/ni1181
78. Xavier MN, Winter MG, Spees AM, Nguyen K, Atluri VL, Silva TM, et al. CD4+ T cell-derived IL-10 promotes *Brucella abortus* persistence via modulation of macrophage function. *PLoS Pathog.* (2013) 9:e1003454. doi: 10.1371/journal.ppat.1003454
79. Spera JM, Ugalde JE, Mucci J, Comerci DJ, Ugalde RA. A B lymphocyte mitogen is a *Brucella abortus* virulence factor required for persistent infection. *Proc Natl Acad Sci USA.* (2006) 103:16514–9. doi: 10.1073/pnas.0603362103
80. Kursar M, Koch M, Mittrucker HW, Nouailles G, Bonhagen K, Kamradt T, et al. Regulatory T cells prevent efficient clearance of *Mycobacterium tuberculosis. J Immunol.* (2007) 178:2661–5. doi: 10.4049/jimmunol.178.5.2661
81. Raghavan S, Fredriksson M, Svennerholm AM, Holmgren J, Suri-Payer E. Absence of CD4+CD25+ regulatory T cells is associated with a loss of regulation leading to increased pathology in *Helicobacter pylori*-infected mice. *Clin Exp Immunol.* (2003) 132:393–400. doi: 10.1046/j.1365-2249.2003.02177.x
82. Hori S, Carvalho TL, Demengeot J. CD25+ CD4+ regulatory T cells suppress CD4+ T cell-mediated pulmonary hyperinflammation driven by *Pneumocystis carinii* in immunodeficient mice. *Eur J Immunol.* (2002) 32:1282–91. doi: 10.1002/1521-4141(200205)32:5<1282::AID-IMMU1282>3.0.CO;2-#
83. Guilliams M, Oldenhove G, Noel W, Herin M, Brys L, Loi P, et al. African trypanosomiasis: naturally occurring regulatory T cells favor trypanotolerance by limiting pathology associated with sustained type 1 inflammation. *J Immunol.* (2007) 179:2748–57. doi: 10.4049/jimmunol.179.5.2748
84. Ko J, Splitter GA. Molecular host-pathogen interaction in brucellosis: current understanding and future approaches to vaccine development for mice and humans. *Clin Microbiol Rev.* (2003) 16:65–78. doi: 10.1128/CMR.16.1.65-78.2003
85. Moreno E, Moriyon I. *Brucella melitensis*: a nasty bug with hidden credentials for virulence. *Proc Natl Acad Sci USA.* (2002) 99:1–3. doi: 10.1073/pnas.022622699
86. Barquero-Calvo E, Chaves-Olarte E, Weiss DS, Guzman-Verri C, Chacon-Diaz C, Rucavado A, et al. *Brucella abortus* uses a stealthy strategy to avoid activation of the innate immune system during the onset of infection. *PLoS ONE.* (2007) 2:e631. doi: 10.1371/journal.pone.0000631

87. Tumurkhuu G, Koide N, Takahashi K, Hassan F, Islam S, Ito H, et al. Characterization of biological activities of *Brucella melitensis* lipopolysaccharide. *Microbiol Immunol.* (2006) 50:421–7. doi: 10.1111/j.1348-0421.2006.tb03810.x
88. Lapaque N, Moriyon I, Moreno E, Gorvel JP. *Brucella* lipopolysaccharide acts as a virulence factor. *Curr Op Microbiol.* (2005) 8:60–6. doi: 10.1016/j.mib.2004.12.003
89. Conde-Álvarez R, Arce-Gorvel V, Iriarte M, Manček-Keber M, Barquero-Calvo E, Palacios-Chaves L, et al. The lipopolysaccharide core of *Brucella abortus* acts as a shield against innate immunity recognition. *PLoS ONE.* (2012) 8:e1002675. doi: 10.1371/journal.ppat.1002675
90. Fontana C, Conde-Alvarez R, Stahle J, Holst O, Iriarte M, Zhao Y, et al. Structural studies of lipopolysaccharide-defective mutants from *Brucella melitensis* identify a core oligosaccharide critical in virulence. *J Biol Chem.* (2016) 291:7727–41. doi: 10.1074/jbc.M115.701540
91. Breedveld MW, Miller KJ. Cyclic beta-glucans of members of the family Rhizobiaceae. *Microbiol Rev.* (1994) 58:145–61.
92. Iñón de Iannino N, Briones G, Tolmasky M, Ugalde RA. Molecular cloning and characterization of *cgs*, the *Brucella abortus* cyclic beta(1–2) glucan synthetase gene: genetic complementation of *Rhizobium meliloti* ndvB and *Agrobacterium tumefaciens* chvB mutants. *J Bacteriol.* (1998) 180:4392–400.
93. Briones G, Iñón de Ianninol N, Roset M, Vigliocco A, Silva-Paulo P, Ugalde RA. *Brucella abortus* cyclic b-1,2-glucan mutants have reduced virulence in mice and are defective in intracellular replication in HeLa cells. *Infect Immun.* (2001) 69:44528–35. doi: 10.1128/IAI.69.7.4528-4535.2001
94. Arellano-Reynoso B, Lapaque N, Salcedo S, Briones G, Ciocchini AE, Ugalde R, et al. Cyclic beta-1,2-glucan is a *Brucella* virulence factor required for intracellular survival. *Nat Immunol.* (2005) 6:618–25. doi: 10.1038/ni1202
95. Roset MS, Ibañez AE, de Souza Filho JA, Spera JM, Minatel L, Oliveira SC, et al. *Brucella* cyclic β-1,2-glucan plays a critical role in the induction of splenomegaly in mice. *PLoS ONE.* (2014) 9:e101279. doi: 10.1371/journal.pone.0101279
96. Martirosyan A, Pérez-Gutiérrez C, Banchereau R, Dutartre H, Lecine P, Dullaers M, et al. *Brucella* β1,2 cyclic glucan is an activator of human and mouse dendritic cells. *PLoS Pathog.* (2012) 8:e1002983. doi: 10.1371/journal.ppat.1002983
97. Martínez-Núñez C, Altamirano-Silva P, Alvarado-Guillén F, Moreno E, Guzman-Verri C, Chaves-Olarte E. The two-component system BvrR/BvrS regulates the expression of the type IV secretion system VirB in *Brucella abortus. J Bacteriol.* (2010) 192:5603–8. doi: 10.1128/JB.00567-10
98. Pizarro-Cerdá J, Meresse S, Parton RG, van der Goot G, Sola-Landa A, Lopez-Goñi I, et al. *Brucella abortus* transits through the autophagic pathway and replicates in the endoplasmic reticulum of nonprofessional phagocytes. *Infect Immun.* (1998) 66:5711–24.
99. Guzman-Verri C, Manterola L, Sola-Landa A, Parra A, Cloeckaert A, Garin J, et al. The two-component system BvrR/BvrS essential for *Brucella abortus* virulence regulates the expression of outer membrane proteins with counterparts in members of the Rhizobiaceae. *Proc Natl Acad Sci USA.* (2002) 99:12375–80. doi: 10.1073/pnas.192439399
100. Lamontagne J, Butler H, Chaves-Olarte E, Hunter J, Schirm M, Paquet C, et al. Extensive cell envelope modulation is associated with virulence in *Brucella abortus. J Proteome Res.* (2007) 6:1519–29. doi: 10.1021/pr060636a
101. Manterola L, Moriyon I, Moreno E, Sola-Landa A, Weiss DS, Koch MHJ, et al. The lipopolysaccharide of *Brucella abortus* BvrS/BvrR mutants contains lipid A modifications and has higher affinity for bactericidal cationic peptides. *J Bacteriol.* (2005) 187:5631–9. doi: 10.1128/JB.187.16.5631-5639.2005
102. Ke Y, Wang Y, Li W, Chen Z. Type IV secretion system of *Brucella* spp. and its effectors. *Front Cell Infec Microbiol.* (2015) 5:72. doi: 10.3389/fcimb.2015.00072
103. Chen B, Liu B, Zhao Z, Wang G. Evaluation of a DNA vaccine encoding *Brucella* BvrR in BALB/c mice. *Mol Med Rep.* (2019) 19:1302–8. doi: 10.3892/mmr.2018.9735
104. Broxton CN, Culotta VC. SOD enzymes and microbial pathogens: surviving the oxidative storm of infection. *PLoS Pathog.* (2016) 12:e1005295. doi: 10.1371/journal.ppat.1005295
105. Pratt AJ, DiDonato M, Shin DS, Cabelli DE, Bruns CK, Belzer CA, et al. Structural, functional, and immunogenic insights on Cu,Zn superoxide dismutase pathogenic virulence factors from *Neisseria meningitidis* and *Brucella abortus. J Bacteriol.* (2015) 197:3834–47. doi: 10.1128/JB.00343-15
106. Tatum FM, Detilleux PG, Sacks JM, Halling SM. Construction of Cu-Zn superoxide dismutase deletion mutants of *Brucella abortus*: analysis of survival *in vitro* in epithelial and phagocytic cells and *in vivo* in mice. *Infect Immun.* (1992) 60:2863–9.
107. Dorneles EMS, Sriranganathan N, Lage AP. Recent advances in *Brucella abortus* vaccines. *Vet Res.* (2015) 2015:46:76. doi: 10.1186/s13567-015-0199-7
108. Olsen SC, Stoffregen WS. Essential role of vaccines in brucellosis control and eradication programs for livestock. *Exp Rev Vaccines.* (2005) 4:915–28. doi: 10.1586/14760584.4.6.915
109. Avila-Calderón ED, Lopez-Merino A, Sriranganathan N, Boyle SM, Contreras-Rodríguez A. A history of the development of *Brucella* vaccines. *Biomed Res Int.* (2013) 2013:743509. doi: 10.1155/2013/743509
110. Nicoletti P. Brucellosis: past, present and future. *Prilozi.* (2010) 31:21–32.
111. Schurig GG, Sriranganathan N, Corbel MJ. Brucellosis vaccines: past, present and future. *Vet Microbiol.* (2002) 90:479–96. doi: 10.1016/S0378-1135(02)00255-9
112. Pandey A, Cabello A, Akoolo L, Rice-Ficht A, Arenas-Gamboa A, McMurray D, et al. The case for live attenuated vaccines against the neglected zoonotic diseases brucellosis and bovine tuberculosis. *PLoS Negl Trop Dis.* (2016) 10:e0004572. doi: 10.1371/journal.pntd.0004572
113. Vemulapalli R, Contreras A, Sanakkayala N, Sriranganathan N, Boyle SM, Schurig GG. Enhanced efficacy of recombinant *Brucella abortus* RB51 vaccines against *B. melitensis* infection in mice. *Vet Microbiol.* (2004) 102:237–45. doi: 10.1016/j.vetmic.2004.07.001
114. Vemulapalli R, McQuiston JR, Schurig GG, Sriranganathan N, Halling SM, Boyle SM. Identification of and IS711 element interrupting the *wboA* gene of *Brucella abortus* vaccine strain RB51 and a PCR assay to distinguish strain RB51 from other *Brucella* species and strains. *Clin Diagn Lab Immunol.* (1999) 6:760–4.
115. Vemulapalli R, He Y, Cravero S, Sriranganathan N, Boyle SM, Schurig GG. Overexpression of protective antigen as a novel approach to enhance vaccine efficacy of *Brucella abortus* strain RB51. *Infect Immun.* (2000) 68:3286–9. doi: 10.1128/IAI.68.6.3286-3289.2000
116. Vemulapalli R, He Y, Buccolo LS, Boyle SM, Sriranganathan N, Schurig GG. Complementation of *Brucella abortus* RB51 with a functional *wboA* gene results in O antigen synthesis and enhanced vaccine efficacy but no change in rough phenotype and attenuation. *Infect Immun.* (2000) 68:3927–32. doi: 10.1128/IAI.68.7.3927-3932.2000
117. Dabral N, Burcham GN, Jain-Gupta N, Sriranganathan N, Vemulapalli R. Overexpression of wbkF gene in *Brucella abortus* RB51WboA leads to increased O-polysaccharide expression and enhanced vaccine efficacy against *B. abortus* 2308, *B. melitensis* 16M, and *B. suis* 1330 in a murine brucellosis model. *PLoS ONE.* (2019) 14:e0213587. doi: 10.1371/journal.pone.0213587
118. Dabral N, Jain-Gupta N, Seleem MN, Sriranganathan N, Vemulapalli R. Overexpression of *Brucella* putative glycosyltransferase WbkA in *B. abortus* RB51 leads to production of exopolysaccharide. *Front Cell Infect Microbiol.* (2015) 5:54. doi: 10.3389/fcimb.2015.00054
119. Monreal D, Grillo MJ, Gonzalez D, Marin CM, de Miguel MJ, Lopez-Goñi I, et al. Characterization of *Brucella abortus* O Polysaccharide and core lipopolysaccharide mutants and demonstration that a complete core is required for rough vaccines to be efficient against *Brucella abortus* and *Brucella ovis* in the mouse model. *Infect Immun.* (2003) 71:3261–71. doi: 10.1128/IAI.71.6.3261-3271.2003
120. Godfroid F, Taminiau B, Danese I, Denoel PA, Tibor A, Weynants VE, et al. Identification of the perosamine synthetase gene of *Brucella melitensis* 16M and involvement of lipopolysaccharide O side chain in *Brucella* survival in mice and in macrophages. *Infect Immun.* (1998) 66:5485–93.
121. Zhang M, Han X, Liu H, Tian M, Ding C, Song J, et al. Inactivation of the ABC transporter ATPase gene in *Brucella abortus* strain 2308 attenuated the virulence of the bacteria. *Vet Microbiol.* (2013) 164:322–9. doi: 10.1016/j.vetmic.2013.02.017
122. Trant CGMC, Lacerda TLS, Carvalho NB, Azevedo V, Rosinha GMS, Salcedo SP, et al. The *Brucella abortus* phosphoglycerate kinase mutant is highly attenuated and induces protection superior to that of vaccine strain in immunocompromised and immunocompetent mice. *Infect immun.* (2010) 78:2283–91. doi: 10.1128/IAI.01433-09

123. Arenas-Gamboa AM, Ficht TA, Kahl-McDonagh MM, Gomez G, Rice-Ficht AC. The *Brucella abortus* S19 DeltavjbR live vaccine candidate is safer than S19 and confers protection against wild-type challenge in BALB/c mice when delivered in a sustained-release vehicle. *Infect Immun.* (2009) 77:877–84. doi: 10.1128/IAI.01017-08
124. Khalaf OH, Chaki SP, Garcia-Gonzalez DG, Ficht TA, Arenas-Gamboa AM. NOD-scid IL2ry^{null} mouse model is suitable to study osteoarticular brucellosis and vaccine safety. *Infect Immun.* (2019) 87:e00901-18. doi: 10.1128/IAI.00901-18
125. Arenas-Gamboa AM, Rice-Ficht AC, Fan Y, Kahl-McDonagh MM, Ficht TA. Extended safety and efficacy studies of the attenuated *Brucella* vaccine candidates 16MΔ*vjbR* and S19Δ*vjbR* in the immunocompromised IRF-1$^{-/-}$ mouse model. *Clin Vaccine Immunol.* (2012) 19:249–60. doi: 10.1128/CVI.05321-11
126. Yang X, Becker T, Walters N, Pascual DW. Deletion of *znuA* virulence factor attenuates *Brucella abortus* and confers protection against wild-type challenge. *Infect Immun.* (2006) 74:3874–9. doi: 10.1128/IAI.01957-05
127. Yang X, Clapp B, Thornburg T, Hoffman C, Pascual DW. Vaccination with a Δ*norD* Δ*znuA* *Brucella abortus* mutant confers potent protection against virulent challenge. *Vaccine.* (2016) 34:5290–7. doi: 10.1016/j.vaccine.2016.09.004
128. Pontes DS, Dorella FA, Ribeiro LA, Miyoshi A, Loir YL, Gruss A, et al. Induction of partial protection in mice after oral administration o flactococcus lactis producing *Brucella abortus* L7/L12 antigen. *J Drug Target.* (2003) 11:489–93. doi: 10.1080/10611860410001670035
129. Sáez D, Fernández P, Rivera A, Andrews E, Oñate A. Oral immunization of mice with recombinant *Lactococcus lactis* expressing Cu,Zn superoxide dismutase of *Brucella abortus* triggers protective immunity. *Vaccine.* (2012) 30:1283–90. doi: 10.1016/j.vaccine.2011.12.088
130. Kim WK, Moon JY, Kim S, Hur J. Comparison between immunization routes of live attenuated *Salmonella Typhimurium* strains expressing BCSP31, Omp3b, and SOD of *Brucella abortus* in murine model. *Front Microbiol.* (2016) 7:550. doi: 10.3389/fmicb.2016.00550
131. Lalsiamthara J, Lee JH. Immunization of guinea pigs with *Salmonella* delivered anti-*Brucella* formulation reduces organs bacterial load and mitigates histopathological consequences of *Brucella abortus* 544 challenge. *Vet Immunol Immunopathol.* (2018) 195:40–5. doi: 10.1016/j.vetimm.2017.11.006
132. Lalsiamthara J, Senevirathne A, Lee JH. Partial protection induced by *Salmonella* based *Brucella* vaccine candidate in pregnant guinea pigs. *Vaccine.* (2019) 37:899–902. doi: 10.1016/j.vaccine.2019.01.020
133. Moustafa D, Garg VK, Jain N, Sriranganathan N, Vemulapalli R. Immunization of mice with gamma-irradiated *Brucella neotomae* and its recombinant strains induces protection against virulent *B. abortus, B melitensis,* and *B suis* challenge. *Vaccine.* (2011) 29:784–94. doi: 10.1016/j.vaccine.2010.11.018
134. Dabral N, Moreno-Lafont M, Sriranganathan N, Vemulapalli R. Oral immunization of mice with gamma-irradiated *Brucella neotomae* induces protection against intraperitoneal and intranasal challenge with virulent *B. abortus* 2308. *PLoS ONE.* (2014) 9:e107180. doi: 10.1371/journal.pone.0107180
135. Clapp B, Yang X, Thornburg T, Walters N, Pascual DW. Nasal vaccination stimulates CD8+ T cells for potent protection against mucosal *Brucella melitensis* challenge. *Immunol Cell Biol.* (2016) 94:496–508. doi: 10.1038/icb.2016.5
136. Izadjoo MJ, Bhattacharjee AK, Paranavitana CM, Hadfield TL, Hoover DL. Oral vaccination with *Brucella melitensis* WR201 protects mice against intranasal challenge with virulent *Brucella melitensis* 16M. *Infect Immun.* (2004) 72:4031–9. doi: 10.1128/IAI.72.7.4031-4039.2004
137. Mailybayeva A, Yespembetov B, Ryskeldinova S, Zinina N, Sansyzbay A, Renukaradhya GJ, et al. Improved influenza viral vector-based *Brucella abortus* vaccine induces robust B and T-cell responses and protection against *Brucella melitensis* infection in pregnant sheep and goats. *PLoS ONE.* (2017) 12:e0186484. doi: 10.1371/journal.pone.0186484
138. Díaz AG, Quinteros DA, Gutiérrez SE, Rivero MA, Palma SD, Allemandi DA, et al. Immune response induced by conjunctival immunization with polymeric antigen BLSOmp31 using a thermoresponsive and mucoadhesive *in situ* gel as vaccine delivery system for prevention of ovine brucellosis. *Vet Immunol Immunopathol.* (2016) 178:50–6. doi: 10.1016/j.vetimm.2016.07.004
139. Delpino MV, Estein SM, Fossati CA, Baldi PC. Partial protection against *Brucella* infection in mice by immunization with non-pathogenic alphaproteobacteria. *Clin Vaccine Immunol.* (2007) 14:1296–301. doi: 10.1128/CVI.00459-06
140. Abkar M, Fasihi-Ramandi M, Kooshki H, Lotfi AS. Oral immunization of mice with Omp31-loaded *N*-trimethyl chitosan nanoparticles induces high protection against *Brucella melitensis* infection. *Int J Nanomed.* (2017) 12:8769–78. doi: 10.2147/IJN.S149774
141. Avila-Calderón ED, Lopez-Merino A, Jain N, Peralta H, López-Villegas EO, Sriranganathan N, et al. Characterization of outer membrane vesicles from *Brucella melitensis* and protection induced in mice. *Clin Dev Immunol.* (2012) 201:352493. doi: 10.1155/2012/352493
142. Schurig GG, Roop IIRM, Bagchu T, Boyle S, Buhrman D, Sriranganathan N. Biological properties of RB51; a stable rough strain of *Brucella abortus. Vet Microbiol.* (1991) 28:171–88 doi: 10.1016/0378-1135(91)90091-S
143. He Y, Vemulapalli R, Zeytun A, Schurig GG. Induction of specific cytotoxic lymphocytes in mice vaccinated with *Brucella abortus* RB51. *Infect Immun.* (2001) 69:5502–8. doi: 10.1128/IAI.69.9.5502-5508.2001
144. Simpson GJG, Mercotty T, Rouille E, Chilundo A, Letteson JJ, Godfroid J. Immunological response to *Brucella abortus* strain 19 vaccination of cattle in a communal area in South Africa. *J S Afr Vet Assoc.* (2018) 89:e1–7. doi: 10.4102/jsava.v89i0.1527
145. Kumar DR, Sivalingam J, Mishra SK, Kumar A, Vineeth MR, Chaudhuri P, et al. Differential expression of cytokines in PBMC of Bos indicus and Bos Taurus ^{x} Bos indicus cattle due to *Brucella abortus* S19 antigen. *Anim. Biotechnol.* (2019) 5:1–7. doi: 10.1080/10495398.2018.1555167
146. Moriyón I, Grillo MJ, Monreal D, González D, Marín C, López-Goñi I, et al. Rough vaccines in animal brucellosis: structural and genetic basis and present status. *Vet Res.* (2004) 35:1–38. doi: 10.1051/vetres:2003037
147. Ivanov AV, Salmakov KM, Olsen SC, Plumb GE. A live vaccine from *Brucella abortus* strain 82 for control of cattle brucellosis in the Russian Federation. *Anim Health Res Rev.* (2011) 12:113–21. doi: 10.1017/S1466252311000028
148. Zabalza-Baranguá A, San-Román B, Chacón-Díaz C, de Miguel MJ, Muñoz PM, Iriarte M, et al. GFP tagging of *Brucella melitensis* Rev1 allows the identification of vaccinated sheep. *Transbound Emerg. Dis.* (2019) 66:505–16. doi: 10.1111/tbed.13053
149. Holmgren J, Czerkinsky C. Mucosal immunity and vaccines. *Nat Med.* (2005) 11:S45–S53. doi: 10.1038/nm1213
150. Czerkinsky C, Holmgren J. Vaccines against enteric infections for the developing world. *Philos Trans R Soc Lond B Biol Sci.* (2015) 370:20150142. doi: 10.1098/rstb.2015.0142
151. Czerkinsky C, Holmgren J. Enteric vaccines for the developing world: a challenge for mucosal immunology. *Mucosal Immunol.* (2009) 2:284–7. doi: 10.1038/mi.2009.22
152. Neutra MR, Kozlowski PA. Mucosal vaccines: the promise and the challenge. *Nat Rev Immunol.* (2006) 6:148–58. doi: 10.1038/nri1777
153. Yu Q, Zhu L, Kang H, Yang Q. Mucosal *Lactobacillus* vectored vaccines. *Hum Vaccin Immunother.* (2013) 9:805–7. doi: 10.4161/hv.23302
154. Pouwels PH, Leer RJ, Shaw M, Heijne den Bak-Glashouwer MJ, Tielen FD, Smit E, et al. Lactic acid bacteria as antigen delivery vehicles for oral immunization purposes. *Int J Food Microbiol.* (1998) 41:155–67.
155. Inic-Kanada A, Stojanovic M, Marinkovic E, Becker E, Stein E, Lukic I, et al. A probiotic adjuvant *Lactobacillus rhamnosus* enhances specific immune responses after ocular mucosal immunization with chlamydial polymorphic membrane protein C. *PLoS ONE.* (2016) 11:e0157875. doi: 10.1371/journal.pone.0157875
156. Ribeiro LA, Azevedo V, Le Loir Y, Oliveira SC, Dieye Y, Piard JV, et al. Production and targeting of the *Brucella abortus* antigen L7/L12 in *Lactococcus lactis*: a first step towards food-grade live vaccines against brucellosis. *Appl Environ Microbiol.* (2002) 68:910–6. doi: 10.1128/AEM.68.2.910-916.2002
157. Bermúdez-Humarán LG, Langella P, Cortes-Perez NG, Gruss A, Tamez-Guerra RS, Oliveira SC, et al. Intranasal immunization with recombinant *Lactococcus lactis* secreting murine interleukin-12 enhances antigen-specific Th1 cytokine production. *Infect Immun.* (2003) 71, 1887–1896.

158. Lalsiamthara J, Senevirathne A, So MY, Lee JH. Safety implication of *Salmonella* based *Brucella* vaccine candidate in mice and *in vitro* human cell culture. *Vaccine*. (2018) 36:1837–45. doi: 10.1016/j.vaccine.2018.02.069
159. Lalsiamthara J, Lee JH. Immuno-profiles of BALB/c mice inoculated with *Salmonella* vector delivering B-cell mitogen hydroxyproline epimerase. *Mol Immunol*. (2018) 95:114–21. doi: 10.1016/j.molimm.2018.02.004
160. Wang Z, Wu Q. Research progress in live attenuated Brucela vaccine development. *Curr Pharm Biotchnol*. (2013) 14:887–96. doi: 10.2174/1389201014666131226123016
161. Yang X, Skyberg JA, Cao L, Clapp B, Thornburg T, Pascual DW. Progress in *Brucella* vaccine development. *Front Biol*. (2013) 8:60–7. doi: 10.1007/s11515-012-1196-0
162. Rosas G, Fragoso G, Ainciart N, Esquivel-Guadarrama F, Santana A, Bobes RJ, et al. *Brucella* spp. lumazine synthase: a novel adjuvant and antigen delivery system to effectively induce oral immunity. *Microbes Infect*. (2006) 8:1277–86. doi: 10.1016/j.micinf.2005.12.006
163. Estein SM, Fiorentino MA, Paolicchi FA, Clausse M, Manazza J, Cassataro J, et al. The polymeric antigen BLSOmp31 confers protection against *Brucella ovis* infection in rams. *Vaccine*. (2009) 27:6704–11. doi: 10.1016/j.vaccine.2009.08.097
164. Avila-Calderón ED, Araiza-Villanueva MG, Cancino-Diaz JC, López-Villegas EO, Sriranganathan N, Boyle SM, et al. Roles of bacterial membrane vesicles. *Arch Microbiol*. (2015) 197:1–10. doi: 10.1007/s00203-014-1042-7

6

Junin Virus Triggers Macrophage Activation and Modulates Polarization According to Viral Strain Pathogenicity

María F. Ferrer[1], Pablo Thomas[1], Aída O. López Ortiz[1,2], Andrea E. Errasti[3], Nancy Charo[2], Victor Romanowski[1,4], Juan Gorgojo[5], María E. Rodriguez[5], Eugenio A. Carrera Silva[2†] and Ricardo M. Gómez[1,4*†]*

[1] Laboratorio de Virus Animales, Instituto de Biotecnología y Biología Molecular, CONICET-Universidad Nacional de La Plata, La Plata, Argentina, [2] Laboratorio de Trombosis Experimental, Instituto de Medicina Experimental, CONICET-Academia Nacional de Medicina, Buenos Aires, Argentina, [3] Facultad de Medicina, Instituto de Farmacologia, University of Buenos Aries, Buenos Aires, Argentina, [4] Global Viral Network, Baltimore, MD, United States, [5] Centro de Investigación y Desarrollo en Fermentaciones Industriales, CONICET-Universidad Nacional de La Plata, La Plata, Argentina

Correspondence:
Eugenio A. Carrera Silva
carrerasilva@yahoo.com.ar
Ricardo M. Gómez
rmg1426@gmail.com

† These authors have contributed equally to this work

The New World arenavirus Junin (JUNV) is the etiological agent of Argentine hemorrhagic fever (AHF). Previous studies of human macrophage infection by the Old-World arenaviruses Mopeia and Lassa showed that while the non-pathogenic Mopeia virus replicates and activates human macrophages, the pathogenic Lassa virus replicates but fails to activate human macrophages. Less is known in regard to the impact of New World arenavirus infection on the human macrophage immune response. Macrophage activation is critical for controlling infections but could also be usurped favoring immune evasion. Therefore, it is crucial to understand how the JUNV infection modulates macrophage plasticity to clarify its role in AHF pathogenesis. With this aim in mind, we compared infection with the attenuated Candid 1 (C#1) or the pathogenic P strains of the JUNV virus in human macrophage cultures. The results showed that both JUNV strains similarly replicated and induced morphological changes as early as 1 day post-infection. However, both strains differentially induced the expression of CD71, the receptor for cell entry, the activation and maturation molecules CD80, CD86, and HLA-DR and selectively modulated cytokine production. Higher levels of TNF-α, IL-10, and IL-12 were detected with C#1 strain, while the P strain induced only higher levels of IL-6. We also found that C#1 strain infection skewed macrophage polarization to M1, whereas the P strain shifted the response to an M2 phenotype. Interestingly, the MERTK receptor, that negatively regulates the immune response, was down-regulated by C#1 strain and up-regulated by P strain infection. Similarly, the target genes of MERTK activation, the cytokine suppressors SOCS1 and SOCS3, were also increased after P strain infection, in addition to IRF-1, that regulates type I IFN levels, which were higher with C#1 compared with P strain infection. Together, this differential activation/polarization pattern of macrophages elicited by P strain suggests a more evasive immune response and may have important implications in the pathogenesis of AHF and underpinning the development of new potential therapeutic strategies.

Keywords: junin virus, human macrophages, TAM receptors, macrophage activation, macrophage polarization, IFN-I

INTRODUCTION

Junin virus (JUNV) is the etiological agent of Argentine hemorrhagic fever (AHF), an endemoepidemic disease mainly affecting agricultural workers in Argentina. The infection is usually acquired through small abrasions in the skin or through aspiration of particles contaminated with urine, saliva, or blood from carrier rodents. The AHF incubation period ranges from 6 to 12 days, ending with the onset of fever. During first 7 days, patients are commonly associated with a flu-like syndrome and the fever persists until the second week, when hemorrhagic or neurological signs of varied severity may be present. The 80% of patients improve after the second week. AHF diagnosis is based on clinical and laboratory data, the latter mainly based on platelet counts below 100,000/mm^3 in combination with white blood cell counts under 2,500/mm^3. Early diagnosis is important, because the early use of immune plasma from convalescent patients reduces mortality rates from 20 to 1%. Candid #1 (C#1) is a live attenuated vaccine against AHF, which is licensed in Argentina and has been administered to several hundred thousand persons in endemic areas for more than 20 years, with a major impact on the incidence of the disease. However, since the first description of the disease in the 1950s, uninterrupted annual outbreaks have been observed in a progressively expanding region in north-central Argentina, to the point that more than 5 million individuals are today considered to be at risk of AHF (1).

JUNV belongs to the clade B New World (NW) of genus mammarenavirus that together with genus reptarenavirus form the *Arenaviridae* family (2). Most mammarenavirus are associated with rodent infections. The Old World (OW) choriomeningitis lymphocytic virus (LCMV) infects *Mus musculus*, and this explains its global distribution. In contrast, other strains of mammarenavirus infect rodents with a circumscribed geographical distribution that explains their endemicity (3). In their natural rodent host, mammarenavirus usually produce a persistent asymptomatic infection that may occasionally be transmitted to humans where it can cause severe hemorrhagic fever (HF). In addition to JUNV, other strains of mammarenavirus associated with HF are the NW Machupo (MACV) and Chapare (CHPV) viruses in Bolivia, Sabiá (SABV) in Brazil and the OW Lassa virus (LASV) in Africa. In contrast, other members such as the NW Tacaribe (TCRV) and Pichindé (PICV) or the OW Mopeia (MOPV) viruses do not cause disease (4). The mammarenavirus are etiological agents of emergent diseases because human activity facilitates contact with wild rodents in new ecological niches and, therefore, new isolates should be expected in the future (3).

Like other members of the same family, JUNVs are enveloped virions, ~120 nm in diameter, with a capsid of helicoidal symmetry that includes a variable number of ribosomes. The virions contain a bi-segmented single-stranded RNA genome, with both segments employing an ambisense coding strategy. The L segment contains genes encoding the RNA-dependent RNA polymerase (L) and the matrix protein (Z). However, the smaller S segment encodes the nucleoprotein (N) and the glycoprotein precursor (GPC) which, after post-translational cleavage, yields mature virion glycoproteins (G) G1, G2 and the stable signal peptide SSP that together will constitute the spikes that decorate the virus surface (5).

Macrophages are the most functionally diverse (plastic) cells of the hematopoietic system. Macrophages are found in all tissues and their main function is to respond to pathogens and modulate the adaptive immune response through antigen processing and presentation (6, 7). Macrophage activation has emerged as a key area of study in immunology, tissue homeostasis, disease pathogenesis and inflammation resolution (8). To accomplish such diverse functions, they mature under the influence of signals from the local microenvironment into either classical M1 or alternatively M2 activated macrophages. M1 macrophages are characterized by the production of high levels of pro-inflammatory cytokines, an ability to mediate resistance to pathogens, strong microbicidal properties, high production of reactive nitrogen and oxygen intermediates and promotion of Th1 responses. In contrast, M2 activated macrophages are characterized by their involvement in parasite control, resolution of inflammation, tissue remodeling, immune regulation, and Th2 promotion responses (6, 9).

In this study, we aimed to characterize the infection of macrophages using two strains of the same arenavirus with different pathogenic properties. For this purpose, we studied the infection of human macrophages by the attenuated C#1 and the pathogenic P strains of JUNV, using an *in vitro* model represented by human macrophage cell cultures.

MATERIALS AND METHODS

Cells

BHK-21 and Vero-76 cells (ATCC, USA) were maintained as monolayers, as previously described (10). Peripheral blood mononuclear cells (PBMCs) were obtained from healthy volunteer donors who had not taken any non-steroidal anti-inflammatory drugs for 10 days prior to sampling as previously described (11). This study was approved by the Institutional Ethics Committee, National Academy of Medicine, Argentina. Written consent was obtained from all subjects. Human monocyte-derived macrophages (HMDM) were obtained as previously reported (12). Briefly, PBMCs from healthy donors were isolated by Ficoll-Hypaque (GE, Chicago, IL, USA) density gradient centrifugation, and positive selection of CD14$^+$ monocytes was performed using an EasySep^{TM} Human CD14 Positive Selection Kit (StemCell Tech, Vancouver, Canada). Macrophage differentiation was carried out by plating 2.5 $\times$ 10^5 CD14$^+$ monocytes in 48-well plates containing 500 µL of RPMI 1640 plus 10% Fetal Bovine Serum (FBS) and 1% penicillin/streptomycin (PS) in the presence of rM-CSF (40 ng/ml) and cultured for 7 days. In selected experiments, 24-well plates were used with a double quantity of cells and medium.

Virus

A virulent strain of JUNV, originally isolated from an AHF patient (P3441), as well as the attenuated Candid 1 (C#1) have been already described (13). The preparation of viral stocks in BHK-21 cells and infectivity titration using the Vero-76 cell line has been previously described (13). All work with the infective P strain was performed in a BSL/3 facility by vaccinated personal.

Reagents

MEM, RPMI, and FBS were purchased from Invitrogen (Buenos Aires, Argentina). rM-CSF was acquired from R&D Systems (Minneapolis, MN, USA). Anti JUNV antibodies were obtained from BEI resources, USA. Anti CD71, CD14, CD86, CD80, HLA-DR, CD11b, CD11c, CD64, CD163, CD206 were obtained from BioLegend (San Diego, CA, USA). Anti-human APC-MERTK (mouse IgG1), Biotin-AXL (goat IgG) and isotype controls were obtained from R&D Systems (Minneapolis, MN, USA). Anti-TYRO3 (rabbit IgG) was obtained from Novus Biological (Littleton, CO, USA). DAPI was purchased from Invitrogen (Buenos Aires, Argentina). ELISA kits (Ready-SET-Go kits) for TNF-α, IL-1β, IL-6, IL-10, and IL-12p70 were obtained from eBioscience, Fisher scientific, Pittsburgh, PA, USA. Cytofix/Cytoperm kit was purchased from BD Bioscience (San Diego, CA, USA).

Cell Infection

For viral infection, cells were washed with PBS twice before incubating with the virus at a multiplicity of infection (MOI) of 1 in serum free medium. After 1 h of incubation at 37°C, cells were washed with PBS twice again and supplemented with a complete culture medium. Mock infection was performed by adding the same volume of BHK-21 cell culture supernatant, instead of JUNV, to the cell monolayer. Cells were observed daily using an inverted microscope with an Olympus SP-320 camera and images were further processed with Photoshop 6.0 software.

Plaque Formation Assay

Ten-fold dilutions of the macrophage-JUNV infected culture supernatants were added to 24-well plates with a 40–50% confluence monolayer of Vero E6 cells. The plate was then incubated at 37°C for 1 h with gentle rocking. Following adsorption, the inoculum was removed and overlaid with 2 ml of MEM containing 0.8% methylcellulose and 2% FBS and further incubated at 37°C in a humid atmosphere with 5% CO_2. Plaques were allowed to develop for either 4–6 days before being fixed (4% w/v paraformaldehyde) and stained with a 1% Crystal Violet in 20% ethanol and $_dH_2O$.

Indirect Immunofluorescence Studies

Cells were cultured on 12 mm diameter glass inserts before viral infection. At the indicated time-point after infection, the inserts were fixed with 4% paraformaldehyde (PFA) for 20 min and permeabilized with 0.1% Tween for 10 min. The slides were incubated overnight at 4°C with a pool of specific monoclonal antibodies against JUNV (13). FITC-conjugated anti mouse Igs were then applied to the PBS-washed slides for 30 min at room temperature (RT). Antibodies were diluted with PBS containing 5% FBS and 5% goat serum as blocking reagents. The slides were counterstained with DAPI and examined under a Nikon E200 microscope equipped with fluorescence filters and a 100-W mercury lamp. Images were acquired with a Tucsen TCC 5.0 refrigerated camera under the control of IS listen software and further processed using Photoshop 6.0 software.

Flow Cytometry Analysis

The viability assay on macrophages culture was performed after 72 h of JUNV infection using Annexin V (AnnV) (Immunotools, Gladiolenweg, Friesoythe, Gemany) together with Fixable viability dye (eBioscience, USA). Briefly, cell harvesting was performed by a 20-min incubation with PBS plus 2% FBS (PBSF) and 1 mM EDTA on ice, followed by up and down pipetting. The harvested cells were washed once with PBSF and then stained with fixable viability dye efluor 780 diluted in PBS for 30 min. After washing cells, they were stained with AnnV following manufacturer's instruction. After final washing, the cells were fixed with a Cytofix/Cytoperm Kit (BD Biosciences, USA).

The surface staining for CD11b, CD64, CD206, CD14 (phenotypic characterization of macrophages) or CD11b, HLA-DR, CD86, and CD80 (activation status) was performed following a standard protocol. Briefly, the harvested cells were washed with PBS and blocked in PBSF on ice for 30 min. The cells were washed with PBS and the respective antibody cocktails (prepared in PBSF) were added to the cell pellet and incubated for 30 min on ice. A fixable viability dye was used according to the manufacturer's instructions to gate on live cells. After washing, the cells were fixed with a Cytofix/Cytoperm Kit, washed again and analyzed in a FACS Canto I (Becton Dickinson, Franklin Lakes, NJ, USA) or Partec-Sysmex CyFlow flow cytometer (Görlitz, Germany). All analysis was carried out with FlowJo software (Tree Star). Intracellular staining was performed following manufacturer's recommendation for the Cytofix/Cytoperm Kit. The preparation of blockage and cocktail antibodies was performed with PBSF. We have used fluorescent minus one (FMO) to set the threshold for each marker.

Enzyme Linked Immunosorbent Assay (ELISA)

IL-6, IL-12p70, TNF-α, and IL-10 levels were assessed in culture supernatants with ELISA Ready-SET-Go kits (e-Bioscience) according to the manufacturer's protocol.

RNA Isolation, RT-PCR, and Real-Time PCR

For gene expression analysis, cultured cells were washed and then harvested with Trizol (Life Technologies, Carlsbad, CA, USA) and total RNA was obtained following the manufacturer's instructions. Reverse transcription was performed using 100 ng of RNA by employing an iScript cDNA synthesis kit (Bio-Rad, Hercules, CA, USA). qPCR reactions were assessed using 1 μl of cDNA and using Sso Advanced Universal mix with Sybr Green and CFX-Connect equipment (Bio-Rad). Primers used in this study are listed in **Table S1**. The reaction was normalized to housekeeping gene expression levels and the specificity of the amplified products was checked through analysis of dissociation curves.

Statistical Analysis

Each experiment was performed with 3–7 different donors. All results are graphed as the median (min-max, horizontal line indicates the median) and non-parametric one-way analysis of variance (ANOVA) (Kruskal–Wallis) followed by Dunn's multiple comparison test was used to detect significant differences between groups. In all cases, P-values lower than 0.05 were considered statistically significant. All statistical analyses were performed using Prism 6 software (GraphPad).

RESULTS

JUNV Strains Replicate Similarly in Human Macrophages

Human monocyte-derived macrophages (HMDM) cells were infected at a multiplicity of infection (MOI) = 1 with the attenuated C#1 or the pathogenic P strains of JUNV. HMDM cells showed clear morphological changes, such as becoming more flattened and extended, as early as 24 h post-infection (hpi) with both JUNV strains (**Figure 1A**). Infectious virus released to the cell culture supernatants were measured over 6 days by plaque formation assay. Infection with both viral strains led to similar levels of infectious viruses, peaking at 3 days post-infection (dpi) and declining until the end of the study (**Figure 1B**). Viral antigen was studied at 3 dpi by immunofluorescence (IF) and flow cytometry (FC) analysis. Viral protein staining was similarly positive with both strains (**Figure 1C**). As expected, FC analysis confirmed these results showing that 58% of HMDM cells were infected with C#1 strain meanwhile 57.6% were positive for the P strain (**Figure 1D**).

JUNV Strains Differentially Enhances the Expression of CD71

Viruses exploit fundamental cellular processes to gain entry into cells and deliver their genetic cargo. Virus entry pathways are largely defined by the interactions between virus particles and their receptors at the cell surface. These interactions determine the mechanisms of virus attachment and, ultimately, penetration into the cytosol. In contrast to LASV and other OW arenaviruses, which use α-dystroglycan to infect cells, the NW arenaviruses, including JUNV, use human transferrin receptor 1 (hTFR1 or CD71) (14). We have previously shown that JUNV infection enhances the expression of hTFR1 in the precursor $CD34^+$ cells, suggesting that JUNV infection promotes its own dissemination (15). Compared with other cell types, mature macrophages may be atypical regarding the requirements for hTFR1 expression levels (16), and for that reason, we explored the expression pattern in HMDM infected cells. In this sense, our results showed that JUNV infection enhances CD71 expression in human macrophages, but with the highest value associated with P strain infection (**Figures 2A–C**).

JUNV Strains Differentially Activate Macrophages and Cytokine Production

We have analyzed the expression pattern of co-stimulatory markers such as CD80 and CD86, and the antigen presentation surface marker (HLA-DR). Our results indicate a differential expression when infected with one or other viral strain. A significantly higher percentage of $CD14^+CD86^+$ cells were observed after C#1 strain infection, while CD80 did not show significant differences between infected cells. On the other hand, P strain-infected macrophages showed the highest percentage of $CD14^+$ $HLA\text{-}DR^{++}$ cells revealing a differential expression pattern after infection with C#1 or P strain (**Figures 3A,B**).

Considering the observed macrophage activation induced by JUNV infection, we next analyzed the level of several cytokines in the supernatants of HMDM at 3 dpi. We found a clear distinctive profile, since higher levels of TNF-α, IL-10, and IL-12 were detected in the supernatants of C#1 strain-infected macrophages, but only IL-6 was significantly increased using the P strain. Interestingly, no difference in IL-1 production was observed compared with mock conditions, suggesting no activation of the inflammasome pathway (**Figures 3C–G**). The percentage of viable cells does not showed significant differences comparing Mock, C#1 and P (90.2, 88.25, and 83.5, respectively) although small increase in AnnV+ cells were observed with P when compared to C#1 and Mock (**Supplementary Information S1**).

JUNV Selectively Skews Macrophage Polarization

Taking into account the fact that JUNV modulates macrophage activation depending on which strain was used, we next evaluated different surface markers to distinguish M1/M2 polarization in HMDM after JUNV infection. The percentage of $CD64^+$ (M1), $CD206^+$, and $CD163^+$ (M2) cells expressed in $CD11b^+$ cells were analyzed by flow cytometry. $CD11b^+CD64^+CD206^-$ cells were increased when cells were infected with C#1 strain as compared to Mock and the P strain with an average of 18 vs. 8% and 3.2%, respectively. However, the M2 phenotype $CD11b^+CD206^+CD64^-$ was significantly higher after P infection as compared C#1 strain or to Mock with an average of 34 vs. 10.1%, and 17.5%, respectively. This indicates that JUNV modulates polarization according to viral strain pathogenicity (**Figures 4A,B**). Additionally, another M2 phenotype analyzed as a double positive, $CD206^+/CD163^+$ cells, showed a clear tendency toward an increased percentage after infection with P strain as compared to Mock and C#1 strain infection (44.2 vs. 29.9% and 33.9%, respectively, see **Supplementary Information S2**).

The Expression of MERTK Was Differentially Modulated With JUNV Variants

The TAM family tyrosine kinase receptors TYRO3, AXL, and MERTK (TAM) receptors have been assigned to have a prominent role in the following: regulating the innate immune response (17); phagocytosis and macrophage polarization by acting in coordination with cytokine signaling (18); and in several aspects of the host response to viral infection (19, 20). Considering our observation that JUNV modulates macrophage polarization and that AXL and MERTK are differentially expressed in pro-inflammatory M1 and anti-inflammatory

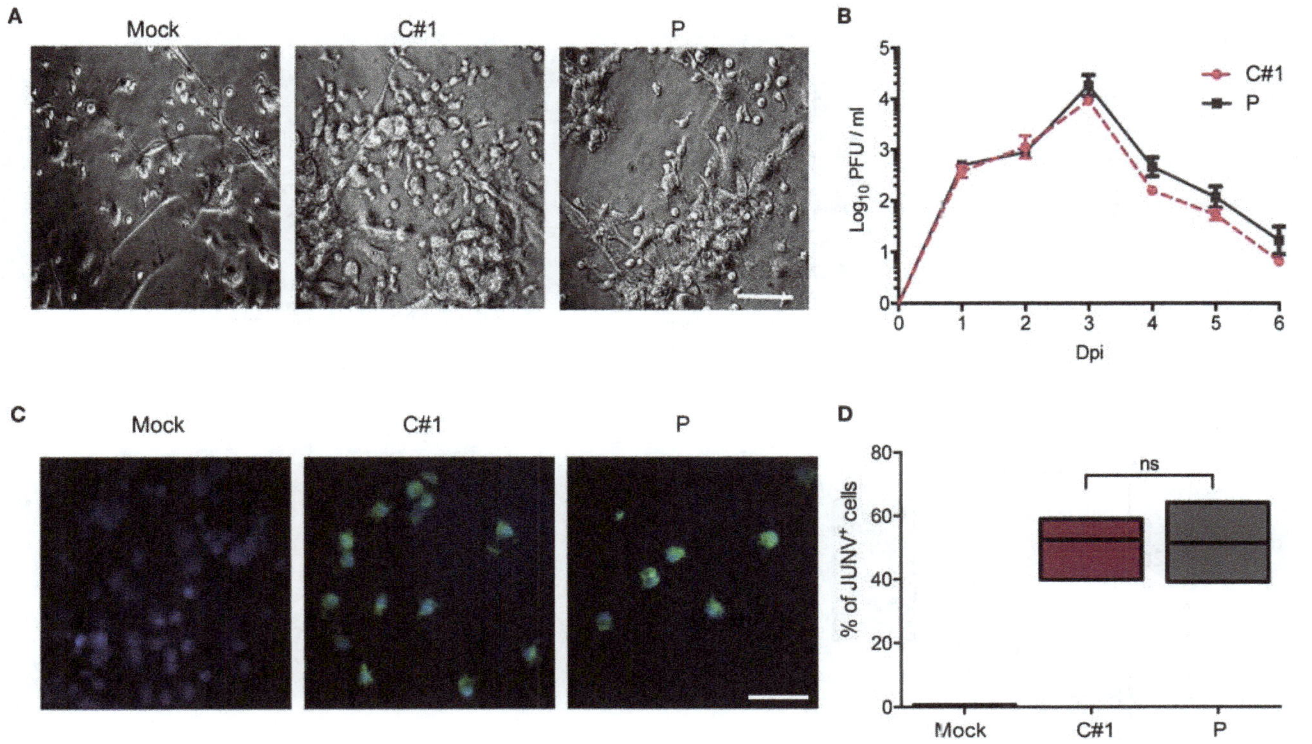

FIGURE 1 | Human macrophages are equally susceptible to both JUNV variants. Human monocyte-derived macrophages (HMDM) cells were infected at a multiplicity of infection (MOI = 1) with the attenuated C#1 or the pathogenic P strains of JUNV. **(A)** Morphological observation of the cells. JUNV-infected cells become more flattened and extended. **(B)** Infective titration of cell supernatants was performed in Vero cells for 6 days by a standard PFU method. **(C)** Viral antigens were detected by immunofluorescence with a pool of antibodies and anti-JUNV-FITC, and nuclei were counterstained with DAPI. **(D)** HMDM cells were infected with C#1 or P strains and at 3 dpi cells were stained with anti-JUNV-FITC and the percentage of viral antigen positive cells were analyzed by flow cytometry. The percentage of infected cells was compared using the Non-parametric One-way ANOVA followed by Dunn's multiple comparison test. The results are graphed as the median (min-max, horizontal line indicates the median). At least three independent donors were used in each assay.

M2 macrophages, respectively (21), we next evaluated TAM expression in HMDM after infection with both strains. Our results showed that while TYRO3$^+$ or AXL$^+$ macrophages showed a similar response to infection with the two strains, the percentage of MERTK$^+$ cells was down-regulated by C#1 strain and up-regulated by P strain infection, highlighting again a differential macrophage response depending on virus strain (**Figures 5A,B**).

Since activation of MERTK triggers the induction of the suppressor of cytokine signaling 1 (SOCS1) and SOCS3, we next analyzed the transcription level of these genes by RT-qPCR. We also analyzed interferon regulatory factor 1 (IRF-1) as a target gene of infection and a member of the interferon regulatory factor family (22). As expected, we observed higher transcription levels of IRF-1, SOCS1, and SOCS3 concomitant with lower levels of IFN-β in macrophages infected with P strain as compared with mock conditions after 24 hpi (**Figures 6A–D**).

DISCUSSION

In the present study, we showed that both attenuated C#1 and pathogenic P JUNV strains induced a phenotypic change in primary human macrophages as early as 1 dpi, that was interpreted as macrophage maturation and/or activation. In addition, we observed similar infectivity titers in the supernatants and a comparable percentage of infected monolayer cells. This stands in contrast with the reported minimal replication of JUNV-XJ (pathogenic) and XJ-Cl3 (attenuated) strains in macrophage cells from adult rats (23), a fact that may be attributed that macrophages were from a different donor species.

Previous studies of human macrophage infection by mammarenavirus have been shown that the non-pathogenic MOPV both replicates and activates macrophages (24) whereas pathogenic LASV replicates, but fails to activate macrophages (25). The lack of activation of LASV-infected macrophages was later associated with sequence differences in viral protein N (26) and involved CXCL10 (27). On the other hand, it has been reported that the non-pathogenic TCRV replicates less efficiently in macrophages than the pathogenic JUNV, but induces a cytokine release not observed in JUNV-infected cells (28). More recently, a differential inhibition of macrophage activation by LCMV and PICV, mediated by the N-terminal domain (NTD) of viral Z protein, has been reported (29). Moreover, LCMV Z NTD leads to increased viral replication and inhibition of IFN responses in macrophages (30), a fact that has been more

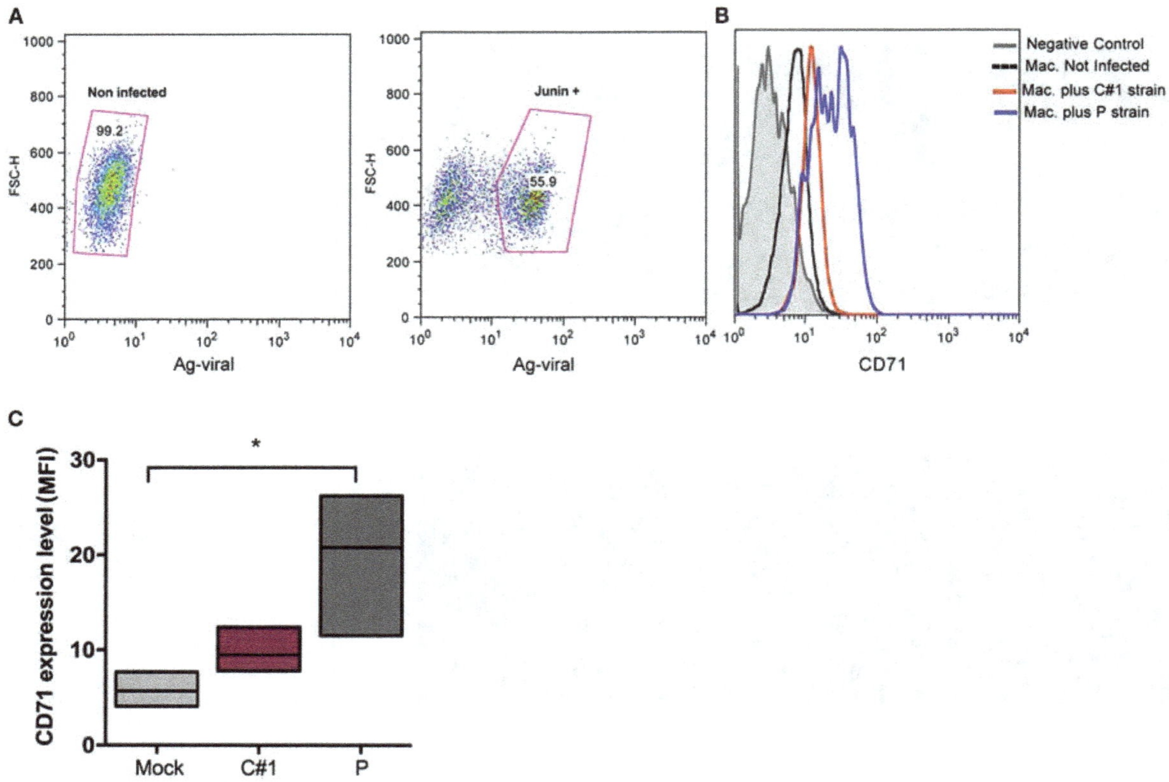

FIGURE 2 | JUNV enhances CD71 expression in human macrophages with P showing the highest values. HMDM cells were infected at a multiplicity of infection (MOI = 1) with C#1 or P strains of JUNV. After 3 dpi, cells were double stained with anti-JUNV and anti-CD71 and analyzed by flow cytometry. **(A)** Representative dot-plots showing positive signal for viral antigen in macrophages. **(B)** Representative histogram showing CD71 expression after gating in positive cells for JUNV antigen and negative controls. **(C)** Expression level of CD71 analyzed as mean fluorescent intensity (MFI) in graph. Non-parametric One-way ANOVA followed by Dunn's multiple comparison test was used to detect significant differences between groups; $^{*}P < 0.05$. The results are graphed as the median (min-max, horizontal line indicates the median) of at least four independent donors in each assay.

recently assigned to the Z protein from pathogenic arenaviruses only (31).

Our results partially support to the hypothesis that OW and NW arenaviruses may have different pathogenic mechanisms, at least in macrophages cells (4, 32).

We have previously shown that JUNV infection up-regulates TfR1 in $CD34^{+}$ hematopoietic stem cells (15). Here, we show that both JUNV strains also increased the expression of CD71 in infected HMDM, with P showing higher values. This supports the hypothesis that JUNV promotes its own dissemination not only in undifferentiated hematopoietic cells but also in a differentiated lineage and that P exploits this mechanism more.

The observed differential maturation and activation markers and the cytokine expression profile depending on which JUNV strain infects the macrophages strongly support the notion that C#1 and P strains are able to elicit differential immune responses. In this sense, a higher level of pro-inflammatory cytokines (IL-12 and TNF-α) together with an increased level of a co-stimulatory marker (CD86) demonstrates the ability of the C#1 strain to mount an adequate inflammatory response. This allows the generation of protective immunity against the virus in the absence of disease in the host. By contrast, the pathogenic P strain elicits a more attenuated activation state of macrophages by decreasing the prototypical pro-inflammatory cytokines. However, it also remarkably induces higher levels of IL-6, a cytokine also associated with immunomodulation (33), and increases the percentage of $CD14^{+}HLA\text{-}DR^{++}$, two signals that indicate an anti-inflammatory response that might allow early immune evasion, facilitating viral dissemination in the host and subsequent disease.

It has been demonstrated that most of the acute viral infections of pathogenic viruses are associated with macrophage activation to a M1 status promoting inflammation (34). Regarding M2, the first studies were carried out with viruses associated with chronic infections, and the first accepted paradigm was that viral infection activates macrophages inducing a M1 profile during the acute phase and an M2 profile emerged during the eventual chronic phase of the disease (34, 35). In many of these studies, the M2-prone response related to an enhanced production of IL-10, which indirectly exerts potent immunosuppressive effects (36–38). Moreover, some viruses, such as herpesviruses and poxviruses, encode functional orthologs of IL-10 (vIL-10s) (39) or IL-6 (33). The viral IL-6 could

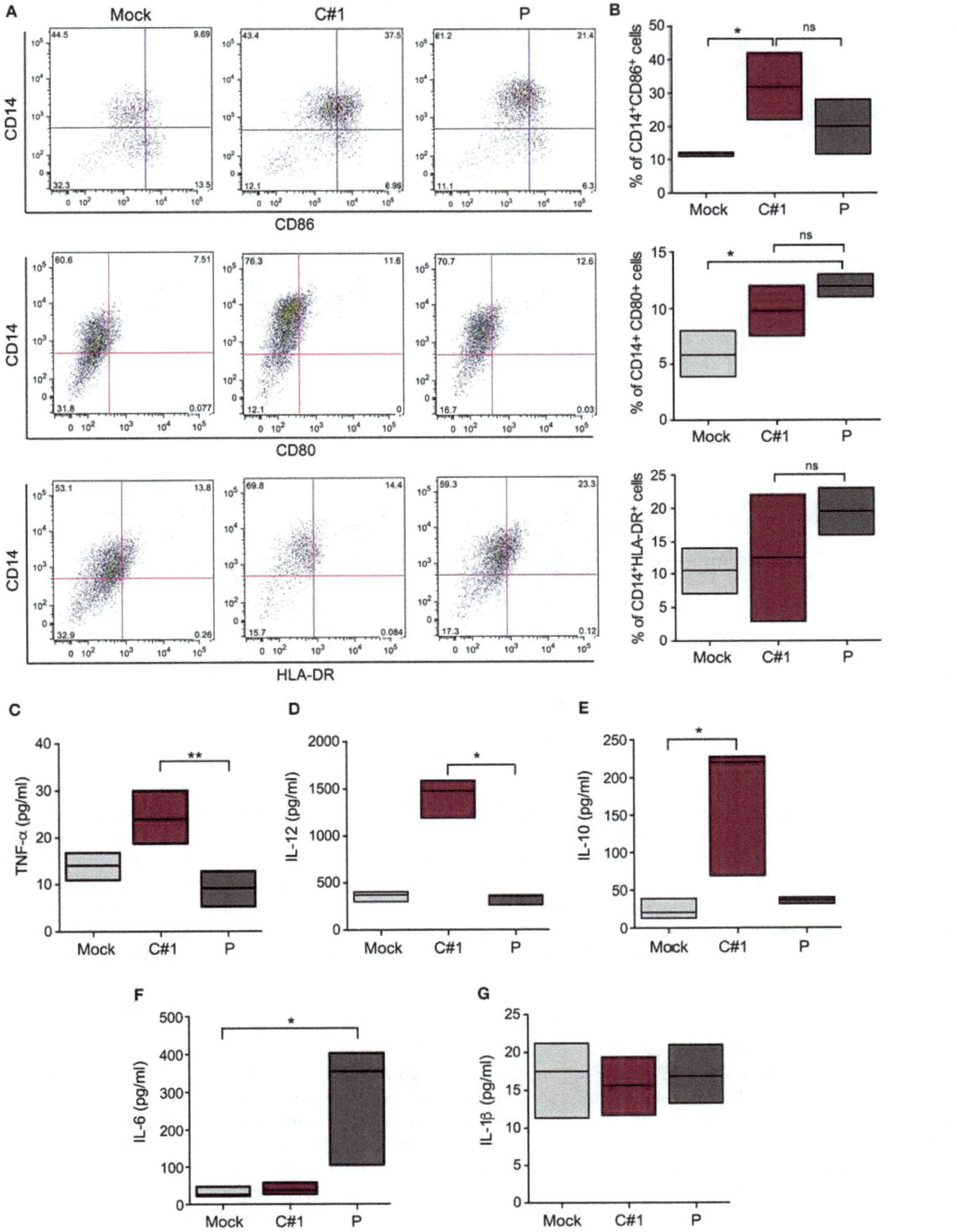

FIGURE 3 | JUNV activates human macrophages and selectively modulates cytokine production. HMDM cells were infected with C#1 or P strains of JUNV (MOI =1) and at 3 dpi the activation and co-stimulation CD80, CD86, or antigen presentation HLA-DR expression were evaluated in CD14+ cells by flow cytometry. **(A)** Representative dot-plots showing CD14+ and each marker are shown. **(B)** The percentage of double positive CD14+CD86+, CD14+CD80+, and

(Continued)

FIGURE 3 | $CD14^{+}HLA\text{-}DR^{++}$ are graphed. We had set the threshold for each marker based on the FMO. The expression level of TNF-α and IL-1β **(C)**, IL-12 **(D)**, IL-10 **(E)**, IL-6 **(F)**, and IL-1β **(G)** were measured in the supernatant of infected macrophages after 72 h, employing commercial ELISA kits. Non-parametric One-way ANOVA followed by Dunn's multiple comparison test was used to detect significant differences between groups, $^{*}P < 0.05$, $^{**}P < 0.01$. The results are graphed as the median (min-max, horizontal line indicates the median) of at least four independent donors in each assay.

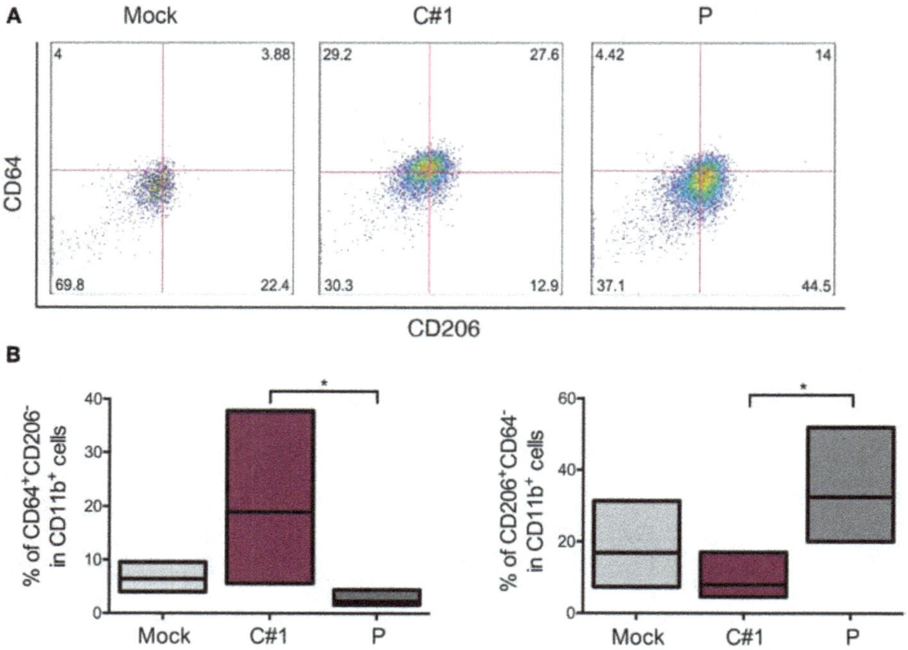

FIGURE 4 | JUNV modulates macrophage M1/M2 polarization. HMDM cells were infected with C#1 or P strains of JUNV (MOI =1) and at 3 dpi the cells expressing $CD64^{+}$ (M1) and $CD206^{+}$ (M2) on $CD11b^{+}$ were evaluated by flow cytometry. **(A)** Representative dot-plots of CD64 vs. CD206 after gating in CD11b of each condition are shown. **(B)** Independent data are graphed showing a shift to M1 after C#1 infection and to M2 after P infection. Non-parametric One-way ANOVA followed by Dunn's multiple comparison test was used to detect significant differences between groups; $^{*}P < 0.05$. The results are graphed as the median (min-max, horizontal line indicates the median) of five independent donors. We had set the quadrant threshold based on the FMO of each marker.

also inhibit antiviral immunity through inhibition of type I IFN, which allows HHV8 to evade immune detection (40).

Our results clearly show a potent pro-inflammatory response was elicited when macrophages were infected with C#1 strain, concordant with a M1 phenotype. However, the P strain elicited a more anti-inflammatory M2 response, associated with a higher level of IL-6, but not IL-10, an increase in $CD11b^{+}CD206^{+}$ and HLA-DR cell expression suggesting that the P strain shifts the macrophage response to a regulatory program (41). In macrophages, IL-10 as well as pro-inflammatory cytokines (TNF-α, IL-12 and IL-6) are produced in response to activation of TLRs 2, 3, 4, 7, and 9, via MyD88 or TRIF, NF-kB, and MAPK pathways (42). The strain P did not stimulate the production of IL-10 neither pro-inflammatory ones such as IL-12 or TNF-α, instead of that, a large amount of IL-6, a cytokine also associated with immunomodulation, was specifically induced by P and not by C#1 strain. Interestingly, in a different model, the IL-6 cytokine has recently been associated with the promotion of the M2 phenotype (43) and described as a potent inducer of SOCS3 (33). Furthermore, the generation of human immunosuppressive myeloid cell populations in human IL-6 transgenic NOG mice has been demonstrated (44).

Very little is known about M2 macrophage polarization during acute viral infection since the early anti-viral response is normally associated with a pro-inflammatory immune response (45). In this regard, a recently transcriptomic analysis of macrophages infected with attenuated or virulent influenza virus strains showed an early and clear profile of genes associated with the M2 phenotype triggered by a pathogenic influenza virus (46).

It has been shown that AXL and MERTK receptors are differentially modulated in cytokine-induced M1 and M2 macrophages, where enhanced levels of MERTK were associated with M2 polarization (21). IRF-1 was initially described as a regulator of type I IFN and MHC-I expression by binding to regulatory regions of their promoters (47). However, IRF-1 is one of the most important IFN-stimulated genes for innate and adaptive antiviral immunity, making a complex network with other transcription factors to finally have a specific response (48–50). In this sense, IRF-2 and 8 can both inhibit IRF-1–mediated induction of transcription competing by promoter binding sites (51, 52), or by blocking protein:protein interactions (53, 54), supporting the hypothesis that viruses can manipulate the induction of IFN and ISGs to enhance their replication. In this sense, the selective modulation of the MERTK, as

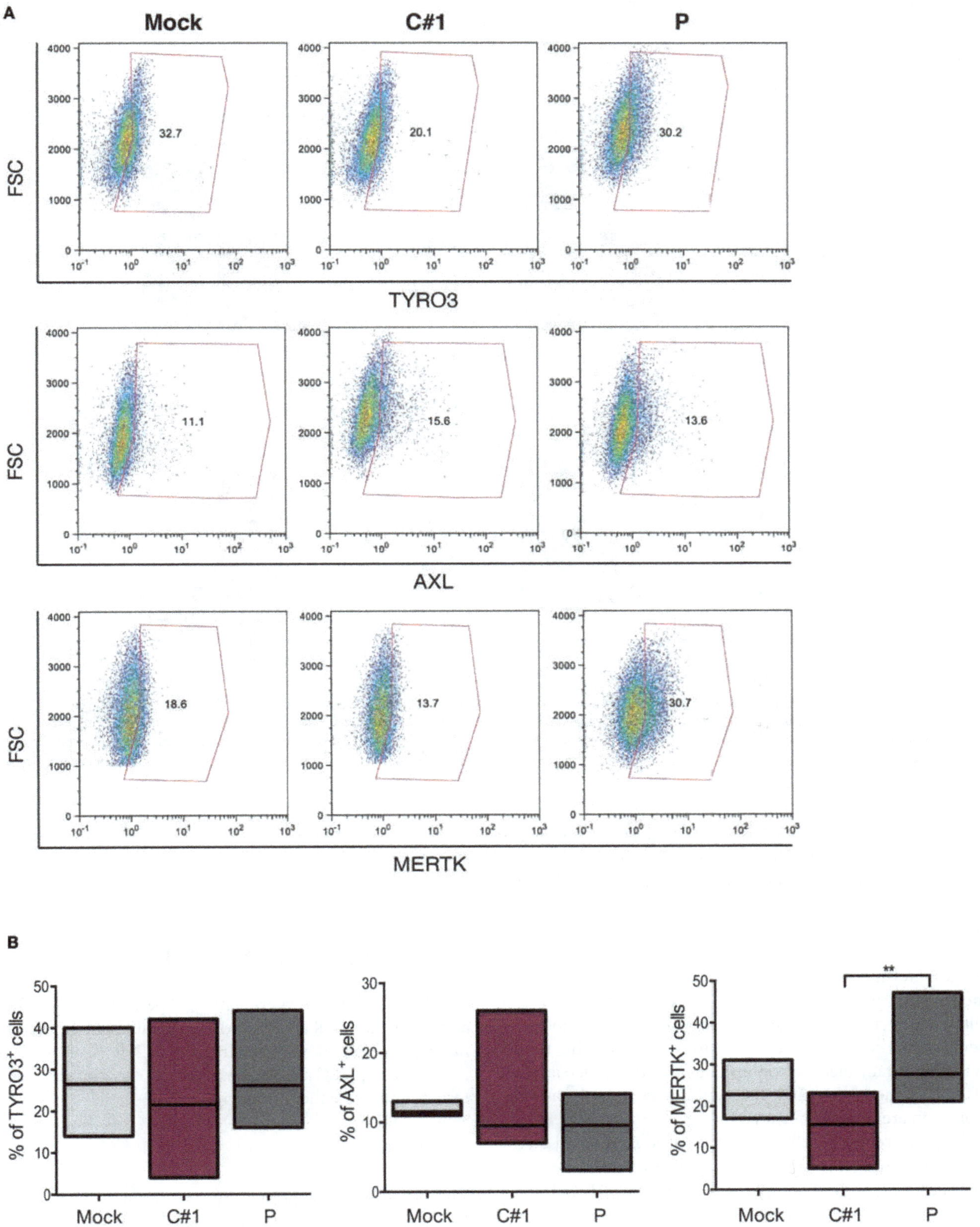

FIGURE 5 | JUNV selectively modulates TAM expression in human macrophages. HMDM cells were infected with C#1 or P strains of JUNV (MOI =1) and at 3 dpi the expression level of TYRO3, AXL, and MERTK receptors was evaluated by flow cytometry. **(A)** Representative dot plot of each receptor is shown and the percentage of macrophages expressing TYRO3, AXL, and MERTK receptors are graphed in **(B)**. Non-parametric One-way ANOVA followed by Dunn's multiple comparison test was

(Continued)

FIGURE 5 | Used to detect significant differences between groups; $^{**}P < 0.01$. The results are graphed as the median (min-max, horizontal line indicates the median) of seven independent donors. We had set the threshold based on the FMO of each receptor.

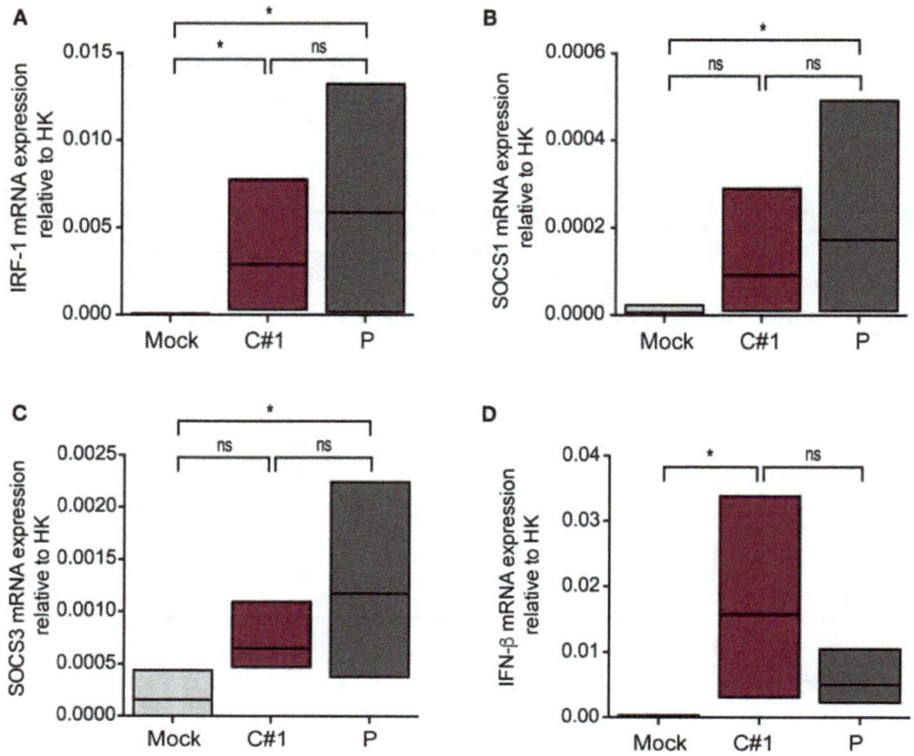

FIGURE 6 | JUNV P enhances transcription levels of IRF-1, IFN-β, SOCS1, and SOCS3. HMDM cells were infected with C#1 or P strains of JUNV (MOI =1) and after 1 dpi the transcription levels of **(A)** IRF-1, **(B)** SOCS1, **(C)** SOCS3, and **(D)** IFN-β, were studied by RT-qPCR. The Comparative Ct method ($2^{-\Delta CT}$) was used to analyze the expression level of the target genes. Non-parametric One-way ANOVA followed by Dunn's multiple comparison test was used to detect significant differences between groups; $^{*}P < 0.05$. The results are graphed as the median (min-max, horizontal line indicates the median) of five independent donors.

well as higher levels of IRF-1, SOCS1, and SOCS3 during P strain infection highlight not only the skewing property of this strain, but also its ability to usurp immunomodulatory pathways (TAM/SOCS1 and 3) and potentially use them for immune evasion.

Our results show that JUNV triggers differential macrophage activation and modulates polarization according to viral strain pathogenicity, inducing distinct cell responses that might facilitate correct immune surveillance or viral evasion and dissemination events that end in disease. Thus, the results provide important mechanistic insights into the understanding of JUNV pathogenesis and the multi-faceted host immune responses in arenavirus infection.

Taking our results together with the above-mentioned recent findings by others, it may be speculated that in some acute viral infections, subversion of the conventional M1 pro-inflammatory response to a M2 anti-inflammatory response by acute pathogenic viruses will be more frequent than previously described, and thus is deserving of further study since this may allow the development of potential new candidates for therapeutic targets.

AUTHOR CONTRIBUTIONS

MF did most of the experiments. PT performed IF studies. AL and NC made qPCR analysis. AE participated in the generation of macrophages and flow cytometry analysis. VR, JG, and MR edited the manuscript. EC and RG designed the experiments, discussed results, and wrote the manuscript.

FUNDING

This work was supported by the grants PICT 2016-1740 (RG), PICT 2015-2573 (EC), and PICT 2016-2608 (MF) from the Agencia Nacional de Promoción Científica y Tecnológica (ANPCyT), Roemmers 2017 (RG), PPID X037 (MF), and P11/X854 (VR) from UNLP, PIP 2015-0567 (AE) and PIP 0680 (VR) from Consejo Nacional de Investigaciones Científicas y

Técnicas (CONICET), Argentina. The funders had no role in study design, data collection and interpretation, or in the decision to submit the work for publication.

ACKNOWLEDGMENTS

We thank C. Lopez, L. Cayuela, S. Tongiani, and P. Gimenez for technical assistance and L. Vasquez for assistance in preparation and maintenance of cellular cultures.

REFERENCES

1. Gomez RM, Jaquenod De Giusti C, Sanchez Vallduvi MM, Frik J, Ferrer MF, Schattner M. Junin virus. A XXI century update. *Microbes Infect.* (2011) 13:303–11. doi: 10.1016/j.micinf.2010.12.006
2. Radoshitzky SR, Bao Y, Buchmeier MJ, Charrel RN, Clawson AN, Clegg CS, et al. Past, present, and future of arenavirus taxonomy. *Arch Virol.* (2015) 160:1851–74. doi: 10.1007/s00705-015-2418-y
3. Charrel RN, De Lamballerie X. Zoonotic aspects of arenavirus infections. *Vet Microbiol.* (2010) 140:213–20. doi: 10.1016/j.vetmic.2009.08.027
4. Kerber R, Reindl S, Romanowski V, Gomez RM, Ogbaini-Emovon E, Gunther S, et al. Research efforts to control highly pathogenic arenaviruses: a summary of the progress and gaps. *J Clin Virol.* (2015) 64:120–7. doi: 10.1016/j.jcv.2014.12.004
5. Bederka LH, Bonhomme CJ, Ling EL, Buchmeier MJ. Arenavirus stable signal peptide is the keystone subunit for glycoprotein complex organization. *MBio.* (2014) 5:e02063. doi: 10.1128/mBio.02063-14
6. Mosser DM, Edwards JP. Exploring the full spectrum of macrophage activation. *Nat Rev Immunol.* (2008) 8:958–69. doi: 10.1038/nri2448
7. Ginhoux F, Schultze JL, Murray PJ, Ochando J, Biswas SK. New insights into the multidimensional concept of macrophage ontogeny, activation and function. *Nat Immunol.* (2016) 17:34–40. doi: 10.1038/ni.3324
8. Murray PJ, Allen JE, Biswas SK, Fisher EA, Gilroy DW, Goerdt S, et al. Macrophage activation and polarization: nomenclature and experimental guidelines. *Immunity.* (2014) 41:14–20. doi: 10.1016/j.immuni.2014.06.008
9. Tarique AA, Logan J, Thomas E, Holt PG, Sly PD, Fantino E. Phenotypic, functional, and plasticity features of classical and alternatively activated human macrophages. *Am J Respir Cell Mol Biol.* (2015) 53:676–88. doi: 10.1165/rcmb.2015-0012OC
10. De Giusti CJ, Ure AE, Rivadeneyra L, Schattner M, Gomez RM. Macrophages and galectin 3 play critical roles in CVB3-induced murine acute myocarditis and chronic fibrosis. *J Mol Cell Cardiol.* (2015) 85:58–70. doi: 10.1016/j.yjmcc.2015.05.010
11. Carestia A, Mena HA, Olexen CM, Ortiz Wilczynski JM, Negrotto S, Errasti AE, et al. Platelets promote macrophage polarization toward pro-inflammatory phenotype and increase survival of septic mice. *Cell Rep.* (2019) 28:896–908.e5. doi: 10.1016/j.celrep.2019.06.062
12. Kusne Y, Carrera-Silva EA, Perry AS, Rushing EJ, Mandell EK, Dietrich JD, et al. Targeting aPKC disables oncogenic signaling by both the EGFR and the proinflammatory cytokine TNFalpha in glioblastoma. *Sci Signal.* (2014) 7:ra75. doi: 10.1126/scisignal.2005196
13. Negrotto S, Mena HA, Ure AE, Jaquenod De Giusti C, Bollati-Fogolin M, Vermeulen EM, et al. Human plasmacytoid dendritic cells elicited different responses after infection with pathogenic and nonpathogenic junin virus strains. *J Virol.* (2015) 89:7409–13. doi: 10.1128/JVI.01014-15
14. Radoshitzky SR, Abraham J, Spiropoulou CF, Kuhn JH, Nguyen D, Li W, et al. Transferrin receptor 1 is a cellular receptor for New World haemorrhagic fever arenaviruses. *Nature.* (2007) 446:92–6. doi: 10.1038/nature05539
15. Pozner RG, Ure AE, Jaquenod De Giusti C, D'atri LP, Italiano JE, Torres O, et al. Junin virus infection of human hematopoietic progenitors impairs *in vitro* proplatelet formation and platelet release via a bystander effect involving type I IFN signaling. *PLoS Pathog.* (2010) 6:e1000847. doi: 10.1371/journal.ppat.1000847
16. Ponka P, Lok CN. The transferrin receptor: role in health and disease. *Int J Biochem Cell Biol.* (1999) 31:1111–37. doi: 10.1016/S1357-2725(99)00070-9
17. Rothlin CV, Carrera-Silva EA, Bosurgi L, Ghosh S. TAM receptor signaling in immune homeostasis. *Ann Rev Immunol.* (2015) 33:12.11–37. doi: 10.1146/annurev-immunol-032414-112103
18. Bosurgi L, Cao YG, Cabeza-Cabrerizo M, Tucci A, Hughes LD, Kong Y, et al. Macrophage function in tissue repair and remodeling requires IL-4 or IL-13 with apoptotic cells. *Science.* (2017) 356:1072–6. doi: 10.1126/science.aai8132
19. Miner JJ, Daniels BP, Shrestha B, Proenca-Modena JL, Lew ED, Lazear HM, et al. The TAM receptor Mertk protects against neuroinvasive viral infection by maintaining blood-brain barrier integrity. *Nat Med.* (2015) 21:1464–72. doi: 10.1038/nm.3974
20. Schmid ET, Pang IK, Carrera Silva EA, Bosurgi L, Miner JJ, Diamond MS, et al. AXL receptor tyrosine kinase is required for T cell priming and antiviral immunity. *Elife.* (2016) 5:e12414. doi: 10.7554/eLife.12414
21. Zagorska A, Traves PG, Lew ED, Dransfield I, Lemke G. Diversification of TAM receptor tyrosine kinase function. *Nat Immunol.* (2014) 15:920–8. doi: 10.1038/ni.2986
22. Dou L, Liang HF, Geller DA, Chen YF, Chen XP. The regulation role of interferon regulatory factor-1 gene and clinical relevance. *Hum Immunol.* (2014) 75:1110–4. doi: 10.1016/j.humimm.2014.09.015
23. Blejer JL, Remesar MC, Lerman GD, Nejamkis MR. Macrophage maturity and modulation of response to Junin virus in infected rats. *J Infect Dis.* (1986) 154:478–82. doi: 10.1093/infdis/154.3.478
24. Pannetier D, Faure C, Georges-Courbot MC, Deubel V, Baize S. Human macrophages, but not dendritic cells, are activated and produce alpha/beta interferons in response to Mopeia virus infection. *J Virol.* (2004) 78:10516–24. doi: 10.1128/JVI.78.19.10516-10524.2004
25. Baize S, Kaplon J, Faure C, Pannetier D, Georges-Courbot MC, Deubel V. Lassa virus infection of human dendritic cells and macrophages is productive but fails to activate cells. *J Immunol.* (2004) 172:2861–9. doi: 10.4049/jimmunol.172.5.2861
26. Carnec X, Baize S, Reynard S, Diancourt L, Caro V, Tordo N, et al. Lassa virus nucleoprotein mutants generated by reverse genetics induce a robust type I interferon response in human dendritic cells and macrophages. *J Virol.* (2011) 85:12093–7. doi: 10.1128/JVI.00429-11
27. Pannetier D, Reynard S, Russier M, Carnec X, Baize S. Production of CXC and CC chemokines by human antigen-presenting cells in response to Lassa virus or closely related immunogenic viruses, and in cynomolgus monkeys with lassa fever. *PLoS Negl Trop Dis.* (2014) 8:e2637. doi: 10.1371/journal.pntd.0002637
28. Groseth A, Hoenen T, Weber M, Wolff S, Herwig A, Kaufmann A, et al. Tacaribe virus but not junin virus infection induces cytokine release from primary human monocytes and macrophages. *PLoS Negl Trop Dis.* (2011) 5:e1137. doi: 10.1371/journal.pntd.0001137
29. Xing J, Chai Z, Ly H, Liang Y. Differential inhibition of macrophage activation by lymphocytic choriomeningitis virus and pichinde virus is mediated by the Z protein N-terminal domain. *J Virol.* (2015) 89:12513–7. doi: 10.1128/JVI.01674-15
30. Xing J, Ly H, Liang Y. The Z proteins of pathogenic but not nonpathogenic arenaviruses inhibit RIG-I-like receptor-dependent interferon production. *J Virol.* (2015) 89:2944–55. doi: 10.1128/JVI.03349-14
31. Brisse ME, Ly H. Hemorrhagic fever-causing arenaviruses: lethal pathogens and potent immune suppressors. *Front Immunol.* (2019) 10:372. doi: 10.3389/fimmu.2019.00372

32. Schattner M, Rivadeneyra L, Pozner RG, Gomez RM. Pathogenic mechanisms involved in the hematological alterations of arenavirus-induced hemorrhagic fevers. *Viruses.* (2013) 5:340–51. doi: 10.3390/v5010340
33. Hunter CA, Jones SA. IL-6 as a keystone cytokine in health and disease. *Nat Immunol.* (2015) 16:448–57. doi: 10.1038/ni.3153
34. Sang Y, Miller LC, Blecha F. Macrophage polarization in virus-host interactions. *J Clin Cell Immunol* 6:311. doi: 10.4172/2155-9899.1000311
35. Zink W, Ryan L, Gendelman HE. Macrophage-virus interactions. In: Burke B, Lewis C, editors. *The Macrophage.* Oxford: Oxford University Press (2002). p. 138–209.
36. Wilson EB, Brooks DG. The role of IL-10 in regulating immunity to persistent viral infections. *Curr Top Microbiol Immunol.* (2011) 350:39–65. doi: 10.1007/82_2010_96
37. Richter K, Perriard G, Behrendt R, Schwendener RA, Sexl V, Dunn R, et al. Macrophage and T cell produced IL-10 promotes viral chronicity. *PLoS Pathog.* (2013) 9:e1003735. doi: 10.1371/journal.ppat.1003735
38. Zdrenghea MT, Makrinioti H, Muresan A, Johnston SL, Stanciu LA. The role of macrophage IL-10/innate IFN interplay during virus-induced asthma. *Rev Med Virol.* (2015) 25:33–49. doi: 10.1002/rmv.1817
39. Ouyang P, Rakus K, Van Beurden SJ, Westphal AH, Davison AJ, Gatherer D, et al. IL-10 encoded by viruses: a remarkable example of independent acquisition of a cellular gene by viruses and its subsequent evolution in the viral genome. *J Gen Virol.* (2014) 95:245–62. doi: 10.1099/vir.0.058966-0
40. Chatterjee M, Osborne J, Bestetti G, Chang Y, Moore PS. Viral IL-6-induced cell proliferation and immune evasion of interferon activity. *Science.* (2002) 298:1432–5. doi: 10.1126/science.1074883
41. Martinez FO, Gordon S. The M1 and M2 paradigm of macrophage activation: time for reassessment. *F1000Prime Rep.* (2014) 6:13. doi: 10.12703/P6-13
42. Saraiva M, O'garra A. The regulation of IL-10 production by immune cells. *Nat Rev Immunol.* (2010) 10:170–81. doi: 10.1038/nri2711
43. Sanmarco LM, Ponce NE, Visconti LM, Eberhardt N, Theumer MG, Minguez AR, et al. IL-6 promotes M2 macrophage polarization by modulating purinergic signaling and regulates the lethal release of nitric oxide during *Trypanosoma cruzi* infection. *Biochim Biophys Acta.* (2017) 1863:857–69. doi: 10.1016/j.bbadis.2017.01.006
44. Hanazawa A, Ito R, Katano I, Kawai K, Goto M, Suemizu H, et al. Generation of human immunosuppressive myeloid cell populations in human interleukin-6 transgenic NOG mice. *Front Immunol.* (2018) 9:152. doi: 10.3389/fimmu.2018.00152
45. Mills CD. Anatomy of a discovery: m1 and m2 macrophages. *Front Immunol.* (2015) 6:212. doi: 10.3389/fimmu.2015.00212
46. Zhang N, Bao YJ, Tong AH, Zuyderduyn S, Bader GD, Malik Peiris JS, et al. Whole transcriptome analysis reveals differential gene expression profile reflecting macrophage polarization in response to influenza A H5N1 virus infection. *BMC Med Genomics.* (2018) 11:20. doi: 10.1186/s12920-018-0335-0
47. Miyamoto M, Fujita T, Kimura Y, Maruyama M, Harada H, Sudo Y, et al. Regulated expression of a gene encoding a nuclear factor, IRF-1, that specifically binds to IFN-beta gene regulatory elements. *Cell.* (1988) 54:903–13. doi: 10.1016/S0092-8674(88)91307-4
48. Brien JD, Daffis S, Lazear HM, Cho H, Suthar MS, Gale M Jr, et al. Interferon regulatory factor-1 (IRF-1) shapes both innate and CD8(+) T cell immune responses against West Nile virus infection. *PLoS Pathog.* (2011) 7:e1002230. doi: 10.1371/journal.ppat.1002230
49. Xu L, Zhou X, Wang W, Wang Y, Yin Y, Laan LJ, et al. IFN regulatory factor 1 restricts hepatitis E virus replication by activating STAT1 to induce antiviral IFN-stimulated genes. *FASEB J.* (2016) 30:3352–67. doi: 10.1096/fj.201600356R
50. Abou El Hassan M, Huang K, Eswara MB, Xu Z, Yu T, Aubry A, et al. Properties of STAT1 and IRF1 enhancers and the influence of SNPs. *BMC Mol Biol.* (2017) 18:6. doi: 10.1186/s12867-017-0084-1
51. Harada H, Willison K, Sakakibara J, Miyamoto M, Fujita T, Taniguchi T. Absence of the type I IFN system in EC cells: transcriptional activator (IRF-1) and repressor (IRF-2) genes are developmentally regulated. *Cell.* (1990) 63:303–12. doi: 10.1016/0092-8674(90)90163-9
52. Hida S, Ogasawara K, Sato K, Abe M, Takayanagi H, Yokochi T, et al. CD8(+) T cell-mediated skin disease in mice lacking IRF-2, the transcriptional attenuator of interferon-alpha/beta signaling. *Immunity.* (2000) 13:643–55. doi: 10.1016/S1074-7613(00)00064-9
53. Sgarbanti M, Borsetti A, Moscufo N, Bellocchi MC, Ridolfi B, Nappi F, et al. Modulation of human immunodeficiency virus 1 replication by interferon regulatory factors. *J Exp Med.* (2002) 195:1359–70. doi: 10.1084/jem.20010753
54. Harman AN, Lai J, Turville S, Samarajiwa S, Gray L, Marsden V, et al. HIV infection of dendritic cells subverts the IFN induction pathway via IRF-1 and inhibits type 1 IFN production. *Blood.* (2011) 118:298–308. doi: 10.1182/blood-2010-07-297721

7

Changes in the NK Cell Repertoire Related to Initiation of TB Treatment and Onset of Immune Reconstitution Inflammatory Syndrome in TB/HIV Co-infected Patients

Carmem Beatriz Wagner Giacoia-Gripp[1], Andressa da Silva Cazote[1], Tatiana Pereira da Silva[1], Flávia Marinho Sant'Anna[2], Carolina Arana Stanis Schmaltz[2], Tania de Souza Brum[3], Juliana Arruda de Matos[4], Júlio Silva[5], Aline Benjamin[2], José Henrique Pilotto[1,3], Valeria Cavalcanti Rolla[2], Mariza Gonçalves Morgado[1] and Daniel Scott-Algara[6]*

[1] Laboratory of AIDS and Molecular Immunology, Oswaldo Cruz Institute (FIOCRUZ), Rio de Janeiro, Brazil, [2] Clinical Research Laboratory on Mycobacteria, National Institute of Infectious Diseases Evandro Chagas (FIOCRUZ), Rio de Janeiro, Brazil, [3] HIV Clinical Research Center, Nova Iguaçu General Hospital (HGNI), Rio de Janeiro, Brazil, [4] Clinical Research Laboratory on Health Surveillance and Immunization, National Institute of Infectious Diseases Evandro Chagas (FIOCRUZ), Rio de Janeiro, Brazil, [5] Platform for Clinical Research, National Institute of Infectious Diseases Evandro Chagas (FIOCRUZ), Rio de Janeiro, Brazil, [6] Unit of Lymphocyte Cell Biology, Pasteur Institute, Paris, France

****Correspondence:***
Carmem Beatriz Wagner Giacoia-Gripp
cbwggripp@gmail.com

Tuberculosis (TB) is the most common comorbidity and the leading cause of death among HIV-infected individuals. Although the combined antiretroviral therapy (cART) during TB treatment improves the survival of TB/HIV patients, the occurrence of immune reconstitution inflammatory syndrome (IRIS) in some patients poses clinical and scientific challenges. This work aimed to evaluate blood innate lymphocytes during therapeutic intervention for both diseases and their implications for the onset of IRIS. Natural killer (NK) cells, invariant NKT cells (iNKT), $\gamma\delta$ T cell subsets, and *in vitro* NK functional activity were characterized by multiparametric flow cytometry in the following groups: 33 TB/HIV patients (four with paradoxical IRIS), 27 TB and 25 HIV mono-infected subjects (prior to initiation of TB treatment and/or cART and during clinical follow-up to 24 weeks), and 25 healthy controls (HC). Concerning the NK cell repertoire, several activation and inhibitory receptors were skewed in the TB/HIV patients compared to those in the other groups, especially the HCs. Significantly higher expression of CD158a ($p = 0.025$), NKp80 ($p = 0.033$), and NKG2C ($p = 0.0076$) receptors was detected in the TB/HIV IRIS patients than in the non-IRIS patients. Although more NK degranulation was observed in the TB/HIV patients than in the other groups, the therapeutic intervention did not alter the frequency during follow-up (weeks 2–24). A higher frequency of the $\gamma\delta$ T cell population was observed in the TB/HIV patients with inversion of the $V\delta2^+/V\delta2^-$ ratio, especially for those presenting pulmonary TB, suggesting an expansion of particular $\gamma\delta$ T subsets during TB/HIV co-infection. In conclusion, HIV infection impacts the frequency of circulating NK cells and $\gamma\delta$ T cell subsets in TB/HIV patients. Important modifications of the NK cell repertoire were observed after anti-TB treatment (week 2) but not during the cART/TB follow-up (weeks 6–24). An increase of CD161$^+$ NK cells was related to an unfavorable outcome. Despite the low number of cases, a more preserved NK cell profile was detected in IRIS patients previous to treatment, suggesting a role for these cells in IRIS onset. Longitudinal evaluation of the NK repertoire showed the impact of TB treatment and implicated these cells in TB pathogenesis in TB/HIV co-infected patients.

Keywords: TB/HIV Co-infection, NK cell repertoire, IRIS, innate immune cells, clinical outcomes

INTRODUCTION

Tuberculosis (TB) is one of the world's deadliest diseases and affects ~10.0 million people worldwide. A total of 1.3 million deaths occurred in 2017, and almost one-fourth of the global population is infected with the infectious agent of TB, *Mycobacterium tuberculosis* (*Mtb*) (1). TB is a leading killer of HIV-infected people (TB/HIV co-infection) worldwide (2). Brazil is a World Health Organization high-burden country for TB and TB/HIV-associated comorbidities (1). In 2017, almost 70.0 thousand TB cases were registered in the country, of which 6,501 (~9.4%) were TB/HIV cases. A total of 9.4% of these cases occurred in the city of Rio de Janeiro, which is ranked as the second Brazilian state capital in terms of the number of TB/HIV cases and is considered a TB-endemic region (3–5). Indeed, estimates from 2016 showed a higher TB incidence rate in Rio de Janeiro city than the national incidence (99 vs. 33.5 TB cases/100,000 hab) (3–5). TB/HIV co-infection poses enormous clinical, scientific, and public health challenges. Although the use of combined antiretroviral therapy (cART) during TB treatment improves patient survival, particularly by restoring immune functions, simultaneous management of cART and anti-TB drugs is not easy due to pharmacological interactions. Moreover, the appearance of an inflammatory syndrome called immune reconstitution inflammatory syndrome (IRIS) in some patients and early mortality are adverse events of cART initiation and represent challenges for the management of TB/HIV patient care (6, 7). IRIS has been associated with lower CD4$^+$ T cell counts at cART initiation followed by a dramatic improvement in these cell counts and a rapid plasma viral load decay that lead to partial restoration of overall immune functions, and the presence of opportunistic pathogens (8–11); however, the immunopathogenesis of this syndrome and the major clinical and laboratory factors associated with IRIS onset are not clearly understood (12). In TB/HIV IRIS patients, elevated concentrations of proinflammatory serum mediators have been detected at IRIS onset, including C-reactive protein and cytokines, such as IL-6, IL-12, and TNF (13–15). Following cART initiation, recovery of CD4 Th1 responses to mycobacterial antigens is reported, and these increased responses have been associated with IRIS (16–18). Indeed, in a previous study by our group, an increase in immune responses was observed in TB/HIV IRIS patients compared with those of non-IRIS patients, as was a marked increase in IFN-γ production by T cells from IRIS patients in response to PPD and other *Mtb* antigens (19).

Given their importance in antigen processing and pathogen trafficking, cells of the innate immune system are a focus of increasing interest in IRIS physiopathology. $\gamma\delta$ T cells appear to play a predominant role against *Mtb* infection, and one study demonstrated reduced numbers of inhibitory natural killer (NK) receptors on mycobacteria-specific V$\delta 2^+$ $\gamma\delta$ T cells in TB/HIV IRIS patients (17). Moreover, studies have examined NK cell function in the development of IRIS among TB/HIV patients. In a study of unmasking IRIS, these cells were found to express increased levels of activation markers (20). In a longitudinal study with a TB/HIV co-infected group in Cambodia, NK cells isolated from paradoxical IRIS patients had higher expression of the degranulation marker CD107a than those of non-IRIS patients prior to IRIS onset at a time point 2 weeks after initiating TB treatment but before starting cART (21). The authors hypothesized that increased NK cell-mediated lysis of *Mtb*-infected cells might increase the antigen load and the risk of IRIS occurrence. Therefore, the physiopathology of TB/HIV coinfection and the occurrence of IRIS might be explained by an exaggerated innate immune response, implicating the participation of different players as Toll-like receptors, inflammasomes, NK cells, monocytes/macrophages, neutrophils, cytokines, among others (21–26).

Moreover, among TB patients, HIV infection is a risk factor for extrapulmonary TB, which sometimes require a high index of suspicion for diagnosis. Although TB is acquired by inhalation of contaminated droplets, it can produce disease in any organ system in addition to the lungs, which are usually the initial site of infection. In the context of TB/HIV co-infection, an increase in the number of reported cases of extrapulmonary TB is observed, accounting for ~20% of TB cases in HIV-uninfected patients and 53–62% of TB cases among HIV-infected patients (27). In our previous studies, ~56% of extrapulmonary TB cases were registered in our cohort of TB/HIV patients, including disseminated cases (19, 28). Although the association between HIV and overall TB (including pulmonary TB) is well-characterized (29), the relationship between extrapulmonary TB and HIV is less clear; the mechanisms related to the escape of *Mtb* to TB sites out of the lungs are not yet fully clarified, although extrapulmonary TB is very likely due to the reduction of CD4$^+$ T cell counts in HIV-infected patients, since CD4$^+$ T-helper cells are important for controlling of *Mtb* infection (30–34).

In this scenario, we hypothesized that the association between the exaggerated responses of NK cells before TB treatment and cART and the increased risk of IRIS after starting both therapies, as observed in the TB/HIV patients from Cambodia (21), would also be found in populations with different genetic backgrounds, such as patients from Rio de Janeiro city, Brazil. We also hypothesized a differential implication of innate immunological parameters in the pathogenesis of extrapulmonary TB, affecting lymph nodes and disseminated TB cases. Therefore, this study aimed to explore the implications of innate immune responses, specifically NK cell responses, in the evolution of TB/HIV co-infection.

METHODS AND PATIENTS

Study Population

The primary study population consisted of 33 HIV-infected patients diagnosed with TB (TB/HIV) who started cART 2 weeks (W2) after TB treatment according to the Brazilian Guidelines for HIV/AIDS Treatment and the National Tuberculosis Program (Ministry of Health) at the time of the study (35, 36). Briefly, 4-drugs TB regimen containing rifampicin, isoniazid, pyrazinamide, and ethambutol, followed by the first line HIV treatment with two nucleoside reverse transcriptase inhibitors (NRTI) + non-nucleoside reverse transcriptase inhibitors (NNRTI) (35–37). Tuberculosis diagnosis was made when suggestive clinical symptoms, and radiological findings were present. In some cases, microbiological methods confirmed the diagnosis: Ziehl-Neelsen staining for the detection of acid-fast bacilli in sputum smears and biopsy specimens, Xpert MTB/RIF® in sputum for MTB and rifampicin resistance detection, mycobacteria culture of sputum, and biopsy samples in Löwenstein-Jensen medium and/or Mycobacteria Growth Indicator Tube (MGIT) (36). HIV infection was determined by rapid test and confirmed by conventional serology testing and western blot, and then, molecular detection of RNA viral load (35). As inclusion criteria, the TB/HIV patients were naïve for HIV drugs and presented $CD4^+$ T cell counts below 200 cells/mm^3. The TB/HIV patients were evaluated at the introduction of anti-TB therapy at the baseline visit (D0), at the initiation of cART (W2) and during the clinical follow-up visits at weeks 6, 10, 14, and 24. Four TB/HIV patients developed paradoxical IRIS defined as a documented clinical worsening of TB signs or symptoms during anti-TB treatment, after cART initiation, not explained by any other diseases or by an adverse effect of drug therapy; lymph node enlargement with inflammatory signs temporally related to cART introduction was considered IRIS in this study (37–39). Each case of IRIS was validated in this study by the members of the clinical coordination team to discard opportunistic disease diagnosis, drug-resistant TB, low adherence, or adverse effects of cART. The TB/HIV patients were also analyzed according to their TB clinical presentations as pulmonary (PTB), lymph node TB (LNTB), and disseminated TB (DTB) (when two non-contiguous sites were affected) (37). Moreover, in the context of clinical outcomes, the patient outcomes were evaluated as favorable (TB treatment responders) or unfavorable (death) at the end (usually 6 months) of TB therapy under cART. In parallel to the TB/HIV patients, three control groups were also studied: HIV mono-infected subjects (HIV; $n = 25$), who were evaluated previous to cART; HIV-seronegative TB patients (TB; $n = 27$), who were evaluated previous to TB treatment; and volunteer healthy controls (HC, $n = 25$). The diagnosis of HIV infection was discarded by conventional serology and HIV RNA viral quantification in TB and HC groups, while TB infection was ruled out by the clinic and radiological examination in HIV and HC groups. However, if healthy participants had any sign or symptom, Xpert MTB/RIF® in sputum for MTB and rifampicin resistance detection and mycobacteria culture of sputum samples in Löwenstein-Jensen medium and/or MGIT were performed. All participants, including the HC, who agreed to participate in this study were enrolled after signing the informed consent form. Participant recruitment started in August 2014 and extended until December 2016 at the Instituto Nacional de Infectologia Evandro Chagas (INI), which is the clinical research unit for adult care in infectious diseases of the Oswaldo Cruz Foundation, and at the Hospital Geral de Nova Iguacu (HGNI), which is a general hospital from the Brazilian Ministry of Health. HGNI is located in the outskirts of Rio de Janeiro, and is a referral center for HIV and TB care in 13 municipalities. This protocol was approved by the local institutional Ethics Committee (Instituto Oswaldo Cruz Research Ethics Committee) and the Brazilian National Ethics Committee—CONEP (CAAE: 04514012.1.1001.5248).

Phenotypic Innate Lymphoid Cell Studies

NK cells, invariant NKT cells (iNKT) and $\gamma\delta$ T cell subsets were characterized from fresh whole blood through multiparametric flow cytometry (Gallios flow cytometer and Kaluza Version 3.0 analysis software, Beckman-Coulter, Kendon, FL, USA). NK cells were identified as $CD3^-CD56^{+/-}CD16^{+/-}$ within the gated lymphocyte population previously defined in the FSC/SSC dot plot. The same strategy was used to define the iNKT cells, which were identified using the monoclonal antibody 6B11, specific to the conserved CDR3 region of the canonical hallmark T cell receptor (TCR)-invariant chain Vα24Jα18 (40–42) and defined as $CD3^+CD56^{+/-}V\alpha24J\alpha18^+$ lymphocytes, as detailed in the **Supplementary Figure 1A**. In its turn, the $\gamma\delta$ T cell subsets were identified as $CD3^+CD56^+Pan\gamma\delta^+$ lymphocytes coexpressing or not the Vδ2 chain. The NK repertoire receptors were evaluated using monoclonal antibodies based on the CAPRI NK study results (21), including the KIR family (CD158a, CD158b1/b2,j, CD158d, CD158e, CD158e1/e2, and CD158i), NCR receptors (NKp30, NKp44, and NKp46), NKG family (2A, 2C, and 2D), CD94, CD85j, CD160, CD161, NKp80, DNAM-1, CD244, and activation marker CD69 (from Beckman-Coulter; BD Biosciences, San Jose, CA, USA; R&D Systems, Minneapolis, MN, USA; and BioLegend, San Diego, CA, USA).

Cytokine Assays and Cytolytic NK Cell Activity

CD107a expression on NK cells and the intracellular cytokine staining (ICS)-based assay were used to measure cytotoxic activity (degranulation) and cytokine expression as described previously with some modifications (21, 43). Briefly, mononuclear cells (PBMCs) isolated from fresh whole blood were incubated overnight at 37°C with 5% CO_2 at 1:1 ratio with the K562 cell line, which was used as target cells, in the presence of a CD107a monoclonal antibody, brefeldin A (5 μg/mL;

Sigma-Aldrich, St. Louis, MO, USA) and monensin (6 μg/mL; Sigma-Aldrich), which were added concomitantly to the cells. Spontaneous basal degranulation and cytokine production were measured by incubating PBMCs under the same conditions without target cells. After incubation, anti-CD3, anti-CD56, and anti-CD16 were added, followed by antibodies for the ICS-based assay (IFN-γ, TNF, TGF-β, and IL-10; Beckman-Coulter and BD Biosciences). These evaluations were assessed by multiparametric flow cytometry using the XL-MCL and Gallios equipment from Beckman-Coulter.

Statistical Analysis

The HIV viral load and immunological parameters, including $CD4^+$ T cells, NK cells (receptor repertoire, CD107a expression, and cytokine levels), iNKT and the γδ T innate cell subsets, were assessed in the TB/HIV patients during follow-up and in the control group at baseline (D0). Descriptive analyses of clinical and demographic characteristics were performed for the patients and controls. The Wilcoxon *t*-test, Mann-Whitney *U* test, and Kruskal-Wallis test were used to evaluate quantitative variables, whereas Fisher's exact test and Pearson's chi-square test were used for categorical variables. A p-value < 0.05 was considered significant. The slope of the $CD4^+$ T cell absolute count and HIV viral load was estimated by a non-linear least squares method for a five-parameter sigmoidal curve (44). Briefly, the slope indicates the growth/degrowth rate of an indicator during the "window of linearity," which is the highest linearity region of the curve. The maximum and minimum points of the second derivate curve were used as boundaries for this region. The statistical analysis was performed using the Stata software version 11.0 (STATA Corp. College Station, TX, USA), and the GraphPad Prism version 6.0 software (GraphPad Software, La Jolla, CA, USA) was used to generate the graphics. Sigmoidal fitting was performed using R version 3.0.3 (2014-03-06—"Warm Puppy").

RESULTS

Demographic Characteristics of the Studied Groups

The clinical and sociodemographic characteristics obtained from all participants in the study are presented in **Table 1**. No differences in age, gender, race or tuberculosis presentation were observed in the distribution of participants among the groups, although a trend for a higher frequency of TB occurrence was observed for males. The basal $CD4^+$ T cell absolute counts were extremely low among the TB/HIV and HIV patients compared to those of the other participants ($p = 0.0001$). As expected, the basal CD4/CD8 ratios were also lower among these patients than in the TB and HC groups ($p = 0.0001$). Interestingly, the TB/HIV group presented HIV viral loads that were significantly higher than those of the HIV group ($p = 0.0077$). The major TB presentation was pulmonary regardless of the presence of HIV coinfection, followed by lymph node TB. Disseminated TB was diagnosed in 15.1% of the TB/HIV patients, whereas no case was detected in the TB group. Among the 33 TB/HIV recruited participants, only 4 (12.1%) developed symptoms consistent with IRIS after beginning cART, which was in agreement with the frequency of IRIS observed in our previous studies (28, 45). The IRIS onset was observed from 1–3 weeks after cART initiation and was clinically diagnosed as defined above. In general, the patients presented worsening of the signs/symptoms related to TB, like fever and enlargement of the right or the left cervical/submandibular lymph nodes, which were either self-resolving, or the patients were treated with corticoid-based therapy, such as Prednisone (**Supplementary Table 1**). At D0, the IRIS and non-IRIS TB/HIV patients presented similar $CD4^+$ T cell absolute counts (data not shown). Concerning the HIV viral load, higher levels were observed for the IRIS patients at the D0 than for the non-IRIS TB/HIV participants ($p = 0.0088$). As defined previously, 26 (78.8%) of the 33 TB/HIV patients were classified as having a favorable outcome, 5 (15.1%) were defined as having an unfavorable outcome, and outcome information were missing for 2 (6.1%) at the end of the study follow-up.

Virological and Immune Responses to TB and/or cART Treatment During Follow-Up

The $CD4^+$ T cells and HIV viral load were also evaluated for the TB/HIV group at starting TB treatment (D0), at cART initiation 2 weeks later (W2), and during the follow-up visits (W6, 10, 14, and 24) (**Figure 1**). The TB/HIV patients showed a significant increment of $CD4^+$ T cells after the first month of cART (at week 6), and this increase was sustained over the follow-up (**Figure 1A**; *Slope* = 36.59). Notably, a higher slope was detected for the $CD4^+$ T cell increment for the TB/HIV IRIS patients (**Figure 1B**; *Slope* = 95.53) than for the non-IRIS patients (**Figure 1C**; *Slope* = 24.31), which indicated the higher increase in $CD4^+$ T cell counts among the IRIS patients. As expected, the HIV viral load significantly declined from weeks two to six, for which a negative slope of 0.95 was observed, and this decay was continuous during the follow-up (**Figure 1D**). A similar response was observed when the TB/HIV non-IRIS patients were assessed separately, implying the development of fast control of HIV replication with cART in these patients, whereas less prominent control of the viral load was detected in the IRIS patients (**Figure 1E**: IRIS *Slope* = −0.35, **Figure 1F**: non-IRIS *Slope* = −1.01).

Circulating Innate Immune Cells and the NK Cell Repertoire Profile Before Clinical Intervention

To characterize the circulating NK, iNKT and γδ T cell profiles, fresh whole blood samples collected from all participants were investigated at the D0. The TB/HIV patients presented a lower frequency of $CD56^{+/-}CD16^{+/-}CD3^-$ NK cells than the healthy controls ($p = 0.037$) and TB patients ($p = 0.015$), showing the negative impact of HIV infection on circulating NK cells (**Figure 2A**). Concerning the iNKT cells, no difference in the frequencies of $CD3^+CD56^+V\alpha24J\alpha18^+$ cells was identified among the TB/HIV patients and the other groups (**Figure 2A**). The same scenario was observed when the $CD3^+V\alpha24J\alpha18^+$ iNKT population was analyzed among the groups (**Supplementary Figure 1B**). Moreover, higher percentages of circulating γδ T cells were observed in the TB/HIV patients compared to those of the HC participants ($p = 0.0027$; **Figure 2A**). The frequencies of γδ T cells expressing the Vδ2 chain ($V\delta2^+$) were decreased in the TB/HIV and

TABLE 1 | Clinical and sociodemographic characteristics of the TB/HIV, HIV, and TB patients and HC volunteers.

Characteristic	TB/HIV ($N = 33$)	HIV ($N = 25$)	TB ($N = 27$)	HC ($N = 25$)	*P*-value*
Age (years), median (IQR)	35 (32–42)	36 (27–43)	36 (27–48)	44 (34–49)	0.1433[a]
Gender, *n* (%)					
Male	24 (72.7)	17 (68.0)	17 (63.0)	10 (40.0)	0.063[b]
Female	9 (27.3)	8 (32.0)	10 (37.0)	15 (60.0)	–
Race, *n* (%)					
Black	6 (18.2)	4 (16.0)	4 (14.8)	3 (12.0)	0.102[c]
Brown	16 (48.5)	15 (60.0)	11 (40.7)	9 (36.0)	–
White	11 (33.3)	6 (24.0)	12 (44.4)	13 (52.0)	–
Site of tuberculosis, *n* (%)					
Pulmonary	20 (60.6)	na	20 (74.1)	na	0.213[c]
Lymph node	6 (18.2)	na	5 (18.1)	na	–
Extrapulmonary	2 (6.1)	na	2 (7.4)	na	–
Disseminated	5 (15.1)	na	–	na	–
IRIS, *n* (%)					
Yes	4 (12.1)	na	na	na	–
No	29 (87.9)	na	na	na	–
Clinical outcomes, *n* (%)[e]					
Favorable	26 (78.8)	na	27 (100)	na	–
Unfavorable	5 (15.5)	na	–	na	–
Missed	2 (6.1)	na	–	na	
Baseline CD4 (cells/mm^3), median (IQR)	57 (17–144)	42 (23–139)	745 (537–980)	1118 (872–1,320)	0.0001[a]
Baseline CD4/CD8 ratio median (IQR)	0.08 (0.04–0.17)	0.11 (0.05–0.19)	1.41 (1.00–2.07)	1.88 (1.57–2.38)	0.0001[a]
Baseline HIV-1 viral load ($\log_{10}$ copies/ml), median (IQR)	5.64 (5.22–5.88)	5.28 (4.99–5.59)	na	na	0.0077[d]

N, number of cases; IQR, Interquartile ranges (75th–25th percentiles); IRIS, Immune Reconstitution Inflammatory Syndrome; na, not applicable.
[a]*Kruskall-Wallis test.*
[b]*Chi-square test.*
[c]*Fisher's exact test.*
[d]*Mann-Whitney U-test.*
[e]*Clinical outcomes analysis is only related to TB.*
$^*p < 0.05$.

HIV-infected patients compared to those in the HCs and TB patients. As expected, γδ T cells expressing other Vδ chains (Vδ2$^-$) were the predominant subset among the TB/HIV and HIV mono-infected patients, with a very low Vδ2$^+$/Vδ2$^-$ ratio (**Figure 2B**; $p < 0.0001$).

Concerning the NK cell repertoire, we tested 20 different receptors. The results for those presented statistically significant differences among the TB/HIV patients and the other groups are depicted in **Figure 3**. Except for CD158d and CD69, generally, the TB/HIV patients showed lower frequencies of these selected NK receptors than the other studied groups. These alterations targeted important activating and inhibitory molecules indistinctly and showed the impact of both comorbidities on the NK cell repertoire. Medians and interquartile ranges for all investigated receptors for all groups are presented in **Supplementary Table 2**.

Analysis of NK Subsets in IRIS Patients

The impacts of the NK subsets on the inflammatory process were assessed in the TB/HIV IRIS patients despite the low number of confirmed IRIS cases. Prior to TB treatment, the non-IRIS patients presented a lower frequency of NK cells than the HC ($p = 0.009$), and a trend for a lower frequency compared to that of the IRIS patients ($p = 0.055$). Conversely, the IRIS patients and HCs had more similar NK cell frequencies (**Figure 4A**). Interestingly, three NK receptors (NKG2C, NKp80, and CD158a, **Figures 4B–D**) were decreased in the non-IRIS patients but were expressed at similar levels between the IRIS patients and HC. At IRIS onset, no significant difference was found in the NK cell subsets between the patients with and without IRIS (data not shown). Despite the limited number of IRIS cases, these observations suggest a more preserved NK cell profile among the IRIS patients, similar to the HC. The iNKT and γδ T cells were also evaluated, but no significant differences were observed for these populations between the IRIS and non-IRIS patients at study entry.

Frequencies of Innate Immune Cells in TB/HIV Patients According to the TB Clinical Presentation

The innate lymphocyte subsets were also analyzed in the context of the TB clinical presentation regardless of the onset of IRIS. TB/HIV patients with PTB presented higher γδ T cell frequencies than either the HC (**Figure 5A**; $p = 0.0005$) or TB/HIV patients presenting LNTB ($p = 0.022$), whereas no

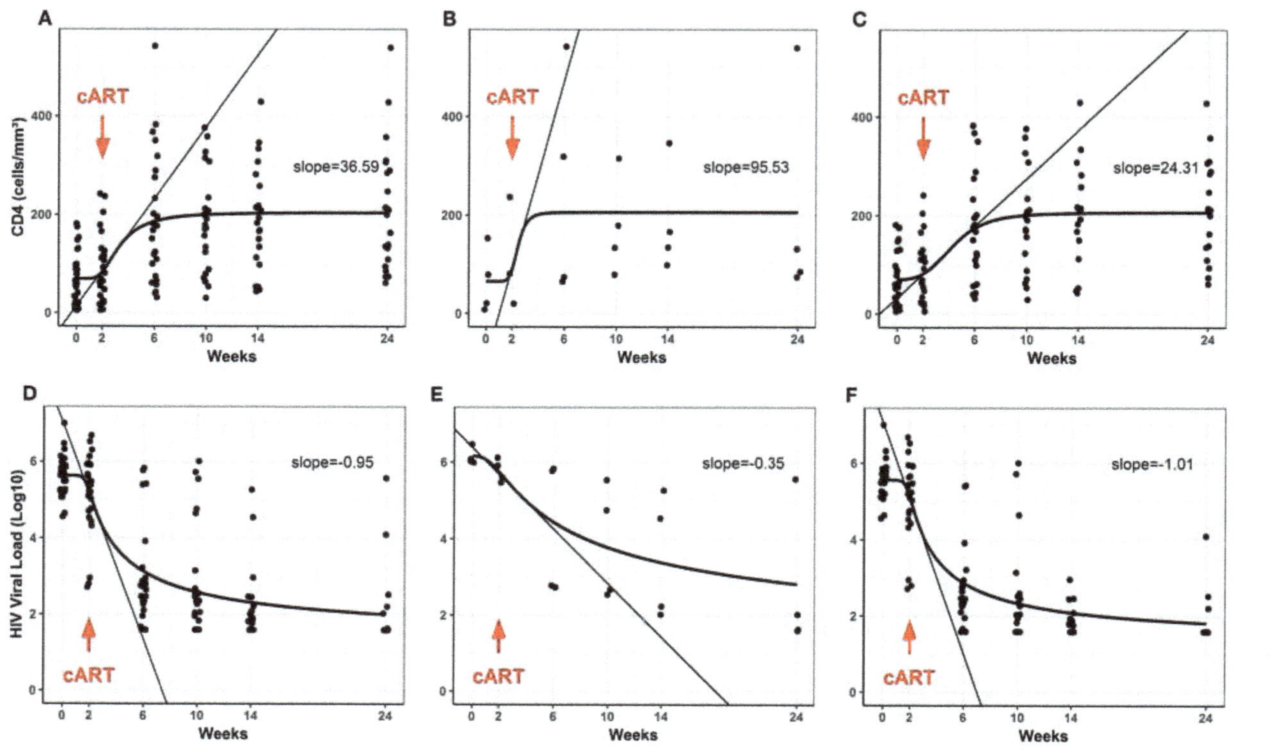

FIGURE 1 | Blood CD4+ T counts and plasma HIV viral loads in the TB/ HIV patients during follow-up. **(A–C)** Evolution of CD4+ T cell counts (absolute values) and **(D–F)** the HIV viral load (Log_{10} copies/mL) after starting cART (red arrows) in the TB/HIV **(A,D)**, IRIS **(B,E)**, and non-IRIS **(C,F)** patients. The results are presented as the slopes of the CD4+ T cell (cells/mm^3) increase and HIV viral load (Log_{10} copies/mL) decrease.

difference was observed in those with DTB (**Figure 5A**). These differences were not detected between the TB patients presenting with PTB and LNTB. A trend for a higher γδ T cell frequency was observed in the TB/HIV patients compared to that of the TB patients (**Figure 5A**; $p = 0.056$) with PTB. These observations suggested that γδ T cell expansion occurred in cases of co-infected patients with PTB presentation. Concerning the NK cell frequency, a decrease was observed for PTB cases among the TB/HIV patients compared to that of the HC ($p = 0.033$) and the TB patients presenting with PTB (**Figure 5B**; $p = 0.005$). The NKp44+ NK cell frequency tended to be higher in the TB/HIV patients presenting with PTB than with LNTB, suggesting that more *in vivo* activation of NK cells occurred in this group of patients (**Figure 5C**; $p = 0.056$). The same findings were not observed between the TB PTB and LNTB groups, reinforcing the role of HIV infection in NK cell activation. No significant differences were observed in either iNKT cells or other profiles of NK subsets when they were analyzed according to the TB clinical presentation (data not shown).

Potential for NK Cell Degranulation and Cytokine Production

The potential for NK cell degranulation and cytokine production was also investigated among the groups. NK cell degranulation was addressed through CD107a expression; the results are shown in **Figure 5**. A significantly higher percentage of NK cells expressing CD107a was observed in the TB/HIV patients at D0 than among the HIV, TB, and HC groups (**Figure 6A**). However, when we analyzed the degranulation capacity of NK cells according to the development of IRIS, no difference was observed between the IRIS patients and the other groups. Moreover, no difference was observed in CD107a-expressing NK cells in the TB/HIV patients regardless of the TB clinical presentation (data not shown). We also analyzed CD107a expression on NK cells under stimulated and non-stimulated conditions. *In vitro* stimulation with the target cell line was able to significantly increase the frequency of CD107a+ NK cells in all groups compared to that of the non-stimulated condition (**Figure 6B**; $p < 0.0001$). Furthermore, significantly higher CD107a+ NK cell percentages were detected in the TB/HIV patients under the non-stimulated condition than in the other groups, indicating *in vivo* NK cell activation. Interestingly, this higher CD107a expression without stimulation was not observed more frequently in IRIS patients (**Figure 6C**; $p = 0.01$). Both the IRIS and non-IRIS patients had similarly increased CD107a+ NK cell frequencies when stimulated *in vitro* by target cells (**Figure 6C**).

Intracellular IFN-γ, TNF, TGF-β, and IL-10 cytokine production by NK cells was assessed after *in vitro* stimulation with target cells. As shown in **Figure 7A**, the TB/HIV patients presented a decrease in IFN-γ and TNF staining compared to

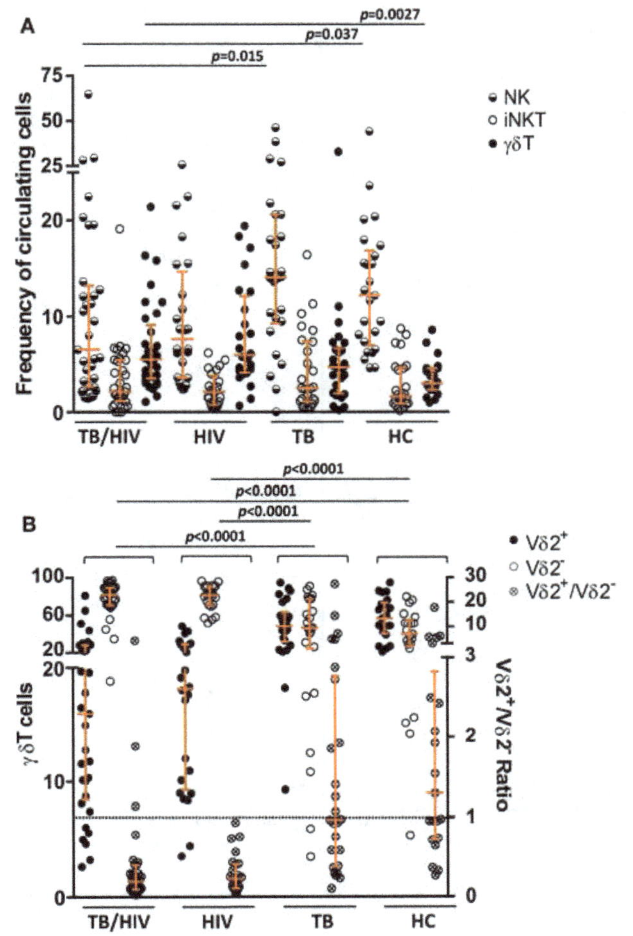

FIGURE 2 | NK, iNKT, and γδ T cell subset phenotyping. The NK, iNKT, and the γδ T cell subsets were analyzed prior to TB treatment and/or cART. The frequencies of **(A)** the circulating NK, iNKT ($CD3^+CD56^+$ $V\alpha24J\alpha18^+$) and γδ T cell populations, **(B)** the $V\delta2^+$ and $V\delta2^-$ T cell subsets, and the $V\delta2^+/V\delta2^-$ ratio for TB patients co-infected with HIV (TB/HIV, $n = 33$), HIV mono-infected individuals (HIV, $n = 25$), TB-only patients (TB, $n = 27$), and healthy controls (HC, $n = 25$) at D0. The results are expressed as the % of total lymphocytes **(A)** or γδ T cells **(B)**. Histograms represent the median and interquartiles (25th–75th percentile) for each group. A dashed line indicates the $V\delta2^+/V\delta2^-$ ratio = 1.0. The data were analyzed using the Mann-Whitney *U* test. Significant *p*-values ($p < 0.05$) are indicated.

that of the HC and the HIV, TB, and HC groups, respectively. On the other hand, the frequency of TGF-β-producing NK cells in the TB/HIV group was significantly higher than that in the HIV mono-infected and TB patients. Despite the very low frequencies of IL-10^+ NK cells observed in all groups, higher production was observed in TB- and/or HIV-infected patients compared to that of the HC. No differences were observed when intracellular cytokine production was compared between the IRIS and non-IRIS patients (not shown). By contrast, lower IFN-γ and TNF production were detected in the PTB and LNTB TB/HIV patients than in the HC (**Figure 7B**), whereas the PTB and DTB TB/HIV patients had higher levels of IL-10^+ NK cells than the HC. Furthermore, IFN-γ- and TNF-producing NK cells were also significantly lower in the LNTB-TB/HIV patients than in the LNTB-TB and the PTB and LNTB TB/HIV patients, respectively. No specific TGF-β production profile was observed regardless of the TB clinical presentation.

Impacts of TB Treatment on the NK Repertoire

Despite a satisfactory virological response and quantitative recovery of $CD4^+$ T cells, no significant recovery of circulating NK, iNKT, and γδ T cells, including the $V\delta2^+$ and $V\delta2^-$ subsets, was detected during the follow-up (data not shown). However, significant alterations were observed in the NK cell repertoire after the first 2 weeks of TB treatment (W2) and prior to cART for almost all receptors, except for NKG2C, which also presented significant changes throughout the 24 weeks of follow-up, as presented in **Figure 8**. Some receptor frequencies were also altered with cART, including CD158e1/e2, which presented significant changes in its frequency only after cART initiation. No differences were observed during the follow-up in TB/HIV patients evaluated according to the TB clinical forms (data not shown).

NK Cell Subsets Associated With an Unfavorable Clinical Outcome

We hypothesized that some association would exist between the NK cell repertoire changes at W2 of TB treatment and the patients' clinical outcomes. The TB/HIV patient outcomes were classified as favorable in cases of TB treatment responders or unfavorable in cases of death, which were the two clinical outcomes observed in our study group. Then, we calculated the delta between D0 and W2 (Δ_{W2-D0}) for all NK cell receptors according to the clinical outcomes. A significant difference was only observed for the circulating $CD161^+$ NK cell subset, which presented a significantly higher Δ_{W2-D0} in the TB/HIV patients with an unfavorable clinical outcome (**Figure 9**).

NK Cell Degranulation and Cytokine Production During Treatment Follow-Up

Higher frequencies of $CD107a^+$ NK cells were observed in TB/HIV patients after stimulation with target cells at all follow-up visits compared to those of the HIV, TB and HC groups at D0 despite TB treatment and cART ($p < 0.05$, data not shown). As observed at D0, *in vitro* stimulation of NK cells with target cells induced higher $CD107a^+$ NK cell expression at all follow-up visits (**Figure 10**). CD107a expression in cultures without stimulation tended to be lower during the follow-up and became significantly different at W24 (**Figure 10**; $p = 0.02$) compared to that at D0. TB and/or cART treatment did not appear to impact significantly the NK granulation capacity after stimulation, at least during the first 24 weeks. Finally, longitudinal analysis of the ICS frequency among the TB/HIV patients revealed no changes during follow-up (data not shown).

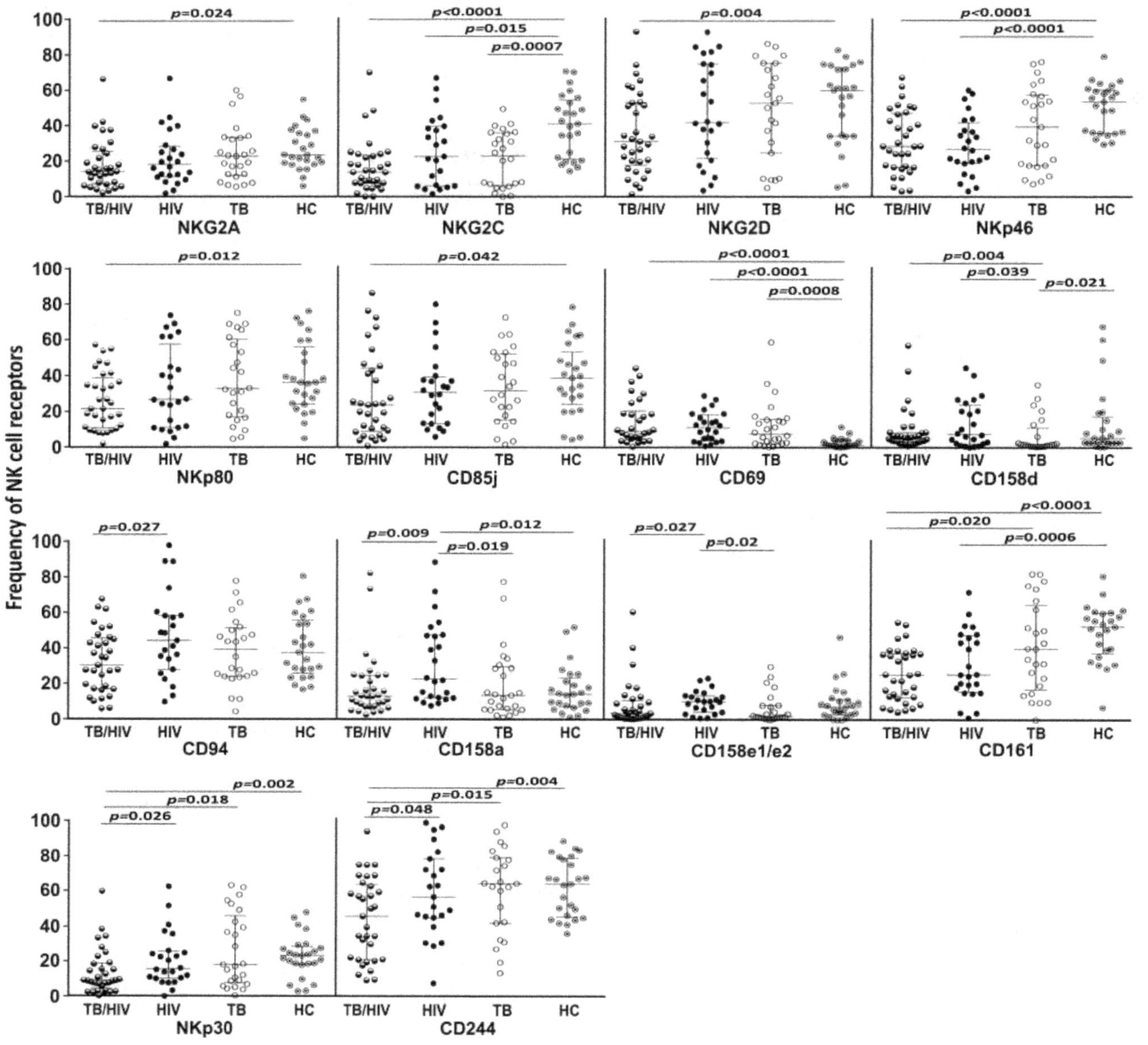

FIGURE 3 | NK cell repertoire before TB and/or cART treatment according to the groups. The results are shown as frequencies of NK cell receptors among the total NK cell population of TB patients co-infected with HIV (TB/HIV, $n = 33$), HIV mono-infected individuals (HIV, $n = 25$), TB-only patients (TB, $n = 27$) and healthy controls (HC, $n = 25$) at D0. The study receptors were C-type lectin receptors (NKG2A, NKG2C, NKG2D, NKp80, CD94, CD69, and CD161), natural cytotoxicity receptors (NKp30 and NKp46), killer cell immunoglobulin-like receptors (CD158d, CD158a and CD158e1/e2), immunoglobulin-like transcript receptor CD85j, and the costimulatory CD244 molecule. The results are presented as the median and interquartiles (25th–75th percentile). The data were analyzed using the Mann-Whitney *U* test. Significant *p*-values ($p < 0.05$) are indicated.

DISCUSSION

In the present work, we investigated the innate blood lymphocyte profile, specifically NK cells, in TB/HIV patients residing in Rio de Janeiro city, Brazil, who were cART naive and evaluated the implications for IRIS development, TB clinical presentation, and clinical outcomes. The HIV/TB association poses enormous clinical challenges, starting with an early, and accurate diagnosis, especially for extrapulmonary cases. Additionally, this association includes the provision of effective anti-TB treatment, use of concurrent cART, management of drug cytotoxicity and IRIS, including its treatment in some cases (46).

In the absence of therapeutic intervention, the NK cell repertoire is impacted by co-infection, since TB/HIV patients present alterations in several NK cell receptors that mainly include decreases in expression. A skewed NK repertoire has been observed in HIV infection, and these alterations have even been associated with HIV-1 pathogenesis and disease progression

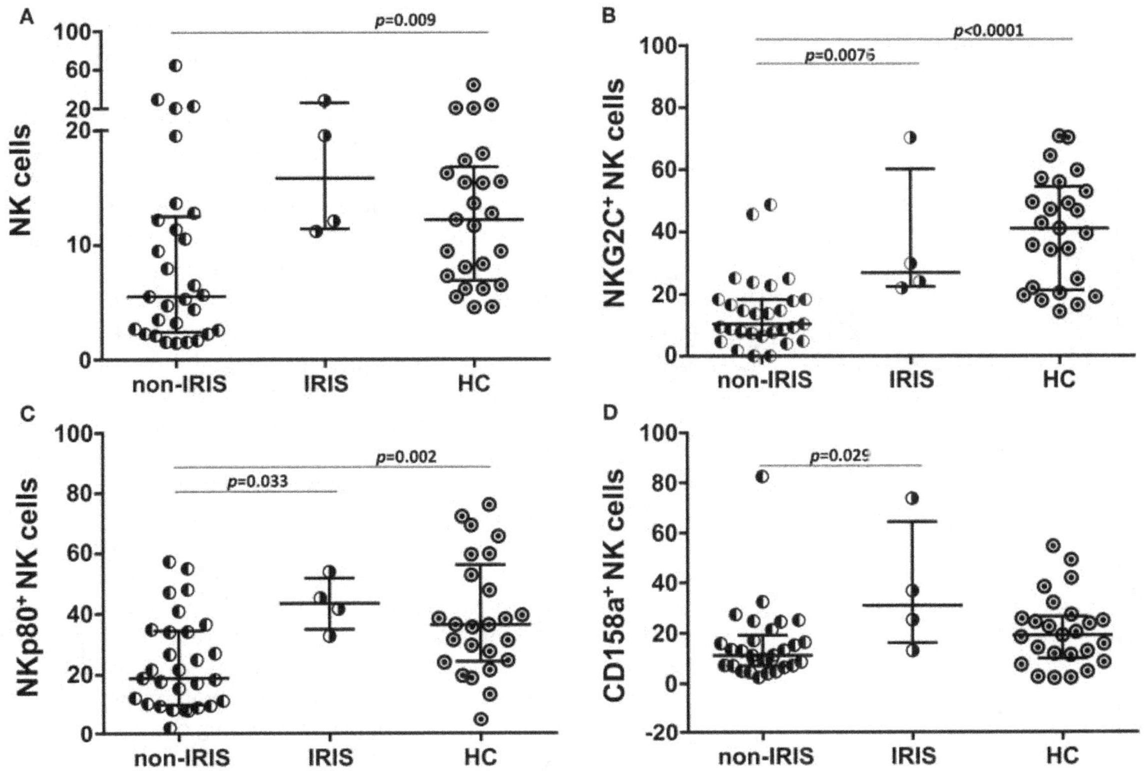

FIGURE 4 | Expression of NK cell receptors in IRIS and non-IRIS patients prior to TB treatment and cART. Different frequencies observed between the TB/HIV IRIS ($n = 4$) and non-IRIS ($n = 29$) patients for **(A)** circulating NK cells and NK subsets expressing **(B)** NKG2C, **(C)** NKp80, and **(D)** CD158a compared to those of the healthy control (HC, $n = 25$) group. The results are presented as the median and interquartiles (25th–75th percentile). The data were analyzed using the Mann-Whitney *U* test. Significant *p*-values ($p < 0.05$) are indicated.

(47, 48). We also observed an impact of HIV infection, since HIV mono-infected patients also presented alterations in the NK repertoire frequencies compared with those of the healthy controls. As reported previously (49–52), modifications in the NK cell repertoire were observed in HIV-seronegative TB patients. These results highlighted the complex interactions of NK cells during TB and/or HIV infection.

In our cohort of TB/HIV patients, only four of 33 (12.1%) patients developed paradoxical IRIS after cART initiation despite their severe immunodeficiency (median $CD4^+$ T cell absolute count: 57 cells/mm^3; IQR: 17–144), and high HIV viral loads (median: 5.64 Log_{10} copies/mL; IQR: 5.22–5.88) at study inclusion, besides the early initiation of cART after starting TB therapy, which are considered significant risk factors for IRIS development (53, 54). The IRIS frequency in this study is in accordance with that reported in our previous studies (28, 45), but differs from the frequencies observed in other populations. This finding reinforces the concept that the IRIS incidence varies according to the geographic region (11), and can be explained by the inclusion of patients with different genetic backgrounds.

Although many studies of HIV/TB patients who developed IRIS have led to the determination of the most prominent risk factors for development of this syndrome, such as a low $CD4^+$ T count before cART initiation followed by a successful $CD4^+$ T cell increase (55, 56), the underlying mechanisms responsible for IRIS have not been clearly defined. One of the most explored mechanisms is its association with the expansion of antigen-specific Th1 $CD4^+$ T cells shortly after cART initiation (16), although subsequent studies questioned whether this association could be considered truly causal (9). However, elements of the innate immune system, such as monocytes/macrophages, dendritic cells (DCs), neutrophils, γδ T lymphocytes, NK cells, and related soluble factors have also been implicated in the onset of IRIS, and have been the focus of important investigations (17, 21, 22, 24, 26, 57).

One clinical trial in Cambodia reported a significantly higher NK cell degranulation capacity in IRIS patients before cART and after 2 weeks of TB treatment than in non-IRIS patients, followed by decreased expression of NK cell activating receptors (NKp30, NKp46, and NKG2D) at IRIS onset (21). Although we diagnosed a small number of IRIS cases, we also identified alterations in the NK cell profile between the IRIS and non-IRIS patients. A decrease in the frequency of NK cells expressing NKp80 and NKG2C was observed in the TB/HIV non-IRIS patients, whereas these receptors were expressed at normal levels in the IRIS patients compared to those of the healthy controls. Moreover, the non-IRIS patients also presented a reduction of NK cells expressing the KIR receptor CD158a.

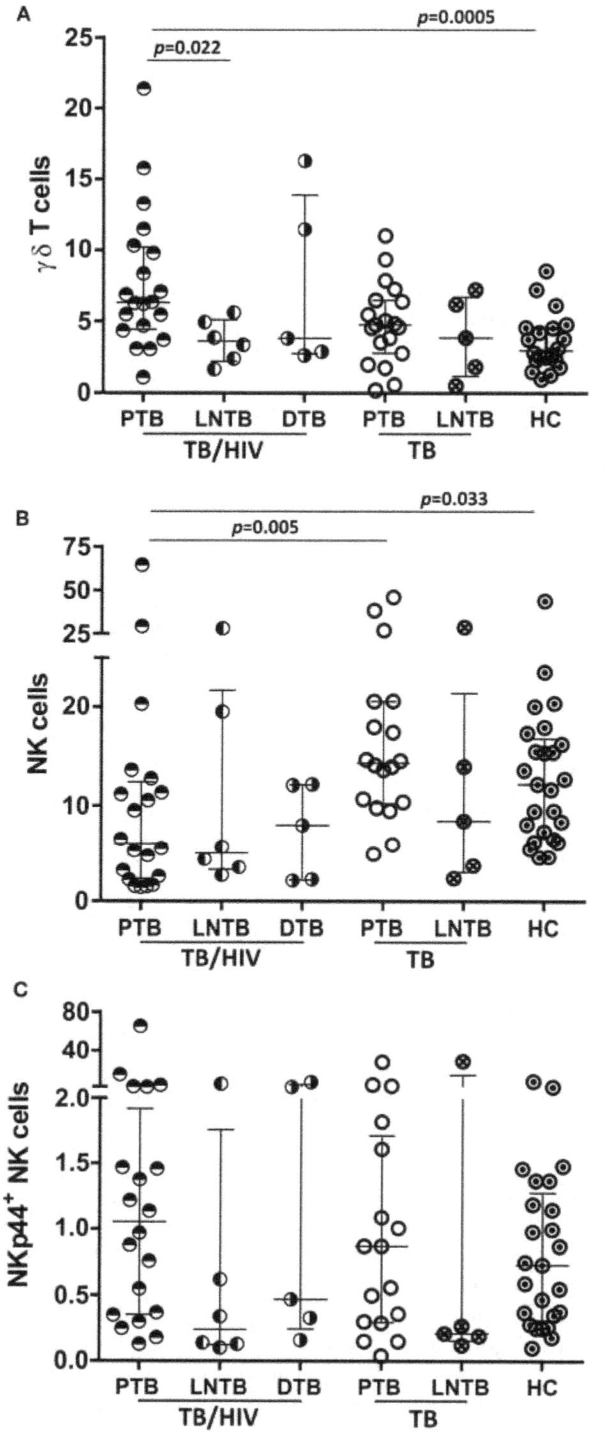

FIGURE 5 | Frequencies of NK and γδ T cells according to the TB clinical presentation. Percentages of **(A)** circulating γδ T cells **(B)** NK cells and **(C)** the NKp44$^+$ NK subset (among the total NK cells) in the TB/HIV and TB groups according to pulmonary (PTB: TB/HIV, $n = 20$; TB, $n = 20$), lymph node (LNTB: TB/HIV, $n = 6$; TB, $n = 5$) or disseminated (DTB: TB/HIV, $n = 5$) clinical presentations of tuberculosis and compared to those of the healthy controls (HC, $n = 25$). The results are presented as the median and interquartiles (25th–75th percentile). The data were analyzed using the Mann-Whitney *U* test. Significant *p*-values ($p < 0.05$) are indicated.

Recently, NKp80 expression was closely related to NK cell functional maturity in secondary lymphocyte tissues, suggesting an important regulatory role for this receptor during the maturation process at those sites that were potentially related to the acquisition of NK cell functionality (cytotoxicity and/or cytokine production) (58). Thus, a loss of this marker could be related to lower NK cell functions in non-IRIS patients. However, we did not find a correlation between the degranulation capacity of NK cells, and expression of the NKp80 marker in the non-IRIS patients (results not shown). NK cells expressing the NKG2C activating receptor have been described as an NK memory-like population against multiple viral infections, especially cytomegalovirus but also viruses such as simian immunodeficiency virus (59–62). Moreover, the NKG2C$^+$ NK population has been suggested to have adaptive properties against *Mtb* and to be able to discriminate between latent and active tuberculosis (increased proportions in latent tuberculosis) (63). The decrease in NKG2C$^+$ NK cells observed in the non-IRIS patients suggests lower NK cell recognition of HIV- and/or TB-infected cells. When considered together with the decrease in NKp46 expression, the NK cell receptors implicated in lysis of TB-infected target cells (64) could explain the lower inflammatory response in this group of patients. In turn, the CD158a/KIR2DL1 receptor acquires its inhibitory function during the developmental licensing process of NK cells, and the absence of this type of receptor during NK cell development has been associated with less functional competence to respond to the lack of HLA ligands on a target cell (65, 66). By contrast, the expression levels of the above-cited receptors in IRIS patients are similar to those observed in the HC group (higher than in the non-IRIS patients) and might suggest a more preserved NK cell repertoire in IRIS patients, who could mount an increased inflammatory response.

In the present study, we also identified alterations in γδ T cells in TB/HIV patients similar to those observed in untreated individuals with chronic HIV-1 infections (67). Higher γδ T cell frequencies were observed in TB/HIV patients than in the healthy controls, with the expansion of the γδ T cell subset expressing the Vδ chain rather than Vδ2 and a low Vδ2$^+$/Vδ2$^-$ ratio. Although not observed in the present study, a higher frequency of Vδ2$^+$ T cells was shown in TB/HIV IRIS patients compared to that of non-IRIS patients (17). Interestingly, when we analyzed γδ T cells and their relationship with the clinical presentations of TB, we identified greater mobilization of γδ T cells in TB/HIV patients presenting pulmonary TB that was not observed with either TB/HIV lymph node TB presentation or in the HCs and was almost higher than that in the HIV-seronegative TB patients. γδ T cells, especially Vδ2$^+$ T cells, have been widely reported to play an important role in protective immune responses to *Mtb* infection. These cells are expanded early during *Mtb* infection and are inclusive in recently acquired latent infection (68–70). In non-human primates, these cells even attenuate TB pathology and contain lesions primarily in the infection site of the lung, with no or reduced TB dissemination (71). However, in our study, the γδ T population in the TB/HIV patients was predominantly composed of Vδ2$^-$ cells, as previously reported. In our study, these cells may be engaged in the immune response

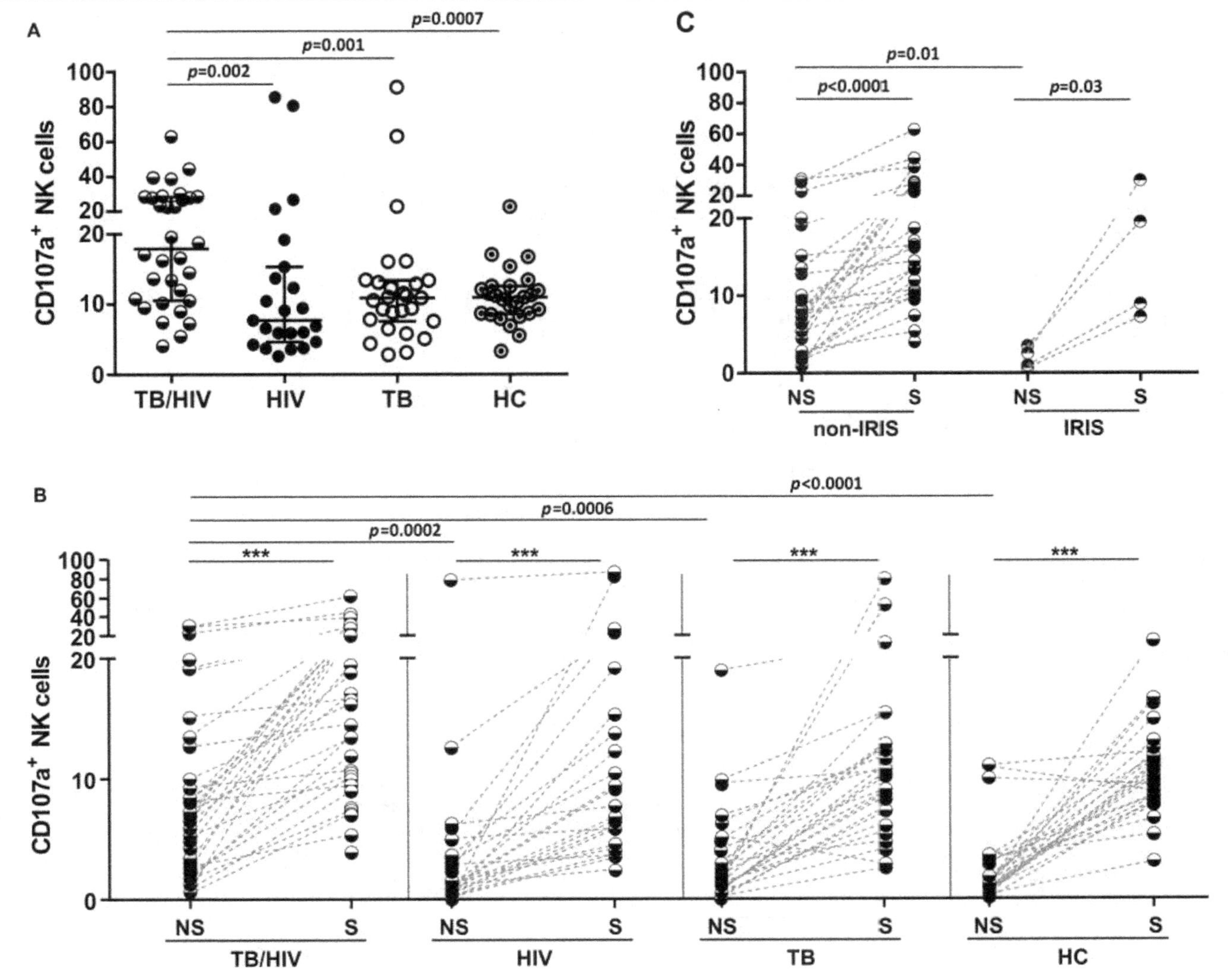

FIGURE 6 | Degranulation capacity of NK cells before TB and/or cART treatment. Frequencies of $CD107a^+$ NK cells at D0 in **(A)** TB/HIV co-infected patients, HIV mono-infected (HIV) patients, TB cases (TB) and healthy controls (HCs) after stimulation with the target cell line, **(B)** in TB/HIV IRIS and non-IRIS patients, and **(C)** under non-stimulated (NS) and stimulated (S) conditions with K562 target cells. The results are shown as **(A)** the median and interquartiles (25th–75th percentile). The data were analyzed using the Mann-Whitney *U* test, for intergroup analysis or the Wilcoxon *t*-test for intragroup analysis. Significant *p*-values ($p < 0.05$) are indicated. $^{***}p < 0.0001$.

against pulmonary TB presentation and may be important innate immune players involved in containment of *Mtb* infection in the lungs in the absence of therapeutic intervention.

In relation to another important lymphocyte population involved in regulatory/effector functions, the iNKT cells (40–42, 72), no significant differences were observed in the present study when TB/HIV patients were compared with the control groups (TB, HIV and HC), as well among the TB clinical forms, onset of IRIS, TB outcomes, or throughout the 6 month of follow-up under TB-treatment and cART, differing from previous studies showing reduced frequency of iNKT cells in HIV, TB or TB/HIV patients compared with healthy controls (73, 74), and between IRIS and non-IRIS cases (74). Historically, the iNKT cells were originally identified with the Vα24 and Vβ11 mAb (75, 76), but it was later shown that the combination of these two selective reactivities did not formally define this population accurately (71, 77). In the present study, iNKT cells were accurately analyzed as $V\alpha24J\alpha18^+$ cells, using the monoclonal antibody 6B11, in the context of the $CD3^+CD56^+$ population, as supported by vast literature (40–42, 78). However, it has been further shown that not all iNKT cells are $CD56^+$ (72). In this sense, we re-analyzed the $V\alpha24J\alpha18^+$ cells in the context of the $CD3^+$ population and, similarly, the obtained results did not show significant differences in the frequency of this population among the studied groups and/or clinical conditions.

We also investigated the *in vitro* degranulation and cytokine production potential of NK cells from TB/HIV patients. We observed a higher degranulation capacity in TB/HIV patients

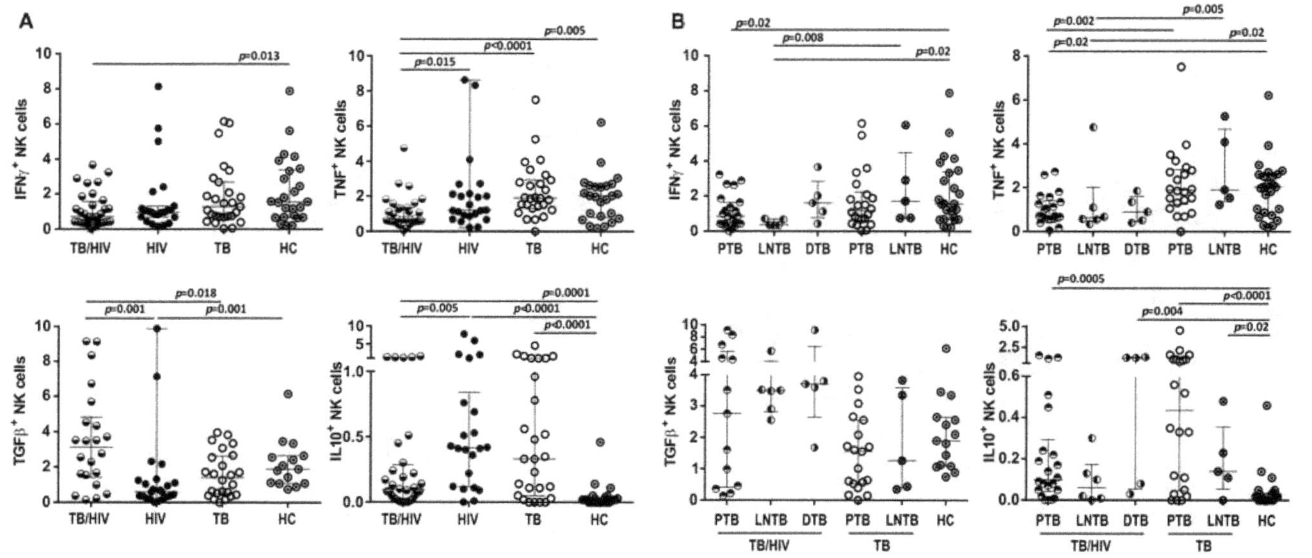

FIGURE 7 | Frequencies of NK cells producing intracellular cytokines under *in vitro* stimulation. Percentages of IFN-γ^+, TNF$^+$, TGF-β^+, and IL-10^+ NK cells after stimulation with target cells at D0 in **(A)** the TB/HIV co-infected, HIV mono-infected (HIV), TB-only (TB) and healthy control (HC) groups, **(B)** according to the TB clinical presentation as pulmonary (PTB), lymph node (LNTB), and disseminated TB in TB/HIV co-infected patients and for PTB and LNTB in the TB-only patients. The results are presented as the median and interquartiles (25th–75th percentile). The data were analyzed using the Mann-Whitney *U* test. Significant *p*-values ($p < 0.05$) are indicated.

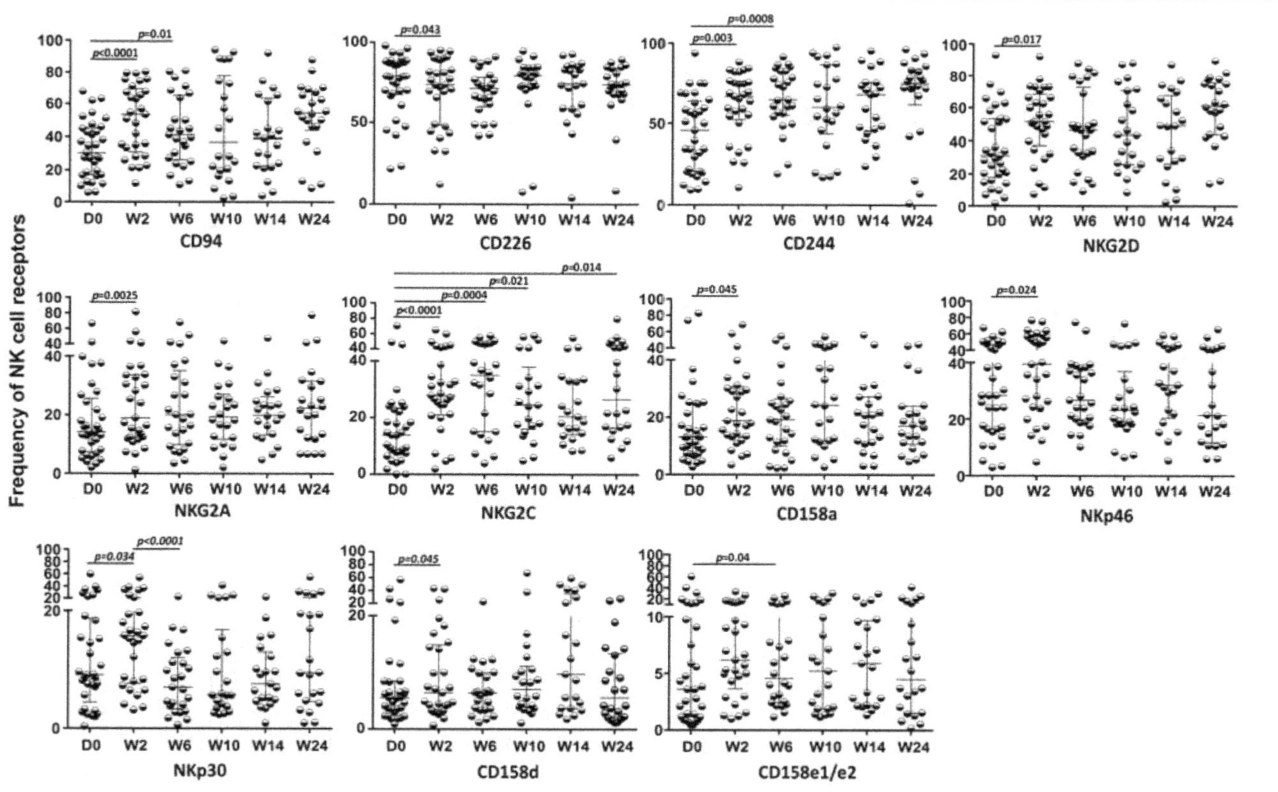

FIGURE 8 | Expression of NK cell receptors during follow-up in the TB/HIV co-infected patients. Expression of different NK receptors in the TB/HIV patients before and after treatment intervention (anti-TB at day 0 and cART at week 2) and at weeks (W) 2, 6, 10, 14, and 24. The results are represented as the median and interquartiles (25th–75th percentile). The data were analyzed using the Wilcoxon *t*-test. Significant *p*-values ($p < 0.05$) are indicated.

than in the other groups. Different from the results obtained in the study in Cambodia (21), we did not observe differences in the CD107a$^+$ NK cell frequencies between the IRIS and non-IRIS patients after *in vitro* stimulation with a target cell line or not. However, the results from Cambodia were obtained after 2 weeks of TB treatment and before cART initiation, whereas in our study, the degranulation capacity was assessed before any treatment intervention. Moreover, we did not detect an increase in degranulation capacity of NK cells after 2 weeks of TB treatment or later (during the follow-up under cART and TB treatment). Although *in vivo* NK cell activation was observed in our study groups (based on an increase in some activation markers and degranulation without any activation) similar to that in the Capri NK study (21), we should consider other factors, such as differences either on genetic backgrounds and/or local endemic pathogens able to stimulate innate immunity. Interestingly, spontaneous CD107a$^+$ expression was significantly lower in the IRIS than in the non-IRIS patients. The spontaneous NK cell degranulation observed in the non-IRIS TB/HIV patients may result from a skewed NK repertoire. Consistent with this observation, the lower frequency of CD158a$^+$ NK cells observed in these patients could be related to a more immature profile among these individuals compared to the more regulated and lower CD107a$^+$ NK cell expression levels detected in the IRIS patients.

Although NK cells regulate immune responses through cytokines secretion (79), there are few reports describing the NK regulatory cytokine secretion patterns in TB/HIV patients (80). In our study, TB/HIV patients showed a lower frequency of intracellular IFN-γ-producing NK cells compared to the HC group, as well as of TNF- compared to HIV, TB, and HC groups. On the other hand, the frequency TGF-β- or IL-10-producing NK cells in the TB/HIV group was significantly higher than that in the HIV and TB patients. These results reflect the interplay between pro-inflammatory and regulatory cytokines in TB/HIV patients and could indicate the establishment of regulatory mechanisms to control the exacerbated inflammatory response by the innate immune system in TB/HIV patients. Similar to our results, lower frequency of NK intracellular pro-inflammatory cytokines, IFN-γ and TNF-, were observed in TB/HIV patients from India compared to healthy controls (80).

We observed that several NK cell receptors were enhanced during the two first weeks of TB treatment. There is no report of NK cell repertoire modifications after 2 weeks of TB treatment in patients infected with TB/HIV or TB alone. Only one communication has studied modifications of NK receptors after 6 months of TB treatment in pulmonary TB (51). Although recovery of NK cell function was observed, perturbations of the NK cell repertoire were still present at the endpoint of the study (51). We do not have a full explanation for this discrepancy, but genetic factors may be differently implicated in these cohorts. For the TB/HIV study group, cART was started in the second week of TB treatment, and the patients were followed in the study until the end of TB treatment at week 24. Despite the CD4$^+$ T cell recovery and control of HIV-1 replication, cART had a low or no impact on the NK cell repertoire. Similarly, other reports were not able to show the recovery of NK cells despite

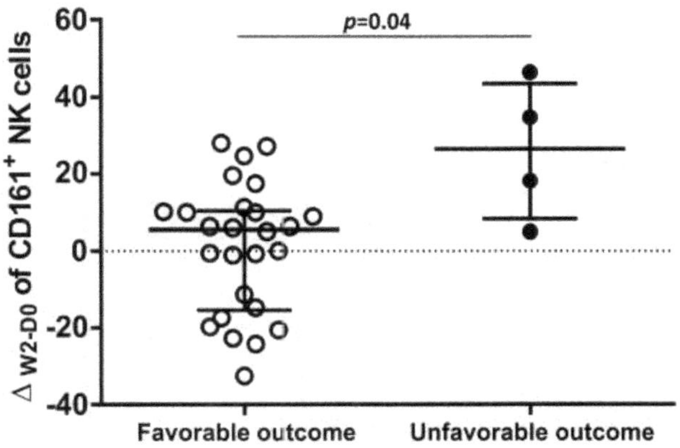

FIGURE 9 | Distribution of Δ_{W2-D0} for CD161$^+$ NK cells. Frequencies obtained for the differences in CD161$^+$ NK cell expression between D0 and week 2 (W2) in TB/HIV patients analyzed based on favorable (n = 26) or unfavorable (n = 5) clinical outcomes. The results are presented as the median and interquartiles (25th–75th percentile). The data were analyzed using the Mann-Whitney U test. A significant p-value ($p < 0.05$) is indicated.

the long cART follow-up period (up to 85 months), with viral replication suppression and increased levels on CD4$^+$ T counts (9). Moreover, recovery of the NK cell repertoire during cART has been described (81), but the restoration takes more time than the recovery of CD4$^+$ T cells, in particular when the CD4$^+$ T- counts are very low, like in our study. Our limited follow-up did not allow us the observation of late modifications in the NK cell repertoire and functions. However, early modifications induced during TB treatment alone showed that patients with an unfavorable outcome presented a higher frequency of CD161$^+$ NK cells than patients with a favorable TB recovery outcome. CD161 is a marker of human IL-17-producing T cell subsets, and its expression marks pro-inflammatory NK cells with high cytokine responsiveness that may contribute to inflammatory disease pathogenesis (82–84). Induction of modifications such as those reported here was observed after IL-10 treatment of PBMCs, including induction of higher CD161 marker expression on NK cells (84, 85). Although the treatment schedule used in this study was related to a reduced risk of death (52), five of the 33 HIV/TB patients presented this unfavorable outcome, and the NK cells with a pro-inflammatory profile observed in these TB/HIV patients could have participated in this process.

Our study has some limitations. The main limitation was the low numbers of IRIS TB/HIV patients, patients with lymph node and disseminated TB presentation, and unfavorable outcomes/death, which possibly were due to the low number of TB/HIV patients recruited during the study period even though the city of Rio de Janeiro is an endemic region for tuberculosis. Indeed, the recruitment of a larger number of the TB/HIV patients, as initially planned, was not achieved along the period of the study support, possibly due to the implementation by the Brazilian Ministry of Health of the free early access to antiretrovirals in the recent years, independently of the CD4$^+$ T-cell counts and clinical conditions, and also INH prophylaxis for some HIV-infected patients, restricting

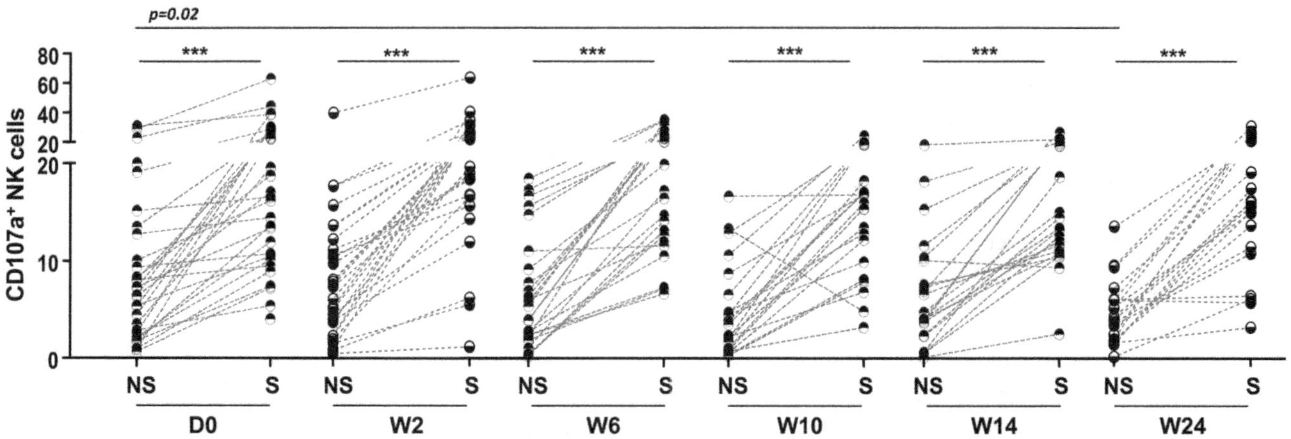

FIGURE 10 | Degranulation capacity of NK cells during the study follow-up. Frequencies of $CD107a^+$ NK cells detected in TB/HIV co-infected patients before and after treatment intervention under non-stimulated (NS) or stimulated (S) conditions with K562 target cells. The data were analyzed using the Wilcoxon *t*-test. Significant *p*-values ($p < 0.05$) are indicated. $^{***}p < 0.0001$.

our access to participants with $CD4^+$ T-cell counts <200 cells/mm^3, a inclusion criteria to the TB/HIV and the HIV patients (86). Because of the sample size, multivariate analyses were not carried out, which restricted the statistical analysis to univariate analyses. Future investigations are necessary to prove the concepts observed and discussed here, such as the association of IRIS development in TB/HIV patients with a more conserved and specialized NK cell profile, the relationship of $\gamma\delta$ T cells with the immune response in patients with pulmonary TB presentation, and the involvement of pro-inflammatory NK cells with an unfavorable outcome of TB/HIV coinfection.

AUTHOR CONTRIBUTIONS

CG-G, JP, MM, and DS-A conceptualized and designed the study and also contributed to the experimental design and provided intellectual input. CG-G, AC, and TdS performed sample processing and clinical data analysis and provided intellectual input. CG-G and AC performed the experiments. VR, JP, TB, FS, and CS enrolled the patients and provided clinical data. CG-G, JdM, and JS performed the statistical analysis. AB provided ethical and regulatory support. CG-G, MM and DS-A analyzed the data and wrote the manuscript. All authors reviewed and approved the final version of the manuscript.

ACKNOWLEDGMENTS

We thank the patients who participated in the study and all staff from the blood collection sectors from the National Institute of Infectious Diseases Evandro Chagas and Nova Iguaçu General Hospital. We also thank Michelle das Neves and Priscilla Guimarães from the CD4 count and viral load clinical services of the Laboratory of AIDS and Molecular Immunology, IOC-Fiocruz. Finally, we thank Thaize Quiroga, MSc from the Flow Cytometry Sorting Core Facility, IOC-FIOCRUZ, and the Flow Cytometry Core of the Central Laboratory from the National Institute of Infectious Diseases Evandro Chagas—FIOCRUZ.

SUPPLEMENTARY MATERIAL

Supplementary Figure 1 | Definition of iNKT ($V\alpha24J\alpha18^+$) cells on $CD3^+$ T lymphocytes and on the $CD56^+CD3^+$ cells. **(A)** An initial gate defined the lymphocytes, in a forward scatter (FSC) vs. side scatter (SSC) dot plot. Then, a $CD3^+$ gate was established in a $CD56^{+/-}$ vs. $CD3^+$ dot plot, and used to define the $CD3^+$ iNKT cells in the $V\alpha24J\alpha18^+$ *vs.* $CD3^+$ dot plot. In parallel, the same $CD3^+$ gate was used to gate the $CD3^+CD56^+$ cells, from which the $CD3^+CD56^+$ vs. $V\alpha24J\alpha18^+$ dot plot defined the iNKT cells. **(B)** analysis of iNKT cells among the TB/HIV ($n = 33$), HIV ($n = 25$), TB ($n = 27$), and HC ($n = 25$) groups, before any therapeutic intervention, based on the $CD3^+CD56^+V\alpha24J\alpha18^+$ or $CD3^+$ $V\alpha24J\alpha18^+$ populations.

Supplementary Table 1 | Clinical characteristics of the TB/HIV IRIS patients.

Supplementary Table 2 | Medians and interquartile ranges (IQRs) of the circulating NK cell repertoire frequencies.

REFERENCES

1. WHO. *Global Tuberculosis Report.* (2018). Vol. 69. Available online at: https://www.who.int/tb/publications/global_report/en/ (accessed February 15, 2019).
2. *WHO Fact Sheets on TB.* (2018). Available online at: https://www.who.int/news-room/fact-sheets/detail/tuberculosis (accessed February 16, 2019).
3. *Boletim Epidemiológico 2008-2016.* (2016). Available online at: http://www.prefeitura.rio/documents/73801/181dbb1c-78db-4a95-a709-5888f93bdfd2 (accessed February 21, 2019).
4. Boletim Epidemiológico, Secretaria de Vigilância em Saúde, Ministério da Saúde. *Coinfecção TB-HIV No Brasil: Panorama Epidemiológico E Atividades Colaborativas.* (2017). Available online at: http://www.aids.gov.br/pt-br/pub/2017/coinfeccao-tb-hiv-no-brasil-panorama-epidemiologico-e-atividades-colaborativas-2017 (accessed February 25, 2019).
5. Boletim Epidemiológico 37. *Secretaria de Vigilância Em Saúde, Ministério Da Saúde. v. 49.* (2018). Available online at: http://portalarquivos2.saude.gov.br/images/pdf/2018/setembro/05/2018-041.pdf (accessed February 26, 2019).

6. Cohen K, Meintjes G. Management of individuals requiring antiretroviral therapy and TB treatment. *Curr Opin HIV AIDS.* (2010) 5:61–9. doi: 10.1097/COH.0b013e3283339309
7. Ravimohan S, Tamuhla N, Steenhoff AP, Letlhogile R, Nfanyana K, Bellamy SL, et al. Immunological profiling of tuberculosis-associated immune reconstitution inflammatory syndrome and non-immune reconstitution inflammatory syndrome death in HIV-infected adults with pulmonary tuberculosis starting antiretroviral therapy: a prospective obse. *Lancet Infect Dis.* (2015) 15:429–38. doi: 10.1016/S1473-3099(15)70008-3
8. Worodria W, Menten J, Massinga-Loembe M, Mazakpwe D, Bagenda D, Koole O, et al. TB-IRIS Study Group. Clinical spectrum, risk factors and outcome of immune reconstitution inflammatory syndrome in patients with tuberculosis-HIV coinfection. *Antivir Ther.* (2012) 17:841–8. doi: 10.3851/IMP2108
9. Lai RP, Nakiwala JK, Meintjes G, Wilkinson RJ. The Immunopathogenesis of the HIV tuberculosis immune reconstitution inflammatory syndrome. *Eur J Immunol.* (2013) 43:1995–2002. doi: 10.1002/eji.201343632
10. Luetkemeyer AF, Kendall MA, Nyirenda M, Wu X, Ive P, Benson CA, et al. Tuberculosis immune reconstitution inflammatory syndrome in A5221 STRIDE: timing, severity, and implications for HIV-TB programs. *J Acquir Immune Defic Syndr.* (2014) 65:423–8. doi: 10.1097/QAI.0000000000000030
11. Walker NF, Scriven J, Meintjes G, Wilkinson RJ. Immune reconstitution inflammatory syndrome in HIV-infected patients. *HIV/AIDS.* (2015) 7:49–64. doi: 10.2147/HIV.S42328
12. Walker NF, Stek C, Wasserman S, Wilkinson RJ, Meintjes G. The tuberculosis-associated immune reconstitution inflammatory syndrome: recent advances in clinical and pathogenesis research. *Curr Opin HIV AIDS.* (2018) 13:512–21. doi: 10.1097/COH.0000000000000502
13. Ruhwald M, Ravn P. Immune reconstitution syndrome in tuberculosis and HIV-co-infected patients: Th1 explosion or cytokine storm? *AIDS.* (2007) 21:882–4. doi: 10.1097/QAD.0b013e3280b079c8
14. Conesa-Botella A, Meintjes G, Coussens AK, Van Der Plas H, Goliath R, Schutz C, et al. Corticosteroid therapy, vitamin D status, and inflammatory cytokine profile in the HIV-tuberculosis immune reconstitution inflammatory syndrome. *Clin Infect Dis.* (2012) 55:1004–11. doi: 10.1093/cid/cis577
15. Barber DL, Andrade BB, McBerry C, Sereti I, Sher A. Role of IL-6 in *Mycobacterium avium*-associated immune reconstitution inflammatory syndrome. *J Immunol.* (2013) 192:676–82. doi: 10.4049/jimmunol.1301004
16. Bourgarit A, Carcelain G, Martinez V, Lascoux C, Delcey V, Gicquel G, et al. Explosion of tuberculin-specific Th1-responses induces immune restoration syndrome in tuberculosis and HIV co-infected patients. *AIDS.* (2006) 20:F1–7. doi: 10.1097/01.aids.0000202648.18526.bf
17. Bourgarit A, Carcelain G, Samri A, Parizot C, Lafaurie M, Abgrall S, et al. Tuberculosis-associated immune restoration syndrome in HIV-1-infected patients involves tuberculin-specific CD4 Th1 cells and KIR-negative T cells. *J Immunol.* (2009) 183:3915–23. doi: 10.4049/jimmunol.0804020
18. Meintjes G, Wilkinson KA, Rangaka MX, Skolimowska K, Van Veen K, Abrahams M, et al. Type 1 helper T cells and FoxP3-positive T cells in HIV-tuberculosis- associated immune reconstitution inflammatory syndrome. *Am J Respir Crit Care Med.* (2008) 178:1083–9. doi: 10.1164/rccm.200806-858OC
19. Silva TP, Giacoia-Gripp CBW, Schmaltz CA, Sant'Anna FM, Saad MH, de Matos JA, et al. Risk factors for increased immune reconstitution in response to *Mycobacterium tuberculosis* antigens in tuberculosis HIV-infected, antiretroviral-naïve patients. *BMC Infect Dis.* (2017) 17:606. doi: 10.1186/s12879-017-2700-6
20. Conradie F, Foulkes AS, Ive P, Yin X, Roussos K, Glencross DK, et al. Natural killer cell activation distinguishes *Mycobacterium tuberculosis*-mediated immune reconstitution syndrome from chronic HIV and HIV/MTB coinfection. *J Acquir Immune Defic Syndr.* (2011) 58:309–18. doi: 10.1097/QAI.0b013e31822e0d15
21. Pean P, Nerrienet E, Madec Y, Borand L, Laureillard D, Fernandez M, et al. Natural killer cell degranulation capacity predicts early onset of the immune reconstitution inflammatory syndrome (IRIS) in HIV-infected patients with tuberculosis. *Blood.* (2012) 119:3315–20. doi: 10.1182/blood-2011-09-377523
22. Andrade BB, Singh A, Narendran G, Schechter ME, Nayak K, Subramanian S, et al. Mycobacterial antigen driven activation of CD14++CD16- monocytes is a predictor of tuberculosis-associated immune reconstitution inflammatory syndrome. *PLoS Pathog.* (2014) 10:e1004433. doi: 10.1371/journal.ppat.1004433
23. Lai RPJ, Meintjes G, Wilkinson KA, Graham CM, Marais S, Van der Plas H, et al. HIV-Tuberculosis-associated immune reconstitution inflammatory syndrome is characterized by toll-like receptor and inflammasome signalling. *Nat Commun.* (2015) 6:8451. doi: 10.1038/ncomms9451
24. Tan HY, Yong YK, Andrade BB, Shankar E, Ponnampalavanar S, Omar S, et al. Plasma interleukin-18 levels are a biomarker of innate immune responses that predict and characterize tuberculosis-associated immune reconstitution inflammatory syndrome. *AIDS.* (2015) 29:421–31. doi: 10.1097/QAD.0000000000000557
25. Tan HY, Yong YK, Shankar EM, Paukovics G, Ellegård R, Larsson M, et al. aberrant inflammasome activation characterizes tuberculosis-associated immune reconstitution inflammatory syndrome. *J Immunol.* (2016) 196:4052–63. doi: 10.4049/jimmunol.1502203
26. Nakiwala, JK, Walker NF, Diedrich CR, Worodria W, Meintjes G, Wilkinson RJ, et al. Neutrophil activation and enhanced release of granule products in HIV-TB immune reconstitution inflammatory syndrome. *J Acquir Immune Defic Syndr.* (2018) 77:221–9. doi: 10.1097/QAI.0000000000001582
27. Raviglione MC, Narain JP, Kochi A. HIV-associated tuberculosis in developing countries: clinical features, diagnosis, and treatment. *Bull World Health Organ.* (1992) 70:515–26.
28. Silva TP, Giacoia-Gripp CBW, Schmaltz CA, Sant' Anna FM, Rolla V, Morgado MG. T cell activation and cytokine profile of tuberculosis and HIV-positive individuals during antituberculous treatment and efavirenz-based regimens. *PLoS ONE.* (2013) 8:e0066095. doi: 10.1371/journal.pone.0066095
29. WHO. *Tuberculosis Fact Sheet.* (2015). Available online at: http://www.who.int/mediacentre/factsheets/fs104/en/http://www.who.int/mediacentre/facsheets/fs104/en/ (accessed March 3, 2019).
30. Krishnan N, Robertson BD, Thwaites G. The mechanisms and consequences of the extra-pulmonary dissemination of *Mycobacterium tuberculosis. Tuberculosis.* (2010) 90:361–6. doi: 10.1016/j.tube.2010.08.005
31. Leeds IL, Magee MJ, Kurbatova EV, Rio C, Blumberg HM, Leonard MK, et al. Site of extrapulmonary tuberculosis is associated with HIV infection. *Clin Infect Dis.* (2012) 55:75–81. doi: 10.1093/cid/cis303
32. Ayed HB, Koubaa M, Marrakchi C, Rekik K, Hammami F, Smaoui F, et al. Extrapulmonary tuberculosis: update on the epidemiology, risk factors and prevention strategies. *Int J Trop Dis.* (2018) 1:006. doi: 10.23937/ijtd-2017/1710006
33. Cantres-Fonseca OJ, Rodriguez-Cintrón W, Olmo-Arroyo FD, Baez-Corujo S. *Extra Pulmonary Tuberculosis: An Overview, Role of Microbes in Human Health and Diseases (December 10th 2018), Nar Singh Chauhan.* IntechOpen (2018). Available online at: https://www.intechopen.com/books/role-of-microbes-in-human-health-and-diseases/extra-pulmonary-tuberculosis-an-overview. doi: 10.5772/intechopen.81322
34. Yang D, Kong Y. The bacterial and host factors associated with extrapulmonary dissemination of *Mycobacterium tuberculosis. Front Biol.* (2015) 10:252–61. doi: 10.1007/s11515-015-1358-y
35. Ministério da Saúde. *Protocolo Clínico E Diretrizes Terapêuticas Para O Manejo Da Infecção Pelo HIV Em Adultos.* (2018). Available online at: http://www.aids.gov.br/pt-br/pub/2013/protocolo-clinico-e-diretrizes-terapeuticas-para-manejo-da-infeccao-pelo-hiv-em-adultos (accessed March 9, 2019).
36. Ministério da Saúde, Comitê Técnico Assessor do Programa Nacional de Controle da Tuberculos. *Manual de Recomendações para o Controle da Tuberculose no Brasil. Ministério da Saúde, Secretaria de Vigilância em Saúde, Departamento de Vigilância Epidemiológica.* (2011). 284p. Available online at: http://bvsms.saude.gov.br/bvs/publicacoes/manual_recomendacoes_controle_tuberculose_brasil.pdf (accessed March 30, 2019).
37. Demitto FO, Schmaltz CAS, Sant'Anna FM, Arriaga MB, Andrade BB, Rolla VC. Predictors of early mortality and effectiveness of antiretroviral therapy in TB-HIV patients from Brazil. *PLoS ONE.* (2019) 14:e0217014. doi: 10.1371/journal.pone.0217014
38. Robertson J, Meier M, Wall J, Ying J, Fichtenbaum CJ. Immune reconstitution syndrome in HIV: validating a case definition and identifying clinical predictors in persons initiating antiretroviral therapy. *Clin Infect Dis.* (2006) 42:1639–46. doi: 10.1086/503903

39. Meintjes G, Lawn SD, Scano F, Maartens G, French MA, Worodria W, et al. Tuberculosis-associated immune reconstitution inflammatory syndrome: case definitions for use in resource-limited settings. *Lancet Infect Dis.* (2008) 8:516–23. doi: 10.1016/S1473-3099(08)70184-1
40. Montoya CJ, Pollard D, Martinson J, Kumari K, Wasserfall C, Mulder CB, et al. Characterization of human invariant natural killer t subsets in health and disease using a novel invariant natural killer T cell-clonotypic monoclonal antibody, 6B11. *Immunology.* (2007) 122:1–14. doi: 10.1111/j.1365-2567.2007.02647.x
41. Exley MA, Hou R, Shaulov A, Tonti E, Dellabona P, Casorati G, et al. Selective activation, expansion, and monitoring of human iNKT cells with a monoclonal antibody specific for the TCR alpha-chain CDR3 loop. *Eur J Immunol.* (2008) 38:1756–66. doi: 10.1002/eji.200737389
42. Lenart M, Gruca A, Mueck A, Rutkowska-Zapała M, Surman M, Szaflarska A, et al. Comparison of 6B11 mAb and α-GalCer-loaded CD1d dextramers for detection of iNKT cells by flow cytometry. *J Immunol Methods.* (2017) 446:1–6. doi: 10.1016/j.jim.2017.03.016
43. Alter G, Malenfant JM, Altfeld M. CD107a as a functional marker for the identification of natural killer cell activity. *J Immunol Methods.* (2004) 294:15–22. doi: 10.1016/j.jim.2004.08.008
44. Spiess AN, Feig C, Ritz C. Highly accurate sigmoidal fitting of real-time PCR data by introducing a parameter for asymmetry. *BMC Bioinformatics.* (2008) 9:221. doi: 10.1186/1471-2105-9-221
45. Serra FC, Hadad D, Orofino RL, Marinho F, Lourenço C, Morgado M, et al. Immune Reconstitution syndrome in patients treated for HIV and tuberculosis in Rio de Janeiro. *Braz J Infect Dis.* (2007) 11:462–5. doi: 10.1590/S1413-86702007000500004
46. Lawn SD, Meintjes G, McIlleron H, Harries AD, Wood R. Management of HIV-associated tuberculosis in resource-limited settings: a state-of-the-art review. *BMC Med.* (2013) 11:253. doi: 10.1186/1741-7015-11-253
47. Mavilio D, Benjamin J, Daucher M, Lombardo G, Kottilil S, Planta MA, et al. Natural killer cells in HIV-1 infection: dichotomous effects of viremia on inhibitory and activating receptors and their functional correlates. *Proc Natl Acad Sci USA.* (2003) 100:15011–6. doi: 10.1073/pnas.2336091100
48. Wong AHW, Williams K, Reddy S, Wilson D, Giddy J, Alter G, et al. Alterations in natural killer cell receptor profiles during HIV type 1 disease progression among chronically infected South African adults. *AIDS Res Hum Retroviruses.* (2010) 26:459–69. doi: 10.1089/aid.2009.0176
49. Vankayalapati R, Garg A, Porgador A, Griffith DE, Klucar P, Safi H, et al. Role of NK cell-activating receptors and their ligands in the lysis of mononuclear phagocytes infected with an intracellular bacterium. *J Immunol.* (2005) 175:4611–7. doi: 10.4049/jimmunol.175.7.4611
50. Méndez A, Granda H, Meenagh A, Contreras S, Zavaleta R, Mendoza MF, et al. Study of KIR genes in tuberculosis patients. *Tissue Antigens.* (2006) 68:386389. doi: 10.1111/j.1399-0039.2006.00685.x
51. Bozzano F, Costa P, Passalacqua G, Dodi F, Ravera S, Pagano, et al. Functionally relevant decreases in activatory receptor expression on NK cells are associated with pulmonary tuberculosis *in vivo* and persist after successful treatment. *Int Immunol.* (2009) 21:779–91. doi: 10.1093/intimm/dxp046
52. Pydi SS, Sunder SR, Venkatasubramanian S, Kovvali S, Jonnalagada S, Valluri VL. Killer cell immunoglobulin like receptor gene association with tuberculosis. *Hum Immunol.* (2013) 74:85–92. doi: 10.1016/j.humimm.2012.10.006
53. Blanc FX, Sok T, Laureillard D, Borand L, Rekacewicz C, Nerrienet E, et al. Earlier versus later start of antiretroviral therapy in HIV-infected adults with uberculosis. *N Engl J Med.* (2011) 365:1471–81. doi: 10.1056/NEJMoa 1013911
54. Abay SM, Deribe K, Reda AA, Biadgilign S, Datiko D, Assefa T, et al. The effect of early initiation of antiretroviral therapy in TB/HIV-coinfected patients: a systematic review and meta-analysis. *J Int Assoc Provid AIDS Care.* (2105) 14:560–70. doi: 10.1177/2325957415599210
55. Manabe YC, Campbell JD, Sydnor E, Moore RD. Immune reconstitution inflammatory syndrome: risk factors and treatment implications. *J Acquir Immune Defic Syndr.* (2007) 46:456–62. doi: 10.1097/QAI.0b013e3181 594c8c
56. Grant PM, Komarow L, Andersen J, Sereti Sanne I, Pahwa S, Lederman MM, et al. Risk factor analyses for immune reconstitution inflammatory syndrome in a randomized study of early vs. deferred ART during an Opportunistic Infection. *PLoS ONE.* (2010) 5:e11416. doi: 10.1371/journal.pone.0011416
57. Tan DBA, Lim A, Yong YK, Ponnampalavanar S, Omar S, Kamarulzaman A, et al. TLR2-induced cytokine responses may characterize HIV-infected patients experiencing mycobacterial immune restoration disease. *AIDS.* (2011) 25:1455–60. doi: 10.1097/QAD.0b013e328348fb18
58. Freud AG, Keller KA, Scoville SD, Mundy-Bosse BL, Cheng S, Youssef Y, et al. NKp80 defines a critical step during human natural killer cell development. *Cell Rep.* (2016) 16:379–91. doi: 10.1016/j.celrep.2016.05.095
59. Guma M, Budt M, Saez A, Brckalo T, Hengel H, Angulo A, et al. Expansion of CD94/NKG2C NK cells in response to human cytomegalovirus-infected fibroblasts. *Blood.* (2006) 107:3624–31. doi: 10.1182/blood-2005-09-3682
60. Bayard C, Lepetitcorps H, Roux A, Larsen M, Fastenackels S, Salle V, et al. Coordinated expansion of both memory T cells and NK cells in response to CMV infection in humans. *Eur J Immunol.* (2016) 46:1168–79. doi: 10.1002/eji.201546179
61. Wagner JA, Fehniger TA. Human adaptive natural killer cells: beyond NKG2C. *Trends Immunol.* (2016) 37:351–3. doi: 10.1016/j.it.2016.05.001
62. Ram DR, Manickam C, Hueber B, Itell HL, Permar SR, Varner V, et al. Tracking KLRC2 (NKG2C)+ memory-like NK cells in SIV+ and rhCMV+ rhesus macaques. *PLoS Pathog.* (2018) 14:e1007104. doi: 10.1371/journal.ppat.1007104
63. Garand M, Goodier M, Owolabi O, Donkor S, Kampmann B, Sutherland JS. Functional and phenotypic changes of natural killer cells in whole blood during *Mycobacterium tuberculosis* infection and disease. *Front Immunol.* (2018) 9:257. doi: 10.3389/fimmu.2018.00257
64. Vankayalapati R, Wizel B, Weis SE, Safi H, Lakey DL, Mandelboim O, et al. The NKp46 receptor contributes to NK cell lysis of mononuclear phagocytes infected with an intracellular bacterium. *J Immunol.* (2014) 168:3451–7. doi: 10.4049/jimmunol.168.7.3451
65. Anfossi N, André P, Guia S, Falk CS, Roetynck S, Stewart CA, et al. Human NK cell education by inhibitory receptors for MHC class I. *Immunity.* (2006) 25:331–42. doi: 10.1016/j.immuni.2006.06.013
66. Brodin P, Höglund P. Beyond licensing and disarming: a quantitative view on NK-cell education. *Eur J Immunol.* (2008) 38:2934–7. doi: 10.1002/eji.200838760
67. Bhatnagar N, Girard PM, Lopez-Gonzalez M, Didier C, Collias L, Jung C, et al. Potential role of Vδ2+ γδT cells in regulation of immune activation in primary HIV infection. *Front Immunol.* (2017) 8:1189. doi: 10.3389/fimmu.2017.01189
68. Chen ZW. Protective immune responses of major Vγ2Vδ2 T-cell subset in *M. tuberculosis* infection. *Curr Opin Immunol.* (2016) 42:105–12. doi: 10.1016/j.coi.2016.06.005
69. Janis EM, Kaufmann SHE, Schwartz RH, Pardoll DM. Activation of γδ T cells in the primary immune response to *Mycobacterium tuberculosis. Science.* (1989) 244:713–6. doi: 10.1126/science.2524098
70. Vorkas CK, Wipperman MF, Li K, Bean J, Bhattarai SK, Adamow M, et al. Mucosal-associated invariant and γδ T cell subsets respond to initial *Mycobacterium tuberculosis* infection. *JCI Insight.* (2018). 3:121899. doi: 10.1172/jci.insight.121899
71 Qaqish A, Huang D, Chen CY, Zhang Z, Wang R, Li S, et al. Adoptive transfer of phosphoantigen-specific γδ T cell subset attenuates *Mycobacterium tuberculosis* infection in nonhuman primates. *J Immunol.* (2017) 198:4753–63. doi: 10.4049/jimmunol.1602019
72. Berzins SP, Smyth MJ, Baxter AG. Presumed guilty: natural killer T cell defects and human disease. *Nat Rev Immunol.* (2011) 11:131–42. doi: 10.1038/nri2904
73. Montoya CJ, Cataño JC, Ramirez Z, Rugeles MT, Wilson SB, Landay AL. Invariant NKT cells from HIV-1 or *Mycobacterium tuberculosis*-infected patients express an activated phenotype. *Clin Immunol.* (2008) 127:1–6. doi: 10.1016/j.clim.2007.12.006
74. Walker NF, Opondo C, Meintjes G, Jhilmeet N, Friedland JS, Elkington PT, et al. Invariant natural killer T cell dynamics in HIV-associated tuberculosis. *Clin Infect Dis.* (2019) doi: 10.1093/cid/ciz501. [Epub ahead of print].
75. Porcelli S, Yockey CE, Brenner MB, Balk SP. Analysis of T cell antigen receptor (TCR) expression by human peripheral blood CD4-8- alpha/beta T cells demonstrates preferential use of several V beta genes and an invariant TCR alpha chain. *J Exp Med.* (1993) 178:1–16. doi: 10.1084/jem.178.1.1

76. Dellabona P, Padovan E, Casorati G, Brockhaus M, Lanzavecchia A. An invariant V alpha 24-J alpha Q/V beta 11 T cell receptor is expressed in all individuals by clonally expanded CD4-8- T cells. *J Exp Med.* (1994) 180:1171–6. doi: 10.1084/jem.180.3.1171
77. Godfrey DI, Hammond KJ, Poulton LD, Smyth MJ, Baxter AG. NKT cells: facts, functions and fallacies. *Immunol Today.* (2000) 21:573–83. doi: 10.1016/S0167-5699(00)01735-7
78. Fereidouni M, Jabbari AF, Mahmoudi M, Varasteh A, Farid HR. Comparison of two flow cytometric methods for detection of human invariant natural killer Q18 T cells (iNKT). *Iran J Immunol.* (2010) 7:1–7.
79. Perussia B. Lymphokine-activated killer cells, natural killer cells and cytokines. *Curr Opin Immunol.* (1991) 3:49–55. doi: 10.1016/0952-7915(91)90076-D
80. Ramana Rao PV, Rajasekaran S, Raja A. Natural killer cell-mediated cytokine response among HIV-positive south Indians with pulmonary tuberculosis. *J Interferon Cytokine Res.* (2010) 30:33–42. doi: 10.1089/jir.2009.0018
81. Frias M, Rivero-Juarez A, Gordon A, Camacho A, Cantisan S, Cuenca-Lopez F, et al. Persistence of pathological distribution of NK cells in HIV-infected patients with prolonged use of HAART and a sustained immune response. *PLoS ONE.* (2015) 10:e0121019. doi: 10.1371/journal.pone.0121019
82. Mikulak J, Oriolo F, Zaghi E, Di Vito C, Mavilio D. Natural killer cells in HIV-1 infection and therapy. *AIDS.* (2017) 31:2317–30. doi: 10.1097/QAD.0000000000001645
83. Maggi L, Santarlasci V, Capone M, Peired A, Frosali F, Crome SQ, et al. CD161 is a marker of all human IL-17-producing T-cell subsets and is induced by RORC. *Eur J Immunol.* (2010) 40:2174–81. doi: 10.1002/eji.200940257
84. Kurioka A, Cosgrove C, imoni Y, van Wilgenburg B, Geremia A, Björkander S, et al. CD161 defines a functionally distinct subset of pro-inflammatory natural killer cells. *Front Immunol.* (2018) 9:486. doi: 10.3389/fimmu.2018.00486
85. Parato KG, Kumar A, Badley AD, Sanchez-Dardon JL, Chambers KA, Young CD, et al. Normalization of natural killer cell function and phenotype with effective anti-HIV therapy and the role of IL-10. *AIDS.* (2002) 16:1251–6. doi: 10.1097/00002030-200206140-00007
86. Boletim Epidemiológico, Secretaria de Vigilância em Saúde, Ministério da Saúde. *HIV/AIDS 2018.* (2018). Available online at: http://www.aids.gov.br/pt-br/pub/2018/boletim-epidemiologico-hivaids-2018.~ (accessed July 10, 2019).

8

The Potential Protective Role of Vitamin D Supplementation on HIV-1 Infection

*Natalia Alvarez, Wbeimar Aguilar-Jimenez and Maria T. Rugeles**

Grupo Inmunovirología, Facultad de Medicina, Universidad de Antioquia (UdeA), Medellín, Colombia

***Correspondence:**
Maria T. Rugeles
maria.rugeles@udea.edu.co

HIV infection remains a global and public health issue with the incidence increasing in some countries. Despite the fact that combination antiretroviral therapy (cART) has decreased mortality and increased the life expectancy of HIV-infected individuals, non-AIDS conditions, mainly those associated with a persistent inflammatory state, have emerged as important causes of morbidity, and mortality despite effective antiviral therapy. One of the most common comorbidities in HIV-1 patients is Vitamin D (VitD) insufficiency, as VitD is a hormone that, in addition to its physiological role in mineral metabolism, has pleiotropic effects on immune regulation. Several reports have shown that VitD levels decrease during HIV disease progression and correlate with decreased survival rates, highlighting the importance of VitD supplementation during infection. An extensive review of 29 clinical studies of VitD supplementation in HIV-infected patients showed that regardless of cART, when VitD levels were increased to normal ranges, there was a decrease in inflammation, markers associated with bone turnover, and the risk of secondary hyperparathyroidism while the anti-bacterial response was increased. Additionally, in 3 of 7 studies, VitD supplementation led to an increase in CD4+ T cell count, although its effect on viral load was inconclusive since most patients were on cART. Similarly, previous evidence from our laboratory has shown that VitD can reduce the infection of CD4+ T cells *in vitro*. The effect of VitD supplementation on other HIV-associated conditions, such as cardiovascular diseases, dyslipidemia or hypertension, warrants further exploration. Currently, the available evidence suggests that there is a potential role for VitD supplementation in people living with HIV-1, however, comprehensive studies are required to define an adequate supplementation protocol for these individuals.

Keywords: HIV, vitamin D supplementation, comorbidities, immune modulation, metabolic homeostasis, antibacterial response, parathyroid hormone, bone turnover

INTRODUCTION

Human immunodeficiency virus 1 (HIV-1) infection is one of the most important public health problems worldwide, affecting approximately 38 million people and having caused over 32 million deaths. In 2018, 1.7 million people became infected, whereas 1 million died due to HIV-related causes (1). CD4+ T lymphocytes are the primary target cells of HIV, followed by dendritic cells, monocytes, and macrophages. The acute infection is characterized by the destruction of gut-associated lymphoid tissue (GALT) that harbors a high number of CD4+ effector memory cells. Destruction leads to both anatomical and functional alterations of the gut mucosal barrier, facilitating the passage of commensal microorganisms into the circulation system, which in turn, promotes continuous immune activation. This process leads to immune exhaustion, or the inability to respond to infection leading to the destruction of the immune system and uncontrolled viral replication, resulting in increased tumor rates and opportunistic infections characteristic of acquired immunodeficiency syndrome (AIDS) (2, 3).

HIV-1 infection has also been associated with several metabolic disorders, including vitamin D (VitD) deficiency. Different studies have reported insufficient VitD levels [calcidiol serum levels <30 ng/mL (4–6)] in up to 100% of HIV-1 infected individuals and VitD deficiency [calcidiol serum levels <20 ng/mL (4–6)] in at least 30% of infected individuals (3). Even with combination Antiretroviral Therapy (cART), decreased VitD levels have been associated with comorbidities such as osteoporosis, cardiovascular diseases, type II diabetes mellitus, and infections (i.e., tuberculosis) (3, 7–10) all of which can be explained by looking at the immunomodulatory, anti-inflammatory, and antimicrobial properties of this hormone (11–13).

Alterations in VitD metabolism during HIV-1 infection is associated with an increase in proinflammatory cytokines which block the effect of the parathyroid hormone (PTH) and the hydroxylation of calcidiol in the kidney, preventing the synthesis of active VitD (14–17). Furthermore, certain non-nucleoside reverse transcriptase inhibitors (NNRTIs) and protease inhibitors (PIs) affect the function of hydroxylase enzymes from the Cytochromes P450 (CYP450) complex, inducing a marked decrease in calcitriol production, the active form of VitD (7).

Several trials have explored the beneficial effects of VitD supplementation in VitD deficient HIV-1 infected patients, focusing on the role of immune activation in HIV pathogenesis as well as the modulatory role of VitD. Therefore, this work aims to review the causes and comorbidities related to hypovitaminosis D during infection, with an emphasis on VitD supplementation in HIV-1 infected individuals. Consequently, we conducted a search using different databases such as PubMed, Scopus, Web of Science and Science Direct, with the search terms HIV-1 with vitamin D supplementation, cholecalciferol dose, vitamin D trial, cholecalciferol supplementation, and 25-Hydroxyvitamin supplementation. We excluded case reports, studies with <15 individuals, studies which supplemented with several micronutrients at once or did not report on VitD supplementation, as well as those that were conducted in a non-HIV population. In addition, to control for variability, a supplementation trial was also excluded due to low patient adherence (18).

COMORBIDITIES DURING HIV-1 INFECTION

While the current use of cART has dramatically decreased AIDS-related morbidity and mortality, its long-term use does not lead to viral eradication (19, 20) and is associated with side-effects (21) and viral drug-resistance (22), making long-term management of HIV-1 infection challenging to achieve. Moreover, persons living with HIV-1 often develop complications related to infection and treatment, with increased risk of complications associated with patient lifestyle, aging, and persistent inflammation (characteristic of HIV-1 infection). Complications include diabetes mellitus, chronic kidney disease, cardiovascular disease, and dyslipidemia (23), loss of bone mineral density (24), as well as a higher susceptibility to bacterial infections (such as Tuberculosis, a leading cause of death among people with HIV) (25, 26). However, to date, despite global efforts, interventions to effectively reduce HIV-related inflammation and comorbidities beyond effective and safer cART remain elusive.

The immunological component in HIV-1 pathophysiology suggests that endogenous immunomodulators, such as VitD, may have a beneficial impact on the infection. VitD is a hormone that, in addition to its physiological role on mineral metabolism, has pleiotropic effects on immune regulation. Indeed, one of the most frequent comorbidities during HIV-1 infection is VitD deficiency, highlighting a niche for a potential intervention which could significantly improve patients, health.

VITAMIN D

Metabolism and Function

Around 90% of VitD is obtained from UVB sunlight, with the remaining amount obtained from diet or nutritional supplementation (6). As was widely explained by a recent review by Jiménez-Sousa et al. (27), the natural process of VitD synthesis occurs in the skin by transforming 7-Dihydrocholesterol into vitamin D3 or cholecalciferol. Subsequently, cholecalciferol is hydroxylated to 25-hydroxycholecalciferol or calcidiol (25OHD) in the liver by the enzyme 25-hydroxylase, which is encoded by the CYP2R1 and CYP27A1 genes. Within the kidney, 1α-hydroxylase, encoded by the CYP27B1 gene, then transforms calcidiol into 1,25-dihydroxycholecalciferol (1,25 (OH) 2D), the physiologically active form of vitamin D (i.e., calcitriol). On the other hand, the enzyme 1,25-dihydroxyvitamin D3 24-hydroxylase, encoded by the CYP24A1 gene, is responsible for initiating calcitriol degradation and regulation.

Calcitriol is the ligand for the VitD receptor (VDR), which is located in the cytosol. Once calcitriol binds the VDR, the complex is translocated into the nucleus where it forms a secondary complex with the retinoid X receptor (RXR). Together, this complex acts as a transcription factor binding specifics sites within the DNA, known as VitD response elements (VDRE), which are located in a significant number of genes, emphasizing their essential role in gene expression regulation (16, 28–30).

VitD function is associated with mineral metabolism as well as bone maintenance. In these processes, VitD directly suppresses PTH release and regulates osteoblast and bone resorption (31). It also improves the absorption of calcium and phosphorus, promoting bone matrix mineralization. Clinical trials have demonstrated an essential role for VitD in preventing osteoporosis, bone breakage, and rickets (32).

Studies have also shown that VDR is expressed on pancreatic β cells as well as on adipocytes indicating a role for calcitriol in insulin secretion and insulin resistance (33). In *in vitro* and *in vivo* cancer therapy experiments, calcitriol has been reported to delay metastasis development by blocking the cell cycle, stimulating DNA repair, and inducing apoptosis (34, 35). VitD also plays a role in cardiovascular diseases, as VDR and CYP27B1 are expressed on myocytes and heart fibroblasts and the inhibition of VDR in mice has been correlated to cardiac hypertrophy (36).

Effects of Vitamin D on the Immune System

VitD influences both the innate and adaptive immune responses through the expression of its receptor on various immune cells such as monocytes, dendritic cells, and lymphocytes (37–40). VitD modulates the immune system by regulating transcription factors such as NF-AT and NF-kB, and by directly binding VDRE. During the innate response, VitD improves the antimicrobial effects of macrophages and monocytes by promoting transcription of antimicrobial peptides such as defensins (DEF) and cathelicidin (CAMP) (11). Recent research shows enhanced phagocytic and cytolytic activity in VitD-treated macrophages and NK cells, respectively (12, 41).

In addition, during the adaptive response, VitD decreases dendritic cell maturation, reducing the expression of MHC class II and their co-stimulatory molecules (CD40, CD80, and CD86) decreasing their ability for antigen presentation and T cell activation. Therefore, VitD promotes a tolerogenic immune status with a lower inflammatory response, indirectly influencing the polarization of T cells (13). In fact, VitD decreases IL-12 and IFN-gamma production, while increasing IL-10, favoring the development of Th2 and Treg cells over Th1 and Th17 (42, 43). As a result, it has been proposed that VitD promotes tolerance and controls exacerbated immune responses.

Effects of Vitamin D Deficiency During HIV-1 Infection

Low VitD levels affect individuals of all ages in the general population and is a global issue. Indeed, it has been reported that over 75% of the US population has VitD deficiency (42, 44). Although the VitD deficit is widespread, people living with HIV-1 are more susceptible to hypovitaminosis D, with up to 100% prevalence reported in some HIV-1 infected cohorts across the world; a condition that has been correlated with comorbidities in seropositive individuals (9). In this population, osteopenia and osteoporosis have also been associated with hypovitaminosis D in up to 60 and 20% of infected individuals, respectively (45). Likewise, VitD may also contribute to the increased risk of cardiovascular disease (CVD) reported among HIV-1 infected patients (46). A similar finding has been reported in individuals with diabetes mellitus (10, 47). Lastly, in HIV+ individuals with tuberculosis, VitD deficiency has been associated with a worse clinical outcome (48).

Even though previous studies have associated the levels of VitD with CD4+ T cell recovery in individuals on cART (9, 49), the relationship between VitD deficiency and CD4+ T cell count remains unclear. Moreover, HIV-1 viral load and disease progression have been positively associated with low levels of VitD. Therefore, it is plausible that VitD supplementation may have a beneficial effect on immune recovery, which could decrease comorbidities among HIV-1 infected individuals (50).

VITAMIN D SUPPLEMENTATION IN HIV-1 INFECTED INDIVIDUALS

Characteristics of the 29 VitD supplementation trials included in this review are listed in **Table 1**. These studies were carried out in HIV-1 infected individuals, mainly of African-American or Afro-descendants, followed by Caucasians, and had a greater representation of men (60%). The number of individuals recruited for each trial ranged from 17 to 365, all of which were supplemented orally with cholecalciferol (Vitamin D3), except in the study by Falasca et al. in which individuals were also administered supplements via the intramuscular route (59). In approximately half (55%) of the studies, individuals were adherent to a cART regimen, while in the remaining studies, more than 65% of individuals were under a cART regimen and had an undetectable viral load. Prior to supplementation, the average VitD levels were <20 ng/mL, supporting that HIV infected individuals usually suffer severe hypovitaminosis D.

The variables that had the most heterogeneity among study populations were geographic origin and age, although most of the studies were carried out in America and Europe with little representation of the African and Asian continents (**Table 1**). All age groups were represented, but several trials were focused on infected children and youth due to the expectation that the infection would last longer leading to chronic and more profound immune dysfunction. The main objective in most trials was to determine whether VitD supplementation allowed individuals to attain normal VitD levels in serum. In most of the studies (93%), the effect on comorbidities and the association with CD4+ T cell count and viral load was also evaluated.

Safe and Efficient Doses of Supplementation

Despite the fact that most HIV-1 infected individuals suffer from hypovitaminosis D, no optimal, and safe supplementation dose has yet been established for this population. Generally, a healthy person should consume between 400 and 600 IU (International Units) of VitD daily to maintain sufficiency. However, currently, the Institute of Medicine recommends a standard dose of 600 IU to maintain the requirements of 97.5% of the population, with 4000 IU as the maximum daily dose (51). The North American Endocrine Society recommends three times the standard dose for cART-adhering individuals living with HIV (6). However, nine trials exceeded the maximum limits without adverse effects or associated toxicity (**Table 1**). Supplementation represents a risk when an individual has calcidiol (25 (OH) D) levels higher than 100 ng/mL or when serum calcium levels exceed 2.70 mmol/L (51). Usually, in these instances, the skeletal system, cell membrane permeability, and nerve impulses are affected, leading to muscle weakness or spasms, constant fatigue, kidney conditions, as well as digestive symptoms such as nausea

TABLE 1 | Vitamin D supplementation studies in HIV-1 infected individuals.

References	Age [mean (range)]	(n)	The dose used in the study. (*Normalized to daily dose*). (IU)	Control group	%Subjects on cART/ virological status	Country	Ethnic group	Efficacy of VitD to restore levels	Main results	Topic of interest
Schall et al. (51)	20 (9–25)	58	7,000 daily for 52 weeks	Placebo and before vs. after supplementation	>76/–	USA	84% Black, 16% Hispanic	High	Supplementation was efficient in most participants	Supplementation
Havens et al. (52)	(18–25)	169	50,000 monthly (1,667 daily) for 12 weeks	Placebo and before vs. after supplementation	100	USA	Black 52%, White 22%, Mixed 26%	High	Supplementation was efficient regardless of the cART regimen	Supplementation
Longenecker et al. (53)	47 (39–55)	45	4,000 daily for 12 weeks	Placebo and before vs. after supplementation	100/78% undetectable	USA	78% Black, 15% White, 4% Hispanic, 3% other	Low	Individuals had severe VitD deficiency and did not reach sufficient calcidiol levels. FMD did not change, while PTH levels decreased	Cardiovascular
Muhammad et al. (54)	33 (25–47)	165	4,000 daily for 48 weeks	Placebo and before vs. after supplementation	100 recently	USA	27% Black, 20% Hispanic, 31% White	High	Supplementation did not change the lipid or glucose profile after starting therapy	Metabolic dysregulation
van den Bout-van den Beukel et al. (55)	>18	20	2,000 daily for 14 weeks, then 1,000 daily 48 weeks	Before vs. after supplementation	90	Netherlands	–	High	Insulin sensitivity and PTH levels decreased at week 24 but then returned to baseline levels	Metabolic dysregulation
Chun et al. (56)	<25	102	4,000 or 7,000 daily for 12 weeks	Placebo and before vs. after supplementation	75/50% undetectable	USA	–	High	CAMP expression increased but only 52 weeks after follow-up	Antibacterial response
Lachmann et al. (57)	35	17	200,000 once (6,667 daily) for 4 weeks	Before vs. after supplementation. cART-Naïve and uninfected individuals	65/–	England	18% Black, 63% White, 9% Asian, 9% Indian	High	The levels of CAMP and MIP-β, associated with an anti-HIV-1 effect, increased. Supplementation modestly reduced CD38+ T-cell frequency in HIV-infected patients on cART	Antibacterial response, Immune modulation
Noe et al. (58)	46	243	20,000 weekly (2,857 daily) for 52 weeks	Before vs. after supplementation	100/–	Germany	–	42 –78%	Between 42 and 78% of the individuals reached sufficient VitD levels after supplementation. There was no change in CD4 T cell counts	Immune modulation
Falasca et al. (59)	45 (34–56)	153	300,000 intramuscular every ten months (1,017 daily) or 25,000 oral monthly (892 daily), for 40 weeks	Supplemented vs. unsupplemented individuals	100/–	Italy	White	30–50%	Oral supplementation was more efficient than intramuscular administration; there was no change in CD4 T cell counts	Immune modulation
Fabre-Mersseman et al. (60)	49 (41–54)	53	100,000 every 14 days (7,142 daily) for 48 weeks	Before vs. after supplementation and deficient vs. sufficient individuals	100/–	France	–	High	The activation levels decreased, and the CD4/CD8 T cell ratio increased	Immune modulation

(Continued)

TABLE 1 | Continued

References	Age [mean (range)]	(n)	The dose used in the study. (*Normalized to daily dose*). (IU)	Control group	%Subjects on cART/ virological status	Country	Ethnic group	Efficacy of VitD to restore levels	Main results	Topic of interest
Eckard et al. (61)	20 (15–22)	51	18,000 (642), 60,000 (2,142) or 120,000 (4,285) monthly for 52 weeks	Before vs. after supplementation	100/–	USA	86% Black	71–92%	High doses diminished immune activation and exhaustion	Immune modulation
Stallings et al. (62)	(5–25)	58	7,000 daily per 48 weeks	Placebo and before vs. after supplementation	76/–	USA	85% Black	33–40%	RNA viral load decreased with increasing 25(OH)D, and CD4% and Th naive% were increased; NK% decreased short-term	Immune modulation
Dougherty et al. (63)	19 (8–24)	44	4,000 or 7,000 daily, for 12 weeks	Before vs. after supplementation	82/47% undetectable	USA	Predominantly Black	81%	There was a minimal increase in % CD4+ T cell, a decrease in viral load and the activation profile of CD8+ T cells in individuals receiving cART	Immune modulation
Kakalia et al. (64)	11 (7–15)	53	5,600 or 11,200 weekly (800 or 1600 daily), for 24 weeks	Before vs. after supplementation and Supplemented vs. no supplemented individuals	79/–	Canada	64% Black	67%	67% of the individuals reached sufficient VitD levels after supplementation, but there was no effect on CD4 T cell counts	Immune modulation
Giacomet et al. (65)	19 (14–23)	48	100,000 every 3 months (1,190 daily) for 48 weeks	Placebo and Before vs. after supplementation	85/81% undetectable	Italy	Predominantly white. Black were excluded	80%	There was no effect on CD4+ T cell count. However, the Th17/Tregs ratio decreased	Immune modulation
Coelho et al. (50)	45 (38–50)	97	100,000 weekly (14,285 daily) per 5 weeks; then 16,000 weekly (2,285 daily) for 19 weeks	Before vs. after supplementation and deficient vs. sufficient individuals	100/–	Brazil	53% White	83%	There was an association between CD4+ T cell recovery and VitD increase. Efavirenz use was associated with a higher increase in VitD levels	Immune modulation, Supplementation in cART
Steenhoff et al. (66)	19 (5–60)	60	4,000 or 7,000 daily for 12 weeks	Before vs. after supplementation	100/81% undetectable	Batswana	Black	80%	Only two individuals exhibited hypercalcemia after supplementation. Higher levels of VitD were achieved in individuals treated with efavirenz or nevirapine, compared with individuals treated with PI	Supplementation in cART
Lake et al. (67)	49 (41–55)	122	50,000 twice per week (14,285 daily) for 5 weeks; then 2,000 daily for seven weeks	Before vs. after supplementation	100/–	USA	60% White	81%	Tenofovir use did not affect levels reached after 24 weeks of treatment	Supplementation in cART

(Continued)

TABLE 1 | Continued

References	Age [mean (range)]	(n)	The dose used in the study. (*Normalized to daily dose*). (IU)	Control group	%Subjects on cART/ virological status	Country	Ethnic group	Efficacy of VitD to restore levels	Main results	Topic of interest
Lerma-Chippirraz et al. (68)	47 (41–52)	300	16,000 weekly or every 2 weeks (2,285 or 1,142 daily) for 104 weeks	Before vs. after supplementation	95/–	Spain	84,3% White, 9% Hispanic, Black 3%	82%	In 67% of individuals with secondary hyperparathyroidism, PTH levels decreased	PTH levels
Bañón et al. (69)	44 (22–75)	365	16,000 monthly (533 daily) for 36 weeks	Before vs. after supplementation and Supplemented vs. no supplemented individuals	98/–	Spain	90% White, 1% Black, 9% Hispanic	81%	The risk of secondary hyperparathyroidism decreased	PTH levels
Pepe et al. (70)	50	60	600,000 once (5,357 daily) for 16 weeks	Before vs. after supplementation	100	Italy	White	High	PTH levels decreased, and VitD levels increased regardless of the cART regimen	PTH levels
Havens et al. (71)	(18–25)	169	50,000 monthly (1,667 daily) for 12 weeks	Placebo and before vs. after supplementation	100/–	USA	Black 52%, White 22%, Mixed 26%	High	PTH and bone turnover markers (BAP and CTX) decreased only in individuals supplemented with VitD while on tenofovir	PTH levels and Bone composition
Quirico et al. (72)	46 (35–57)	79	3,200 daily for 96 weeks	Before vs. after supplementation	100/–	Italy	White	100%	Supplementation did not affect the bone mass but decreased PTH levels	PTH levels and Bone turnover
Puthanakit et al. (73)	(12–20)	24	400 daily for 24 weeks	Before vs. after supplementation	100/–	Thailand	Asian	Low	There was an increase in the BMDZ-score	Bone turnover
Overton et al. (74)	33 (25–47)	165	4,000 daily for 48 weeks	Placebo and before vs. after supplementation	100/ recently	USA	33% Black, 37% White, 25% Hispanic	High	Supplementation plus the start of cART attenuated the increase in bone turnover markers	Bone turnover
Piso et al. (75)	43 (34–52)	96	300,000 once (3,500 daily) for 12 weeks	Before vs. after supplementation	76	Switzerland	–	High	Bone replacement markers (BAP, PYR and DPD) decreased	Bone turnover
Etminani-Esfahani et al. (76)	40 (31–49)	98	300,000 once (3,500 daily) for 12 weeks	Before vs. after supplementation	100/–	Iran	–	100%	Osteocalcin increased in Efavirenz-treated individuals indicating improvement of bone formation	Bone turnover
Arpadi et al. (77)	10 (6–16)	56	100,000 every 2 months (1,785 daily) for 48 weeks	Placebo and before vs. after supplementation	–/36% undetectable	USA	64% Black, 36% Hispanic	High	Supplementation with calcium and cholecalciferol did not affect bone mass accumulation, despite a significant increase in serum calcidiol levels	Bone turnover
Rovner et al. (78)	21 (5–25)	54	7,000 daily for 48 weeks	Placebo and before vs. after supplementation	76/–	USA	86% Black	Low	No change in bone composition in infected children and youth	Bone turnover

IU, International Units; cART, Combination Antiretroviral Therapy; VitD, Vitamin D; PTH, Parathyroid Hormone; FMD, Flow Mediated Brachial Artery Dilation; CAMP, Cathelicidin; HBD, Human Beta Defensins; MIP-1β, Macrophage Inflammatory Protein beta; PI, Protease Inhibitor; BAP, Bone-Specific Alkaline Phosphatase; CTX, Carboxy-terminal Collagen Crosslinks; BMDZ-score, Body Mass index Z-Scores; PYR, Pyridinolines; DPD, Deoxypyridinium.

and vomiting. Nonetheless, all of the supplementation studies reported herein were shown to be safe.

In the studies reported in this review, the supplementation schemes varied regarding the dose and frequency of administration. To make the data more homogeneous for ease of comparison, daily doses were calculated according to the equivalent in weeks or months used in each trial (**Table 1**). The daily dose ranged from approximately 400 to 14,000 IU, with 4,000 and 7,000 IU as the most common doses. The duration of each trial varied from 4 to 104 weeks. Although most of the doses increased VitD levels, sufficiency was challenging to achieve due to the severe deficiency suffered by the HIV-1 infected population. The use of 7000 IU daily was the most effective dose (51, 56, 60, 63, 66, 78), and restored sufficiency [defined as calcidiol serum levels >30 ng/mL (4)] in 80% of treated individuals with higher levels seen following 12 months of treatment (61). Only 2 of the 215 individuals treated with this regimen had calcidiol levels >90 ng/mL and hypercalcemia (66). Once sufficiency is attained, a maintenance dose guaranteeing stable circulatory VitD levels should be established. Since the follow-up period was short during each of the trials, the long term effects of supplementation are still unclear; therefore, further studies will be required to evaluate the safety of long-term use.

VitD supplementation trials can be confounded by several aspects such as the season in which the study is carried out (78) or skin pigmentation since sunlight can affect vitamin levels. A study performed by Dougherty et al. showed that calcidiol basal levels were lower in individuals in winter than in other seasons (63). Additionally, in a healthy population, individuals with darker skin were reported to require higher doses of cholecalciferol (up to 2000 UI/day) to achieve VitD sufficiency (79). Ancestry may also play a key role in affecting the efficacy of supplementation since a study from Botswana reported that the VitD binding protein (DBP) was lower in plasma of individuals of African descent (1.8 umol/L) (66) compared to those which had an Afro-American background (3.3 umol/L) (80). Other factors, such as drug use as well as malabsorption syndromes and other unknown side effects associated with HIV-1 infection can also affect the results of VitD supplementation. Of note, no ethnic bias was identified during the review of the aforementioned studies as most of the results were obtained in trials which included individuals with varying ethnicities.

The Effect of Vitamin D Supplementation on CD4+ T Lymphocyte Count and Viral Load

CD4+ T cell counts and viral load are essential indicators for determining the clinical course of HIV-1 infection. However, since the mechanisms by which VitD influences HIV-1 disease progression, morbidity, and mortality are poorly understood, further investigations are required.

Currently, studies have shown that in HIV-1 infected individuals, VitD insufficiency is associated with low CD4+ T cell counts. In Coelho et al. 88% of individuals who had a CD4+ nadir count <50 cells/mm^3 had VitD insufficiency, while only 6% of participants with a similar nadir had VitD levels within normal range (50). In the same study, 1 ng/mL of calcidiol (25(OH) D) was shown to increase CD4 cell count by 3,3 cells/mm3, suggesting a beneficial role of VitD supplementation on immune recovery. Eckard and Dougherty reported similar results, showing a significant increase in CD4+ count after supplementation (11, 63). Likewise, Stallings et al. reported a reduction in viral load following supplementation (62). However, in other studies, VitD supplementation did not affect CD4+ T cell counts (58, 59, 64, 66).

It is important to note that in supplementation trials in which an increase in the CD4+ T lymphocyte count was observed, participants had remained on a cART regimen; therefore, it has been challenging to establish a causal relationship between VitD supplementation, immune recovery, and virological control. However, in a supplementation study in which 9 of the individuals were not on cART, an increase in CD4+ T cell count and differences in virological control were not seen (63). Although these findings still need to be corroborated, this evidence suggests that VitD may enhance immune recovery and viral control in combination with cART and may serve as an adjuvant to current therapy. Furthermore, none of the supplementation trials reviewed herein reported secondary side effects, supporting the safety of VitD treatment.

Supplementation Effects on Immune Activation

HIV-1 infected individuals have significantly higher levels of immune activation, even with cART, compared to their uninfected counterparts (81). Additionally, hypovitaminosis D has been associated with an increase in inflammatory markers, both in the general population, and in HIV-1 infected individuals (82, 83), therefore VitD insufficiency may facilitate the persistence of systemic immune activation. Taking into account that immune activation is the main mechanism associated with HIV progression and its associated comorbidities, it is necessary to continue the search for immunomodulators that can return the host to an immune quiescent state. Accordingly, it is interesting to speculate the role that VitD may play in this regard since it has been shown to promote the differentiation of naive T cells into Tregs or Th2 cells, inhibiting the development of Th1, and Th17 cells (13, 84). In fact, Fabre-Mersseman et al. reported that, after supplementing VitD insufficient patients with a dose of 7000 IU daily, immune activation levels, determined by measuring the expression of CD38 and Ki67 in CD8+ T lymphocytes, were reduced and there was an increase in the CD4+/CD8+ T cell ratio (60).

Similarly, in a trial by Eckard et al. looking at different doses of VitD supplementation, CD4+ and CD8+ T cell activation, frequency of inflammatory monocytes (CD14+ CD16+), and expression of PD1+ (an exhaustion marker) in CD4+ T cells decreased significantly in individuals treated with 4000 IU daily for 52 weeks (61). These results are in agreement with those reported by Dougherty et al. which showed a decrease in the percentage of activated cytotoxic T cells (CD8+ CD38+ HLA DR+) following a daily dose of 4000 or 7000 IU of VitD for 12 weeks, (63). These results support VitD supplementation as an adjuvant during routine clinical care of HIV-1 infected patients.

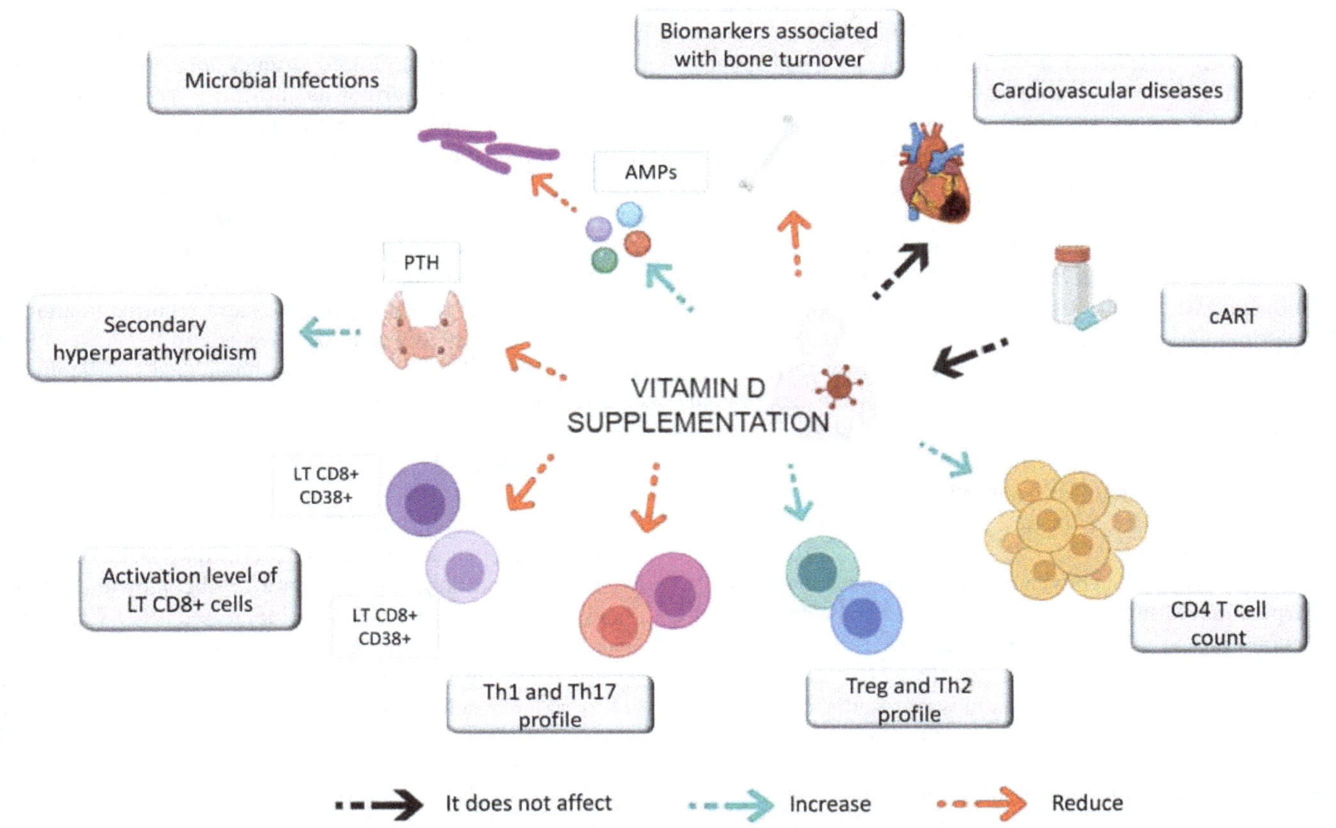

FIGURE 1 | Effect of vitamin D supplementation on clinical and immunological aspects associated with HIV-1 infection. VitD supplementation in HIV-1 infected individuals reduces PTH levels that promotes secondary hyperparathyroidism. It also induces the expression of AMPs (antimicrobial peptides) such as CAMP and HBD and improve bone formation while decrease biomarkers associated with bone turnover. VitD supplementation seems not impact CVD, and the VitD repletion success did not depend on the cART regimen. In addition, supplementation with this hormone seems also to increases CD4 T cell count, promoting their differentiation toward a Th2 and Treg profile while decreasing the Th1 and Th17 profiles and the activation levels of CD8 + T cells.

The Effect of Antiretroviral Therapy on the Response to VitD Supplementation

Although there is evidence suggesting that some antiretrovirals affect VitD metabolism, little is known regarding the effect of VitD supplementation on cART. Non-nucleoside Reverse Transcriptase Inhibitors (NNRTI) have been associated with lower levels of VitD. For example, efavirenz has been suggested to increase VitD catabolism and disrupt 25(OH)D synthesis through the modulation of the cytochrome p450 system, which controls VitD hydroxylation (85–88). However, other trials do not support this hypothesis. Indeed, a study comparing several cART regimens showed that after receiving a daily dose of 4000 or 7000 UI of VitD for 12 weeks, VitD levels were 20 ng/mL higher among individuals on efavirenz compared to all other therapeutic regimens (63). In another study using a similar timeline and supplementation dose schedule, individuals treated with efavirenz reached VitD sufficiency. Of note, variations in baseline VitD levels were not associated with any antiretroviral drug (66). These results suggest that, although efavirenz has been associated with low VitD levels, it is possible to reach sufficient concentrations following supplementation. Moreover, once sufficient levels are reached, efavirenz could have additional benefits related to bone mass, as reported in a supplementation trial in South Africans children (89).

Conversely, zidovudine, a Nucleoside Reverse Transcriptase Inhibitor (NRTI), has been associated with lower levels of vitamin D, while tenofovir has not been associated with deficiency nor insufficiency and neither NRTI has shown significant effects during supplementation trials (9, 59, 90). The Protease inhibitors (PIs) have not yet been correlated with baseline VitD levels or with success or failure to achieve sufficient levels after supplementation (17, 91). No data is currently available for the effect of integrase inhibitors or CCR5 inhibitors on supplementation. In summary, according to previous evidence, the use of cART, even including efavirenz, does not limit the achievable objective of increasing levels of VitD during supplementation trials.

The Effect of Vitamin D Supplementation on HIV-1 Associated Comorbidities

Hypovitaminosis D has been associated with various comorbidities associated with HIV-1 disease progression resulting in higher mortality rates among infected individuals (92, 93). These individuals have an increased risk of osteomalacia and osteoporosis, notable weight loss, low bone mineral density, and a reduction in muscle mass (78). In contrast, individuals with sufficient VitD levels have a low tendency for skeletal affections; however, the ideal level to minimize risk remains unknown (63).

Although a study in HIV-1 infected individuals with vitamin D deficiency showed a significant reduction in the risk of hypocalcemia after supplementation (58), 3 out of the 5 trials that evaluated bone composition found that, despite an increase in VitD levels following supplementation, bone mass did not change in children and adults (72, 78), even with the addition of calcium (89). In contrast, two studies showed that VitD supplementation decrease biomarkers associated with bone turnover (71, 75) while Etminani-Esfahani et al. reported an increase in Osteocalcin, biomarker associated with bone formation following a single high dose of VitD. Similar results were also noted in other studies (73, 94), where VitD supplementation was found to improve bone composition among HIV-1 infected individuals, albeit, this process might require more time than that seen in previously reported studies.

On the other hand, hypovitaminosis D is related to secondary hyperparathyroidism, a reversible state associated with excessive secretion (>65 pg/mL) of PTH (68), a known cause of decreased bone mineral density (95). Consequently, PTH can be an early indicator of vitamin D deficiency and is an essential criterion for determining if a person requires supplementation (65). Studies evaluating secondary hyperparathyroidism in HIV-1 infected persons are scarce, and as a result, there is little data on the impact of this condition on their clinical status. However, five supplementation trials evaluating PTH levels showed that while VitD levels increased, the levels of PTH decreased during the initial phases of the trials (53, 63, 65, 66, 72, 95).

Finally, although some studies have linked VitD deficiency to hypertension, cardiovascular disease, myocardial infarction, and metabolic syndromes in HIV infected individuals, few studies have evaluated the effect of VitD supplementation on these conditions. In a trial by Chris T Longenecker et al., VitD supplementation in HIV-1 infected patients with hypovitaminosis D did not affect endothelial function, measured by flow-mediated brachial artery dilation (FMD). Furthermore, changes in serum 25(OH)D or FMD were not correlated in the treatment group, although they had not reached sufficient levels of VitD. In Muhammad et al. the authors concluded that VitD supplementation is unlikely to be an effective strategy to attenuate metabolic dysregulation following cART initiation, since lipid and glucose profiles did not improve during treatment (54). These results suggest that VitD supplementation is not enough to avoid the development of these comorbidities, and cannot achieve vitamin sufficiency to improve health conditions (53).

Vitamin D and Bacterial Infections

VitD plays a key role in the effector activity of innate immune cells in response to microbial infections. During monocytes and macrophages activation, the VDR and the enzyme 1α-hydroxylase (CYP27B1), an activator of vitamin D, are expressed. During the intracrine conversion of the VitD precursor (25(OH)D) to its active form (1,25(OH)2D), it is possible to stimulate the expression of antimicrobial peptides such as cathelicidin (CAMP) and human beta defensins (HBD) (96). Some studies reported that VitD affects autophagy, supporting its anti-microbial properties, for example by promoting *Mycobacterium tuberculosis* clearance and antiviral responses (i.e., inhibiting HIV replication) (97). In a supplementation trial, treatment of HIV-1 infected individuals with VitD promoted CAMP expression, despite requiring longer treatment periods compared to uninfected individuals (56). Similarly, an increase in CAMP and macrophage inflammatory protein beta (MIP-1β) production was also reported in another trial (57). Further studies are needed to evaluate other antimicrobial molecules that can be modulated by vitamin D, such as β-defensin 2 or hepcidin.

CONCLUSION

VitD supplementation in HIV-1 infected individuals leads to an increase in VitD serum levels, regardless of cART, geographical location, and ethnicity of the individual being administered the supplementation. Increased VitD levels may have positive effects on several clinical and immunologic aspects which are summarized in **Figure 1.** Among them, the most striking results included the potential reduction in the likelihood of secondary hyperparathyroidism and microbial infections such as tuberculosis, as well as an increase in CD4+ T lymphocytes count and a decrease in biomarkers associated with bone turnover and chronic inflammation. However, the effect of VitD supplementation on viral load has not yet been established since the current guidelines for HIV patient management indicate initiation of therapy as soon as individuals are diagnosed, making it impossible to evaluate. Furthermore, the effect of VitD supplementation on the incidence of other comorbidities associated with hypovitaminosis D, such as metabolic syndromes has not yet been carried out.

Overall, evidence suggests that VitD supplementation may be a good adjuvant to cART. However, it is important to emphasize that the effects greatly depend on the dose quantity and duration of which the supplementation is given. In general, the dosages which showed the most success were 4000 and 7000 IU daily for at least 12 weeks. Studies with larger sample sizes are required to confirm the beneficial effects of VitD and to establish optimal supplementation and maintenance doses in the context of HIV-1 infection.

AUTHOR CONTRIBUTIONS

NA contributed with the literature search and reading and writing and correcting the manuscript. WA-J contributed with writing and suggestions and corrections. MR contributed to reviewing the manuscript and writing.

ACKNOWLEDGMENTS

We acknowledge to Universidad de Antioquia UdeA and COLCIENCIAS (code 111574455024) for the financial support.

REFERENCES

1. UNAIDS. *Data 2019*. Jt United Nations Program HIV/AIDS. Geneva (2019). p. 1–468. Available online at: https://www.unaids.org/sites/default/files/media_asset/2019-UNAIDS-data_en.pdf
2. Alcamí J, Coiras M. Inmunopatogenia de la infección por el virus de la inmunodeficiencia humana. *Enferm Infecc Microbiol Clin.* (2011) 29:216–26. doi: 10.1016/j.eimc.2011.01.006
3. Barbosa N, Costa L, Pinto M. Vitamin D and HIV Infection : a systematic review. *Immunod Disord.* (2014) 3:1. doi: 10.4172/2324-853X.1000107
4. Thacher TD, Clarke BL. Vitamin D insufficiency. *Mayo Clin Proc.* (2011) 86:50–60. doi: 10.4016/26528.01
5. Holick MF. Vitamin D Status : measurement, interpretation, and clinical application. *Elsevier.* (2009) 19:73–8. doi: 10.1016/j.annepidem.2007.12.001
6. Holick MF, Binkley NC, Bischoff-Ferrari HA, Gordon CM, Hanley DA, Heaney RP, et al. Evaluation, treatment, and prevention of vitamin D deficiency: an endocrine society clinical practice guideline. *J Clin Endocrinol Metab.* (2011) 96:1911–30. doi: 10.1210/jc.2011-0385
7. Conesa-Botella A, Florence E, Lynen L, Colebunders R, Menten J, Moreno-Reyes R. Decrease of vitamin D concentration in patients with HIV infection on a non nucleoside reverse transcriptase inhibitor-containing regimen. *AIDS Res Ther.* (2010) 7:40. doi: 10.1186/1742-6405-7-40
8. Sudfeld CR, Wang M, Aboud S, Giovannucci EL, Mugusi FM, Fawzi WW. Vitamin D and HIV progression among Tanzanian adults initiating antiretroviral therapy. *PLoS ONE.* (2012) 7:e40036. doi: 10.1371/journal.pone.0040036
9. Lake JE, Adams JS. Vitamin D in HIV-infected patients. *Curr HIV/AIDS Rep.* (2011) 8:133–41. doi: 10.1007/s11904-011-0082-8
10. Pinzone MR, Di Rosa M, Malaguarnera M, Madeddu G, Focà E, Ceccarelli G, et al. Vitamin D deficiency in HIV infection: an underestimated and undertreated epidemic. *Eur Rev Med Pharmacol Sci.* (2013) 17:1218–32. Available online at: https://www.europeanreview.org/article/4071
11. Prietl B, Treiber G, Pieber TR, Amrein K. Vitamin D and immune function. *Nutrients.* (2013) 5:2502–21. doi: 10.3390/nu5072502
12. Radovic J, Markovic D, Velickov A, Djordjevic B, Stojnev S. Vitamin D immunomodulatory effect. *Acta Med Med.* (2012) 51:58–64. doi: 10.5633/amm.2012.0409s
13. Baeke F, Takiishi T, Korf H, Gysemans C, Mathieu C. Vitamin D: modulator of the immune system. *Curr Opin Pharmacol.* (2010) 10:482–96. doi: 10.1016/j.coph.2010.04.001
14. Beard JA, Bearden A, Striker R. Vitamin D and the anti-viral state. *J Clin Virol.* (2011) 50:194–200. doi: 10.1016/j.jcv.2010.12.006
15. Ross AC, McComsey GA. The role of vitamin D deficiency in the pathogenesis of osteoporosis and in the modulation of the immune system in HIV-infected patients. *Clin Rev Bone Miner Metab.* (2012) 10:277–87. doi: 10.1007/s12018-012-9131-0
16. Conrado T, Miranda-Filho DDB, Bandeira F. Vitamin D deficiency in HIV-infected individuals: one more risk factor for bone loss and cardiovascular disease? *Arq Bras Endocrinol Metabol.* (2010) 54:118–22. doi: 10.1590/S0004-27302010000200006
17. Orkin C, Wohl DA, Williams A, Deckx H. Vitamin D deficiency in HIV: a shadow on long-term management? *AIDS Rev.* (2014). 16:59–74. Available online at: https://www.aidsreviews.com/resumen.php?id=1258&indice=2014162&u=unp
18. Benguella L, Arbault A, Fillion A, Blot M, Piroth C, Denimal D, et al. Vitamin D supplementation, bone turnover, and inflammation in HIV-infected patients. *Med Mal Infect.* (2018) 48:449–56. doi: 10.1016/j.medmal.2018.02.011
19. Arco A, Teira R, Bachiller P, Pedrol E, Domingo P, Mariño A, et al. Late initiation of HAART among HIV-infected patients in spain is frequent and related to a higher rate of virological failure but not to immigrant status. *HIV Clin Trials.* (2011) 12:1–8. doi: 10.1310/hct1201-1
20. Piconi S, Trabattoni D, Gori A, Parisotto S, Magni C, Meraviglia P, et al. Immune activation, apoptosis and Treg activity are associated with persistently reduced CD4 R T-cell counts during antiretroviral therapy. *AIDS.* (2010) 24:1991–2000. doi: 10.1097/QAD.0b013e32833c93ce
21. Waal D, Cohen K, Maartens G. Systematic review of antiretroviral-associated lipodystrophy : lipoatrophy, but not central fat gain, is an antiretroviral adverse drug reaction. *PLoS ONE.* (2013) 8:e63623. doi: 10.1371/journal.pone.0063623
22. Maggiolo F, Airoldi M, Kleinloog HD, Callegaro A, Ravasio V, Arici C, et al. Effect of adherence to HAART on virologic outcome and on the selection of resistance-conferring mutations in NNRTI- or PI-treated patients. *HIV Clin Trials.* (2007) 8:282–92. doi: 10.1310/hct0805-282
23. Perturbations I. HIV and cardiovascular disease : role of immunometabolic perturbations. *Physiology.* (2018) 33:74–82. doi: 10.1152/physiol.00028.2017
24. Mirza FS, Luthra P, Chirch L. Endocrinological aspects of HIV infection. *J Endocrinol Invest.* (2018) 41:881–99. doi: 10.1007/s40618-017-0812-x
25. Shahcheraghi SH, Ayatollahi J, Niri MD, Fazilati A. The most common bacterial infections in HIV-infected patients Addressing the issue of shortage of oral cholera vaccines on the global front. *Medical Journal of Dr. D.Y. Patil University.* (2016) 9:773–4. doi: 10.4103/0975-2870.194234
26. Currier JS, Havlir D V. CROI 2018 : complications of HIV infection and antiretroviral therapy. *Top Antivir Med.* (2018) 26:22–9. Available online at: https://www.iasusa.org/wp-content/uploads/2010/04/18-2-57.pdf
27. Jiménez-sousa MÁ, Martínez I, Medrano LM. Vitamin D in human immunodeficiency virus infection: influence on immunity and disease. *Front Immunol.* (2018) 9:458. doi: 10 3389/fimmu.2018.00458
28. Christakos S, Dhawan P, Verstuyf A, Verlinden L, Carmeliet G. Vitamin D: metabolism, molecular mechanism of action, and pleiotropic effects. *Physiol Rev.* (2016) 96:365–408. doi: 10.1152/physrev.00014.2015
29. Cooper C, Thorne A. Vitamin D supplementation does not increase immunogenicity of seasonal influenza vaccine in HIV-infected adults. *HIV Clin Trials.* (2011) 12:275–6. doi: 10.1310/hct1205-275
30. Christakos S, Ajibade D V., Dhawan P, Fechner AJ, Mady LJ. Vitamin D: metabolism. *Endocrinol Metab Clin North Am.* (2010) 39:243–53. doi: 10.1016/j.ecl.2010.02.002
31. Escaffi FMJ, Miranda CM, Alonso KR, Cuevas M. A. Dieta mediterránea y Vitamina d como potenciales factores preventivos del deterioro cognitivo. *Rev Médica Clínica Las Condes.* (2016) 27:392–400. doi: 10.1016/j.rmclc.2016.06.012
32. Bikle DD. Vitamin D metabolism, mechanism of action, and clinical applications. *Chem Biol.* (2014) 21:319–29. doi: 10.1016/j.chembiol.2013.12.016
33. Kayaniyil S, Vieth R, Retnakaran R, Knight JA, Qi Y, Gerstein HC, et al. Association of vitamin D with insulin resistance and beta-cell dysfunction in subjects at risk for type 2 diabetes. *Diabetes Care.* (2010) 33:1379–81. doi: 10.2337/dc09-2321
34. Chung M, Lee J, Terasawa T, Lau J, Trikalinos TA. Vitamin D with or without calcium supplementation for prevention of cancer and fractures: an updated meta-analysis for the U.S. preventive services task force. *Ann Intern Med.* (2011) 155:827–38. doi: 10.7326/0003-4819-155-12-201112200-00005
35. Manson JE, Mayne ST, Clinton SK. Vitamin D and prevention of cancer - ready for prime time? *N Engl J Med.* (2011) 364:1385–7. doi: 10.1056/NEJMp1102022
36. Chen S, Law CS, Grigsby CL, Olsen K, Hong TT, Zhang Y, et al. Cardiomyocyte-specific deletion of the vitamin D receptor gene results in cardiac hypertrophy. *Circulation.* (2011) 124:1838–47. doi: 10.1161/CIRCULATIONAHA.111.032680
37. Korf H, Wenes M, Stijlemans B, Takiishi T, Robert S, Miani M, et al. 1,25-Dihydroxyvitamin D3 curtails the inflammatory and T cell stimulatory capacity of macrophages through an IL-10-dependent mechanism. *Immunobiology.* (2012) 217:1292–300. doi: 10.1016/j.imbio.2012.07.018
38. Morán-Auth Y, Penna-Martinez M, Shoghi F, Ramos-Lopez E, Badenhoop K. Vitamin D status and gene transcription in immune cells. *J Steroid Biochem Mol Biol.* (2013) 136:83–5. doi: 10.1016/j.jsbmb.2013.02.005
39. Kongsbak M, Levring TB, Geisler C, von Essen MR. The vitamin D receptor and T cell function. *Front Immunol.* (2013) 4: 148. doi: 10.3389/fimmu.2013.00148
40. Barragan M, Good M, Kolls JK. Regulation of dendritic cell function by vitamin D. *Nutrients.* (2015) 7:8127–51. doi: 10.3390/nu7095383
41. Zasloff M. Antimicrobial peptides of multicellular organisms. *Nature.* (2002) 415:389–95. doi: 10.1038/415389a
42. Adams JS, Hewison M. Update in vitamin D. *J Clin Endocrinol Metab.* (2010) 95:471–8. doi: 10.1210/jc.2009-1773

43. Smolders J, Thewissen M, Peelen E, Menheere P, Tervaert JWC, Damoiseaux J, et al. Vitamin D status is positively correlated with regulatory T cell function in patients with multiple sclerosis. *PLoS ONE.* (2009) 4:8. doi: 10.1371/journal.pone.0006635
44. Palacios C, Gonzalez L. Is vitamin D deficiency a major global public health problem? *J Steroid Biochem Mol Biol.* (2014) 144:138–45. doi: 10.1016/j.jsbmb.2013.11.003
45. Bander D, Parczewski M. Osteoporosis and vitamin D deficiency in HIV-infected patients: genetic and classical factors compared to the HIV-associated ones - review. *HIV AIDS Rev.* (2012) 11:1–4. doi: 10.1016/j.hivar.2011.11.001
46. Lai S, Fishman EK, Gerstenblith G, Brinker J, Tai H, Chen S, et al. Vitamin D deficiency is associated with coronary artery calcification in cardiovascularly asymptomatic African Americans with HIV infection. *Vasc Health Risk Manag.* (2013) 9:493–500. doi: 10.2147/VHRM.S48388
47. Szep Z, Guaraldi G, Shah SS, Lo Re V, Ratcliffe SJ, Orlando G, et al. Vitamin D deficiency is associated with type 2 diabetes mellitus in HIV infection. *AIDS.* (2011) 25:525–9. doi: 10.1097/QAD.0b013e328342fdfd
48. Mansueto P, Seidita A, Vitale G, Gangemi S, Iaria C, Cascio A. Vitamin D deficiency in HIV infection: not only a bone disorder. *Biomed Res Int.* (2015) 2015:735615. doi: 10.1155/2015/735615
49. Aziz M, Livak B, Burke-Miller J, French AL, Glesby MJ, Sharma A, et al. Vitamin D insufficiency may impair CD4 recovery among Women's Interagency HIV Study participants with advanced disease on HAART. *AIDS.* (2013) 27:573–8. doi: 10.1097/QAD.0b013e32835b9ba1
50. Coelho L, Cardoso SW, Luz PM, Hoffman RM, Mendonça L, Veloso VG, et al. Vitamin D3 supplementation in HIV infection: effectiveness and associations with antiretroviral therapy. *Nutr J.* (2015) 14:81. doi: 10.1186/s12937-015-0072-6
51. Schall JI, Hediger ML, Zemel BS, Rutstein RM, Stallings VA. Comprehensive safety monitoring of 12-month daily 7000-IU vitamin D3 supplementation in human immunodeficiency virus-infected children and young adults. *JPEN J Parenter Enteral Nutr.* (2016) 40:1057–63. doi: 10.1177/0148607115593790
52. Havens PL, Mulligan K, Hazra R, Flynn P, Rutledge B, Van Loan MD, et al. Serum 25-hydroxyvitamin D response to vitamin D 3 HIV-1 infection. *J Clin Endocrinol Metab.* (2017) 97:4004–13. doi: 10.1210/jc.2012-2600
53. Longenecker CT, Hileman CO, Carman TL, Ross AC, Seydafkan S, Brown TT, et al. Original article Vitamin D supplementation and endothelial function in vitamin D deficient HIV-infected patients : a randomized placebo-controlled trial. *Antiviral Therapy.* (2012) 17:613–21. doi: 10.3851/IMP1983
54. Muhammad J, Chan ES, Brown TT, Tebas P, Mccomsey GA, Melbourne K, et al. Vitamin D supplementation does not affect metabolic changes seen with ART initiation. *Open Forum Infect Dis.* (2017) 4:14–17. doi: 10.1093/ofid/ofx210
55. van den Bout-van den Beukel CJP, van den Bos M, Oyen WJG, Hermus ARMM, Sweep FCGJ, Tack CJJ, et al. The effect of cholecalciferol supplementation on vitamin D levels and insulin sensitivity is dose related in vitamin D-deficient HIV-1-infected patients. *HIV Med.* (2008) 9:771–9. doi: 10.1111/j.1468-1293.2008.00630.x
56. Chun RF, Liu NQ, Lee T, Schall JI, Denburg MR, Rutstein RM, et al. Vitamin D supplementation and antibacterial immune responses in adolescents and young adults with HIV/AIDS. *J Steroid Biochem Mol Biol.* (2015) 148:290–7. doi: 10.1016/j.jsbmb.2014.07.013
57. Lachmann R, Bevan MA, Kim S, Patel N, Hawrylowicz C, Vyakarnam A, et al. A comparative phase 1 clinical trial to identify anti-infective mechanisms of Vitamin D in people with HIV infection. *AIDS.* (2015) 29:1127–35. doi: 10.1097/QAD.0000000000000666
58. Noe S, Heldwein S, Pascucchi R, Oldenbüttel C, Wiese C, Von Krosigk A, et al. Cholecalciferol 20 000 IU once weekly in HIV-positive patients with low vitamin D levels: result from a cohort study. *J Int Assoc Provid AIDS Care.* (2017) 16:315–20. doi: 10.1177/2325957417702487
59. Falasca K, Ucciferri C, Di Nicola M, Vignale F, Di Biase J, Vecchiet J. Different strategies of 25OH vitamin D supplementation in HIV-positive subjects. *Int J STD AIDS.* (2014) 25:785–92. doi: 10.1177/0956462414520804
60. Fabre-Mersseman V, Tubiana R, Papagno L, Bayard C, Briceno O, Fastenackels S, et al. Vitamin D supplementation is associated with reduced immune activation levels in HIV-1-infected patients on suppressive antiretroviral therapy. *AIDS.* (2014) 28:2677–82. doi: 10.1097/QAD.0000000000000472
61. Eckard AR, O 'riordan MA, Rosebush JC, Lee ST, Habib JG, Ruff JH, et al. Vitamin D supplementation decreases immune activation and exhaustion in HIV-1-infected youth. *Antivir Ther.* (2017) 24:347. doi: 10.3851/IMP3199
62. Stallings VA, Schall JI, Hediger ML, Zemel BS, Tuluc F, Dougherty KA, et al. High-dose vitamin D3 supplementation in children and young adults with HIV: a randomized, placebo-controlled trial. *Pediatr Infect Dis J.* (2015) 34:e32–40. doi: 10.1097/INF.0000000000000483
63. Dougherty KA, Schall JI, Zemel BS, Tuluc F, Hou X, Rutstein RM, et al. Safety and efficacy of high-dose daily vitamin D3 supplementation in children and young adults infected with human immunodeficiency virus. *J Pediatric Infect Dis Soc.* (2014) 3:294–303. doi: 10.1093/jpids/piu012
64. Kakalia S, Sochett EB, Stephens D, Assor E, Read SE, Bitnun A. Vitamin D supplementation and CD4 count in children infected with human immunodeficiency virus. *J Pediatr.* (2011) 159:951–7. doi: 10.1016/j.jpeds.2011.06.010
65. Giacomet V, Vigano A, Manfredini V, Cerini C, Bedogni G, Mora S, et al. Cholecalciferol supplementation in HIV-infected youth with vitamin D insufficiency: effects on vitamin D status and T-cell phenotype: a randomized controlled trial. *HIV Clin Trials.* (2013) 14:51–60. doi: 10.1310/hct1402-51
66. Steenhoff AP, Schall JI, Samuel J, Seme B, Marape M, Ratshaa B, et al. Vitamin D(3)supplementation in Batswana children and adults with HIV: a pilot double blind randomized controlled trial. *PLoS ONE.* (2015) 10:e0117123. doi: 10.1371/journal.pone.0117123
67. Lake JE, Hoffman RM, Tseng C-H, Wilhalme HM, Adams JS, Currier JS. Success of standard dose vitamin d supplementation in treated human immunodeficiency virus infection. *Open Forum Infect Dis.* (2015) 2:ofv068. doi: 10.1093/ofid/ofv068
68. Lerma-Chippirraz E, Güerri-Fernández R, Villar García J, González Mena A, Guelar Grinberg A, Milagros Montero, M, et al. Validation protocol of vitamin D supplementation in patients with HIV-Infection. *AIDS Res Treat.* (2016) 2016:5120831. doi: 10.1155/2016/5120831
69. Bañón S, Rosillo M, Gómez A, Pérez-Elias MJ, Moreno S, Casado JL. Effect of a monthly dose of calcidiol in improving vitamin D deficiency and secondary hyperparathyroidism in HIV-infected patients. *Endocrine.* (2015) 49:528–37. doi: 10.1007/s12020-014-0489-2
70. Pepe J, Mezzaroma I, Fantauzzi A, Falciano M, Salotti A, Di Traglia M, et al. An oral high dose of cholecalciferol restores vitamin D status in deficient postmenopausal HIV-1-infected women independently of protease inhibitors therapy: a pilot study. *Endocrine.* (2016) 53:299–304. doi: 10.1007/s12020-015-0693-8
71. Havens PL, Stephensen CB, Hazra R, Flynn PM, Wilson CM, Rutledge B, et al. Vitamin D3 decreases parathyroid hormone in HIV-infected youth being treated with tenofovir: a randomized, placebo-controlled trial. *Clin Infect Dis.* (2012) 54:1013–25. doi: 10.1093/cid/cir968
72. Quirico M, Valeria R, Lorenza M, Umberto P, Cristina PM, Simona O, et al. Bone mass preservation with high-dose cholecalciferol and dietary calcium in HIV patients following antiretroviral therapy. Is it possible? Bone mass preservation with high-dose cholecalciferol and dietary calcium in HIV patients following antiretroviral therapy. Is it possible? *HIV Clin Trials.* (2018) 19:188–96. doi: 10.1080/15284336.2018.1525841
73. Puthanakit T, Wittawatmongkol O, Poomlek V, Sudjaritruk T, Brukesawan C. Effect of calcium and vitamin D supplementation on bone mineral accrual among HIV-infected Thai adolescents with low bone mineral density. *J Virus Eradic.* (2018) 4:6–11. Available online at: http://viruseradication.com/journal-details/Effect_of_calcium_and_vitamin_D_supplementation_on_bone_mineral_accrual_among_HIV-infected_Thai_adolescents_with_low_bone_mineral_density/
74. Overton ET, Chan ES, Brown TT, Tebas P, McComsey GA, Melbourne KM, et al. Vitamin D and Calcium attenuate bone loss with antiretroviral therapy initiation: a randomized trial. *Ann Intern Med.* (2015) 162:815–24. doi: 10.7326/M14-1409
75. Piso RJ, Rothen M, Rothen JP, Stahl M, Fux C. Per oral substitution with 300000 IU vitamin D (Cholecalciferol) reduces bone turnover markers in HIV-infected patients. *BMC Infect Dis.* (2013) 13:577. doi: 10.1186/1471-2334-13-577
76. Etminani-Esfahani M, Khalili H, Jafari S, Abdollahi A, Dashti-Khavidaki S. Effects of vitamin D supplementation on the bone specific biomarkers in HIV

infected individuals under treatment with efavirenz. *BMC Res Notes.* (2012) 5:204. doi: 10.1186/1756-0500-5-204
77. Arpadi SM, McMahon D, Abrams EJ, Bamji M, Purswani M, Engelson ES, et al. Effect of bimonthly supplementation with oral cholecalciferol on serum 25-hydroxyvitamin D concentrations in HIV-infected children and adolescents. *Pediatrics.* (2009) 123:e121–6. doi: 10.1542/peds.2008-0176
78. Rovner AJ, Stallings VA, Rutstein R, Schall JI, Leonard MB, Zemel BS. Effect of high-dose cholecalciferol (vitamin D3) on bone and body composition in children and young adults with HIV infection: a randomized, double-blind, placebo-controlled trial. *Osteoporos Int.* (2017) 28:201–9. doi: 10.1007/s00198-016-3826-x
79. IOM I of M (US). Dietary reference intakes for calcium and vitamin d. *Pediatrics.* (2011) 130:e1424. doi: 10.1542/peds.2012-2590
80. Powe CE, Evans MK, Wenger J, Zonderman AB, Berg AH, Nalls M, et al. Vitamin D-binding protein and vitamin D status of black americans and white Americans. *N Engl J Med.* (2013) 369:1991–2000. doi: 10.1056/NEJMoa1306357
81. Hunt PW, Cao HL, Muzoora C, Ssewanyana I, Bennett J, Emenyonu N, et al. Impact of CD8 + T-cell activation on CD4+ T-cell recovery and mortality in HIV-infected Ugandans initiating antiretroviral therapy. *AIDS.* (2011) 25:2123–31. doi: 10.1097/QAD.0b013e32834c4ac1
82. Ansemant T, Mahy S, Piroth C, Ornetti P, Ewing S, Guilland JC, et al. Severe hypovitaminosis D correlates with increased inflammatory markers in HIV infected patients. *BMC Infect Dis.* (2013) 13:7. doi: 10.1186/1471-2334-13-7
83. Hyppönen E, Berry D, Cortina-Borja M, Power C. 25-Hydroxyvitamin D and pre-clinical alterations in inflammatory and hemostatic markers: a cross sectional analysis in the 1958 british birth cohort. *PLoS ONE.* (2010) 5:e010801. doi: 10.1371/journal.pone.0010801
84. Sloka S, Silva C, Wang J, Yong VW. Predominance of Th2 polarization by Vitamin D through a STAT6-dependent mechanism. *J Neuroinflammation.* (2011) 8:56. doi: 10.1186/1742-2094-8-56
85. Villamor E. A potential role for vitamin D on HIV infection? *Nutr Rev.* (2006) 64:226–33. doi: 10.1301/nr.2006.may.226-233
86. Gyllensten K, Josephson F, Lidman K, Sääf M. Severe vitamin D deficiency diagnosed after introduction of antiretroviral therapy including efavirenz in a patient living at latitude 59°N [3]. *AIDS.* (2006) 20:1906–7. doi: 10.1097/01.aids.0000244216.08327.39
87. Hariparsad N, Nallani SC, Sane RS, Buckley DJ, Buckley AR, Desai PB. Induction of CYP3A4 by efavirenz in primary human hepatocytes: comparison with rifampin and phenobarbital. *J Clin Pharmacol.* (2004) 44:1273–81. doi: 10.1177/0091270004269142
88. Childs K, Welz T, Samarawickrama A, Post FA. Effects of vitamin D deficiency and combination antiretroviral therapy on bone in HIV-positive patients. *AIDS.* (2012) 26:253–62. doi: 10.1097/QAD.0b013e32834f324b
89. Arpadi SM, McMahon DJ, Abrams EJ, Bamji M, Purswani M, Engelson ES, et al. Effect of supplementation with cholecalciferol and calcium on 2-y bone mass accrual in HIV-infected children and adolescents: a randomized clinical trial. *Am J Clin Nutr.* (2012) 95:678–85. doi: 10.3945/ajcn.111.024786
90. Fox J, Peters B, Prakash M, Arribas J, Hill A, Moecklinghoff C. Improvement in vitamin D deficiency following antiretroviral regime change: results from the MONET trial. *AIDS Res Hum Retroviruses.* (2011) 27:29–34. doi: 10.1089/aid.2010.0081
91. Cervero M, Agud JL, Torres R, García-Lacalle C, Alcázar V, Jusdado JJ, et al. Higher vitamin D levels in HIV-infected out-patients on treatment with boosted protease inhibitor monotherapy. *HIV Med.* (2013) 14:556–62. doi: 10.1111/hiv.12049
92. Mehta S, Giovannucci E, Mugusi FM, Spiegelman D, Aboud S, Hertzmark E, et al. Vitamin D status of HIV-infected women and its association with HIV disease progression, anemia, and mortality. *PLoS ONE.* (2010) 5:e8770. doi: 10.1371/journal.pone.0008770
93. Viard JP, Souberbielle JC, Kirk O, Reekie J, Knysz B, Losso M, et al. Vitamin D and clinical disease progression in HIV infection: results from the EuroSIDA study. *AIDS.* (2011) 25:1305–15. doi: 10.1097/QAD.0b013e328347f6f7
94. Bang UC, Kolte L, Hitz M, Schierbeck LL, Nielsen SD, Benfield T, et al. The effect of cholecalciferol and calcitriol on biochemical bone markers in HIV type 1-infected males: Results of a clinical trial. *AIDS Res Hum Retroviruses.* (2013) 29:658–64. doi: 10.1089/aid.2012.0263
95. Casado JL, Bañon S, Andrés R, Perez-Elías MJ, Moreno A, Moreno S. Prevalence of causes of secondary osteoporosis and contribution to lower bone mineral density in HIV-infected patients. *Osteoporos Int.* (2014) 25:1071–9. doi: 10.1007/s00198-013-2506-3
96. Sudfeld CR, Mugusi F, Aboud S, Nagu TJ, Wang M, Fawzi WW. Efficacy of vitamin D3 supplementation in reducing incidence of pulmonary tuberculosis and mortality among HIV-infected Tanzanian adults initiating antiretroviral therapy: study protocol for a randomized controlled trial. *Trials.* (2017) 18:66. doi: 10.1186/s13063-017-1819-5
97. Campbell GR, Spector SA. Vitamin D inhibits human immunodeficiency virus type 1 and Mycobacterium tuberculosis infection in macrophages through the induction of autophagy. *PLoS Pathog.* (2012) 8:5 doi: 10.1371/journal.ppat.1002689

9

Live Attenuated *Salmonella enterica* Expressing and Releasing Cell-Permeable Bax BH3 Peptide Through the MisL Autotransporter System Elicits Antitumor Activity in a Murine Xenograft Model of Human B Non-hodgkin's Lymphoma

*Armando Alfredo Mateos-Chávez[1], Paola Muñoz-López[1,2], Elayne Irene Becerra-Báez[1,2], Luis Fernando Flores-Martínez[1], Diego Prada-Gracia[3], Liliana Marisol Moreno-Vargas[3], Guillermina Juliana Baay-Guzmán[1], Uriel Juárez-Hernández[1,4], Bibiana Chávez-Munguía[5], Lourdes Cabrera-Muñóz[6] and Rosendo Luria-Pérez[1]**

[1] Unit of Investigative Research on Oncological Diseases, Children's Hospital of Mexico Federico Gomez, Mexico City, Mexico, [2] Posgrado en Biomedicina y Biotecnología Molecular, Escuela Nacional de Ciencias Biológicas, Instituto Politécnico Nacional, Mexico City, Mexico, [3] Research Unit on Computational Biology and Drug Design, Children's Hospital of Mexico Federico Gomez, Mexico City, Mexico, [4] Department of Molecular Biomedicine, Center for Research and Advanced Studies of the National Polytechnic Institute, Mexico City, Mexico, [5] Department of Infectomics and Molecular Pathogenesis, Center for Research and Advanced Studies of the National Polytechnic Institute, Mexico City, Mexico, [6] Department of Clinical and Experimental Pathology, Children's Hospital of Mexico Federico Gomez, Mexico City, Mexico

***Correspondence:**
Rosendo Luria-Pérez
rluria@himfg.edu.mx

The survival of patients with non-Hodgkin's lymphoma (NHL) has substantially improved with current treatments. Nevertheless, the appearance of drug-resistant cancer cells leads to patient relapse. It is therefore necessary to find new antitumor therapies that can completely eradicate transformed cells. Chemotherapy-resistant cancer cells are characterized by the overexpression of members of the anti-apoptotic B-cell lymphoma 2 (Bcl-2) protein family, such as Bcl-$_{XL}$, Bcl-2, and Mcl-1. We have recently shown that peptides derived from the BH3 domain of the pro-apoptotic Bax protein may antagonize the anti-apoptotic activity of the Bcl-2 family proteins, restore apoptosis, and induce chemosensitization of tumor cells. In this study, we investigated the feasibility of releasing this peptide into the tumor microenvironment using live attenuated *Salmonella enterica*, which has proven to be an ally in cancer therapy due to its high affinity for tumor tissue, its ability to activate the innate and adaptive antitumor immune responses, and its potential use as a delivery system of heterologous molecules. Thus, we expressed and released the cell-permeable Bax BH3 peptide from the surface of *Salmonella enterica* serovar Typhimurium SL3261 through the MisL autotransporter system. We demonstrated that this recombinant bacterium significantly decreased the viability and increased the apoptosis of Ramos cells, a human B NHL cell line. Indeed, the intravenous administration of this recombinant *Salmonella enterica* elicited antitumor activity and extended survival in a xenograft NHL murine model. This antitumor activity was mediated by apoptosis and an inflammatory response. Our approach may represent an eventual alternative to treat relapsing or refractory NHL.

Keywords: non-Hodgkin's lymphoma, *Salmonella enterica*, cancer, Bax BH3 peptide, apoptosis, immunotherapy, MisL autotransporter

INTRODUCTION

Cancer is a worldwide primary health problem, with an annual mortality rate of over 8 million individuals (1). Within the broad malignancy spectrum, non-Hodgkin's lymphoma (NHL) represents 90% of all lymphomas and is one of the most frequent neoplasias in the world (1, 2). NHL arises from the malignant transformation of immature and mature immune cells, compromising B lymphocytes in 86% of cases, and T and NK lymphocytes in 14% (3). Fortunately, chemotherapy, radiotherapy, and immunotherapy have increased patient overall survival to over 80% at 5 years (4, 5). However, complete treatment success is limited by the development of drug resistance, a situation with a dire prognosis and with limited possibilities of a cure (6). It is therefore necessary to find new antitumor therapies that can completely eradicate drug-resistant transformed cells (7).

One of the mechanisms of drug resistance in cancer is the modification of the genes and proteins controlling the mitochondrial pathway of apoptosis, such as members of the B-cell lymphoma 2 (Bcl-2) family (8, 9). This family includes pro-apoptotic BH3-only proteins (Bid, Bim, Puma, Noxa, Bad, Bmf, Hrk, and Bik), anti-apoptotic proteins (Bcl-2, Bcl-$_{XL}$, Bcl-w, Mcl-1, and A1), and effector pro-apoptotic proteins (Bax, Bak, and Bok). Overexpression of anti-apoptotic proteins such as Bcl-2, Bcl-$_{XL}$, and Mcl-1 has been associated with drug resistance in human tumor cell lines (10–12), including NHL cells (13–16). Structural analysis of proteins in the Bcl-2 family has shown an interaction between them via a hydrophobic groove formed by the BH domains (17–19), and the overexpression of anti-apoptotic proteins promotes binding to the pro-apoptotic effector proteins Bax or Bak and inhibits their polymerization on the mitochondrial membrane, thus precluding the release of cytochrome c and the initiation of apoptosis (20, 21). Interaction of these proteins has led to the proposal of eliminating tumor cells that are resistant to apoptosis by blocking the activity of anti-apoptotic proteins with peptides derived from the BH3 domain of pro-apoptotic proteins such as Bak, Bax, Noxa, and Bid that once bound to the Bcl-$_{XL}$, Bcl-2, and Mcl-1 proteins, antagonizing their function (22–24). *In vitro* assays using hydrophobic peptides from the BH3 domain of the proteins Bax, Bad, and Bak, once coupled to the fusogenic peptide of the antennapedia protein (to make them permeable to head and neck squamous cell carcinoma tumor cells), antagonized the Bcl-$_{XL}$ and Bcl-2 activity and restored the apoptosis (25). Furthermore, the small molecules that mimic the function of the BH3-only proteins have been tested in clinical trials, and even the inhibitor of Bcl-2 activity, Venotoclax/ABT-199, was recently approved by the U.S. Food and Drug Administration (FDA) for the treatment of chronic lymphocytic leukemia (CLL) (26, 27).

In spite of their efficacy and promising results, BH3 domain peptides and the molecules mimicking the BH3 domain still need to be specifically and selectively directed toward the tumor microenvironment in order to decrease side effects. Several strategies have been attempted to overcome this problem, so in this study, we have suggested the use of a live attenuated bacterial vector, *Salmonella enterica* serovar Typhimurium strain SL3261, which has been proven to be an ally in the therapy of cancer due to its high affinity for tumor tissue (28, 29), its ability to activate the innate and adaptive antitumor immune responses (30), and its potential use as a delivery system, since once in the tumor microenvironment, it becomes a true factory of heterologous molecules (31, 32). We recently demonstrated the ability of *Salmonella enterica* to carry and transfer plasmids into tumor cells (bactofection). Transferred plasmid encoding a peptide from the BH3 domain of the pro-apoptotic Bax protein antagonized the anti-apoptotic activity of the Bcl-2 family proteins, restored apoptosis, and induced chemosensitization of tumor cells (33). In this study, we evaluated the feasibility for the cell-permeable Bax BH3 peptide [Tag peptide (T) bound to Bax BH3 peptide (X) and the fusogenic peptide (P)] expressed and released from the surface of *Salmonella enterica* serovar Typhimurium strain SL3261 through the MisL autotransporter system (34) (*Salmonella enterica* L-STXP) to promote apoptosis signaling and the death of NHL tumor cells. Our results demonstrated that *Salmonella enterica* L-STXP significantly decreased the viability and increased apoptosis in Ramos cells, a human B NHL cell line. Indeed, the intravenous administration of this recombinant bacterium elicited antitumor activity and extended survival in a murine xenograft model of human B NHL. This antitumor activity was mediated by apoptosis and an inflammatory response. Taken together, our results suggest that the live attenuated *Salmonella enterica* serovar Typhimurium strain SL3261 expressing and releasing cell-permeable Bax BH3 peptide through the MisL autotransporter system may represent an eventual alternative to treat relapsing or refractory NHL.

MATERIALS AND METHODS

Molecular Modeling by Homology

To generate the model of the L-SXTP chimera [MisL autotransporter system = L (35) (NCBI Reference Sequence NP_462656.1), OmpT cleavage recognition site = S (34), Bax BH3 peptide = X (25), Flag peptide = T (34), and fusogenic peptide = P (34, 36)], we used two independent strategies and then chose the consensus model. On the one hand, we used an assembly of large rigid fragments, including the entire folding, obtained from similar structures aligned by means of their primary and secondary sequences. This methodology cuts and pastes fragments of the peptide skeleton of known structures (SWISS-MODEL) (37, 38). On the other hand, we used modeling for the satisfaction of molecular constraints extracted from databases and similar structures aligned. This method helps produce a set of structures for the A sequence, all of them compatible with the restrictions observed in the templates (MODELER) (39, 40). All subunits (L, S, X, T, and P) were modeled separately using molecular modeling by homology. As templates, we used three-dimensional (3-D) structures from the PDB (http://www.rcsb.org/pdb). The MisL autotransporter system was modeled using a library of segments that contained structural information of the following coordinate files: 4MEE, 3KVN, 3SLJ, 3QQ2, 3AEH, 1UYN, 2QOM, 3ML3, 1DAB, 3H09—all of them with identities in sequence between 13 and 43%. The Bax BH3 peptide, coupled at OmpT peptide, was modeled using the 3-D structure of BCL-2 in complex with a Bax BH3 peptide (PDB code: 2XA0, 2.7 Å resolution) (41) and the Bax BH3-in-Groove dimer (PBD: 4BDU, 2.9 Å resolution) (42). The fusogenic peptide, coupled at Flag peptide, was modeled using the 3-D coordinates deposited in the following ID PDBs: 5FN4, 6IJO, and 5OA1.

Geometry Optimization of the Proposed Models

Once the 3-D models were prepared, hydrogen atoms were added, and side chain orientations were optimized through energy minimization using the steepest descent method, employing 2,000 cycles using the CHARMM27 parameters found in NAMD (43). Next, the complex was assembled and finally was embedded in a biological membrane using the set of CHARM-GUI programs (44, 45). The positioning in the membrane, in terms of inclination angle and hydrophobic thickness, was calculated using the Orientations of Proteins in Membranes (OPM) database (46). We also obtained information on the number of transmembrane secondary structure segments and their composition.

Stereochemical Quality Evaluation of the Models

Coordinate files of the 3-D models were sent to MolProbity (47) to produce a Ramachandran plot (ϕ and ψ angles), reflecting polypeptide chain distortion in the non-allowed region. We also sent the coordinate files to RAMPAGE to identify side chains with less common conformations possibly because of local protein tension (48). The quality of the models was further validated using two additional tools: ProQ3/ProQ3D (49, 50) and QMEAN (51).

Bacterial Strains and Oligonucleotides

The following bacterial strains were used: *Escherichia coli* strain DH5-α (*E. coli* DH5-α) (Gibco, BRL, Gaithersburg, MD, USA) and *Salmonella enterica* serovar Typhimurium strain SL3261, a mutant at Aro A (*Salmonella enterica* SL3261) (34, 52). The employed oligonucleotide sequences used in this study are summarized in **Table 1**. The oligonucleotide sequences encoded the following peptides: fusogenic [P, EAAAAAEAAAAAEAAAAAEAAAAA (34, 36)], Flag [T, DYKDDDDK (34)], Bax BH3 [X, STKKLSECLKRIGDELDSNM (25)], OmpT protease cleavage site [S, KRPGGGGGKRGGGGGPKR (34)].

Oligonucleotide Coupling (Adapters)

The fragments encoding the peptides of interest (adapters) were obtained by coupling 1 pMol of each initiator (forward and reverse) with 200 μM of $MgCl_2$ in a volume of 100 μL. The reaction mixture was heated to 94°C for 15 min and slowly cooled to room temperature. The product of coupling contains the encoding sequence of the peptide of interest flanked by the restriction sites Xba I and BamH I, open to ligation without the need for prior digestion, and the internal sites Nhe I, Sal I, Nsi I, Xho I, in accordance with the initiator's design (**Figure 1**). The primers FP1 and FP2 give origin to the adapter that encodes the fusogenic peptide (P), the primers BAX1 and BAX2 give origin to the adapter that encodes the Bax-BH3 peptide (X), the primers FLAG1 and FLAG2 give origin to the adapter that encodes the Molecular Tag (T), and finally, the primers SCOT1 and SCOT2 give origin to the adapter that encodes the OmpT protease cleavage site (S).

Plasmid Construction

Following the strategy previously reported by Luria-Perez et al. (34) and Ruiz-Pérez et al. (35), the complete β domain (294 amino acids) and a mutated portion of the α domain (210 amino acids) of the MisL autotransporter were used to express the peptides of interest on the surface of *Salmonella enterica* serovar Typhimurium strain SL3261. From the amino region toward the carboxy terminal, the following peptides were cloned: fusogenic, to destabilize the membrane; Bax BH3, to antagonize the activity of anti-apoptotic proteins from the Bcl-2 family; the molecular Tag Flag, to follow the fusion proteins; and finally, the recognition site of the OmpT protease, to release the peptides from the bacterial surface; this peptide complex was coupled to the mutated amino-terminal of the α domain of MisL (Δα-MisL), followed by the β domain of the MisL (β-MisL) autotransporter. The generated plasmids and the expected fusion proteins are shown in **Figure 1A**, and the general strategy in plasmid construction is shown in **Figure 1B**. Plasmid construction was performed in the bacterium *E. coli* DH5-α. Briefly, the plasmid pnirBLTBbMisL (35) was digested with the enzymes Nhe I and BamH I, and a 1,318 bp fragment was obtained, containing the Δα-β domain of the MisL autotransporter; this fragment was purified and stored. The remaining fragment, pnirBLTB (2,627 bp) was used to sequentially insert the adapter fragments encoding the fusogenic peptide (P), the Bax-BH3(X) peptide, the Molecular Tag Flag (T), and the cleavage site of the OmpT protease (S). These adapters contain the external restriction sites Xba I at position 5′ and BamH I at position 3′, open and ready to engage in ligation without the need for prior digestion, and internal sites at position 3′ such as Nhe I, Sal I, Nsi I, or Xho I. Thus, every plasmid adapter may be identified by the loss of an Nhe I site and the gain of new restriction sites at position 3′. Finally, the fragment encoding the Δα-β domain of

TABLE 1 | Oligonucleotides used in this study.

Name	Sequence	Characteristics
FP 1	5′CTAGATGCGAAGCGGCCGCTGCAGCGGAAGCCGCAGCTGCGGCAGAA GCTGCGGCAGCCGCTGAAGCGGCTGCCGCGGCAGCTAGCGTCGACG3′	Forward. Encodes the synthetic fusogenic peptides and *Xba*I, *Nhe*I, *Sal*I, and *BamH*I restriction sites (underlined).
FP 2	5′GATCCGTCGACGCTAGCTGCCGCGGCAGCCGCTTCAGCGGCTGCCGCA GCTTCTGCCGCAGCTGCGGCTTCCGCTGCAGCGGCCGCTTCGCAT3′	Reverse. Encodes the synthetic fusogenic peptides and *Xba*I, *Nhe*I, *Sal*I, and *BamH*I restriction sites (underlined).
FLAG1	5′CTAGAGATTATAAAGATGACGATGACAAAGCTAGCATGCATG3′	Forward. Encodes the molecular Tag Flag and *Xba*I, *Nhe* I, *Nsi*I, and *BamH* I restriction sites (underlined).
FLAG2	5′GATCCATGCATGCTAGCTTTGTCATCGTCATCTTTATAATCT3′	Reverse. Encodes the molecular Tag Flag and *Xba*I, *Nhe*I, *Sal* I and *BamH*I restriction sites (underlined).
BAX 1	5′CTAGAAGCACCAAAAAACTGAGCGAATGCCTGAAACGCATTGGC GATGAACTGGATAGCAACATGGCTAGCCTCGAGG3′	Forward. Encodes the Bax BH3 peptide and *Xba* I, *Nhe* I, *Xho* I, and *BamH* I restriction sites (underlined).
BAX 2	5′GATCCCTCGAGGCTAGCCATGTTGCTATCCAGTTCATCGCC AATGCGTTTCAGGCATTCGCTCAGTTTTTTGGTGCTT3′	Reverse. Encodes the Bax BH3 peptide and *Xba* I, *Nhe* I, *Xho* I and *BamH* I restriction sites (underlined).
SCOT 1	5′CTAGAAAACGCCCGGGCGGTGGCGGTGGCAAACGCGG CGGTGGCGGTGGCCCGAAACGCGCTAGCGTCGACG3′	Forward. Encodes the protease OmpT cleavage site sequence and *Xba*I, *Nhe* I, *Sal*I and *BamH*I restriction sites (underlined).
SCOT 2	5′GATCCGTCGACGCTAGCGCGTTTCGGGCCACCGCCAC CGCCGCGTTTGCCACCGCCACCGCCCGGGCGTTTT3′	Reverse. Encodes the protease OmpT cleavage site sequence and *Xba*I, *Nhe* I, *Sal*I, and *BamH*I restriction sites (underlined).

the MisL autotransporter (L) is inserted. With this strategy, the plasmid that encodes the cell-permeable Bax BH3 peptide that can be expressed and released through the MisL autotransporter system was constructed: pL-SXTP (encoding the Δα-β MisL, the cleavage site of the OmpT protein, the Bax-BH3 peptide, the molecular Tag Flag, and the fusogenic peptide), as well as the control plasmids: pL-XT (encoding the Δα-β MisL, the Bax BH3 peptide, and the molecular Tag Flag), pL-SXT (encoding the Δα-β MisL, the cleavage site of the OmpT protein, the Bax-BH3 peptide, and the molecular Tag Flag), pL-TP (encoding the Δα-β MisL, the molecular Tag Flag, and the fusogenic peptide), pL-XTP (encoding the Δα-β MisL, the Bax-BH3 peptide, the molecular Tag Flag, and the fusogenic peptide). These plasmids gave origin to the recombinant proteins with the same names: L-SXTP, L-XT, L-SXT, L-TP, and L-XTP, respectively. The expression of these recombinant proteins is controlled by the promoter nirB, inducible in anaerobiosis (35).

Bacterial Culture and Induction Conditions

Bacterial cultures and induction conditions of the recombinant protein were conducted with slight modifications to the previously described methods (34). Briefly, the bacteria *E. coli* DH5-α and *Salmonella enterica* SL3261 were transformed by heat shock or electroporation, respectively, with the previously described plasmids and cultured in broth or Brain Heart Infusion (BHI) agar (Bioxon) with 100 μg/ml ampicillin at 37°C. The *Salmonella enterica* SL3261 strains were cultured in medium supplemented with 0.01% 2,3 dihydroxybenzoic acid (DHB) (Sigma-Aldrich). Considering that recombinant protein expression requires anaerobic conditions, since it is controlled by the induction promoter in anaerobiosis *nirB*, a bacterial colony was cultured in 5 ml BHI broth supplemented with DHB and ampicillin at 37°C and shaken at 200 rpm. When an optic density of 1.0–600 nm was obtained, 100 μl was transferred into a 15-ml tube with thioglycollate broth (Sigma-Aldrich) to promote anaerobic environment, incubated for 10–12 h in DHB with ampicillin, at 37°C and shaken at 200 rpm. The recombinant *Salmonellas* received the name of the recombinant protein they express: *Salmonella enterica* L-SXTP, *Salmonella enterica* L-SXT, *Salmonella enterica* L-XT, *Salmonella enterica* L-SXT, *Salmonella enterica* L-TP, and *Salmonella enterica* L-XTP.

Recombinant Protein Expression

Recombinant protein expression was analyzed by Western blot and the translocation of the recombinant proteins to the bacterial surface by immunofluorescence and flow cytometry.

Western Blot Assays

Recombinant protein expression was analyzed with slight modifications to the previously described techniques (34, 35). Briefly, recombinant bacteria, after induction as previously described, were harvested by centrifugation, and 10^9 bacteria were resuspended in 100 μl loading buffer (Tris 0.5 M, pH 6.8, SDS 2%, 2-mercaptoethanol 140 mM, and bromophenol blue 0.1%) and boiled at 94°C for 15 min. Recombinant proteins were analyzed by electrophoresis on 12.0% acrylamide gels under reduction conditions (SDS-PAGE), and the Western blots (WB) were performed as previously described (34). Briefly, the transfer of proteins to the nitrocellulose membrane was conducted by semi-dry transference at 25 V and for 10 min in the Trans-Turbo Blot System (Bio-Rad). Immunodetection of the recombinant proteins was performed with a monoclonal antibody induced in an anti-Flag mouse (1 mg/ml, Sigma-Aldrich), diluted 1:1,000 in PBA 1× (1% BSA in PBS 1×). The membranes were incubated for 2 h with the primary antibody and subsequently for 1 h with the anti-mouse IgG-HRP secondary antibody (1 mg/ml, Abcam) at room temperature, diluted 1:1,000 in PBA 1×. Finally, the membranes were developed in a solution of 4-chloro-α-naphtol (Sigma-Aldrich) in methanol-PBS 1×, pH 7.4, and hydrogen peroxide (J.T. Baker).

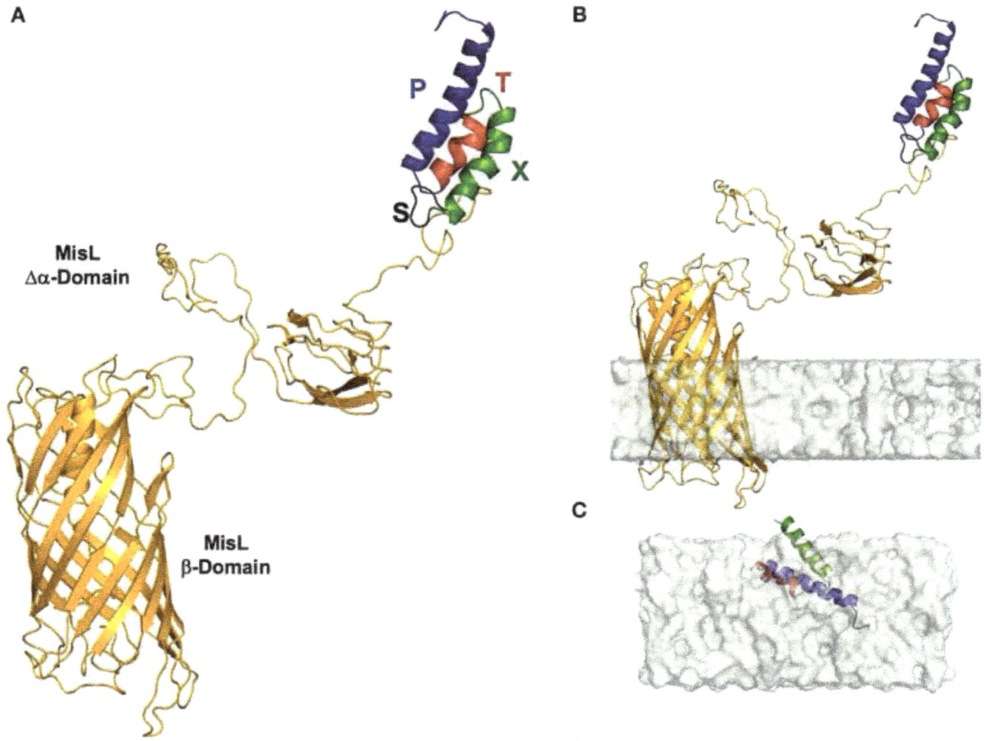

FIGURE 1 | Three-dimensional (3-D) structure of the L-SXTP recombinant protein. **(A)** The MisL autotransporter (L) is observed as a protein composed of two domains. A β-barrel of 12 antiparallel chains (in yellow) and an extracellular α domain that presents to the N-terminal region a combination of several units of secondary structure of β-strands, organized in a specific geometry of β-solenoid architecture. The domains are connected by an α-helical linker, which is embedded within the pore of ~24 Å in diameter of the β-barrel in an extended conformation. The peptides of the fusion core consolidate an α-helical folding and are exposed in the N-terminal region: fusogenic peptide (P) (in blue)-Molecular Tag (T) (in red)-Bax-BH3 peptide (X) (in green)-cleavage site of OmpT protease (S) (in black). **(B)** 3-D structure of L-STXP embedded in a membrane model. We can observe an angle of inclination of 12° with respect to the normal of the membrane and a hydrophobic membrane thickness of 23.8 ± 1.5 Å. Twelve transmembrane segments, in a configuration of antiparallel β-strands, are identified: 1 (312–316), 2 (336–343), 3 (354–362), 4 (385–392), 5 (403–412), 6 (432–443), 7 (452–463), 8 (487–499), 9 (510–520), 10 (545–553), 11 (560–565), 12 (577–584). **(C)** A recreation of the internalization of the fusion core, in a DPPC membrane model, from a theoretical calculation of the membrane internalization propensity of the amino acid residues that constitute the fusion core (data not shown).

Immunofluorescence and Flow Cytometry Assays

Recombinant protein translocation to the bacterial surface via the MisL autotransporter was evaluated by immunofluorescence and flow cytometry, as previously described (34, 35). Briefly, after inducing the expression of the recombinant proteins as described above, 10^8 bacteria were incubated with antibody mouse anti-Flag FITC (1 mg/ml, Sigma-Aldrich) at a dilution of 1:100 in PBA 1× for 2 h, at room temperature, at 100 rpm, in dark conditions. The bacterial suspension was washed in PBS 1× and resuspended in 50 μl PBS 1×, 5 μl of which were used for fluorescent microscopy analysis (Olympus Microscope, model IX73), and the rest was resuspended in 450 μl PBS 1× for flow cytometry analysis in the CytoFLEX system (Beckman Coulter).

Cell Lines and Cell Cultures

The Ramos cell line (Burkitt's lymphoma), a human B NHL cell line, was obtained from the American Type Cell Collection (ATCC, CRL-1923) and cultured in Advanced RPMI 1640 medium (Invitrogen), supplemented with 1% antibiotics-antimycotics containing 10,000 U/ml penicillin G, 10 mg/ml streptomycin, and 25 μg/ml amphotericin B and 4% fetal bovine serum (FBS, Invitrogen). Cultures were permanently maintained at 37°C and 5% CO_2. For the infection assays, the cells were grown with Advanced RPMI 1640 medium (Invitrogen), supplemented with 2% FBS without antibiotics (Invitrogen).

Detection of the Anti-apoptotic Molecules by Western Blot

The detection of the anti-apoptotic molecules was conducted with slight modifications to the technique described by Hernández-Luna et al. (16). A million Ramos cells were lysed with RIPA lysis buffer (Sigma-Aldrich) supplemented with a cocktail of protease inhibitors (Roche). Protein quantification was performed with the bicinchoninic acid kit by ThermoFisher Scientific. For the Western blot, 25 μg of total protein was placed in each well, and an electrophoresis on 12% polyacrylamide-SDS gel was performed. The proteins were then transferred to nitrocellulose membranes (Bio-Rad) with a Trans-Turbo Blot System by Bio-Rad (25 V, 10 min). For the detection of the Bcl-$_{XL}$ and Mcl-1 proteins, we used anti-Bcl-$_{XL}$ and anti-Mcl-1 antibodies (Cell Signaling) induced in rabbits and diluted 1:1,000 in blocking buffer (Li-Cor), and as a secondary antibody, goat anti-rabbit IgG IR Dye 680 cw (Li-Cor) diluted 1:10,000 in blocking buffer (Li-Cor). As a constitutive protein control, we used an anti-β tubulin antibody induced in rabbit and diluted at 1:1,000 in blocking buffer (Li-Cor). Finally, the image was obtained and analyzed in the system for Infrared Fluorescent Imaging, Odyssey CLx (Li-Cor).

Tumor Cell Infection With Recombinant *Salmonella* Strains

Infection of tumor cells with recombinant *Salmonella* strains was conducted as described by Vendrell et al. (53). Briefly, Ramos cells were cultured in 48-well plates (500,000 cells/well) in 1 mL of Advanced RPMI 1640 medium supplemented with 2% FBS without antibiotic. The cells were infected at a Multiplicity of Infection (MOI) of 100 with previously induced recombinant bacteria. After centrifugation at 2,000 rpm for 5 min to foster the interaction between bacteria and cells, they were incubated at 37°C and 5% CO_2 for 2–10 h. Subsequently they were washed twice in base advanced RPMI 1640 medium supplemented with gentamycin (Sigma-Aldrich) 100 µg/mL and finally resuspended in 1 mL of advanced RPMI 1640 medium supplemented with 2% FBS and 50 µg/mL gentamycin and used in the cellular viability and apoptosis detection protocols. Vincristine (Sigma-Aldrich) 0.5 nM diluted in injectable water was used as a positive control in all cases; this drug is used as treatment for NHL.

Cellular Viability Assay by Trypan Blue Dye Exclusion

The viability assays were conducted with slight modifications to the previously described technique (53). Briefly, 500,000 Ramos cells, infected at a MOI of 100 with the previously induced recombinant *Salmonella* strains expressing the peptides of interest via the MisL autotransporter, were incubated for 2–10 h at 37°C and 5% CO_2 and analyzed in an automated cell counter (BioRad) to determine cell viability by trypan blue dye exclusion (Invitrogen). Vincristine (Sigma-Aldrich) 0.5 nM diluted in injectable water was used as a positive control.

Apoptosis Assays

The *in vitro* apoptosis assays were analyzed by flow cytometry and Western blot as follows:

a). Determination of Active Caspase-3 Cells and TUNEL by Flow Cytometry. These assays were performed with modifications to the technique described by Hernández-Luna et al. (16, 33). After treating the Ramos cells (500,000 cells) with the induced recombinant *Salmonella* strains (MOI of 100) during 8 h, cells were washed, fixed, permeabilized (Cytofix/Cytoperm, Becton Dickinson) and stained with the anti-active caspase-3 FITC antibody according to the FITC Active Caspase-3 Apoptosis Kit (BD Pharmingen) instructions; for the TUNEL assay, the enzyme and substrate were added according to the instructions of the *in situ* Cell Death Detection Kit, Fluorescein (Roche, Sigma-Aldrich). Data acquisition and analysis were performed in a CytoFLEX (Beckman Coulter) flow cytometer.

b). Determination of Caspase-3 and Cleaved PARP by Western Blot. The detection of the apoptotic molecules was conducted with slight modifications to the technique described by Hernández-Luna et al. (16). After treating the Ramos cells (6×10^6 cells) with the induced recombinant *Salmonella* strains (MOI of 100) during 8 h, cells were lysed with RIPA lysis buffer (Sigma-Aldrich) supplemented with a cocktail of protease inhibitors (Roche). Protein quantification was performed with the bicinchoninic acid kit by ThermoFisher Scientific. For the Western blot, 15 µg of total protein was placed in each well, and an electrophoresis on 15% polyacrylamide-SDS gel was performed. The proteins were then transferred to nitrocellulose membranes (Bio-Rad) with a Trans-Turbo Blot System by Bio-Rad (25 V, 10 min). For the detection of the complete caspase-3 and cleaved PARP proteins, we used an anti-caspase 3 (Human specific, Abcam) and anti-cleaved PARP-1 (Human specific, Cell Signaling) antibodies induced in rabbits and diluted 1:300 and 1:500, respectively, in blocking buffer (Li-Cor), and as a secondary antibody, goat anti-rabbit IgG IR Dye 680 cw (Li-Cor) diluted 1:10,000 in blocking buffer (Li-Cor). As a constitutive protein control, we used an anti-β tubulin antibody (Abcam), induced in rabbit and diluted at 1:7,000 in blocking buffer (Li-Cor). Finally, the image was obtained and analyzed in the system for infrared fluorescent imaging, Odyssey CLx (Li-Cor).

Mice

Pathogen-free, female athymic BALB/c *nu/nu* mice between the ages of 6 and 8 weeks were obtained from the bioterium of the National Institute of Medical Sciences and Nutrition Salvador Zubiran and kept in an enriched and sterile environment in the bioterium of the Children's Hospital of Mexico Federico Gomez in accordance with the local and federal regulations for the Care and Use of Laboratory Animals. Distress and suffering were avoided as much as possible. All procedures were supervised by a clinical veterinarian.

Murine Xenograft Model

The development of the mouse xenograft model of the human B NHL was performed with slight modifications to the previously described method by Manders et al. (54). Briefly, female athymic BALB/c *nu/nu* mice between 6 and 8 weeks of age were inoculated intraperitoneally with cyclophosphamide (100 mg/kg of body weight), and 24 h later, they were anesthetized in a gas chamber with isoflurane, 100 units (Abbott); they were then subcutaneously inoculated on the right flank with 10^7 Ramos cells in a volume of 100 µl of Opti-MEM reduced serum medium without phenol red (Invitrogen). As soon as the tumors were visible and reached an approximate size of 100–150 mm^3 (approximately after 15 days of inoculation), mice were separated into groups of five to evaluate the antitumor activity of the recombinant *Salmonellas*. The volume of the ellipsoidal tumor was determined with the following formula: volume = 1/6π X length X width X height.

Antitumor Activity of the Recombinant *Salmonella* Strains

These assays were performed with slight modifications to the technique described by Nakase et al. (55). Briefly, groups of five mice with tumors measuring ~100–150 mm^3 received four doses in the tail vein, at intervals of 7 days, of 100 μl with 1 × 10^7 CFU in PBS 1× from each of the different previously induced recombinant *Salmonella* strains. The mice were also administered with 0.6 mg/ml ampicillin in their drinking water. Control mice received 100 μl PBS 1× following the same inoculation protocol. Tumor size was measured with a Vernier caliper and calculated as mentioned previously. Survival was registered daily. After 5 days of last inoculation of recombinant *Salmonella* strains, the mice were euthanized, and the tumor tissue was resected and stored for bacterial culture and immunohistochemistry assays. Serums were collected for inflammatory cytokine determination.

Bacterial Culture From Tumor Tissue: Determination of Colony-Forming Units (CFU)

To demonstrate recombinant *Salmonella* strains tumor targeting, the murine xenograft model of the human B NHL was treated with the recombinant *Salmonella* strains, and then the bacteria were isolated from the tumor tissue; this procedure was performed with slight modifications to the previously described method by Miyake K et al. (56). Briefly, groups of three mice with tumors measuring ~100–150 mm^3 received four doses in the tail vein, at intervals of 7 days, of 100 μl with 1 × 10^7 CFU in PBS 1× from each of the different previously induced recombinant *Salmonella* strains. Mice were also administered with 0.6 mg/ml ampicillin in their drinking water. Control mice received 100 μl PBS 1× following the same inoculation protocol. Five days after last inoculation, mice were euthanized, and the tumors were resected for bacteria culture. The tumor specimens were weighed, homogenized, and suspended in 1 ml PBST (0.05% Tween 20 in PBS 1×). The suspension was diluted five times each up to 1:10,000, then cultured in BHI agar medium in the presence or absence of ampicillin (100 μg/ml) for 12 h. Finally, the colonies were counted and reported as CFU per tissue gram (CFU/g). We also analyzed the presence of the bacteria in the tumor tissue, performing an immunohistochemical assay using as primary antibody an anti-*Salmonella* induced in rabbit.

Detection of Apoptotic Markers in Tumor Tissue by Immunohistochemistry

To demonstrate that the antitumor activity of the recombinant *Salmonella* strains was mediated by an apoptosis mechanism, tumor-bearing mice that previously received four doses in the tail vein of the recombinant *Salmonella* strains, as described previously, were euthanized after 5 days of the last inoculation, and the tumors were resected for immunohistochemical staining of apoptotic markers.

Tumor Histology

The tumors were removed and fixed with absolute ethanol. The tumors were dehydrated and then embedded in paraffin. For histological examination, 4-μm-thick sections were cut on a semi-automated microtome (Leica, USA), placed on glass slides, and deparaffinized. The slides were stained sequentially with hematoxylin and eosin (H&E) to assess the tumor histology. Slides were analyzed under an Olympus BX-40 microscope.

Determination of Apoptotic Markers by Immunohistochemistry Staining

The expression of active Caspase-3, Caspase-8, Ki67, and the presence or absence of *Salmonella* were analyzed in 4-μm tumor slices by immunohistochemistry using specific antibodies as previously described (57). In brief, antigen retrieval was performed by immersing the slides in Antigen Unmasking Solutions Citrate-Based (VECTOR) for 20 min into pressure cooker. Endogenous peroxidase activity was inhibited by immersing the slides in 3% H_2O_2-methanol for 15 min two times, and background nonspecific binding was reduced by incubating with normal horse serum in PBS 1× for 60 min. The slides were incubated 60 min at room temperature with antibody against active Caspase-3 (GeneTex, dilution 1:250), Caspase 8 (GeneTex, dilution 1:1,500), Ki67 (BioSystems, dilution 1:100), and *Salmonella* (1:4000). Finally, the slides were washed two times in PBS 1× 0.1 M pH 7.4 for 5 min. In order to reduce variability. All samples were processed at the same time in a single experiment using a single batch of antibody. After washing, the slides were incubated with the ImmPRESS HRP anti-rabbit IgG polymer system for 30 min at room temperature and then with 3,3′-diaminobenzidine tetra-hydrochloride (DAKO, Carpinteria, CA, USA) for 1–5 min. The reaction was arrested with distilled water, and the slides were counterstained with hematoxylin. Thereafter, the tissues were washed in tap water for 5 min, dehydrated sequentially in 70, 90, and 100% ethanol and xylene and then mounted.

Detection of Apoptosis by Terminal Deoxynucleotidyl Transferase dUTP Nick End Labeling (TUNEL) Assay in Tumor Tissue

The DNA fragmentation in tumor tissue was evaluated by *in situ* TUNEL assay using an *in situ* Cell Death Detection Kit (POD) (Roche Applied Science, Mannheim, Germany) following the manufacturer's instructions in 4-μm tumor slices. Briefly, an Antigen Unmasking Solution Citrate-Based (VECTOR), incubated in a water bath for 20 min, was used for antigen retrieval, and endogenous peroxide activity was blocked with methanol and 3% hydrogen peroxide for 15 min. They were blocked with normal horse serum for 1 h, and the preparations were incubated for 60 min with TUNEL reaction mixture [Terminal transferase (Tdt) diluted in a buffer solution that included fluorescein conjugated oligonucleotides] and subsequently incubated with an anti-fluorescein antibody (Converter-POD) for 30min, both reactions were performed at 37°C in a humidified atmosphere in the dark. Color was generated by adding the substrate 3,3′-diaminobenzidine (DAB) (VECTOR) for 1–2 min, and counterstaining was performed with hematoxylin. The tissues were dehydrated and covered with resin. Finally, the slides were analyzed under light microscopy (Olympus BX-40), and the nuclear positive cells were determined.

In all cases, for digital automated morphometry, the immunohistochemically stained sections were digitizing at 40×

magnification using an Aperio Scanscope CS (Aperio, Vista, CA). The images were reviewed using an ImageScope (Aperio). Once the areas were recorded, they were sent for automated image analysis using the Spectrum Software V11.1.2.752 (Aperio). For the within-tissue intensity, an algorithm was developed to quantify the total protein expression. The output from the algorithm gives a number of quantitative measurements, namely, the intensity of positive staining. The staining intensity was categorized as 0 (no staining), 1+ (weak), 2+ (moderate), and 3+ (strong).

Determination of Inflammatory Cytokines by Cytometric Bead Array (CBA)

After the antitumor activity assays of the murine model of NHL xenotransplantation induced by different recombinant strains of *Salmonella enterica*, as it was previously described, the mice were euthanized, and the serum samples obtained were analyzed by means of the CBA in order to characterize the profile of inflammatory cytokines induced along the treatment. The serum samples were prepared according to the BD™ CBA Mouse Inflammation Kit (Becton Dickinson, BD) specifications. In this assay, six bead populations with distinct fluorescence intensities have been coated with capture antibodies specific for Interleukin-6 (IL-6), Interleukin-10 (IL-10), Interleukin-12p70 (IL-12p70), Monocyte chemoattractant protein-1 (MCP-1); Interferon-γ (IFN-γ), and Tumor necrosis factor-α (TNF-α) proteins. The six bead populations are mixed together to form the BD CBA, which is resolved in a red channel (i.e., FL3 or FL4) of a flow cytometer. The captured beads, PE-conjugated detection antibodies, and recombinant standards or test samples are incubated together to form sandwich complexes. Following the acquisition of sample data using the flow cytometer, the sample results are generated in graphical and tabular format using the BD CBA Analysis Software or FCAP Array™ Software. Briefly, the standards dilutions and the undiluted serums were exposed to a mixture of cytokines (IL-12p70, IL-6, IL-10, TNF-α, IFN-γ, MCP1) together with the PE-coupled detection reagent. The mixture was incubated for 2 h at room temperature in darkness. After that, it was washed with 1 ml of washing buffer and centrifuged at 200 g for 5 min to then remove the supernatant and recovering with 100 μl of washing buffer. The samples were finally analyzed with a BD FACS Canto II flow cytometer, resulting in a total of 500 events per sample. The FCAP Array software of BD (3.0 version) was used for the quantitative analysis of the concentration and Median Fluorescence Intensities (MFI) of each cytokine.

Statistical Analysis

To determine the differences between cells or mice groups treated with the different recombinant *Salmonella* strains, we used one-way analysis of variance (ANOVA) and *post hoc* Bonferroni tests, with a 95% confidence interval. In all cases, the average of three or more independent experiments is presented ± the standard deviation (*SD*). Animal survival was analyzed with the log-rank test on Kaplan-Meier curves. Differences were considered significant at $p \leq 0.05$ in all comparisons. Statistical analysis was performed with GraphPad Prism 5 software.

RESULTS

3-D Structure of the MisL Autotransporter System Carrying the Cell-Permeable Bax BH3 Peptide

Type V autotransporter proteins, the family MisL belongs to, present a diverse variety of functions such as cell adhesion, pathogenesis phenomena, or mediating in the immune response interruption of the host. This is the result of having a rich structural diversity given by its large amount of secondary structures, the geometrical organization of their domains, and the different oligomerization states that these proteins arrange. In our case, because of its function, MisL-SXTP chimera (L-SXTP) has been clearly identified as a molecular carrier. Therefore, and since the fused peptides are located toward the N-terminal region, characterizing the 3-D structure of L-SXTP together with the evaluation of the effect that these peptides may have on its folding and stability are extremely relevant. With this motivation, molecular modeling of the L-SXTP chimera allowed us to obtain a good approximation of the 3-D structure of each of the components of the chimera introduced in this work (**Figure 1A**). The MisL autotransporter is observed as a protein composed of two domains. A first β-barrel domain made up of 12 antiparallel chains with five short handles is internalized toward the periplasmic space, and a second extracellular domain showing at the N-terminal region a combination of several units of β-strands was organized in a specific geometry known as β-solenoid architecture. Inside this former structural motif, chains of amino acids are densely packed in a compact core that was predominantly hydrophobic. Finally, connecting both domains, an α-helical linker extends along the first domain β-barrel pore of ~24 Å diameter. Although the peptides of the fusion core consolidate an α-helical folding and the cleavage site of the OmpT protease is revealed as a flexible loop, these motifs do not induce any unfolding or instability of the 3-D structure of MisL, neither in its global configuration, nor in the proximity to the β-solenoid (**Figure 1A**). The fusion core is exposed in the N-terminal region, and it is the cleavage site of the OmpT protease that facilitates its release by the PgtE protease (data not shown) (58). When predicting the spatial arrangement of our model in a lipid bilayer, a 12° tilt angle with respect to the normal of the membrane can be observed. In addition, 12 transmembrane segments can be identified in a configuration of antiparallel β-strands [1 (312–316), 2 (336–343), 3 (354–362), 4 (385–392), 5 (403–412), 6 (432–443), 7 (452–463), 8 (487–499), 9 (510–520), 10 (545–553), 11 (560–565), 12 (577–584)] embedded in a hydrophobic membrane thickness of 23.8 ± 1.5 Å (**Figure 1B**). The depth of penetration of these structures in the membrane coincides with those reported for other 3-D structures of various autotransporters deposited in the protein data bank. With respect to the fusion core [Tag peptide (T) bound to Bax BH3 peptide (X) and the fusogenic peptide (P)], we hypothesize that after being excised due to proteolytic processing cleavage site of the OmpT, it is released with a helix-loop-helix conformation. When making a theoretical prediction about the internalization of the core in the membrane, we observed that given its amino acid composition and its hydrophobicity, it is possible that it crosses the membrane through a diffusion process (**Figure 1C**).

Construction of the Plasmids *pL-XT*, *pL-SXT*, *pL-TP*, *pL-XTP*, and *pL-SXTP*

The ability of the MisL autotransporter to translocate the proteins on the surface of *Salmonella enterica* SL3261 (*S. enterica* SL3261) and its release from it to the tumoral microenvironment has been previously reported by our group (34, 35, 58). In this work, we designed recombinant proteins, controlled by the promoter *nirB*, inducible in a microaerophilic environment; these proteins contain in their amino terminal portion the signal peptide of heat-labile enterotoxin B subunit (LTB) of enterotoxigenic *E. coli*, necessary to perform the translocation to the periplasmic space through the Sec Dependent System (59). According to the described strategy for the construction of the plasmids, the adapters that encode for each one of the peptides were inserted sequentially downstream from the *nirB* promoter's sequence and the signal peptide LTB sequence, as shown in **Figure 2B**. For the plasmid that encodes the cell-permeable Bax BH3 peptide, which expresses and releases from the MisL autotransporter system, it was first inserted in the adapter that encodes the fusogenic peptide(P) to destabilize the membrane, followed by the adapter for the Bax BH3 peptide (X) to antagonize the activity from the anti-apoptotic proteins of the Bcl-2 family, subsequently, the molecular Tag Flag (T) for the tracking of the recombinant proteins, and finally, the cleavage site of the protease OmpT (S) to release the peptides from the bacterium surface; this peptide complex was linked to the sequence that encodes for the autotransporter $\Delta\alpha$-β MisL (L), and the plasmid received the name *pL-STXP* (4,188 bp) (see **Figure 2B**). Under this same strategy, four plasmid controls were built: *pL-XT* (4,047 bp), which encodes for the Bax BH3 peptide; *pL-SXT*(4,107 bp), which encodes for the cleavage site of the OmpT protease and the Bax BH3 peptide; *pL-TP*(4,062 pb), which encodes for the fusogenic peptide; *pL-XTP* (4,128 pb), which encodes for the Bax BH3 peptide and the fusogenic peptide; all cases encode for the molecular Tag Flag and the autotransporter $\Delta\alpha$-β MisL. All of the constructions were sequenced. These plasmids originated from the recombinant proteins with the same names: L-SXTP, L-XT, L-SXT, L-TP, and L-XTP, respectively (**Figure 2A**).

The Cell-Permeable Bax BH3 Peptide Is Expressed on the Surface of the *S. enterica* Through the MisL Autotransporter System

The expressions of the recombinant protein L-SXTP (express and release the Cell-permeable Bax BH3 Peptide through MisL autotransporter) and the control proteins L-XT, L-SXT, L-TP, and L-XTP were evaluated by Western blot using total extracts obtained from the bacteria *E. coli* DH5-α and *S. enterica* SL3261 that were previously transformed with the different plasmids and cultured in anaerobic conditions during 10–12 h. The Western blot using an anti-Flag antibody revealed the expected protein of ~75 KDa. The inmunofluorescence (IFA) and the flow cytometry showed that all recombinant proteins were expressed on the surface of *S. enterica* SL3261 with a similar expression profile. Transformed *Salmonella* with the different plasmids received the name of the recombinant protein that they expressed (**Figure 3**). In order to reinforce the evidence on the cell-permeable Bax BH3 peptide expression over the *S. enterica* surface through the MisL autotransporter, the *S. enterica* SL3261 (negative control), the *S. enterica* SXTP (containing the cell-permeable Bax BH3 peptide coding plasmid without the MisL autotransporter; thus, only expressed in the cytosol), and the *S. enterica* L-SXTP (containing the cell-permeable Bax BH3 peptide coding plasmid expressed in the surfaced by means of the MisL autotransporter), strains were induced as described previously. After that, the protein expression was evaluated by DotBlot, flow cytometry, and immunoelectron microscopy; in all cases, using a mouse anti-Flag antibody (**Supplementary Figure 1**). As expected, the presence of cell-permeable Bax BH3 peptide, 6 KDa approx., was detected by DOT Blot in the *S. enterica* SXTP strains extracts. And the presence of cell-permeable Bax BH3 peptide coupled to the MisL autotransporter, 75 KDa approx., was detected for *S. enterica* L-SXTP (**Supplementary Figure 1A**). The cell-permeable Bax BH3 peptide expression in the bacterial surface was analyzed by means of flow cytometry in non-permeable conditions. Resulting in an absence of peptides detected over the surface of *S. enterica* SXT given that it lacks the translocation machinery, *S. enterica* SL3261 was used as negative control. The translocation effect is acquired with the genetic coupling to the MisL autotransporter, as it can be observed in the right shift of the *S. enterica* L-SXTP histogram (**Supplementary Figure 1B**). To better confirm this observation, immunoelectron microscopy was performed with the recombinant *Salmonellas*. Mouse anti-Flag antibodies were used as the primary antibody, and anti-mouse IgG antibodies coupled to 20 nm gold particles were used as the secondary antibody. The cross sections of bacteria show that the cell-permeable Bax BH3 peptide was only detected on the bacterial surface when coupled to the MisL autotransporter (*S. enterica* L-SXTP). In this former case, the peptide is also detected in the bacterial cytosol as well as in the case of *S. enterica* SXTP and *S. enterica* L-SXTP, as expected (**Supplementary Figure 1C**).

The Cell-Permeable Bax BH3 Peptide Expressed and Released From *S. enterica* Induces Cell Death of NHL Cells

After confirmed expression of the cell-permeable Bax BH3 peptide on the surface of the *S. enterica* L-STXP, and the other controls, we analyzed its effect over the viability of NHL cells. Accordingly, Ramos cells that express anti-apoptotic proteins as Bcl-$_{XL}$ and Mcl-1 (**Figure 4A**) were infected to a MOI of 100, during 2, 4, 6, 8, and 10 h with the recombinant *Salmonella* strains, previously transformed with the different plasmids and cultured in anaerobic conditions during 10 h. As additional controls, we included non-transformed *S. enterica* SL3261 and vincristine 0.5 nM (drug employed as chemotherapy in NHL). After the infection time, the cell viability assays was analyzed by trypan blue exclusion. The **Figure 4B** shows that *S. enterica* L-SXTP, which expresses and releases the cell-permeable Bax BH3 through the MisL autotransporter, reduced dramatically the cellular viability after 8 h of infection to values of 61% ± 2.8, and

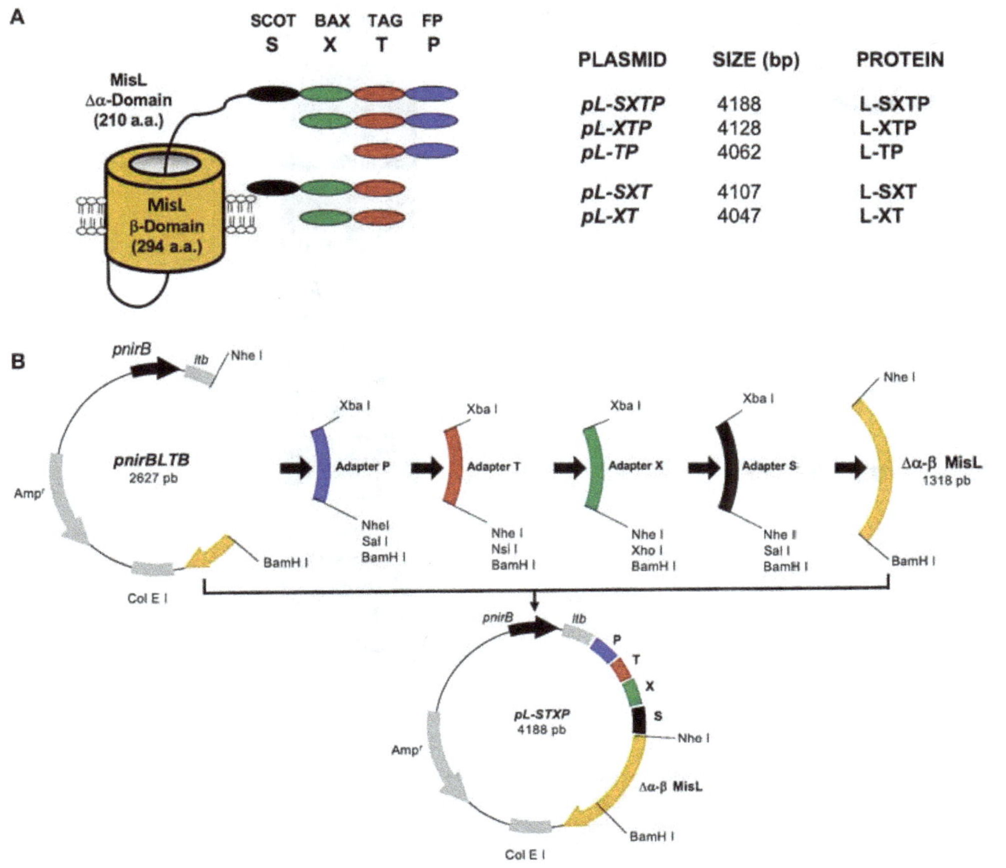

FIGURE 2 | Construction of the recombinant proteins. **(A)** Representative scheme of the expressed and released peptides from the surface of *S. enterica* SL3261 through the misL autotransporter. The β domain of MisL is constituted by 294 amino acids, and the mutated α domain contains 210 amino acids, the peptides of interest are linked to the N terminal portion of the mutated α domain. **(B)** General strategy for the construction of the plasmids. The sequences that encode for the fusogenic peptide (P), the molecular Tag flag (T), the Bax BH3 peptide (X), and the cleavage site for the OmpT protease (S) were inserted in the pnirLTBβMisL plasmid, which contains the signal peptide of heat-labile enterotoxin B subunit (LTB) of enterotoxigenic *E. coli* under the anaerobiosis inducible *nirB* promoter. The sequence of the β MisL autotransporter was extracted from the pnirLTBβMisL plasmid by a double digestion with the Nhe I and BamH I enzymes; this fragment was purified and stored. Later, the adapters that encode for each peptide were inserted in a sequential manner in the *pnirBLTB +P+T...n* plasmid, and finally, the fragment that encodes for the β domain of the MisL autotransporter was reinserted.

this effect was greater 10 h after infection (31% ± 4.3) compared with the non-treated cell control (medium), which remained with viability values above 95% ± 0.5 at all the analyzed times. The treatment with non-transformed *S. enterica* SL3261 reduced the viability of Ramos cells to a 79% ± 4.3 at 8 h and to 64% ± 1.4 at 10 h; these values were very similar to the ones obtained with the *S. enterica* L-XT treatment (82.6% ± 2.3 at 8 h and 63% ± 1.4 at 10 h) and *S. enterica* L-SXT treatment (79.6% ± 1.5 at 8 h and 68.3% ± 1.5 at 10 h). A lesser effect over the viability was observed when the cell was treated with *S. enterica* L-XTP (83.3% ± 0.5 at 8 h and 72.6% ± 7.0 at 10 h) and *S. enterica* L-TP (83% ± 2.6 at 8 h and 79.3% ± 2.5 at 10 h). Vincristine 0.5 nM reduced the viability of Ramos cells to values of 76.3 ± 2.5% at 8 h and to 72 ± 2.0% at 10 h of treatment. The control for the vehicle (water) used to dissolve vincristine showed viability values of 91% ± 2.0 at all analyzed hours in the kinetics. **Figure 4C** shows a representative experiment of the viability of Ramos cells at 8 h after the infection with the recombinant *Salmonella* strains. These results were consistent with the observed data at 8 h of infection in the kinetics: medium and vehicle maintained the celular viability at 90% ± 2.2 values; vincristine 0.5 nM, non-transformed *S. enterica*, and the *Salmonellas* L-XT, L-SXT, L-TP, and L-XTP affected the viability to values from 76.3% ± 1.0 to 82.6% ± 2.7, and the significant reduction in the viability was confirmed when the cells were treated with *S. enterica* L-SXTP (62.6% ± 6.7). **Figure 4D** shows a representative experiment of the viability of Ramos cells at 10 h after the infection with the recombinant *Salmonella* strains. These results were also consistent with the observed data at 10 h of infection in the kinetics: medium and vehicle mantained the cellular viability at 93.5% ± 0.6 values; vincristine 0.5 nM, non-transformed *S. enterica*, and the *Salmonellas* L-XT, L-SXT, L-TP, and L-XTP affected the viability to values from 74.0% ± 5.8 to 67.0% ± 8.1, and the dramatic reduction in the viability was confirmed when the cells were treated with *S. enterica* L-SXTP (33.5% ± 0.5). These data demonstrated that the cell-permeable Bax BH3 peptide, expressed and released by *S. enterica* through the MisL autotransporter, may kill NHL cells.

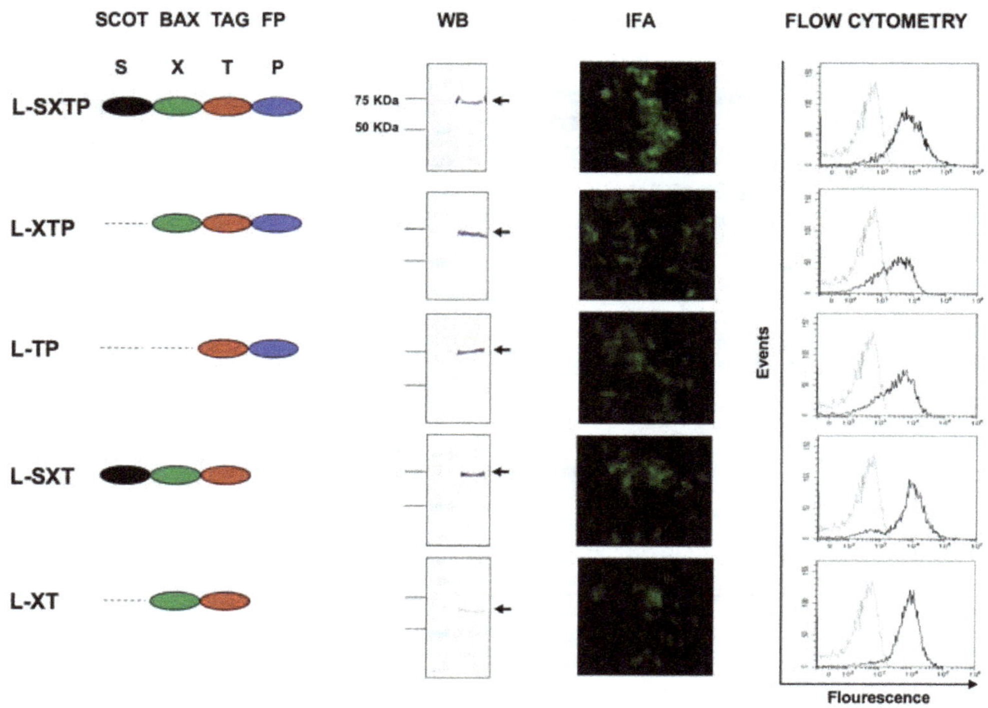

FIGURE 3 | Expression of the recombinant proteins on the surface of *S. enterica*. The expression and translocation of the recombinant proteins on the surface of *S. enterica* was evaluated after 12 h of induction in a thioglycollate medium. From left to right, the Western blots (WB), performed with total bacteria extracts, showed a protein of ~75 KDa. The immunofluorescence (IFA) and the flow cytometry were performed with bacterial suspensions. Controls in the flow cytometry (histogram to the left) are *S. enterica* SL3261 expressing only the autotransporter MisL. In all assays, the immunodetection was performed with monoclonal anti-Flag antibody.

The Cell-Permeable Bax BH3 Peptide Expressed and Released From *S. enterica* Promotes Apoptosis of NHL Cells

In order to determine whether the reduction of the Ramos cells viability, mediated by *S. enterica* L-SXTP, was due to cellular death by apoptosis, promoted by the cell-permeable Bax BH3 peptide, and expressed and released of the MisL autotransporter, Ramos cells were treated during 8 h with the recombinant *Salmonella* strains (MOI of 100) transformed with the different plasmids and cultured in anaerobic conditions for 10 h. As additional controls, we included non-transformed *S. enterica* SL3261 and vincristine 0.5 nM. After the infection, the cells were assessed to determine the caspase-3 activation and DNA fragmentation (TUNEL). As shown in **Figure 5A**, Ramos cells treated with *S. enterica* L-SXTP showed a greater number of active caspase-3 cells (30.4% ± 2.3) compared with the non-transformed *S. enterica* SL3261 controls (16.7% ± 3.8) and the recombinant *S.* strains L-XT (12.3% ± 4.0), L-SXT (13.4% ± 7.9), L-TP (14.7% ± 1.9), and L-XTP (13.7% ± 6.0). High values were also observed for the positive control of vincristine (49.5% ± 5.8) compared with the medium (10.3% ± 2.9) and vehicle controls (11.7% ± 3.6) as expected. These results were consistent with the data from the TUNEL assay, in which Ramos cells treated with *S. enterica* L-SXTP showed up to 51.7% ± 4.0 of TUNEL-positive cells compared with the non-transformed *S. enterica* SL3261 controls (25.9% ± 3.8) and the recombinant *Salmonellas* L-XT (15.9% ± 1.9), L-SXT (20.9% ± 6.7), L-TP (16.5% ± 5.1), and L-XTP (24.9% ± 3.8). In this case, great values of TUNEL-positive were also observed for the positive control of vincristine (31.3% ± 6.2) compared with the medium (9.5% ± 1.9) and vehicle (9.3% ± 1.1) (**Figure 5B**). Similar results were obtained with a TUNEL assay using immunocytochemical staining (**Supplementary Figure 2**). Another characteristic event of apoptosis is the proteolytic cleavage of poly (ADP-ribose) polymerase-1 (PARP-1), a nuclear enzyme involved in DNA repair, DNA stability, and transcriptional regulation. Particularly, caspase-3 and caspase-7 cleave the 116 KDa form of PARP-1 and generate an ~89 and 24 KDa fragment. The cleavage of PARP-1 between Asp214 and Gly215 results in the separation of the two zinc-finger DNA-binding motifs from the automodification and catalytic domains, thus preventing the recruitment of the enzyme to sites of DNA damage. Cleaved PARP-1 has been considered as a hallmark of apoptosis (60). In **Figure 5C**, we analyzed by Western blot the presence of cleaved PARP-1 in the Ramos cells treated during 8 h with the recombinant *Salmonella* strains (MOI of 100). Our finding shows the enhanced presence of cleaved PARP-1 in the cells treated with *S. enterica* L-SXTP as expected; these results are consistent with the high percentaje of Ramos cells with active caspase-3 and TUNEL positivity, described above. Since PARP-1 is a substrate of caspase-3 (32 KDa), we also analyzed this apoptotic molecule by Western blot. The presence of this former protein was detected in the cells treated with vincristine and also in the cells treated with the recombinant

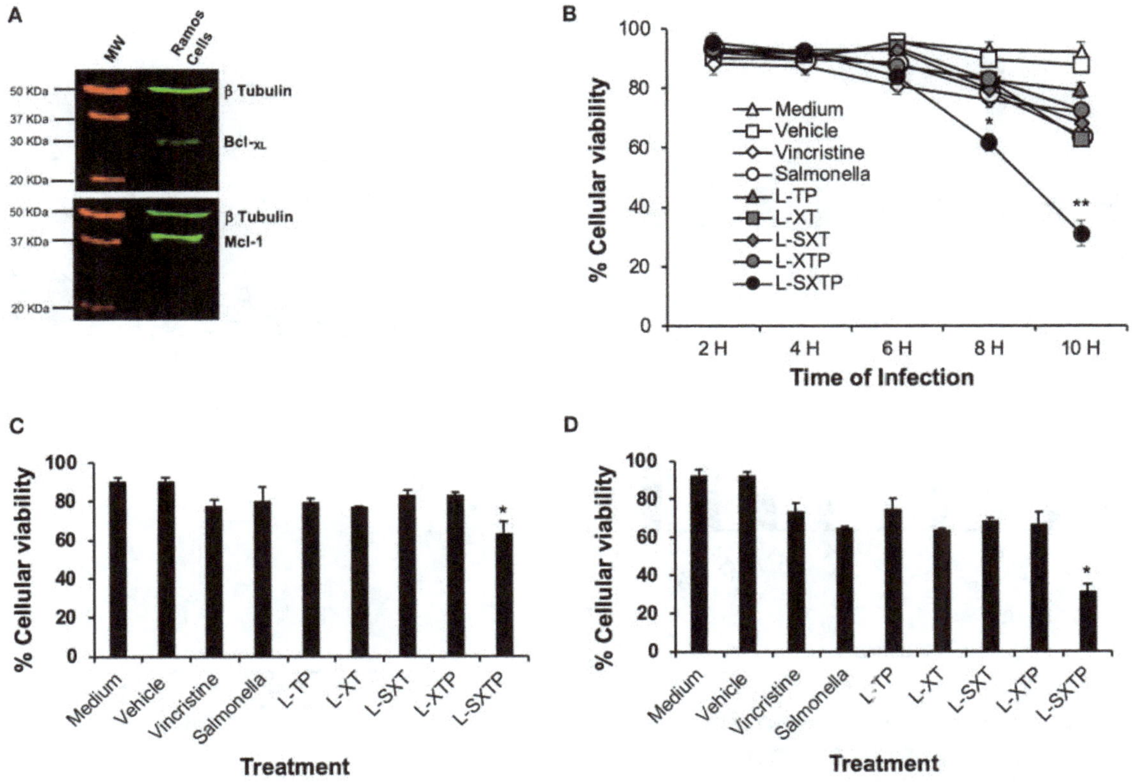

FIGURE 4 | *S. enterica* L-STXP reduces the viability of Ramos cells. **(A)** Expression of the anti-apoptotic proteins Bcl-$_{XL}$ and Mcl-1 in Ramos cells (Burkitt lymphoma, NHL). Proteic extracts of Ramos cells (25 μg per well) were analyzed by Western blot using the anti Bcl-$_{XL}$, anti Mcl-1, and anti β-tubulin antibodies diluted to 1:1,000. As secondary antibody, we used goat antirabbit IgG antibody (IRDye Oddissey) 1:10,000. **(B)** Decrease in the Ramos cells viability to treatment with *S. enterica* L-STXP. Ramos cells were infected to a MOI of 100 with the different recombinant *Salmonella* strains (L-TP, L-XT, L-SXT, L-XTP, and L-SXTP) during 2–10 h. As controls, we used non-treated cells (medium) as a negative control, sterile water as solvent to vincristine (vehicle), non-transformed *S. enterica* SL3261 (*Salmonella*), and vincristine 0.5 nM as a positive control. The viability was analyzed by trypan blue dye exclusion. A representative experiment of the viability of Ramos cells at 8 **(C)** and 10 h **(D)** after the infection with the recombinant *Salmonella* strains confirms the dramatic reduction of the viability of Ramos cells treated with recombinant *Salmonella* L-SXTP compared with controls. In the graphics, the error bars represent the average ± *SD* of measurements in triplicate. The results are representative of three independent experiments. ANOVA test was performed with Bonferroni *post hoc* for the difference between the groups. For **(B)**, $^{*}p < 0.001$, $^{**}p < 0.0001$; for **(C)**, $^{*}p < 0.001$; for **(D)**, $^{*}p < 0.0001$.

Salmonella strains; interestingly, the results showed a complete reduction in the expression of this molecule in the cells treated with *S. enterica* L-SXTP. This observation may be explained because the processing of this molecule toward active caspase-3 was observed in **Figure 5A**. These data suggest that the cell-permeable Bax BH3 peptide, expressed and released by *S. enterica* through the MisL autotransporter, antagonized the activity of the anti-apoptotic proteins in the Ramos cells, restoring the cellular death by apoptosis.

Antitumor Activity of the Cell-Permeable Bax BH3 Peptide Expressed and Released From *S. enterica* in a Murine Xenograft Model of Human B NHL

The antitumor effect of *S. enterica* L-SXTP, which expresses and releases from its surface the cell-permeable Bax BH3 peptide through the MisL autotransporter system, was analyzed in a murine xenograft model of human B NHL. Accordingly, athymic nu/nu female BALB/c mice from 6 to 8 weeks were implanted in the right flank with 10^7 Ramos cells. Once the tumor reached 100–150 mm^3 in size (approximately within 15 days after inoculation), groups of five mice were inoculated in the tail vein (1 × 10^7 CFU) with each one of the previously induced recombinant *Salmonella* strains. Mice received four identical doses of bacteria with a 7-days interval. Control mice received PBS or non-transformed *S. enterica* SL3261 under the same inoculation scheme. The size tumor and survival were registered daily. **Figure 6A** shows that inoculation with recombinant *Salmonella* strains were performed at days 0, 7, 14, and 21. The analysis at day 25 (4 days after the fourth inoculation) shows a maximum reduction or the tumoral size in the mice that received *S. enterica* L-STXP (440 ± 330 mm^3), this size corresponds to only 4% of the tumoral size development from the group that received PBS (9,527 ± 582 mm^3, representing 100% of the size developed by the tumor). Decreased tumor volume, as compared with PBS-treated mice for the control groups were 33% with non-transformed *S. enterica* SL3261, 24% with *S. enterica*

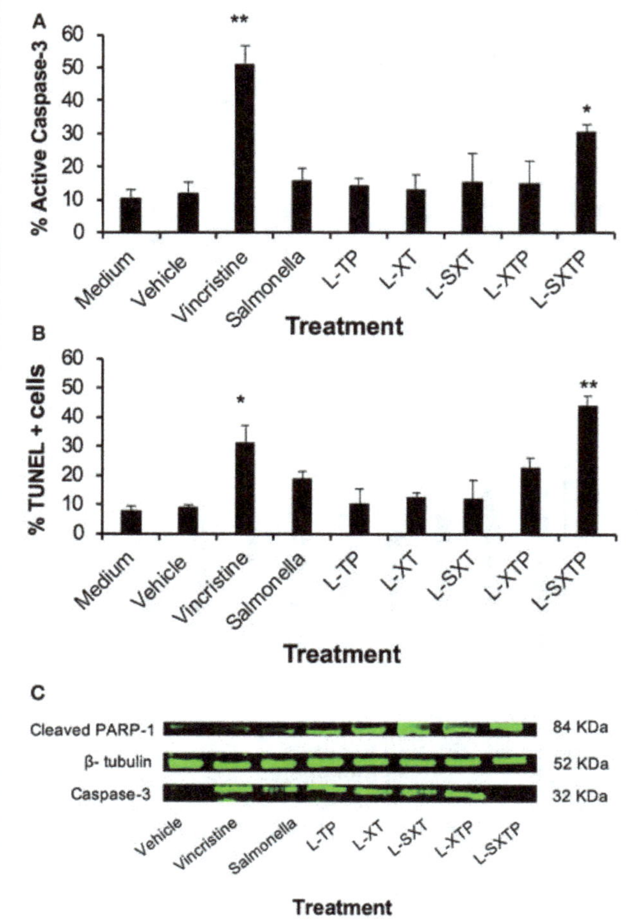

FIGURE 5 | *S. enterica* L-STXP induces the apoptosis of Ramos cells. Ramos cells were infected during 8 h to a MOI of 100 with the different recombinant *Salmonella* strains (L-TP, L-XT, L-SXT, L-XTP, and L-SXTP). As controls, we used non-treated cells (medium) as a negative control, injectable water as solvent to vincristine (vehicle), non-transformed *S. enterica* SL3261 (*Salmonella*) and vincristine 0.5 nM as a positive control. The apoptosis was analyzed by determination of caspase-3-active **(A)** and TUNEL-positive cells **(B)**. **(C)** Infected tumor cells were lysed, and total protein was obtained. The expression of caspase-3 and PARP-1 was examined by Western blotting. β-tubulin was used as the loading control. In the graphics, the error bars represent the average ± *SD* of three independent experiments. ANOVA test was performed with Bonferroni *post hoc* for the difference between the groups. In all cases, $^{*}p < 0.001$, $^{**}p < 0.0001$.

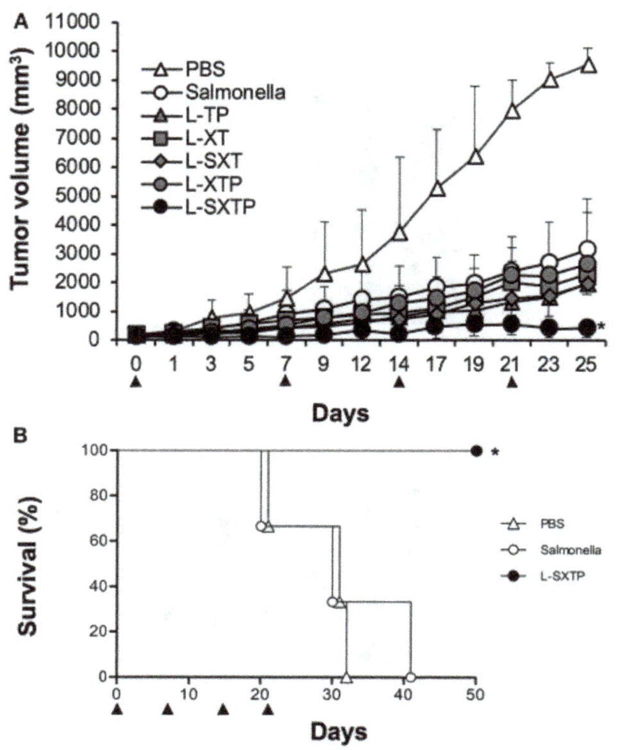

FIGURE 6 | Antitumor activity of *S. enterica* L-STXP in a murine xenograft model of human B NHL. Athymic nu/nu BALB/c mice were subcutaneously injected with 10^7 Ramos cells in the right flank. The treatment of the different groups was initiated when the tumors reached 100–150 mm^3. The mice received 1×10^7 CFU at days 0, 7, 14, and 21 (arrowhead), with each one of the recombinant *Salmonella* strains (L-TP, L-XT, L-SXT, L-XTP, and L-SXTP). Groups of mice treated with PBS 1× and non-transformed *S. enterica* SL3261 (*Salmonella*) were included as additional controls. **(A)** For the kinetics of tumor growth, the tumor size was analyzed daily with a Vernier caliper. In the graphics, the error bars represent the average ± *SD* of the tumor size ($n = 5$ mice/group). The results are representative of two independent experiments. ANOVA test was performed with Bonferroni *post hoc* for the difference between the groups. $^{*}p < 0.0001$. **(B)** Survival curve after the tumor treatment. The data represent the percentage of survival ($n = 3$ mice/group). The results are representative of two independent experiments. $^{*}p = 0.02$ by log-rank test.

L-XT, 20% with *S. enterica* L-SXT, 20% with *S. enterica* L-TP, and 27% with *S. enterica* L-XTP. At day 25, the presence of the different recombinant *Salmonella* strains was also comfirmed in the tumors of the different treated groups; the recovered bacteria still showed the capacity to produce recombinant protein (**Figure 7B**). For the survival analysis, groups of three tumor-bearing mice were inoculated with PBS 1×, non-transformed *S. enterica* SL3261, and previously induced *S. enterica* L-STXP. For this assay, the groups were observed until 50 days. In **Figure 6B**, the extension of the survival is observed for up to 50 days from the mice that received the *S. enterica* L-STXP treatment compared with the group that received PBS 1× (the last mouse died around the 30th day) and the group that received non-transformed *S. enterica* SL3261 (the last mouse died around the 40th day). These findings altogether clearly prove the antitumor and therapeutic effect of the cell-permeable Bax BH3 peptide expressed and released from *S. enterica* through the MisL autotransporter system.

Targeting of Recombinant *Salmonella* Strains to the Murine Xenograft Model of Human B NHL

The targeting of the different recombinant *Salmonella* strains to the murine xenograft model of human B NHL was analyzed by culture in BHI agar (in the presence or absence of ampicillin) of the homogenized xenograft tumor specimen previously treated with the recombinant *Salmonella* strains. Subsequently, the recombinant bacteria isolated in agar BHI with ampicillin were analyzed for protein expression by immunofluorescence assay.

Figure 7A shows the presence of bacteria in all groups of mice inoculated with the recombinant *Salmonella* strains, and these bacteria still have the ability to express the recombinant proteins on its surface, as depicted in **Figure 7B**. To reinforce these findings, we also analyzed the presence of bacteria in tumor tissue. *In situ* immunohistochemical assay was performed using an antibody anti-*Salmonella* induced in rabbit, our results show the presence of 4–10 *Salmonella* bacilli per oil immersion field in all tumor-bearing mice treated with the recombinant *Salmonella* strains. No *Salmonella* bacilli were found in the group treated with PBS 1×. *Salmonella* bacilli were localized in tumor sections with no histological changes (undamaged) and also in sections with necrosis/apoptosis areas (damaged), as observed in **Figure 7C**. These results confirm that the recombinant *Salmonella* strains have targeted the tumor microenvironment of the murine xenograft model of human B NHL.

The Cell-Permeable Bax BH3 Peptide Expressed and Released From *S. enterica* Induces Apoptosis in the Murine Xenograft Model of Human B NHL

The apoptosis induced by *S. enterica* L-SXTP was evaluated in the murine xenograft model of human B NHL that previously received four doses in the tail vein of the recombinant *Salmonella* strains and euthanized after 5 days of the last inoculation. Tumors from those mice were resected and prepared for histological analysis and immunohistochemical staining. **Figure 8** shows representative images of staining tumors from each group. Hematoxylin and eosin staining shows a lymphoid neoplasm in all groups composed of monomorphic medium-sized cells with relatively uniform round to oval nuclei, multiple small nucleoli, and basophilic cytoplasm. These neoplasms also show a high mitotic rate and Ki67 proliferative index around 95% (data not shown). Macrophages and tumor-infiltrating lymphocytes were barely observed. Necrotic areas were detected in groups treated with the recombinant *Salmonellas* strains, but they were more evident in the group treated with *S. enterica* L-SXTP. **Figure 8** also shows active caspase-3 and TUNEL-positive cells in all groups treated with the recombinant *Salmonellas* strains. However, treatment with *S. enterica* L-SXTP elicits the highest apoptosis, as expected. It is important to note that a strong signal of apoptotic markers was found in the necrotic areas. Caspase 8-positive cells were barely detected in the tumor-bearing mice with all treatments. These data confirm the activation of intrinsic apoptosis as the mechanism of antitumor activity mediated by the *S. enterica* L-SXTP in the murine xenograft model of human B NHL.

Inflammatory Cytokines Are Elevated in the Murine Xenograft Model of Human B NHL Treated With *S. enterica* That Expresses and Releases the Cell-Permeable Bax BH3 Peptide

Given that the capacity of *S. enterica* L-SXTP to induce apoptosis in the murine xenograft model of human B NHL has been proven, we can wonder if the intravenous administration of these recombinant *Salmonella* strains has an effect on the inflammatory cytokine production. To approach this question, serum samples of the mice that had previously received four doses in the tail vein with the recombinant *Salmonella* strains and euthanized after 5 days of the last inoculation were analyzed by means of the CBA kit. This kit allows the detection of six inflammatory cytokines: IL-6, IL-10, MCP-1, IFN-γ, TNF-α, and IL-12p70. **Figure 9** shows the comparison between the presence of every cytokine analyzed in the murine xenograft model, which had received the treatment with recombinant *Salmonellas* and the corresponding concentration values found for the control group of mice treated with PBS 1× (low average concentration values ranging from 0.34 to 0.42 pg/ml). The average concentrations of TNF-α observed for the different groups show values in the interval between 96.2 and 93.5 pg/ml, while between 20.4 and 23.1 pg/ml for IL-6, and between 51.1 and 62.3 pg/ml for IL-10. Unexpectedly, the group of mice treated with *S. enterica* L-SXTP showed high concentration values of cytokines as MCP-1 (113.1 pg/ml), IL-12 (72.1 pg/ml), and IFN-γ (148.2 pg/ml) compared with those values obtained from the group treated *S. enterica*: MCP-1 (23.1 pg/ml), IL-12 (27.7 pg/ml), and IFN-γ (89.8 pg/ml). These findings clearly suggest that *S. enterica* L-SXTP stimulates the production of inflammatory cytokines with antitumoral activity, in addition to inducing the expression and the release of the cell-permeable Bax BH3 peptide.

DISCUSSION

In the last years, the survival of patients with NHL has increased substantially (4, 5), nevertheless, the development of drug resistance limits the complete success of the treatments (6) and sets the guidelines for the research and development of new antitumor therapies that can completely eradicate drug-resistant transformed cells (7). The drug resistance has been associated mostly to the aberrant inhibition of the signals of intrinsic apoptosis, in which the genes and proteins of the Bcl-2 family play a very important role (8, 9). In the cells, the balance between survival or death is controlled by the members of the three groups of this family of proteins: the group of multidomain anti-apoptotic proteins (Bcl-2, $Bcl\text{-}_{XL}$, Bcl-w, Mcl-1, and A1) promotes the survival of the cells by inhibiting the pro-apoptotic proteins; the group of multidomain pro-apoptotic proteins (BH1-3) (Bax, Bak, and Bok), which are apoptosis effectors; and the group of pro-apoptotic BH3-only proteins (Bid, Bim, Puma, Noxa, Bad, Bmf, Hrk, and Bik), which are the apoptosis initiators (17–19). In the healthy cells, the anti-apoptotic proteins attach and inhibit the effector proteins Bax or Bak, blocking their polymerization on the mitochondrial surface and avoiding the apoptosis initiation (20). The single BH3-only proteins are induced in response to stress signals and promote the apoptosis binding directly to the effector proteins or to the anti-apoptotic proteins to release the effector proteins (27). According to this balance, the overexpression of this anti-apoptotic proteins in the tumor cells favors the survival of the transformed cell and represents a treatment resistance mechanism (61).

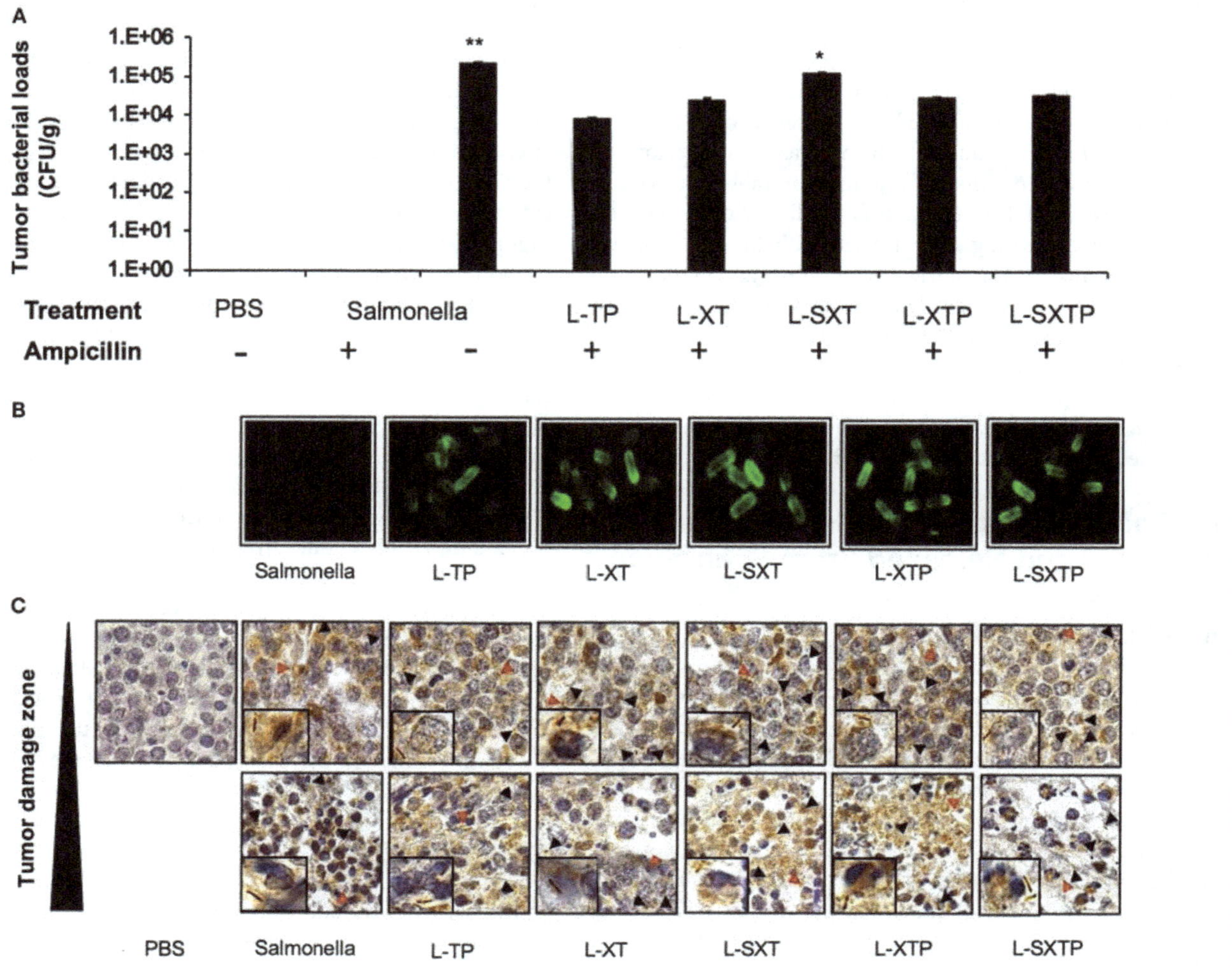

FIGURE 7 | Tumor targeting of recombinant *Salmonella* strains in a murine xenograft model of human B NHL. Tumor-bearing mice were treated with four doses of 1×10^7 colony-forming units (CFU) in the tail vein of the recombinant *Salmonella* strains and evaluated for the antitumor activity (tumor size) and euthanized after 5 days of the last inoculation. Tumors from those mice were resected and analyzed for tumor colonization. **(A)** Tumor suspensions were cultured in BHI agar medium in the presence or absence of ampicillin during 12 h at 37°C. The figure shows the number of colonies counted and reported as CFU per tissue gram (CFU/g). No *Salmonella* bacilli were observed in the group treated with PBS 1×. In the group of *S. enterica*, the bacteria grow only in the absence of ampicillin. **(B)** Subsequently, some recombinant bacteria isolated in agar BHI with ampicillin were analyzed for protein expression by immunofluorescence assay using an antibody anti-Flag-FITC. **(C)** The presence of the bacteria in the tumor tissue was also analyzed by performing an *in situ* immunohistochemical assay using an anti-*Salmonella* induced in rabbit as the primary antibody. The presence of *Salmonella* bacilli in brown color (arrowhead and close up) was detected in tumor sections with no histological changes and also in sections with necrosis/apoptosis areas (damaged zone). Images have 100× magnifications. The results are representative of three independent experiments. ANOVA test was performed with Bonferroni *post hoc* for the difference between the groups. For **(A)**, $^*p = 0.02$, $^{**}p < 0.0001$.

In NHL, it has been documented that the overexpression of anti-apoptotic proteins Bcl-2 (13, 14), Bcl-$_{XL}$ (15, 16), and Mcl-1 (62) is associated to drug-resistant profile. Reverting this resistance mechanism has been possible due to the structural studies that reveal that proteins from the Bcl-2 family interact with each other through a hydrophobic groove formed by their BH domains (17–19), and that peptides derived from the BH3 domain of pro-apoptotic proteins can bind to the anti-apoptotic proteins, antagonizing their function (22–24). *In vitro* assays using hydrophobic peptides from the BH3 domain of the proteins Bax, Bad, and Bak, when binding them to the fusogenic peptide of the antennapedia protein to make them permeable to the tumor cells of head and neck squamous cell carcinoma, antagonized the activity of Bcl-$_{XL}$ and Bcl-2 and restored the apoptosis (25). The concept of eliminating the tumor cells blocking the activity of the anti-apoptotic proteins has also been successful using the small molecules that mimic the function of the BH3-only proteins, as ABT-737(63) and its oral bioavailable derivative ABT-263/Navitoclax) (64), GX15-070/Obatoclax (65), and ABT-199/Venotoclax; this last one was recently approved by the FDA for the treatment of CLL (26, 27) but not for NHL.

Despite its effectiveness and promising results, the peptides from the BH3 domain and the mimetic molecules from BH3 domain still need to be specifically and selectively directed toward the tumor microenvironment in order to decrease side effects. In order to solve this problem, in this work, we propose

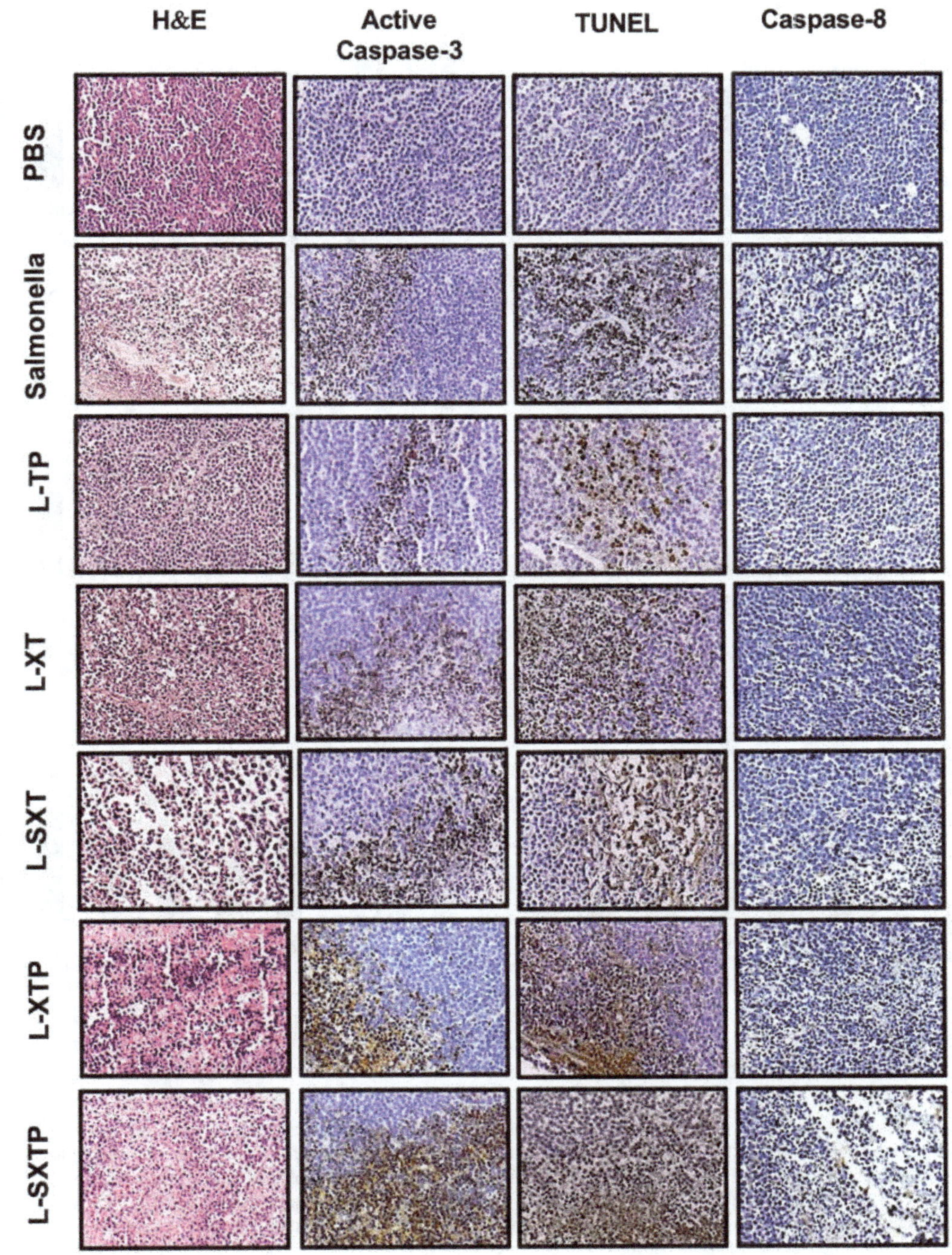

FIGURE 8 | Apoptotic markers detected by immunohistochemistry in tumors treated with the recombinant *Salmonella* strains. Tumor-bearing mice were treated with four doses of 1×10^7 colony-forming units (CFU) in the tail vein of the recombinant *Salmonella* strains and evaluated for the antitumor activity (tumor size) and were euthanized after 5 days of the last inoculation. Tumors from those mice were resected and analyzed for apoptotic markers as active caspase-3, TUNEL, and caspase-8. The column of hematoxylin and eosin staining shows a lymphoid neoplasm in all groups, composed of monomorphic medium-sized cells with a high mitotic rate. Macrophages and tumor-infiltrating lymphocytes were barely observed. Necrosis areas were detected in groups treated with the recombinant *Salmonellas* strains. For apoptotic markers, we used an antibody against active caspase-3 (1:250) and caspase 8 (1:1,500). The *in situ* TUNEL assay was performed following the instructions for the *in situ* Cell Death Detection Kit (Roche). In all cases, brown color represents positive cells. The columns of active caspase-3 and TUNEL shows a strong signal in the group treated with *S. enterica* L-SXTP. A small number of positive cells were observed for caspase-8 staining in all groups. Images have 20× magnification. The results are representative of three independent experiments.

to use a live attenuated bacterium to carry the peptide from the BH3 domain of the Bax protein directly into the tumor microenvironment and allow the access to the cytosol of the NHL tumor cells. *S. enterica* serovar Typhimurium, gram-negative and anaerobic facultative bacteria, is probably the most studied live attenuated bacterium in the therapy against cancer

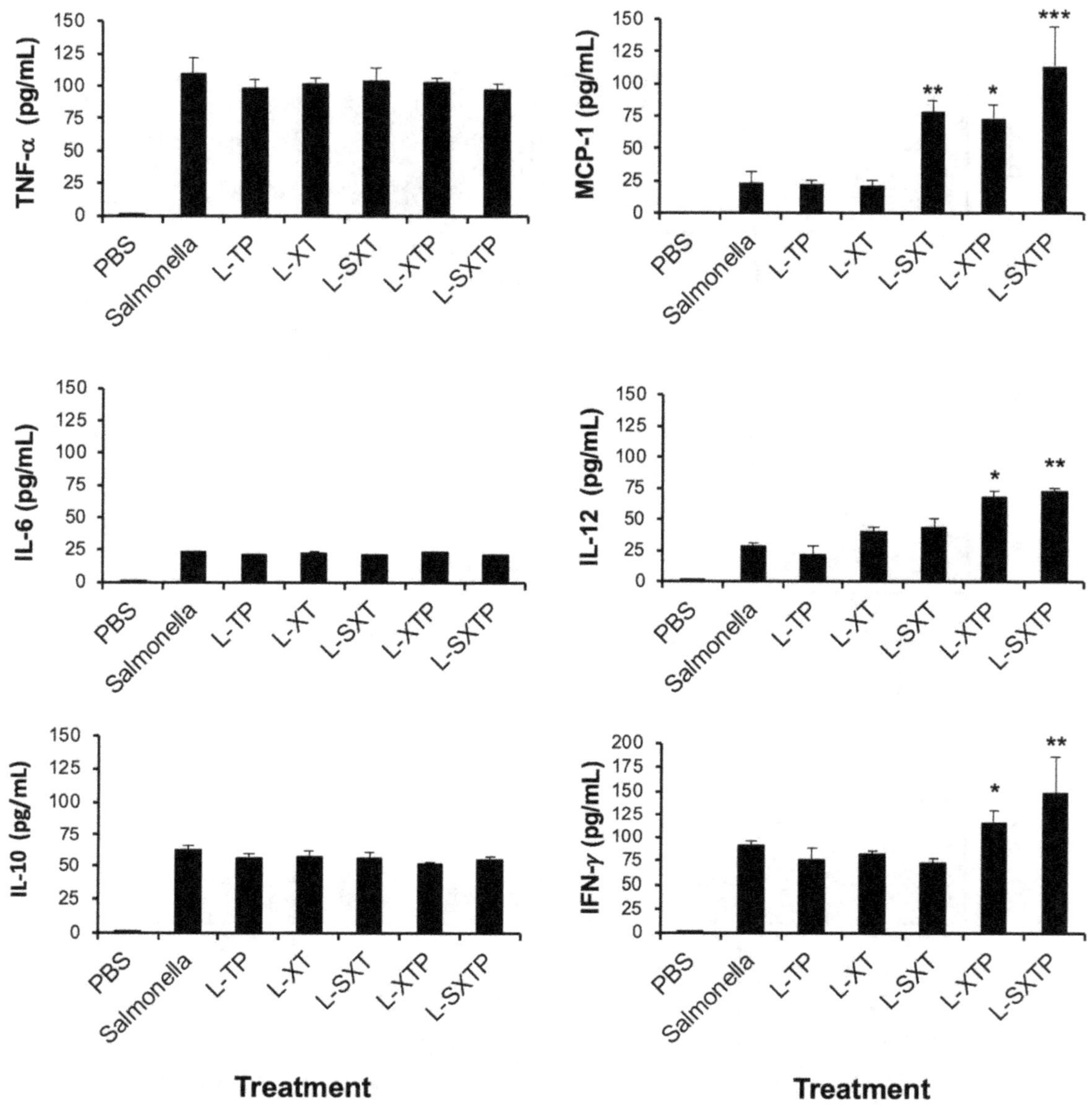

FIGURE 9 | Inflammatory cytokines determined in serum from tumor-bearing mice treated with the recombinant *Salmonella* strains. Tumor-bearing mice were treated with four doses of 1×10^7 colony-forming units (CFU) in the tail vein of the recombinant *Salmonella* strains and evaluated for the antitumor activity (tumor size) and were euthanized after 5 days of the last inoculation. Serum from those mice was analyzed for the presence of inflammatory cytokines as IL-6, IL-10, MCP-1, IFN-γ, TNF-α, and IL-12p70 using the Cytometric Bead Array (CBA) Mouse Inflammation Kit (BD Biosciences). Samples were acquired in the flow cytometry BD FACSCanto II, and the output was processed in the FCAP Array software v3.0. (BD Biosciences). The results are representative of three independent experiments. ANOVA test was performed with Bonferroni *post hoc* for the difference between the groups. For MCP-1, $^{*}p < 0.005$, $^{**}p < 0.001$, $^{***}p < 0.0001$; For IL-12, $^{*}p < 0.009$, $^{**}p < 0.001$; For IFN-γ, $^{*}p < 0.001$, $^{**}p < 0.0002$.

due to its high affinity for tumor tissue (28, 29), favored by hypoxia, acidity, necrosis, and release of metabolites that can act as chemoattractant for this bacterium in solid and semisolids tumors, its great intrinsic antitumor potential (66, 67), its ability to activate the innate and adaptive antitumor immune response (30), and its great capacity of use as delivery system because once it is in the tumor microenvironment, it turns into a true factory of heterologous molecules (31, 32), as cytokines (68–71), chemokines (72), ligands of death (73, 74), pro-apoptotic proteins domains (75), and peptides (76), among others (30). Furthermore, safe strains are available such as *S. enterica* serovar Typhimurium VNP20009, mutant in *msbB* and *pur I* genes, with a reduced toxicity associated with lipopolysaccharide, and this bacterial strain was demonstrated to be safe and tolerable in clinical trials (77). Recently, it has been reported that *S. enterica* SL3261 (Aro A, mutant in the aromatic amino acids) was used to express anti CD20 antibodies and drug converting enzymes to eradicate human lymphomas (78), and our group has shown the success of *S. enterica* SL3261 to carry and transfer plasmids into tumor cells. Transferred plasmid that encodes a peptide from the

BH3 domain of the pro-apoptotic Bax protein antagonized the anti-apoptotic activity of the Bcl-2 family proteins, restored the apoptosis, and induced chemosensitization in tumor cells (33).

In the present study, we evaluated the feasibility of the cell-permeable Bax BH3 peptide (constituted by the Bax-BH3 peptide, bound to the molecular Tag Flag and to the fusogenic peptide) expressed and released from the surface of *S. enterica* SL3261 through the MisL autotransporter system (L-SXTP) to promote apoptosis signaling and death of NHL cells. Previously, we have reported that the MisL autotransporter system can be used to express heterologous molecules on the surface of *S. enterica* (35), and these molecules were released to the microenvironment by a cleavage site of OmpT protease (34, 58).

In this work, using molecular modeling of the L-SXTP complex, we showed for the first time an approximation of the 3-D structure of the MisL autotransporter and each one of the components of the cell-permeable Bax BH3 peptide. This 3-D structure allowed us to confirm that MisL is an autotransporter protein (79) constituted by a β barrel domain of 12 antiparallel chains with five short handles that internalize toward the periplasmic space and one extracellular α domain that presents toward the edge N-terminal a combination of several units of β-strand secondary structure, organized in a specific geometry of β-solenoid architecture, the cell-permeable Bax BH3 peptide consolidates an α-helix folding and the cutting site for the OmpT protease, revealing itself as a flexible loop; these do not induce an unfolding or instability of the 3-D structure of the MisL autotransporter neither in its global configuration nor in the vicinity to the β-solenoid (**Figures 1A,B**). For the theoretical prediction of the internalization of the cell-permeable Bax BH3 peptide in the membrane, we observed that due to its amino acid composition and its hydrophobicity, it is possible that it crosses the membrane through a diffusion process (**Figure 1C**). With this information, and using molecular biology, we obtained the *S. enterica* L-STXP, which expresses and releases from its surface the cell-permeable Bax BH3 peptide through the MisL autotransporter, and we also obtained the controls: *S. enterica* L-XT (control that expresses the Bax-BH3 peptide), *S. enterica* L-SXT (control that expresses and releases the Bax-BH3 peptide), *S. enterica* L-TP (control that expresses the fusogenic peptide), *S. enterica* L-XTP (control that expresses the Bax-BH3 peptide and the fusogenic peptide and keeps it anchored to the bacteria membrane), all the recombinant proteins expressed the molecular Tag flag (T) and the MisL autotransporter (L) (**Figures 2A,B**). The introduction of the plasmids and the induction of the protein did not affect the growth of *S. enterica* (data not shown). As expected, our results showed that the peptides of interest were expressed and translocated to the surface of *S. enterica* through the MisL autotransporter, as shown in the Western blot assays, immunofluorescence, and flow cytometry in **Figure 3**; the immunoelectron microscopy also shows that the recombinant protein L-SXTP was expressed on the surface of the *S. enterica* L-SXTP (**Supplementary Figure 1**). These data confirm the functionality of the MisL autotransporter in its ability to translocate proteins to the surface of *S. enterica* (34, 35, 58) and are consistent with the observations of the molecular modeling in which it described that the addition of the cell-permeable Bax BH3 peptide to the α domain of the MisL autotransporter does not affect its structure.

We further evaluated the effect of the recombinant *Salmonella* strains over the viability of Ramos cells that come from a Burkitt lymphoma, an aggressive human B NHL that expresses Bcl-$_{XL}$ and Mcl-l (**Figure 4A**). With this aim, Ramos cells were treated at different times with the recombinant *Salmonella* strains to a MOI of 100. As depicted in **Figure 4B**, the differential effect can be observed gradually between the 8 and 10 h. In this assay, the recombinant strain of *S. enterica* L-SXTP induced the death of 39% of the NHL cells at 8 h with an increase to almost double at 10 h (69%). Interestingly, the *Salmonella* strain that expresses the cell-permeable Bax BH3 peptide on its surface but does not release it (*S. enterica* L-XTP) induced an even lesser rate of death (16% at 8 h and 27% at 10 h) to the observed values for the non-transformed bacteria *S. enterica* SL3261 (21% at 8 h and 36% at 10 h). This observation suggests that it is necessary to release the cell-permeable Bax BH3 peptide from the bacteria surface for induction of cell death. The other recombinant *Salmonella* strains (L-XT, L-SXT, and L-TP) showed lesser values compared to the ones induced by non-transformed *S. enterica* SL3261. These data were confirmed in the viability assays 8 and 10 h after the treatment of Ramos cells with the different recombinant *Salmonella* strains (**Figures 4C,D**). A slight increase of the cell death observed with non-transformed *S. enterica* SL3261 can be mediated by the intrinsic oncolytic activity of the bacteria (30) due to the release of the nitrate reductase that metabolizes nitrates and nitrites to nitric oxide, a molecule that has the ability to induce cellular apoptosis (80), and by the induction of autophagy due to the increase in proteins such as Beclin-1 and LC3 (81).

The apoptosis assays performed to Ramos cells treated with the different recombinant *Salmonella* strains during 8 h confirm that the cellular death induced by *S. enterica* L-SXTP in the viability assays is due to the restoration of the apoptosis mechanism. As expected, the Ramos cells that received the treatment with *S. enterica* L-SXTP showed twice of active caspase-3 cells and TUNEL positivity than the Ramos cells that received the treatment with the non-transformed *S. enterica* SL3261 and other controls (**Figures 5A,B**). These results were consistent with the increase of cleavage PARP-1 (substrate of caspase-3) in the group treated with *S. enterica* L-SXTP compared with the controls (**Figure 5C**). In this group, complete caspase-3 was not evident (**Figure 5C**), however, and increasing amount of cleavage form of caspase-3, detected as active caspase-3-positive cells, was observed (**Figure 3A**). Interestingly, the high rate of active caspase-3-positive cells observed in the group with vincristine does not induce highest rate of TUNEL-positive cells as expected, these data were consistent with low expression of cleaved PARP-1. The slight increase in the apoptosis, mediated by non-transformed *S. enterica* SL3261, can be due to the intrinsic oncolytic activity of *S. enterica* aforementioned. These results are consistent with previous reports in which the use of Bax-BH3 peptides bound to an antennapedia fusogenic peptide restored the apoptosis in head and neck squamous cell carcinoma and acute leukemia cells (25).

To demonstrate the antitumor effect of the recombinant *Salmonella* strains, we developed a murine xenograft model of human B NHL using Ramos cells, which were implanted in the right flank of athymic nu/nu female BALB/c mice, and after 15 days, when the tumors reached between 100 and 150 mm^3, mice were inoculated in the tail vein (1×10^7 CFU) with each one of the previously induced recombinant *Salmonella* strains. Mice received four identical doses of bacteria with a 7-days interval. Our results showed that the mice that received the treatment with *S. enterica* L-SXTP significantly reduced the tumor size during the 26 days after the first treatment. Interestingly, the groups of mice inoculated with recombinant *Salmonella* strains as control (L-XT, L-SXT, L-TP, and L-XTP) also showed tumor reduction, at intermediate sizes, compared with the group that only received treatment with PBS 1*. This effect could be due to the intrinsic oncolytic activity of *S. enterica* and its ability to activate the innate immunity (30), which is still present in this athymic mice, and can be mediated by the presence of dendritic cells, neutrophils, macrophages, and natural killer tumor-infiltrating cells (66, 82). In the tumor-bearing mice treated with the recombinant *Salmonella* strains, the presence of *Salmonella* bacilli that still produce recombinant proteins at day 26 (**Figures 7A,B**) confirms the *S. enterica* ability to reach the tumor microenvironment, and once there, express the cell-permeable Bax BH3 peptide through the MisL autotransporter system. This observation may be promoted by the capacity of *S. enterica* to infect B lymphocytes (83) and was consistent with studies that claim that these bacteria colonize solid and semisolid tumors (32). In addition, the group that received *S. enterica* L-SXTP also increased the survival in the 50 days that the study lasted (**Figure 6B**) compared with the group that received PBS (31 days) and the group that was treated with non-transformed *S. enterica* SL3261 (41 days). In this last group, the intrinsic oncolytic activity mechanisms and the activation of the innate immune response mediated by *S. enterica* (30) were sufficient to improve 10 more days the mice survival compared with those that received PBS. These findings clearly prove the antitumor and therapeutic effect of the cell-permeable Bax BH3 peptide expressed and released from *S. enterica* through the MisL autotransporter system. The histological analysis of the tumor-bearing mice that received four doses of recombinant *Salmonella* strains and euthanized after 5 days of the last inoculation (day 26) shows a lymphoid neoplasm composed of monomorphic medium sized cells, with scarce macrophages and tumor-infiltrating lymphocytes, with the presence of necrotic areas mostly in the group treated with *S. enterica* L-SXTP. The presence of recombinant bacteria observed in tumor sections with or without histological changes (**Figure 7C**) confirm the targeting of the *S. enterica* strains to the murine xenograft model of human B NHL and is consistent with the tumor targeting of *Salmonella* reported in other murine models of lymphoma (53, 84). The presence of apoptotic marker as active caspase-3 and TUNEL-positive cells was detected in all groups treated with the recombinant *Salmonella* strains; however, the effect was more evident in the tumor treated with *S. enterica* L-SXTP. These *in situ* results (**Figure 8**) are consistent with the *in vitro* assays, where the enhanced active caspase-3-positive cells correlate with higher TUNEL-positive cells and enhanced cleaved PARP-1 (**Figure 5**). The presence of apoptotic markers in the groups treated with the non-transformed *S. enterica* and others controls can be due to the intrinsic oncolytic activity of *S. enterica* aforementioned (30). It is important to mention that caspase-8 was almost negative in all groups (**Figure 8**), suggesting that the extrinsic apoptosis does not play any role in the antitumor activity mediated by the recombinant *Salmonella* strains used as treatment.

Since the histology analysis barely identified some immune cells as macrophages and tumor infiltrating lymphocytes in the murine xenograft model of human B NHL treated with the recombinant *Salmonella* strains, we further analyzed the systemic production of inflammatory cytokines in the serum of the tumor-bearing mice treated with the recombinant *Salmonella* strains. Inflammatory cytokines IL-6, TNF-α, MCP-1, IFN-**γ**, and IL-12p70 that have been associated with antitumor activity were identified (53, 84–86), and also an anti-inflammatory cytokine was detected (IL-10) (85) (**Figure 9**). Surprisingly, the tumor-bearing mice inoculated with *S. enterica* L-SXTP shows more than two-fold concentrations of the MCP-1, IFN-**γ**, and IL-12p70 cytokines compared with the group that received non-transformed *S. enterica* SL3261 and controls. These findings suggest that the antitumor and therapeutic effect of the cell-permeable Bax BH3 peptide expressed and released from *S. enterica* through the MisL autotransporter system may be enhanced with the presence of inflammatory cytokines with antitumor activity, an event that requires further investigation.

Taken together, our findings represent an important step forward in demonstrating the potential of live attenuated *S. enterica* serovar Typhimurium strain SL3261 expressing and releasing cell-permeable Bax-BH3 peptide through the MisL autotransporter system as an eventual alternative to treat relapsed or refractory NHL.

AUTHOR CONTRIBUTIONS

RL-P conceived, supervised the project, designed the experiments, analyzed the data, and wrote the manuscript. AM-C and PM-L generated the recombinant proteins, performed the viability, and apoptosis assays. EB-B, LF-M, and GB-G participated in the in vivo experiments. DP-G and LM-V performed the molecular modeling of the MisL autotransporter system. UJ-H performed the bacteria tumor targeting experiments. BC-M generated the immunoelectron microscopy data. LC-M participated in the histology and immunohistochemical analysis.

ACKNOWLEDGMENTS

The authors would like to thank Marco A. Hernández-Luna, Daniel D. Hernández-Cueto, Omar Ugarte-Alvarez, Jonathan Erik Cocoletzi-Bautista, Marilu Rodriguez-Jimenez, Diego Anaya-Estrada, Raúl Castro-Luna, and Leonel Martínez-Cristóbal, for their excellent technical assistance.

REFERENCES

1. Bray F, Ferlay J, Soerjomataram I, Siegel RL, Torre LA, Jemal A. Global cancer statistics 2018: GLOBOCAN estimates of incidence and mortality worldwide for 36 cancers in 185 countries. *CA Cancer J Clin.* (2018) 68:394–424. doi: 10.3322/caac.21492
2. Miranda-Filho A, Pineros M, Znaor A, Marcos-Gragera R, Steliarova-Foucher E, Bray F. Global patterns and trends in the incidence of non-Hodgkin lymphoma. *Cancer Causes Control.* (2019) 30:489–99. doi: 10.1007/s10552-019-01155-5
3. Swerdlow SH, Campo E, Harris NL, Jaffe ES, Pileri SA, Stein H, Thiele J. *WHO Classification of Tumours of Haematopoietic and Lymphoid Tissues.* Lyon: International Agency for Research on Cancer (2017).
4. Allemani C, Matsuda T, Di Carlo V, Harewood R, Matz M, Niksic M, et al. Global surveillance of trends in cancer survival 2000-14 (CONCORD-3): analysis of individual records for 37 513 025 patients diagnosed with one of 18 cancers from 322 population-based registries in 71 countries. *Lancet.* (2018) 391:1023–75. doi: 10.1016/S0140-6736(17)33326-3
5. Chihara D, Oki Y, Fanale MA, Westin JR, Nastoupil LJ, Neelapu S, et al. Stage I non-Hodgkin lymphoma: no plateau in disease-specific survival ? *Ann Hematol.* (2019) 98:1169–76. doi: 10.1007/s00277-018-3571-7
6. Armitage JO, Gascoyne RD, Lunning MA, Cavalli F. Non-Hodgkin lymphoma. *Lancet.* (2017) 390:298–310. doi: 10.1016/S0140-6736(16)32407-2
7. Barth MJ, Minard-Colin V. Novel targeted therapeutic agents for the treatment of childhood, adolescent and young adult non-Hodgkin lymphoma. *Br J Haematol.* (2019) 182:633–43. doi: 10.1111/bjh.15783
8. Stavrovskaya AA. Cellular mechanisms of multidrug resistance of tumor cells. *Biochemistry Biokhimiia.* (2000) 65:95–106.
9. Johnstone RW, Ruefli AA, Lowe SW. Apoptosis: a link between cancer genetics and chemotherapy. *Cell.* (2002) 108:153–64. doi: 10.1016/S0092-8674(02)00625-6
10. Miyashita T, Reed JC. Bcl-2 oncoprotein blocks chemotherapy-induced apoptosis in a human leukemia cell line. *Blood.* (1993) 81:151–7. doi: 10.1182/blood.V81.1.151.151
11. Bonetti A, Zaninelli M, Leone R, Cetto GL, Pelosi G, Biolo S, et al. bcl-2 but not p53 expression is associated with resistance to chemotherapy in advanced breast cancer. *Clin Cancer Res.* (1998) 4:2331–6.
12. Wesarg E, Hoffarth S, Wiewrodt R, Kroll M, Biesterfeld S, Huber C, et al. Targeting BCL-2 family proteins to overcome drug resistance in non-small cell lung cancer. *Int J Cancer J Int Cancer.* (2007) 121:2387–94. doi: 10.1002/ijc.22977
13. Wallace DJ, Shen D, Reed GF, Miyanaga M, Mochizuki M, Sen HN, et al. Detection of the bcl-2 t(14;18) translocation and proto-oncogene expression in primary intraocular lymphoma. *Invest Ophthal Visual Sci.* (2006) 47:2750–6. doi: 10.1167/iovs.05-1312
14. Goodlad JR, Batstone PJ, Hamilton DA, Kernohan NM, Levison DA, White JM. BCL2 gene abnormalities define distinct clinical subsets of follicular lymphoma. *Histopathology.* (2006) 49:229–41. doi: 10.1111/j.1365-2559.2006.02501.x
15. Habens F, Lapham AS, Dallman CL, Pickering BM, Michels J, Marcusson EG, et al. Distinct promoters mediate constitutive and inducible Bcl-XL expression in malignant lymphocytes. *Oncogene.* (2007) 26:1910–9. doi: 10.1038/sj.onc.1209979
16. Hernandez-Luna MA, Rocha-Zavaleta L, Vega MI, Huerta-Yepez S. Hypoxia inducible factor-1alpha induces chemoresistance phenotype in non-Hodgkin lymphoma cell line via up-regulation of Bcl-(xL). *Leuk Lymph.* (2012) 54:1048–55. doi: 10.3109/10428194.2012.733874
17. Westphal D, Dewson G, Czabotar PE, Kluck RM. Molecular biology of Bax and Bak activation and action. *Biochim Biophys Acta.* (2011) 1813:521–31. doi: 10.1016/j.bbamcr.2010.12.019
18. Renault TT, Manon S. Bax: addressed to kill. *Biochimie.* (2011) 93:1379–91. doi: 10.1016/j.biochi.2011.05.013
19. Petros AM, Olejniczak ET, Fesik SW. Structural biology of the Bcl-2 family of proteins. *Biochim Biophys Acta.* (2004) 1644:83–94. doi: 10.1016/S0167-4889(03)00175-7
20. Hacker G, Weber A. BH3-only proteins trigger cytochrome c release, but how? *Arch Biochem Biophys.* (2007) 462:150–5. doi: 10.1016/j.abb.2006.12.022
21. Adams CM, Clark-Garvey S, Porcu P, Eischen CM. Targeting the Bcl-2 family in B cell lymphoma. *Front Oncol.* (2018) 8:636. doi: 10.3389/fonc.2018.00636
22. Holinger EP, Chittenden T, Lutz RJ. Bak BH3 peptides antagonize Bcl-xL function and induce apoptosis through cytochrome c-independent activation of caspases. *J Biol Chem.* (1999) 274:13298–304. doi: 10.1074/jbc.274.19.13298
23. Moreau C, Cartron PF, Hunt A, Meflah K, Green DR, Evan G, et al. Minimal BH3 peptides promote cell death by antagonizing anti-apoptotic proteins. *J Biol Chem.* (2003) 278:19426–35. doi: 10.1074/jbc.M209472200
24. Czabotar PE, Lee EF, van Delft MF, Day CL, Smith BJ, Huang DC, et al. Structural insights into the degradation of Mcl-1 induced by BH3 domains. *Proc Natl Acad Sci USA.* (2007) 104:6217–22. doi: 10.1073/pnas.0701297104
25. Li R, Boehm AL, Miranda MB, Shangary S, Grandis JR, Johnson DE. Targeting antiapoptotic Bcl-2 family members with cell-permeable BH3 peptides induces apoptosis signaling and death in head and neck squamous cell carcinoma cells. *Neoplasia.* (2007) 9:801–11. doi: 10.1593/neo.07394
26. Souers AJ, Leverson JD, Boghaert ER, Ackler SL, Catron ND, Chen J, et al. ABT-199, a potent and selective BCL-2 inhibitor, achieves antitumor activity while sparing platelets. *Nat Med.* (2013) 19:202–8. doi: 10.1038/nm.3048
27. Merino D, Kelly GL, Lessene G, Wei AH, Roberts AW, Strasser A. BH3-mimetic drugs: blazing the trail for new cancer medicines. *Cancer Cell.* (2018) 34:879–91. doi: 10.1016/j.ccell.2018.11.004
28. Pawelek JM, Low KB, Bermudes D. Tumor-targeted Salmonella as a novel anticancer vector. *Cancer research.* (1997) 57:4537–44.
29. Chávez-Navarro H, Hernández-Cueto DD, Vilchis-Estrada A, Bermúdez-Pulido DC, Antonio-Andrés G, Luria-Pérezn R. *Salmonella enterica*: un aliado en la terapia contra el cáncer. *Bol Med Hosp Infant Mex.* (2015) 72:11. doi: 10.1016/j.bmhimx.2015.02.005
30. Hernandez-Luna MA, Luria-Perez R. Cancer immunotherapy: priming the host immune response with live attenuated *Salmonella enterica*. *J Immunol Res.* (2018) 2018:2984247. doi: 10.1155/2018/2984247
31. Hernandez-Luna MA, Luria-Perez R, Huerta-Yepez S. [Therapeutic intervention alternatives in cancer, using attenuated live bacterial vectors: *Salmonella enterica* as a carrier of heterologous molecules]. *Rev Invest Clin.* (2013) 65:65–73.
32. Forbes NS. Engineering the perfect (bacterial) cancer therapy. *Nat Rev Cancer.* (2010) 10:785–94. doi: 10.1038/nrc2934
33. Hernandez-Luna MA, Diaz de Leon-Ortega R, Hernandez-Cueto DD, Gaxiola-Centeno R, Castro-Luna R, Martinez-Cristobal L, et al. Bactofection of sequences encoding a Bax protein peptide chemosensitizes prostate cancer tumor cells. *Bol Med Hosp Infant Mex.* (2016) 73:388–96. doi: 10.1016/j.bmhimx.2016.10.002
34. Luria-Perez R, Cedillo-Barron L, Santos-Argumedo L, Ortiz-Navarrete VF, Ocana-Mondragon A, Gonzalez-Bonilla CR. A fusogenic peptide expressed on the surface of *Salmonella enterica* elicits CTL responses to a dengue virus epitope. *Vaccine.* (2007) 25:5071–85. doi: 10.1016/j.vaccine.2007.03.047
35. Ruiz-Perez F, Leon-Kempis R, Santiago-Machuca A, Ortega-Pierres G, Barry E, Levine M, et al. Expression of the Plasmodium falciparum immunodominant epitope (NANP)(4) on the surface of *Salmonella enterica* using the autotransporter MisL. *Infect Immun.* (2002) 70:3611–20. doi: 10.1128/IAI.70.7.3611-3620.2002
36. Laus R, Graddis TJ, Hakim I, Vidovic D. Enhanced major histocompatibility complex class I-dependent presentation of antigens modified with cationic and fusogenic peptides. *Nat Biotechnol.* (2000) 18:1269–72. doi: 10.1038/82377
37. Waterhouse A, Bertoni M, Bienert S, Studer G, Tauriello G, Gumienny R, et al. SWISS-MODEL: homology modelling of protein structures and complexes. *Nucleic Acids Res.* (2018) 46(W1):W296–303. doi: 10.1093/nar/gky427
38. Bienert S, Waterhouse A, de Beer TA, Tauriello G, Studer G, Bordoli L, et al. The SWISS-MODEL Repository-new features and functionality. *Nucleic Acids Res.* (2017) 45(D1):D313–D9. doi: 10.1093/nar/gkw1132
39. Sali A, Blundell TL. Comparative protein modelling by satisfaction of spatial restraints. *J Mol Biol.* (1993) 234:779–815. doi: 10.1006/jmbi.1993.1626
40. Eswar N, Webb B, Marti-Renom MA, Madhusudhan MS, Eramian D, Shen MY, et al. Comparative protein structure modeling

using Modeller. *Curr Protoc Bioinformatics.* (2006) 15:5.6.1–5.6.30. doi: 10.1002/0471250953.bi0506s15

41. Ku B, Liang C, Jung JU, Oh BH. Evidence that inhibition of BAX activation by BCL-2 involves its tight and preferential interaction with the BH3 domain of BAX. *Cell Res.* (2011) 21:627–41. doi: 10.1038/cr.2010.149
42. Czabotar PE, Westphal D, Dewson G, Ma S, Hockings C, Fairlie WD, et al. Bax crystal structures reveal how BH3 domains activate Bax and nucleate its oligomerization to induce apoptosis. *Cell.* (2013) 152:519–31. doi: 10.1016/j.cell.2012.12.031
43. Phillips JC, Braun R, Wang W, Gumbart J, Tajkhorshid E, Villa E, et al. Scalable molecular dynamics with NAMD. *J Comput Chem.* (2005) 26:1781–802. doi: 10.1002/jcc.20289
44. Jo S, Kim T, Iyer VG, Im W. CHARMM-GUI: a web-based graphical user interface for CHARMM. *J Comput Chem.* (2008) 29:1859–65. doi: 10.1002/jcc.20945
45. Lee J, Cheng X, Swails JM, Yeom MS, Eastman PK, Lemkul JA, et al. CHARMM-GUI input generator for NAMD, GROMACS, AMBER, OpenMM, and CHARMM/OpenMM simulations using the CHARMM36 additive force field. *J Chem Theory Comput.* (2016) 12:405–13. doi: 10.1021/acs.jctc.5b00935
46. Lomize MA, Lomize AL, Pogozheva ID, Mosberg HI. OPM: orientations of proteins in membranes database. *Bioinformatics.* (2006) 22:623–5. doi: 10.1093/bioinformatics/btk023
47. Chen VB, Arendall WB III, Headd JJ, Keedy DA, Immormino RM, Kapral GJ, et al. MolProbity: all-atom structure validation for macromolecular crystallography. *Acta Crystallogr D Biol Crystallogr.* (2010) 66(Pt 1):12–21. doi: 10.1107/S0907444909042073
48. Lovell SC, Davis IW, Arendall WB III, de Bakker PI, Word JM, Prisant MG, et al. Structure validation by Calpha geometry: phi,psi and Cbeta deviation. *Proteins.* (2003) 50:437–50. doi: 10.1002/prot.10286
49. Uziela K, Shu N, Wallner B, Elofsson A. ProQ3: improved model quality assessments using Rosetta energy terms. *Sci Rep.* (2016) 6:33509. doi: 10.1038/srep33509
50. Uziela K, Menendez Hurtado D, Shu N, Wallner B, Elofsson A. ProQ3D: improved model quality assessments using deep learning. *Bioinformatics.* (2017) 33:1578–80. doi: 10.1093/bioinformatics/btw819
51. Benkert P, Kunzli M, Schwede T. QMEAN server for protein model quality estimation. *Nucleic Acids Res.* (2009) 37:W510–4. doi: 10.1093/nar/gkp322
52. Hoiseth SK, Stocker BA. Aromatic-dependent Salmonella typhimurium are non-virulent and effective as live vaccines. *Nature.* (1981) 291:238–9. doi: 10.1038/291238a0
53. Vendrell A, Gravisaco MJ, Goin JC, Pasetti MF, Herschllik L, De Toro J, et al. Therapeutic effects of Salmonella typhi in a mouse model of T-cell lymphoma. *J Immunother.* (2013) 36:171–80. doi: 10.1097/CJI.0b013e3182886d95
54. Manders JM, Postema EJ, Corstens FH, Boerman OC. Enhancing tumor implantation and growth rate of Ramos B-cell lymphoma in nude mice. *Comp Med.* (2002) 52:36–8.
55. Nakase I, Konishi Y, Ueda M, Saji H, Futaki S. Accumulation of arginine-rich cell-penetrating peptides in tumors and the potential for anticancer drug delivery *in vivo. J Controlled Release.* (2012) 159:181–8. doi: 10.1016/j.jconrel.2012.01.016
56. Miyake K, Murata T, Murakami T, Zhao M, Kiyuna T, Kawaguchi K, et al. Tumor-targeting Salmonella typhimurium A1-R overcomes nab-paclitaxel resistance in a cervical cancer PDOX mouse model. *Arch Gynecol Obstet.* (2019) 299:1683–90. doi: 10.1007/s00404-019-05147-3
57. Baay-Guzman GJ, Bebenek IG, Zeidler M, Hernandez-Pando R, Vega MI, Garcia-Zepeda EA, et al. HIF-1 expression is associated with CCL2 chemokine expression in airway inflammatory cells: implications in allergic airway inflammation. *Respir Res.* (2012) 13:60. doi: 10.1186/1465-9921-13-60
58. Ruiz-Olvera P, Ruiz-Perez F, Sepulveda NV, Santiago-Machuca A, Maldonado-Rodriguez R, Garcia-Elorriaga G, et al. Display and release of the Plasmodium falciparum circumsporozoite protein using the autotransporter MisL of *Salmonella enterica. Plasmid.* (2003) 50:12–27. doi: 10.1016/S0147-619X(03)00047-7
59. Nasr R, Akbari Eidgahi MR. Construction of a synthetically engineered nirb promoter for expression of recombinant protein in *Escherichia coli. Jundishapur J Microbiol.* (2014) 7:e15942. doi: 10.5812/jjm.15942
60. Los M, Mozoluk M, Ferrari D, Stepczynska A, Stroh C, Renz A, et al. Activation and caspase-mediated inhibition of PARP: a molecular switch between fibroblast necrosis and apoptosis in death receptor signaling. *Mol Biol Cell.* (2002) 13:978–88. doi: 10.1091/mbc.01-05-0272
61. Knight T, Luedtke D, Edwards H, Taub JW, Ge Y. A delicate balance - The BCL-2 family and its role in apoptosis, oncogenesis, and cancer therapeutics. *Biochem Pharmacol.* (2019) 162:250–61. doi: 10.1016/j.bcp.2019.01.015
62. Kuramoto K, Sakai A, Shigemasa K, Takimoto Y, Asaoku H, Tsujimoto T, et al. High expression of MCL1 gene related to vascular endothelial growth factor is associated with poor outcome in non-Hodgkin's lymphoma. *Br J Haematol.* (2002) 116:158–61. doi: 10.1046/j.1365-2141.2002.03253.x
63. Oltersdorf T, Elmore SW, Shoemaker AR, Armstrong RC, Augeri DJ, Belli BA, et al. An inhibitor of Bcl-2 family proteins induces regression of solid tumours. *Nature.* (2005) 435:677–81. doi: 10.1038/nature03579
64. Roberts AW, Seymour JF, Brown JR, Wierda WG, Kipps TJ, Khaw SL, et al. Substantial susceptibility of chronic lymphocytic leukemia to BCL2 inhibition: results of a phase I study of navitoclax in patients with relapsed or refractory disease. *J Clin Oncol.* (2012) 30:488–96. doi: 10.1200/JCO.2011.34.7898
65. Hwang JJ, Kuruvilla J, Mendelson D, Pishvaian MJ, Deeken JF, Siu LL, et al. Phase I dose finding studies of obatoclax (GX15-070), a small molecule pan-BCL-2 family antagonist, in patients with advanced solid tumors or lymphoma. *Clin Cancer Res.* (2010) 16:4038–45. doi: 10.1158/1078-0432.CCR-10-0822
66. Zhou S, Gravekamp C, Bermudes D, Liu K. Tumour-targeting bacteria engineered to fight cancer. *Nat Rev Cancer.* (2018) 18:727–43. doi: 10.1038/s41568-018-0070-z
67. Kasinskas RW, Forbes NS. Salmonella typhimurium specifically chemotax and proliferate in heterogeneous tumor tissue *in vitro. Biotechnol Bioeng.* (2006) 94:710–21. doi: 10.1002/bit.20883
68. Loeffler M, Le'Negrate G, Krajewska M, Reed JC. IL-18-producing Salmonella inhibit tumor growth. *Cancer Gene Ther.* (2008) 15:787–94. doi: 10.1038/cgt.2008.48
69. Sorenson BS, Banton KL, Frykman NL, Leonard AS, Saltzman DA. Attenuated Salmonella typhimurium with IL-2 gene reduces pulmonary metastases in murine osteosarcoma. *Clin Orthop Related Res.* (2008) 466:1285–91. doi: 10.1007/s11999-008-0243-2
70. Sorenson BS, Banton KL, Frykman NL, Leonard AS, Saltzman DA. Attenuated Salmonella typhimurium with interleukin 2 gene prevents the establishment of pulmonary metastases in a model of osteosarcoma. *J Pediatric Surg.* (2008) 43:1153–8. doi: 10.1016/j.jpedsurg.2008.02.048
71. Agorio C, Schreiber F, Sheppard M, Mastroeni P, Fernandez M, Martinez MA, et al. Live attenuated Salmonella as a vector for oral cytokine gene therapy in melanoma. *J Gene Med.* (2007) 9:416–23. doi: 10.1002/jgm.1023
72. Loeffler M, Le'Negrate G, Krajewska M, Reed JC. Salmonella typhimurium engineered to produce CCL21 inhibit tumor growth. *Cancer Immunol Immunother.* (2009) 58:769–75. doi: 10.1007/s00262-008-0555-9
73. Loeffler M, Le'Negrate G, Krajewska M, Reed JC. Inhibition of tumor growth using salmonella expressing Fas ligand. *J Natl Cancer Inst.* (2008) 100:1113–6. doi: 10.1093/jnci/djn205
74. Cao HD, Yang YX, Lu L, Liu SN, Wang PL, Tao XH, et al. Attenuated Salmonella typhimurium carrying TRAIL and VP3 genes inhibits the growth of gastric cancer cells *in vitro* and *in vivo. Tumori.* (2010) 96:296–303. doi: 10.1177/030089161009600218
75. Jeong JH, Kim K, Lim D, Jeong K, Hong Y, Nguyen VH, et al. Anti-tumoral effect of the mitochondrial target domain of Noxa delivered by an engineered Salmonella typhimurium. *PLoS ONE.* (2014) 9:e80050. doi: 10.1371/journal.pone.0080050
76. Camacho EM, Mesa-Pereira B, Medina C, Flores A, Santero E. Engineering Salmonella as intracellular factory for effective killing of tumour cells. *Sci Rep.* (2016) 6:30591. doi: 10.1038/srep30591
77. Nemunaitis J, Cunningham C, Senzer N, Kuhn J, Cramm J, Litz C, et al. Pilot trial of genetically modified, attenuated Salmonella expressing the *E. coli* cytosine deaminase gene in refractory cancer patients. *Cancer Gene Ther.* (2003) 10:737–44. doi: 10.1038/sj.cgt.7700634
78. Massa PE, Paniccia A, Monegal A, de Marco A, Rescigno M. Salmonella engineered to express CD20-targeting antibodies and a drug-converting enzyme can eradicate human lymphomas. *Blood.* (2013) 122:705–14. doi: 10.1182/blood-2012-12-474098
79. Dorsey CW, Laarakker MC, Humphries AD, Weening EH, Baumler AJ. *Salmonella enterica* serotype Typhimurium MisL is an intestinal colonization factor that binds fibronectin. *Mol Microbiol.* (2005) 57:196–211. doi: 10.1111/j.1365-2958.2005.04666.x
80. Barak Y, Schreiber F, Thorne SH, Contag CH, Debeer D, Matin A. Role of nitric oxide in Salmonella typhimurium-mediated cancer

cell killing. *BMC Cancer.* (2010) 10:146. doi: 10.1186/1471-2407-10-146

81. Lee CH, Lin ST, Liu JJ, Chang WW, Hsieh JL, Wang WK. Salmonella induce autophagy in melanoma by the downregulation of AKT/mTOR pathway. *Gene Therapy.* (2014) 21:309–16. doi: 10.1038/gt.2013.86
82. Bascuas T, Moreno M, Grille S, Chabalgoity JA. Salmonella immunotherapy improves the outcome of CHOP chemotherapy in non-Hodgkin lymphoma-bearing mice. *Front Immunol.* (2018) 9:7. doi: 10.3389/fimmu.2018.00007
83. Garcia-Gil A, Galan-Enriquez CS, Perez-Lopez A, Nava P, Alpuche-Aranda C, Ortiz-Navarrete V. SopB activates the Akt-YAP pathway to promote Salmonella survival within B cells. *Virulence.* (2018) 9:1390–402. doi: 10.1080/21505594.2018.1509664
84. Grille S, Moreno M, Bascuas T, Marques JM, Munoz N, Lens D, et al. *Salmonella enterica* serovar Typhimurium immunotherapy for B-cell lymphoma induces broad anti-tumour immunity with therapeutic effect. *Immunology.* (2014) 143:428–37. doi: 10.1111/imm.12320
85. Avogadri F, Mittal D, Saccheri F, Sarrafiore M, Ciocca M, Larghi P, et al. Intra-tumoral Salmonella typhimurium induces a systemic anti-tumor immune response that is directed by low-dose radiation to treat distal disease. *Eur J Immunol.* (2008) 38:1937–47. doi: 10.1002/eji.200738035
86. Kim JE, Phan TX, Nguyen VH, Dinh-Vu HV, Zheng JH, Yun M, et al. Salmonella typhimurium suppresses tumor growth via the pro-inflammatory cytokine interleukin-1beta. *Theranostics.* (2015) 5:1328–42. doi: 10.7150/thno.11432

10

Omp19 Enables *Brucella abortus* to Evade the Antimicrobial Activity From Host's Proteolytic Defense System

Karina A. Pasquevich[*†], *Marianela V. Carabajal*[†], *Francisco F. Guaimas, Laura Bruno, Mara S. Roset, Lorena M. Coria, Diego A. Rey Serrantes, Diego J. Comerci and Juliana Cassataro*[*]

Consejo Nacional de Investigaciones Científicas y Técnicas (UNSAM-CONICET), Instituto de Investigaciones Biotecnológicas Dr. Rodolfo A. Ugalde, Universidad Nacional de San Martín, Buenos Aires, Argentina

***Correspondence:**
Karina A. Pasquevich
kpasquevich@iib.unsam.edu.ar
Juliana Cassataro
jucassataro@iib.unsam.edu.ar

[†] *These authors have contributed equally to this work*

Pathogenic microorganisms confront several proteolytic events in the molecular interplay with their host, highlighting that proteolysis and its regulation play an important role during infection. Microbial inhibitors, along with their target endogenous/exogenous enzymes, may directly affect the host's defense mechanisms and promote infection. Omp19 is a *Brucella* spp. conserved lipoprotein anchored by the lipid portion in the *Brucella* outer membrane. Previous work demonstrated that purified unlipidated Omp19 (U-Omp19) has protease inhibitor activity against gastrointestinal and lysosomal proteases. In this work, we found that a *Brucella omp19* deletion mutant is highly attenuated in mice when infecting by the oral route. This attenuation can be explained by bacterial increased susceptibility to host proteases met by the bacteria during establishment of infection. Omp19 deletion mutant has a cell division defect when exposed to pancreatic proteases that is linked to cell-cycle arrest in G1-phase, Omp25 degradation on the cell envelope and CtrA accumulation. Moreover, Omp19 deletion mutant is more susceptible to killing by macrophage derived microsomes than wt strain. Preincubation with gastrointestinal proteases led to an increased susceptibility of Omp19 deletion mutant to macrophage intracellular killing. Thus, in this work, we describe for the first time a physiological function of *B. abortus* Omp19. This activity enables *Brucella* to better thrive in the harsh gastrointestinal tract, where protection from proteolytic degradation can be a matter of life or death, and afterwards invade the host and bypass intracellular proteases to establish the chronic infection.

Keywords: bacterial protease inhibitor, Omp19, gastrointestinal route of infection, brucellosis, intracellular proteases

INTRODUCTION

The intestinal mucosa is the largest interface between the external environment and the tissues of the human body. The first line of defense in the gastrointestinal tract is in the lumen, where microorganisms are degraded in a non-specific fashion by pH and gastric, pancreatic and biliary secretions. Pathogenic microorganisms confront several proteolytic events in the molecular interplay with their host, therefore proteolysis and its regulation play an important role during infection.

Microbes synthetize protease inhibitors to control endogenous proteases. Some inhibitors can also interact with exogenous peptidases produced by other species and thus may directly affect host's defense mechanisms (1). Few works in the literature show the importance of bacterial protease inhibitors activity against host-proteases (2–4). Our hypothesis is that pathogenic bacteria synthesize protease inhibitors to evade the antimicrobial activity from host's proteases.

In our laboratory, we have been working on the use of a conserved *Brucella* spp. protein devoid of its lipid moiety called U-Omp19 as a vaccine against brucellosis (5–7). Omp19 has significant sequence identity with bacterial protease inhibitors from I38 family. Remarkably, recombinant U-Omp19 inhibits gastrointestinal and lysosomal proteases (8, 9). However, the physiological function of Omp19 in *Brucella* is still unknown.

Brucellosis is a worldwide re-emerging zoonotic disease that is transmitted from domestic and wild animals to humans. The human disease, mostly caused by *Brucella abortus* and *B. melitensis,* represents an important cause of morbidity worldwide whereas animal brucellosis is associated with serious economic losses caused mainly by elicited abortions and infertility (10, 11).

Oral infection is one of the principal ways of brucellosis transmission. Animals usually lick tissues from abortions or ingest contaminated pasture and humans acquire often the disease by consumption of infected, unpasteurized dairy products (10, 12–16). Few virulence factors required for food-borne infection by *Brucella* have been described: Urease and cholylglycine hydrolase that confer resistance to gastric acidity and bile salts, respectively (17, 18). Once inside the host, *Brucella* disseminate via infected phagocytic cells to different tissues and organs, developing foci of infection, surviving intracellularly and leading to a chronic disease (19).

Digestive enzymes, primarily proteases, contribute to the non-specific host defense system exerting a toxic action on microorganisms by destruction of their cell wall (20). Omp19 is a lipoprotein anchored in the *Brucella* outer membrane (7). This location together with its protease inhibitor activity suggest that it may play a protective role against host proteases.

In this work, we studied if Omp19 enables *Brucella* to better thrive in the harsh gastrointestinal tract, where protection from proteolytic degradation can be a matter of life or death, and thus promoting host invasion and intracellular infection.

MATERIALS AND METHODS

Ethics Statement

Protocols of this study agreed with international ethical standards for animal experimentation (Helsinki Declaration and amendments, Amsterdam Protocol of welfare and animal protection and NIH guidelines for the Care and Use of Laboratory Animals). Protocols of this study were approved by the Institutional Committee for the Care and Use of Experimentation Animals from UNSAM (CICUAE-UNSAM_N°04/2014).

Bacterial Strains, Media, and Culture Conditions

Brucella strains were derived from the wild type (wt) 2308 biovar and were: (i) smooth virulent wt *B. abortus*; (ii) unmarked *omp19* deletion mutant (Δ*omp19*); and (iii) *omp19* complemented Δ*omp19* mutant (Δ*omp19*pBBR4*omp19*). All strains were grown as described in Czibener and Ugalde (21). When necessary, media were supplemented with the Ampicillin (100 μg/ml) or Nalidixic acid (5 μg/ml). CFU determination from intestine containing samples were performed in medium with following antibiotics to inhibit normal flora growth: Vancomycin (20 μg/ml), Cycloheximide (100 μg/ml), Bacitracin (10 U/ml), and Nalidixic acid. All work with live *Brucella* was performed in BSL3-laboratories and BSL3-animal facility at UNSAM. *Escherichia coli* strains were grown at 37°C in LB with Ampicillin.

Generation of Mutant Strains

(i) Δomp19 Strain

Omp19 (BAB1_1930) unmarked chromosomal mutant was generated as described in Herrmann et al. (22). Briefly, two DNA fragments of ~500 bp containing flanking regions of BAB1_1930 were amplified from *B. abortus* 2308 genomic DNA. Primers used to amplify omp19′s upstream regions were: omp19(EcoRI)_Up_Fw_5′-GAATTCTCGAAGGCT GTTTCGCTATCG-3′ and omp19_Up_Rv_5′- CAGGTTCTCC ATTTGCGCATTT-3′; and omp19_Down_Fw_5′-CAAAT GGAGAACCTGTCTGACCCGGAAACGATGAAC-3′ and omp19(BamHI)_Down_Rv_5′-GGATCCTTGTGCGCCTG ACGATGC-3′ for downstream region. Fragments were ligated by overlapping PCR using omp19(EcoRI)_Up_Fw and omp19(BamHI)_Down_Rv. The resulting fragment was digested with EcoRI and BamHI, cloned into pK18mobSacB (23) and conjugated to *B. abortus* 2308 by biparental mating. Single recombinants selection, selection with sucrose, excision of plasmids, and generation of deletion mutants was performed as described previously described (21). Deletion of BAB1_1930 was confirmed by PCR and sequence analysis and western blot (**Figure S1**).

(ii) Complementation of Δomp19 Mutant

A 1000 bp DNA fragment containing the complete gene (BAB1_1930) and its promotor was amplified using primers Omp19(BamHI)_ATG_5′-ATGGATCCATGGGAATTTCA AAAGCAAGTCTGC-3′ and Omp19(SpeI)_TGA_5′-GAAC TAGTTCAGCGCGACAGCGTCA-3′, digested with BamHI and SpeI and ligated into pBBR4 to generate the plasmid pBBR4*omp19*. This plasmid was electroporated into Δ*omp19* mutant. The resulting complemented strain was called Δ*omp19*pBBR4*omp19*. Complementation was confirmed by PCR and western blot (not shown).

Recombinant Proteins, Enzymes, and Extracts

Mouse intestine- and stomach-extracts were obtained as previously described (8). Briefly, intestines and stomachs extracts were obtained from 6 to 12 weeks old female or male Balb/c mice ($n = 10$). Prior to fluid preparation, mice were fasted for 2.5 h (water ad lib.) and euthanized by CO_2 inhalation. Stomachs and small intestines were resected, homogenized in PBS, and fluid separated by centrifugation (10 min, 13,200 × g at 4°C). Pooled Intestinal or stomach fluids were snap-frozen in liquid nitrogen and stored at −80°C. Protein concentration and proteolytic activity were determined as previously described by Ibañez et al. (8). Microsomes of J774 murine macrophages were obtained as described previously by Coria et al. (9). Pancreatin, Elastase, and Trypsin from pig and α-Chymotrypsin from bovine were from Sigma.

Recombinant U-Omp19 was produced as previously described by Pasquevich et al. (5). For Omp25 production, the complete sequence of *B. abortus* omp25 gene (GenBank_X79284.1) (24) was synthetized and subcloned into pET22(b)+ (Novagen) in frame with 6×His-tag (genscript). Expression and purification was performed as described in Goel and Bhatnagar (25).

Infection of Mice

Six to eight-week-old female BALB/c mice were bred at IIB-UNSAM. Five mice/group were inoculated (i) wt, (ii) Δ*omp19*, or (iii) Δ*omp19*pBBR4*omp19 Brucella* strains either by gavage (i.g.) with 1 × 10^9 CFU in 0.2 ml PBS (18, 26) or with 1 × 10^{10} CFU directly into the oral cavity as previously described by von Bargen et al. (27). Infected mice were kept in cages within a BSL3 facility. At different times post-infection mice were euthanized by CO_2 inhalation and organs were aseptically collected, homogenized, and plated for CFU determination. Intestinal samples were plated on TSA supplemented with Vancomycin, Cycloheximide, Bacitracin, and Nalidixic acid. In some experiments tissue samples from duodenum were obtained for immunofluorescence analysis.

Intestinal Tissue Immunofluorescence

Duodenum sections from mice infected i.g. either with wt or Δ*omp19 B. abortus* were excised, fixed (4% paraformaldehyde), immersed in 30%-sucrose buffer, embedded in OCT-medium and frozen (-80°C). Cryosections (10 μm) were mounted on positively charged glass-slides (Biogenex), permeabilized with 0.2% Tween20 and blocked with 1% BSA and 5% horse serum in PBS. *Brucella* detection was performed as previously described (21). RNAse A (10 μg/ml) treated samples were counterstained with Alexa-Fluor555-WGA (ThermoFisher) and TO-PRO®-3 (Invitrogen). Sections were mounted using FluorSave reagent (Calbiochem) and images obtained on an IX-81 Olympus microscope with FV-1000 confocal module. A ROI was set for each treatment, background subtracted and images merged (RGB) (ImageJ software, NIH).

Bacterial Susceptibility to Proteases

(i) Agar Disk-Diffusion Method

Brucella strains (1 × 10^8 CFU) were spread on TSA plates supplemented with Vancomycin, Cycloheximide, Bacitracin, and Nalidixic acid. Five-mm filter disks impregnated with either PBS, intestine- or stomach-extract were placed on the agar surface. After 72 h of incubation (37°C) zones of inhibition were determined.

(ii) Protease Broth-Susceptibility Test

Brucella strains (1 × 10^5 CFU/ml) were incubated in 10% TSB plus buffer, intestine-extract (8.5 mg/ml), pancreatin (2 mg/ml), α-chymotrypsin (50 μM), trypsin (20 μM), pancreatic elastase (5 μM), or microsomes from J774 macrophages (2 mg/ml) for the different periods of time at 37°C. Negative control was buffer supplemented with 10% TSB. Buffer was PBS (intestine extract or microsomes), 0.5% ClNa (pancreatin), 10 mM Tris-HCl, pH7.8 (α-chymotrypsin and trypsin), or 10 mM Tris-HCl pH8.8 (pancreatic elastase). All protease solutions were sterilized by filtration before to incubation with the bacteria. Live bacteria (CFU/ml) were determined at different time points by serial dilutions plating.

Bacterial Growth Analysis

Brucella strains were labeled with TRSE (Invitrogen) as previously described by Brown et al. (28). Bacteria were spotted on 1% agarose pads with 10% TSB plus PBS or pancreatin (2 mg/ml). Images were obtained before and after 24 h of culture on an Olympus IX-81 microscope with FV-1000 confocal module. Images were subtracted the background and merged using RGB format (ImageJ software). Number of total bacteria (N) and initial number of bacteria (N_0, number of labeled or partially labeled bacteria) were enumerated using Spot Detector plugin (ICY software, Institute Pasteur). Three to nine images/condition in duplicates were evaluated (50–150 colonies/condition). Then, assuming exponential growth, the average number of cell divisions (n) was calculated:

$$\textit{Average number of cell divisions} = n = \log_2 \frac{N}{N_0}$$

DNA Content on Individual Bacteria

Brucella in exponential phase (5 × 10^7 CFU/ml) were incubated with or without pancreatin (2 mg/ml). After 1.5–6 h, cells were washed, fixed, incubated with RNase A and labeled with SYTOX-Green (Invitrogen). Samples were analyzed in a FACS ARIA II (BD Biosciences) and analyzed with FlowJo7.6.2 software (Tree Star).

Western Blot

Brucella strains (5 × 10^8 CFU/ml) were cultured with 10% TSB buffer with or without pancreatic elastase (10 μM), washed and boiled in sample buffer (5 min). CFU/ml were determined in a sample taken prior to stop the reaction and 1 × 10^7 CFU/lane were subjected to SDS-PAGE and transferred onto nitrocellulose membranes. Immunoblotting was performed using mouse monoclonal antibodies against Omp1, Omp2b, Omp25, Omp10, Omp16, and Omp19 (29), rabbit polyclonal anti-CtrA (30) or mouse anti-GroEL serum, followed by incubation with anti-mouse-IgG-HRP (Sigma) or anti-mouse-IgG IRDye antibodies (Li-Cor Biosciences). Images were acquired with Odyssey image-scanner and band intensities (RFU) were quantified (Image-Studio-Lite Software). Omp16, Omp10, and GroEL were similar in all treatments and served as loading control. Percentage of digested Omp25 was calculated:

$$\textit{percentage of digested Omp25} = \frac{\textit{Digested Omp25 RFU/lane}}{\textit{Total Omp25 RFU/lane}} \times 100.$$

Omp25 Digestion

Purified Omp25 (1 µM) was incubated with pancreatic elastase (1 µM) or buffer (10 mM Tris-HCl, pH8.8) with or without U-Omp19 (45 µM). Reactions were stopped by sample buffer addition and boiling. Omp25 digestion was followed by western blot.

Cell Culture and Infection Assay

J774 macrophages were maintained in RPMI 1640 supplemented with 5% fetal bovine serum (FBS) and streptomycin (50 µg/ml)-penicillin (50 U/ml) (Gibco Life Technologies) in a humidify 5% CO_2 atmosphere at 37°C. Cells (5×10^4 per well) were seeded on 24-well plates in antibiotic-free medium and were kept for 24 h. *B. abortus* infections were carried out at a multiplicity of infection (MOI) of 500:1 or 100:1. After a 1 h incubation with the bacteria, wells were washed three times with PBS and incubated with fresh medium containing 50 µg/ml of Gentamycin and 100 µg/ml streptomycin to kill non-internalized bacteria. At the indicated time points, infected cells were washed three times with PBS and lysed with 500 µl 0.1% Triton X-100 (Sigma-Aldrich). The intracellular CFU were determined by plating serial dilutions on TSA. In some experiments, prior to the infection of cell the bacteria were incubated at 5×10^7 CFU/ml with or without pancreatin (2 mg/ml) during 2 h. Afterwards bacteria were washed and suspended in medium to infect the cells.

Statistical Analysis

Statistical analysis and plotting were performed using Prism® 7.04 (GraphPad, Inc., USA). CFU data were logarithmically transformed. Unpaired two-tailed Student *t*-test was used for pairwise comparisons between means of two groups or one-way or two-way ANOVA followed by Bonferroni's posttest was used for comparing more than two means. Significance level was set at $p < 0.05$.

RESULTS

Omp19 Expression Is Needed for Oral Acquired *B. abortus* Infection

To investigate the role of Omp19 in *Brucella* infection, a deletion mutant (Δ*omp19*) and its complemented strain (Δ*omp19*pBBR4*omp19*) were constructed in the *B. abortus* wild-type (wt) strain 2308.

Mutant and wt strains had similar growth curves, resistance to low pH and bile salts. Moreover, membrane permeability to hydrophobic substances, expression of main outer membrane proteins (Omps) (Omp1, Omp2b, Omp25, Omp10, and Omp16) and lipopolysaccharide O-antigen were similar between wt and Δ*omp19* strains (**Figures S1A–F**). The authenticity of the mutant was verified by PCR and immunoblot analysis on whole-cell extracts with an anti-Omp19 Mab (**Figures S1E,F**).

To evaluate the role of Omp19 in the establishment of *B. abortus* infection through the digestive tract *in vivo*, BALB/c mice were inoculated intragastrically (i.g.) with wt, Δ*omp19* or Δ*omp19*pBBR4*omp19* and 20 days post-infection bacterial loads at spleens and cervical lymph nodes (CLNs) were assessed. While wt and Δ*omp19*pBBR4*omp19* established infection, there were significant lower numbers of CFUs at spleens and CLNs from Δ*omp19* infected mice ($p < 0.001$ vs. wt) (**Figures 1A,B**).

Upon gavage administration, initial events of bacterial invasion and onset of infection in the oral cavity may be bypassed. Thus, BALB/c mice were administered directly into the oral cavity as described in von Bargen et al. (27) with wt or Δ*omp19*. Twenty days post-infection *B. abortus* were isolated from spleens and CLNs from wt infected mice, whereas almost no CFUs were found in these organs of Δ*omp19* infected mice ($p < 0.05$ and $p < 0.01$ vs. wt, respectively) (**Figures 1C,D**).

Altogether, these results demonstrate that Omp19 plays a crucial role in the establishment of infection by *Brucella* through the oral route in mice.

Brucella abortus Reaches Intestinal Tissues Upon Oral Infection and Requires Omp19 to Evade the Bacteriostatic Action of Intestinal Content

To evaluate if Δ*omp19* attenuation after oral infection is due to higher susceptibility to gastrointestinal content, short-term gavage infection experiments were performed. BALB/c mice were i.g. inoculated with wt or Δ*omp19* strains and at different time points post-infection the stomach and intestinal sections were analyzed. After 15 min equal numbers of bacteria were isolated from the stomachs of both groups (**Figure 2A**). After 1 h both strains were present in the duodenum at the lumen as well as in the epithelium (**Figure 2B**).

Next, *B. abortus* loads in different sections of the small intestine: duodenum, jejunum, ileum and Peyer's patches were evaluated. Almost no differences in wt and Δ*omp19* CFUs were detected at 2 h post-infection with a slight but significant increase in Δ*omp19* CFUs at Ileum (**Figure 2C**) that may not explain the attenuation of this strain when infecting by the oral route. However, when plated undiluted (direct plating from each tissue on TSA + Antibiotics) low-density bacterial growth and small colonies were found in the drops of Δ*omp19*, indicating that the intestine content impaired Δ*omp19* strain's growth. This effect was temporarily and reversible, since upon dilution it disappeared and both, wt and Δ*omp19*, showed similar numbers and phenotype of colonies (**Figure 2D**). These results indicate that the intestine content exerts a bacteriostatic action on Δ*omp19*, suggesting that Omp19 protects *Brucella* from intestinal proteases.

Similar results were obtained when bacteria where inoculated directly at the oral cavity of mice. Both strains, wt and Δ*omp19*, were recovered from intestinal tissues after 1 h of infection (**Figure 2E**), indicating that *Brucella* reaches the intestine after oral infection (by gavage or oral cavity delivery) and there it is exposed to the intestinal content that exerts a bacteriostatic effect.

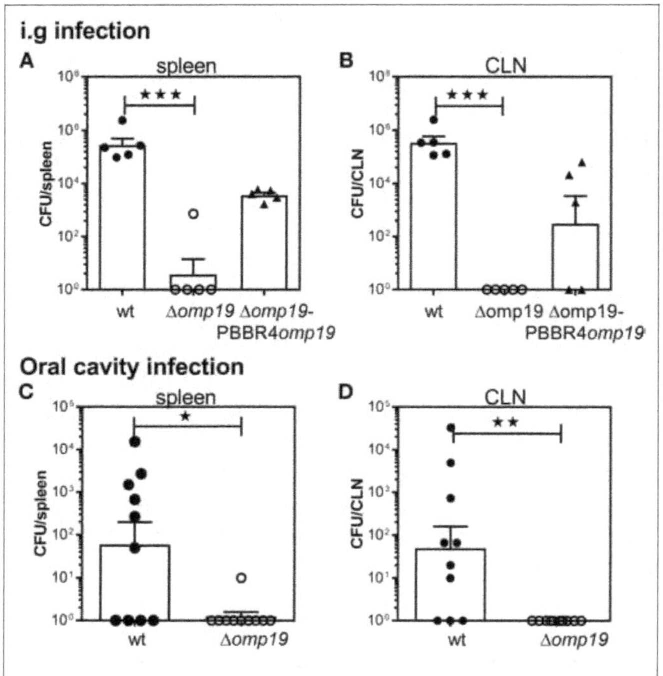

FIGURE 1 | *B. abortus Δomp19* is attenuated after oral infection. **(A,B)** BALB/c mice were i.g. inoculated with 1×10^9 CFU/mouse of wt, *Δomp19* or *Δomp19*pBBR4*omp19 B. abortus* strains. Spleen and CLNs were homogenized and plated for CFU counting at 20 days post-infection (***$p < 0.001$ vs. wt *B. abortus*). Results are representative of three independent experiments with 5 mice per group. **(C,D)** BALB/c mice were inoculated at the oral cavity with wt or *Δomp19 B. abortus* (1×10^{10} CFU/mouse). Twenty days after infection the number of CFU at the spleens and CLNs were quantified (*$p < 0.05$ and **$p < 0.01$ vs. wt *B. abortus*). Pooled data from two independent experiments are shown. Each point represents data from an individual mouse. Horizontal lines and error bars represent the mean ± s.e.m. (For some mice, no live bacteria were recovered from spleens or CLNs. These were arbitrarily assigned with values of 1 CFU).

Omp19 Protects *B. abortus* Against the Action of Pancreatic Proteases

To further assess the role of Omp19 against the action of gastric and gut content, *in vitro* bacterial susceptibility assays were performed.

An agar disk-diffusion test indicated that *Δomp19* is more susceptible to the action of intestine content than the wt strain ($p < 0.01$ vs. wt + intestine extract) (**Figure 3A**), whereas stomach content did not affect bacterial growth.

Incubation with intestine-extract inhibited *Δomp19*'s growth and this action was bacteriostatic, since viable bacteria were recovered by dilution (**Figure 3B**). Viable bacteria determination over time indicated that in presence of intestine-extract *Δomp19* was unable to grow ($p < 0.001$ vs. *wt* + intestine), whereas the wt and the complemented strains grew exponentially after 13 h of culture (**Figure 3C**). Similar results were obtained using pancreatin (a pig pancreatic extract) (**Figure 3D**), supporting that *B. abortus* requires Omp19 to grow when exposed to intestinal content.

As purified U-Omp19 inhibits main gastrointestinal proteases (8), the effect of individual proteases (pancreatic elastase, α-chymotrypsin, trypsin) on wt, *Δomp19* and *Δomp19*pBBR4*omp19* viability was assessed. *Δomp19* was more susceptible *in vitro* to pancreatic elastase action than wt and *Δomp19*pBBR4*omp19* ($p < 0.001$). In contrast, α-chymotrypsin and trypsin did not alter bacterial growth (**Figure 3E**).

These results together demonstrate that *B. abortus* requires the expression of Omp19 to resist the action of intestinal proteases.

Δomp19 B. abortus Stops Cell Division and Cell-Cycle Progression at G1-Phase After Incubation With Pancreatic Proteases

To evaluate if *Δomp19*'s growth impairment when exposed to proteases is due to a cell division defect, *Brucella's* growth was studied by microscopy. *Brucella* Texas-red succinimidyl-ester (TRSE) labeling allows, after growth, the visualization of an unlabeled pole and subsequently unlabeled or partially labeled daughter cells. TRSE-labeled *wt* and *Δomp19* were cultured on TSB-agarose pads containing buffer or pancreatin. After 24 h wt and *Δomp19* in buffer-pads and wt in pancreatin-pads formed microcolonies with many unlabeled cells surrounding partially labeled cells. However, *Δomp19* in pancreatin-pads formed no or small colonies (small chains) with few unlabeled sphere-shaped bacteria (**Figure 4A**), indicating a cell division defect. Quantitative analysis of labeled (or partially labeled) cells and unlabeled cells in each image revealed a significantly lower average number of cell divisions for *Δomp19* in pancreatin-pads ($p < 0.001$ vs. *wt* in pancreatin) (**Figure 4B**).

Cell division requires critical regulation of the cell-cycle to coordinate genome replication and segmentation, therefore cell-cycle progression on individual bacteria was determined. While incubation of wt with pancreatin did not alter its progression along the cell-cycle, *Δomp19* resulted in cell-cycle arrest at G1 (**Figure 4C**), that was evident after 3 h of incubation by the rate of cells accumulated in G1-phase ($p < 0.001$ vs. wt + pancreatin, **Figure 4D**). Besides, expression of cell-cycle master regulator CtrA and chaperonin GroEL were evaluated upon treatment with pancreatic elastase. Pancreatic elastase treatment increased CtrA signal in *Δomp19*, whereas GroEL expression was similar in both strains exposed or not to proteases (**Figure 4E**).

Together, these results reveal that *Δomp19* exposed to pancreatic proteases has a cell division defect that is linked to impaired progression through G1-phase and CtrA accumulation.

Omp19 Protects Omp25 From Pancreatic Elastase Digestion

As cell envelope constitutes the first contact with host-proteases, cell envelope proteins were evaluated in wt and *Δomp19* upon protease treatment. No changes between wt and *Δomp19* were detected upon pancreatic elastase treatment in Omp1, Omp10, or Omp16. On the contrary, in both strains Omp25 presented a lower molecular weight band and reduced Omp2b intensity upon pancreatic elastase incubation that would correspond to digested Omp25 and Omp2b, respectively (**Figure 5A**). While no Omp19-dependent protection of Omp2b digestion was evidenced in wt strain compared to *Δomp19* strain, the percentage of digested Omp25 was higher in *Δomp19* (**Figure 5B**), highlighting

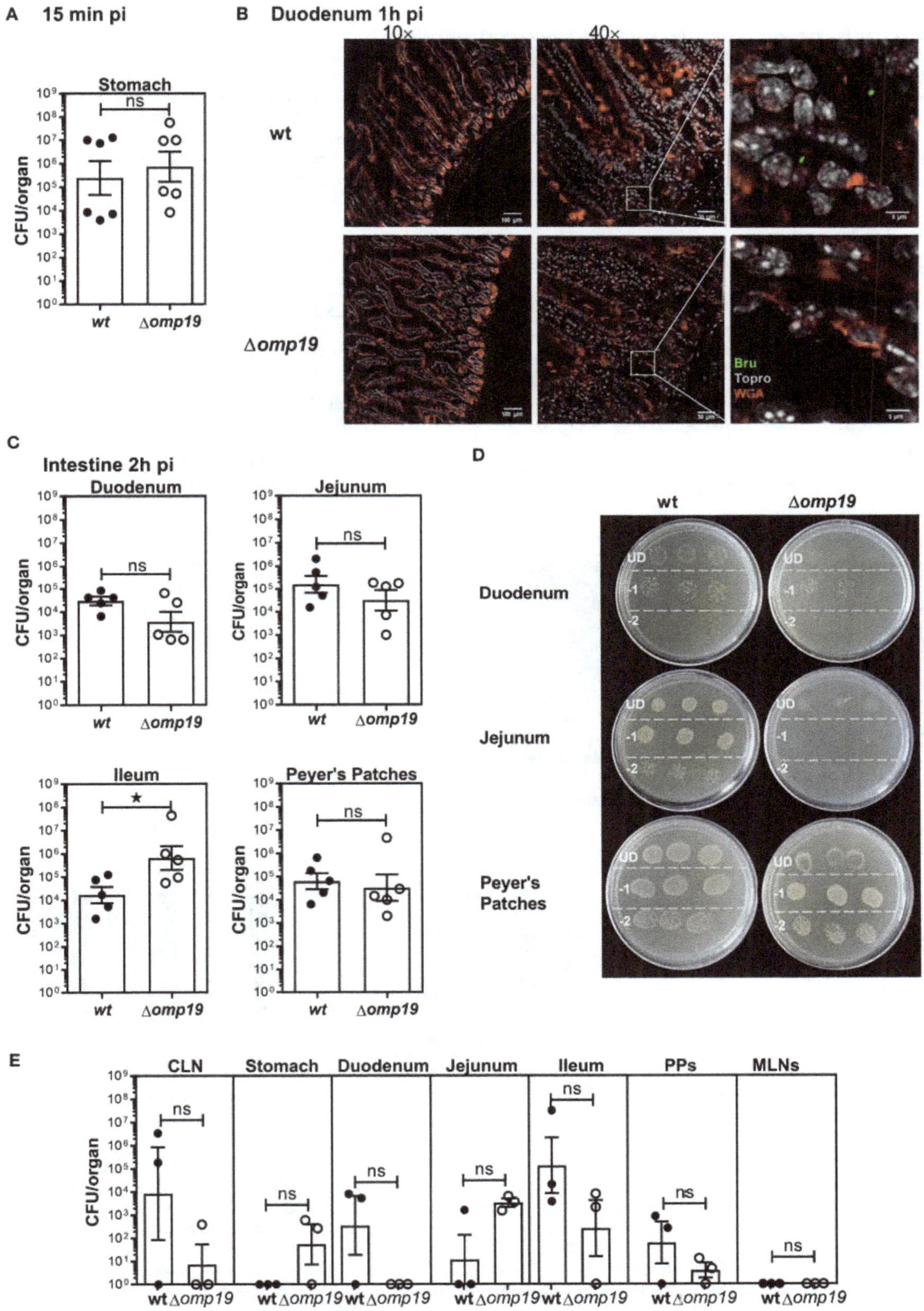

FIGURE 2 | *Brucella abortus* requires Omp19 to evade the bacteriostatic action of intestinal content. BALB/c mice were i.g. inoculated with (1×10^9 CFU) of wt or Δ*omp19 B. abortus* strains. **(A)** Total CFUs per stomach in animals sacrificed at 15 min post-infection. Each point represents an individual mouse, horizontal lines, and *(Continued)*

FIGURE 2 | error bars represent the mean ± s.e.m. **(B)** Confocal microscopy images of duodenum of infected mice at 1 h post-infection. The images correspond to ROI merged signals for *Brucella* (green channel), mucin (WGA) (red channel) and nuclei (TO-PRO-3, NIR channel). The inset region of middle images (40×) was magnified and presented in the right, showing individual Brucellae in the epithelium. Scale bars are: 100 μm (left panels), 30 μm (middle panels) and 5 μm (right panels). **(C)** Total *B. abortus* CFUs recovered from duodenum, jejunum, Ileum or Peyer's Patches from infected mice sacrificed at 2 h post-infection. **(D)** Representative agar plates showing sequential 1:10 dilutions and drop plating from depicted tissues homogenates from wt or Δ*omp19* infected mice. UD (undiluted), −1: 1 to 10 dilution; −2: 1 to 100 dilution. Results are representative of two independent experiments. **(E)** BALB/c mice were inoculated at the oral cavity with wt or Δ*omp19 B. abortus* (1 × 10^{10} CFU/mouse). Two hours after infection the number of CFU at CLNs, Stomach, Duodenum, Jejunum, Ileum, PPs, and MLNs were quantified. Each bar represents the mean CFU/organ (logarithmic sc±ale) and error bars represent the mean ± s.e.m. (For some mice, no live bacteria were recovered, these were arbitrarily assigned with values of 1 CFU). (Statistical analysis was performed by unpaired *t*-test to compare between the indicated groups: $^{ns}p > 0.05$; $^{*}p < 0.05$).

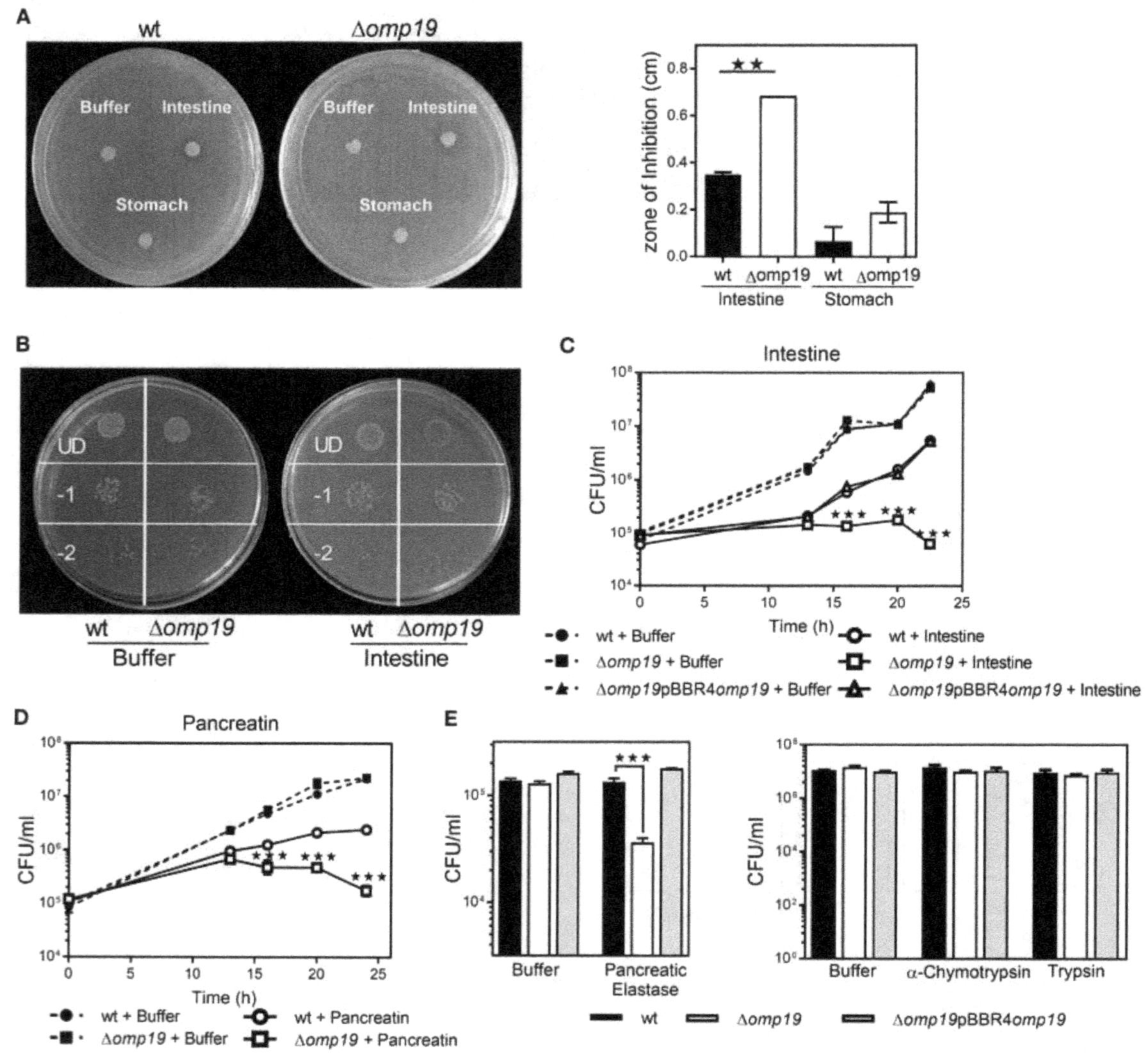

FIGURE 3 | Omp19 protects *B. abortus* against the action of pancreatic proteases. **(A)** 1 × 10^8 CFU of wt and Δ*omp19 B. abortus* were spread on TSA plates supplemented with antibiotics. Five-mm filter-disk were impregnated with either PBS, intestine- or stomach-extract and placed on the agar surface. The plates were incubated at 37°C for 72 h and afterwards the diameter of the zones of inhibition were determined (diameter of no growth zone minus diameter of the disk). ($^{**}p < 0.01$ vs. *wt B. abortus* + intestine extract). **(B)** Representative picture of a plate with *wt* and Δ*omp19 B. abortus* treated with buffer or intestine extract. Plated undiluted (UD) or after serial dilutions: 1/10 (−1) and 1/100 (−2). **(C)** *wt*, Δ*omp19* or Δ*omp19*pBBR4*omp19 B. abortus* strains (1 × 10^5 CFU/ml) were incubated with PBS or intestine extract at 37°C. Live bacteria (CFU/ml) were determined after 12, 16, 20, and 24 h of incubation by serial dilutions plating ($^{***}p < 0.001$ vs. *wt B. abortus* + intestine extract). **(D)** *wt* and Δ*omp19 B. abortus* (1 × 10^5 CFU/ml) were incubated with buffer (0.5% ClNa) or pancreatin (2 mg/ml). Live bacteria (CFU/ml) were determined after 12, 16, 20, and 24 h of incubation by plating serial dilutions on TSA ($^{***}p < 0.001$ vs. *wt B. abortus* + pancreatin at the same time point). **(E)** wt and Δ*omp19 B. abortus* (1 × 10^5 CFU/ml) were incubated with buffer (10 mM Tris-HCl, pH8.8) or pancreatic elastase for 5 h or with buffer (10 mM Tris-HCl, pH7.8), α-chymotrypsin or trypsin for 24 h. Live bacteria (CFU/ml) were determined by plating serial dilutions on TSA ($^{***}p < 0.001$ vs. wt *B. abortus* + pancreatic elastase). Results are representative of two or three independent experiments.

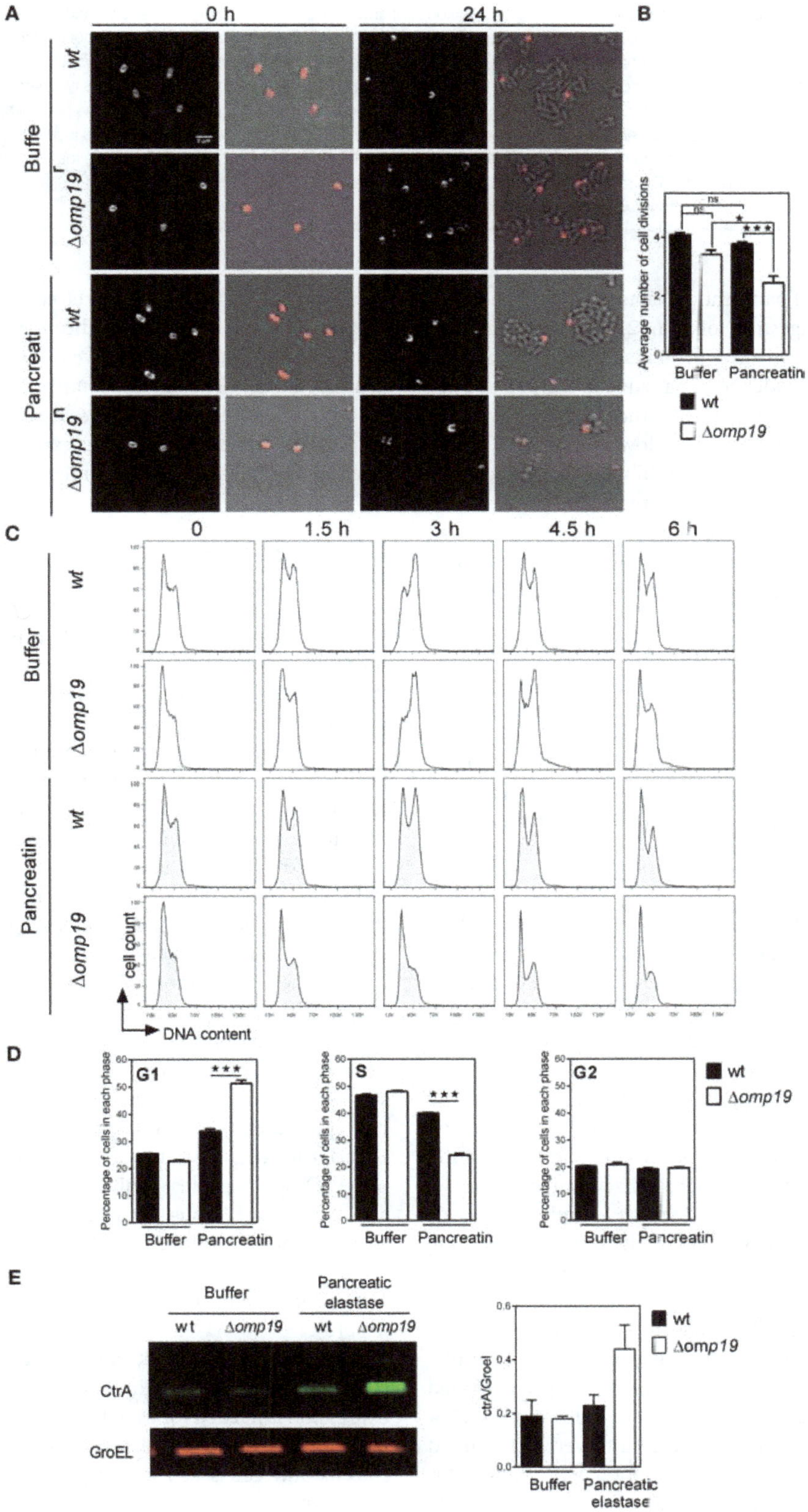

FIGURE 4 | *Δomp19 B. abortus* has a cell division defect and cell cycle arrest upon incubation with pancreatic proteases. TRSE-labeled *wt* and *Δomp19 B. abortus* were dropped on TSB-agarose pads containing buffer or pancreatin and cultured for 24 h at 37°C. **(A)** Representative Texas Red fluorescence (left) and phase

(Continued)

FIGURE 4 | contrast microscopy images (right) from the beginning of incubation (0 h) and after 24 h of incubation are shown. **(B)** Average number of cell divisions after 24 h of culture obtained by quantification of the number of labeled (or partially labeled) cells and unlabeled cells in each individual colony (*$p < 0.05$ and ***$p < 0.001$ vs. *wt B. abortus* strain in pancreatin). Results are representative of two independent experiments. **(C)** Flow cytometry analysis of DNA content on individual bacteria. *wt* and *Δomp19 B. abortus* were incubated in buffer or pancreatin for the indicated time periods and the content of DNA was evaluated by Flow cytometry. Representative histograms are shown. Results are representative of two independent experiments. **(D)** Bar graphs indicate the percentage of cells in each phase of cell cycle after 3 h of culture. (***$p < 0.001$ vs. *wt B. abortus* strain in pancreatin). **(E)** *B. abortus* wt and *Δomp19* strains were incubated with buffer or pancreatic elastase. Equal quantities of bacteria were subjected to SDS-page followed by western blot analysis using specific antibodies for CtrA and GroEL. Images are representative of two independent experiments. The ratio of CtrA and GroEL signals was evaluated by quantitative analysis of western blot images. Bar graph represent the mean ± s.e.m. of pooled results from two independent experiments.

Omp19's inhibitory role of pancreatic elastase. Omp19 inhibition of pancreatic elastase digestion of Omp25 was confirmed *in vitro* using recombinant purified proteins. Pancreatic elastase digestion of rOmp25 was evidenced by a reduced Omp25-specific signal in western blot compared with the signal of rOmp25 without protease. This reduction was lower when U-Omp19 was added, indicating that U-Omp19 inhibits Omp25 digestion by pancreatic elastase (**Figure 5C**). Differences in the digestion pattern between Omp25 expressed on the *Brucella* membrane and recombinant Omp25, may be due to differential accessibility of pancreatic elastase cleavage sites, since in membrane associated Omp25 most cleavage sites are in predicted transmembrane regions or in loops facing the periplasm, only one cleavage site would be accessible to the protease when Omp25 is in the context of the *Brucella* membrane (**Figure 5D**).

These results together indicate that when Omp19 is absent, pancreatic elastase gains access to the membrane following degradation of Omp25, on the contrary under physiologic condition where Omp19 is present, *Brucella* wt can withstand this protease activity.

Omp19 Impairs Macrophage Microsomal Proteolytic Killing of *B. abortus*

Reaching the intracellular replicative niche is the next step for establishment of infection. Therefore, the ability of *Δomp19* mutants to enter cells and replicate intracellularly was studied in professional phagocytes (**Figure 6**). In agreement with previous studies significant lower amounts of *Δomp19* were found after 6, 24, and 48 h of infection in comparison to wt strain (**Figure 6A**). Moreover, *Δomp19* strain was significantly more susceptible to killing by microsomal content than wt or *Δomp19*pBBR4*omp19* ($p < 0.01$ vs. wt + microsomes or *Δomp19*pBBR4*omp19* + microsomes) (**Figure 6B**), suggesting that Omp19 may protect the bacteria from lysosomal proteolysis during intracellular traffic.

When infecting through the oral route *Brucella* will reach the intracellular compartment after facing with gastrointestinal proteases, thus *Δomp19* and *wt* strains were preincubated with pancreatin or buffer for 2 h prior to infection of J774 macrophages and intracellular bacterial counts were determined after 1, 2, or 4 h of infection. Pre-incubation with pancreatin did not affect bacterial internalization, since similar amounts of intracellular bacteria of both strains were recovered after 1 h of infection. After 4 h of infection, preincubation with pancreatin led to an increased susceptibility of *Δomp19* to intracellular killing by macrophages, compared to pancreatin pretreated wt ($p < 0.0001$) or buffer pretreated *Δomp19* ($p < 0.0001$) (**Figure 6C**). These results indicate that the sequential action of intestinal proteases followed by intracellular microsome proteolytic killing has an important effect on hampering *Δomp19* ability to establish an intracellular niche in macrophages. Altogether these results may explain the highly attenuated phenotype of this strain when infection occurs by the oral route.

DISCUSSION

After consumption of infected milk or experimental oral infection, live *Brucella* are detected in fecal samples of natural host like cattle, bison, wolf and marine mammals, indicating that *Brucella* transits and pass the harsh environment of gastrointestinal tract (33).

Our results demonstrate that in mice, after oral infection (either by gavage or inoculation at the oral cavity) *Brucella* reaches the gut. After 1 h of infection brucellae were found at the lumen and epithelium of duodenum. This fast infection capacity of *Brucella* was shown in a calf ligated ileal-loop model, in which *Brucella* bacteremia was detected 30 min after intraluminal inoculation without histopathologic traces of lesions (34). *Brucella* may spread systemically from the digestive tract by transepithelial migration in mucosal epithelial barrier or through M cells (26, 34, 35).

As protease inhibitor activity against main gastrointestinal proteases was demonstrated for U-Omp19 and because of its strategic location on the outer membrane for interacting with host proteases (7–9), we speculated that Omp19 may allow *Brucella* to withstand the gastrointestinal proteolysis and infect orally. Omp19's protease inhibitor broad-specificity (8, 9) would also be advantageous regarding the different proteases that *Brucella* may encounter along infection. Like broad-spectrum serine-protease inhibitor from *Tannerella forsythia*, that may protect it from proteases from other bacteria and from the host (3).

In this work, Omp19's role in virulence in an oral infection murine model was examined. Our results showed that Omp19 expression is needed for establishment of oral acquired *B. abortus* infection. In contrast to wt, *Δomp19* was cleared from the spleens and CLNs at 20 days post infection. Remarkably after intraperitoneal infection of mice, *omp19* deletion resulted in significant loss of virulence but the bacteria were not cleared (36, 37), this difference highlights the importance of Omp19 for *Brucella* oral infection, probably due to the huge amounts of proteases encountered when infecting through this route.

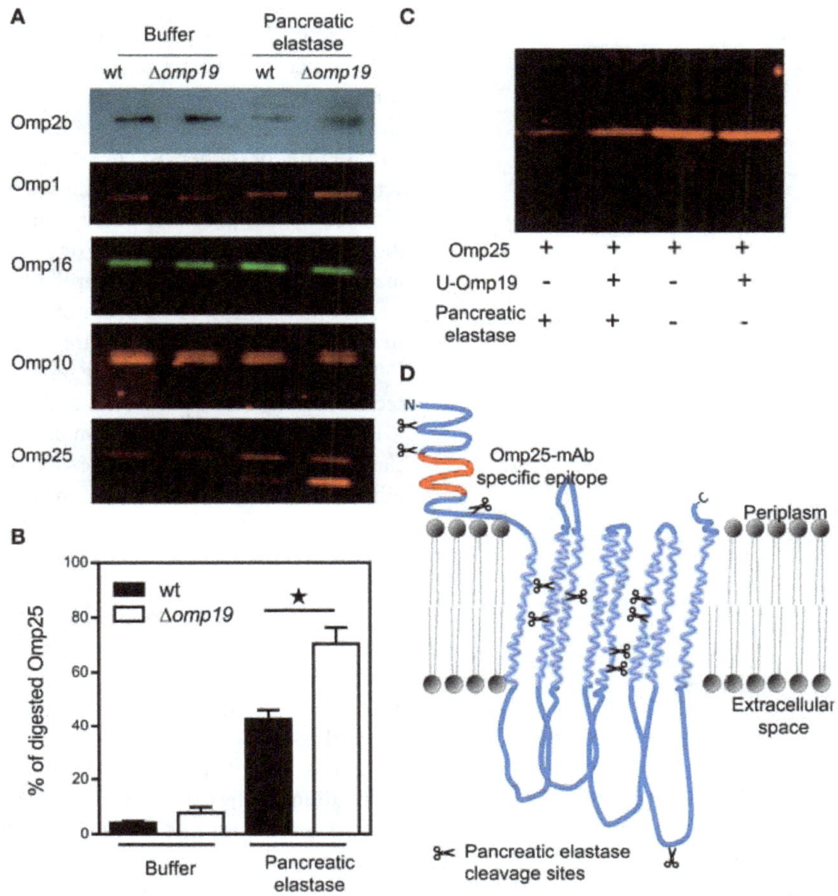

FIGURE 5 | Omp19 on the *B. abortus* membrane protects Omp25 from pancreatic elastase digestion. Wt and Δ*omp19 B. abortus* strains were incubated with buffer (10 mM Tris-HCl, pH8.8) or pancreatic elastase. **(A)** Equal quantities of bacteria were subjected to SDS-page followed by western blot analysis using specific antibodies for cell envelope proteins: Omp2b, Omp1, Omp16, Omp10, and Omp25. Images are representative from two or three independent experiments. **(B)** Percentage of digested Omp25 evaluated by quantitative analysis of western blot images. Data represent pooled results from two independent experiments (*$p < 0.05$ vs. *wt B. abortus* strain in pancreatic elastase). **(C)** Recombinant purified Omp25 was incubated with pancreatic elastase with or without U-Omp19. Following incubation, each mixture of reaction was separated on SDS-PAGE followed by western blot analysis with Omp25 specific antibodies. **(D)** Graphical representation of BOCTOPUS (31) or PRED-TMBB2 (32) transmembrane β-barrel predicted topology for Omp25 with respect to the lipid bilayer representation of the *B. abortus* outer membrane. Scissors indicate predicted pancreatic elastase cleavage sites (AA or AG) on Omp25 sequence. The position of the specific epitope for the anti-Omp25 mAb used is colored in red.

Attenuation upon systemic infection and intracellularly may be due to other host-proteases action, like lysosomal proteases, to which Omp19's inhibitory activity was demonstrated (9).

Intestinal content exerted a bacteriostatic action on Δ*omp19 in vivo* and *in vitro*, revealing a protective role for Omp19 in *Brucella* against intestinal proteases. This is the first work demonstrating *in vivo* a role of a protease inhibitor in acquisition of a bacterial disease by the oral route, therefore these findings are highly relevant for foodborne infections. Interestingly, gut microbiota, that survive in this protease-rich medium, produce protease inhibitors to protect them self from exogenous proteases (38–41).

In vitro experiments with purified proteases shed light into the role of individual proteases in the bacteriostatic action of intestinal content. Δ*omp19's* growth is hampered by the action of pancreatic elastase, indicating that inhibition of this protease by Omp19 on *B. abortus* membrane is important during the initial steps of infection. Trypsin and α-chymotrypsin have been shown to elicit antibacterial activities against *E. coli, Proteus vulgaris, Pseudomonas aeruginosa, S. aureus, Streptococcus pyogenes, and Vibrio cholerae* (42, 43), but have no effect on *B. abortus*. This resistance is Omp19-independent, indicating that it may be mediated by other mechanism.

Pancreatic proteases induce a cell division defect in Δ*omp19* that is linked to cell-cycle arrest in G1-phase. Interestingly, G1 arrest also occurs during intracellular trafficking of *B. abortus* and on starvation in *Sinorhizobium meliloti* (44, 45). Therefore, delaying initiation of DNA replication could be a common feature used by α-proteobacteria in response to harsh conditions such as infection or starvation.

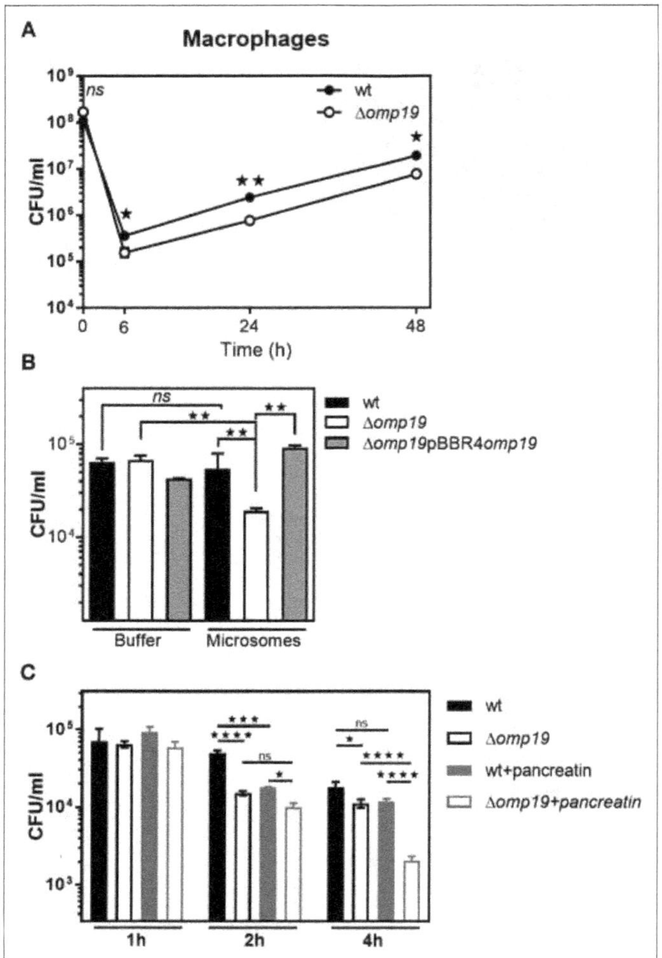

FIGURE 6 | Omp19 impairs macrophage microsomal proteolytic killing of *B. abortus*. **(A)** J774 macrophages were infected (MOI 500:1) with the *B. abortus* wt or *Δomp19* strains. At the indicated time points post-infection intracellular CFUs of *B. abortus* wt or *Δomp19* strains were determined. (Statistical analysis was performed by two-way ANOVA followed by Bonferroni posttest to compare between the indicated groups: $^{ns}p > 0.05$; $^{*}p < 0.05$ or $^{**}p < 0.01$). **(B)** *wt*, *Δomp19* or *Δomp19*pBBR4*omp19 B. abortus* strains (1×10^5 CFU/ml) were incubated with PBS or J774 derived microsomes at 37°C. Live bacteria (CFU/ml) were determined after 8 h by serial dilutions plating (Statistical analysis was performed by one-way ANOVA followed by Bonferroni posttest to compare between the indicated groups: $^{ns}p > 0.05$, $^{**}p < 0.01$). **(C)** *Δomp19* and *wt* strains were preincubated with buffer or pancreatin for 1 h prior to infection of J774 macrophages (MOI 100:1). Intracellular CFUs were determined at 1, 2, or 4 h post-infection. (Statistical analysis was performed by two-way ANOVA followed by Bonferroni posttest to compare between the indicated groups: $^{ns}p > 0.05$; $^{*}p < 0.05$, $^{***}p < 0.001$, $^{****}p < 0.0001$).

In *Caulobacter crescentus*, degradation of the CtrA cell-cycle master regulator occurs at specific points in the cell-cycle. Clearance of active CtrA at the G1/S transition allows the initiation of DNA replication and cell-cycle progression (30, 46). Moreover, expression of a constitutively active stable CtrA derivative results in dominant G1 arrest (30). In *B. abortus*, the essential role of CtrA in cell division was recently confirmed (47). Thus, accumulation of CtrA in *Δomp19* upon pancreatic protease treatment, agrees with the cell-cycle arrest in G1 induced in this strain upon treatment with proteases.

Antimicrobial functions of proteases can be due to the attack of Omps leading to loss of membrane integrity (42, 43, 48, 49). Since outer membrane proteins are exposed on the bacterial surface, they could be targets of pancreatic elastase. Among all Omps evaluated, our results indicate that Omp10, Omp16, and Omp1 of either wt or *Δomp19* were resistant to the action of pancreatic elastase, whereas, Omp2b and Omp25 were digested by this protease. This result is consistent with protease digestion of Omps in *E. coli* or *P. aeruginosa*, in which the major Omps, OmpA, and OmpF, respectively, were degraded, while other Omps remained not affected (48, 49). Although *Brucella* Omp25 does not share identity with *E. coli* OmpA (50), topology predictions suggest that both contain similar secondary structural properties and may play a similar function (51). Notably, Omp19 expression in *Brucella* inhibited pancreatic elastase mediated Omp25 digestion. This role of Omp19 on inhibition of pancreatic elastase mediated Omp25 digestion was confirmed *in vitro* using recombinant purified proteins. Omp19 inhibition of pancreatic elastase digestion of Omp25 may explain the resistance of wt strain to the action of this protease. A similar role was described for the periplasmic protease inhibitor ecotin from *E. coli,* which reduces the bactericidal action of neutrophil elastase by protecting OmpA on the bacterial membrane from neutrophil elastase mediated digestion (2).

In this work, we found that a *Brucella omp19* deletion mutant is highly attenuated in mice after oral infection. This attenuation can be explained by bacterial increased susceptibility to host proteases met by *Brucella* during establishment of infection. *Δomp19* has a cell division defect when exposed to pancreatic proteases that is linked to cell-cycle arrest in G1-phase, Omp25 degradation on the cell envelope and CtrA accumulation. Interestingly, a link between these three molecules was found recently, in which CtrA can bind the promotor of *omp25* and *omp19*. The same work demonstrates that CtrA controls the expression of Omp25 (47), therefore the increment in Omp25 intensity in *Δomp19* upon pancreatic elastase treatment may be explained by the increment in CtrA expression.

Upon entry into mammalian cells, the intracellular pathogen *Brucella abortus* resides within a membrane-bound compartment, the *Brucella*-containing vacuole (BCV), the maturation of which is controlled by the bacterium to generate a replicative organelle derived from the endoplasmic reticulum (ER). BCVs traffic along the endocytic pathway and fuse with lysosomes, and such fusion events are required for further maturation of BCVs into an ER-derived replicative organelle (52). Thus, the role of Omp19 for intracellular survival was studied. In agreement with previous work (36, 37), *Δomp19* was attenuated inside macrophages. This attenuation may be due to increased susceptibility to intracellular proteases when lacking Omp19. This hypothesis is reinforced by the fact that Omp19 is able to inhibit lysosomal proteases (9) and here we demonstrated that *Δomp19* is more susceptible to proteolytic killing by microsomes from macrophages. This increased susceptibility may explain the slight attenuation for systemic infections in mice, in which high persistence of *Δomp19* was shown after 4 weeks of infection (36, 37). An additive effect in increasing susceptibility of *Δomp19* was observed when the strains were preincubated with pancreatic proteases prior to infection of macrophages. This increased susceptibility may account for the high attenuation of Δ*omp19* after *in vivo* oral infection. Therefore, Omp19 would allow *Brucella* spp. to bypass lysosomal destruction thus enabling *Brucella* to survive inside macrophages and start a chronic infection.

Overall, this study demonstrates that the protease inhibitor Omp19 confers *B. abortus* the ability to resist the action of proteases. Together with urease that may protect *Brucella* from stomach low pH (17) and cholylglycine hydrolase that confers resistance to bile salts (18), Omp19 by inhibiting intestinal and intracellular proteases contributes to the establishment of chronic infection through the oral route.

CONTRIBUTION TO THE FIELD STATEMENT

Understanding how infectious pathogens spread is critical to prevent infectious diseases. One of the principal ways in which human and animal Brucellosis is acquired, is the oral route. This implies that Brucellae must survive the harsh conditions along the gastrointestinal tract before reaching the mononuclear phagocytes to form a replicative niche. In this work, we demonstrate that *Brucella* has a lipoprotein, called Omp19, which is a protease inhibitor, that enables it to survive the proteolytical action of gut digestive and microsomal derived proteases. The significance of our research is in identifying a new mechanism involved in virulence in oral acquired Brucellosis, that will enhance our understanding of *Brucella* pathogenesis and would serve as a model for other food-borne diseases.

ETHICS STATEMENT

Protocols of this study agreed with international ethical standards for animal experimentation (Helsinki Declaration and amendments, Amsterdam Protocol of welfare and animal protection and NIH guidelines for the Care and Use of Laboratory Animals). Protocols of this study were approved by the Institutional Committee for the Care and Use of Experimentation Animals from UNSAM (CICUAE-UNSAM_N°04/2014).

AUTHOR CONTRIBUTIONS

KP, MC, and JC designed the experiments. Funding acquisition was done by JC. MC performed most laboratory assays with assistance from KP, FG, LB, DR, and LC. MR performed susceptibility to bile salts assays and some of the J774 macrophage infection assays. KP, JC, and MC performed all statistical analysis. DC provided bacterial strains, materials and, together with JC and KP contributed with their expertise on the subject. KP, MC, and JC interpreted all results. KP and JC wrote the manuscript. All authors reviewed, commented, and approved the manuscript.

FUNDING

This work was supported by grants from the Agencia Nacional de Promoción Científica y Tecnológica (ANPCyT-Argentina): PICT 2013 No 1500, PICT 2016 No 1310 (to JC) and in part by grants from the Bill and Melinda Gates Foundation through the Grand Challenges Explorations Initiative (OPP1060394 and OPP1119024) (to JC). MC was supported by a fellowship of the National Research Council of Argentina (CONICET).

ACKNOWLEDGMENTS

We thank Dr. L. Shapiro (Stanford University, California, USA) for generously providing rabbit polyclonal anti-CtrA serum. We gratefully acknowledge the technical assistance of Valeria Sanchez for performing intestinal cryosections as well as Ariel Billordo for operating the FACSCalibur and FACS ARIA II. We also thank Dr. Xavier De Bolle (University of Namur, Namur, Belgium) for constructive discussions and technical support regarding TRSE labeling of *Brucella*. KP, FG, MR, LC, DC, and JC are members of the National Research Council of Argentina (CONICET).

REFERENCES

1. Kedzior M, Seredynski R, Gutowicz J. Microbial inhibitors of cysteine proteases. *Med Microbiol Immunol.* (2016) 205:275–96. doi: 10.1007/s00430-016-0454-1
2. Eggers T, Murray IA, Delmar VA, Day AG, Craik CS. The periplasmic serine protease inhibitor ecotin protects bacteria against neutrophil elastase. *Biochem J.* (2004) 379 (Pt 1):107–18. doi: 10.1042/bj20031790
3. Ksiazek M, Mizgalska D, Enghild JJ, Scavenius C, Thogersen IB, Potempa J. Miropin, a novel bacterial serpin from the periodontopathogen *Tannerella forsythia*, inhibits a broad range of proteases by using different peptide bonds within the reactive center loop. *J Biol Chem.* (2015) 290:658–70. doi: 10.1074/jbc.M114.601716
4. Stapels DA, Ramyar KX, Bischoff M, von Kockritz-Blickwede M, Milder FJ, Ruyken M, et al. *Staphylococcus aureus* secretes a unique class of neutrophil serine protease inhibitors. *Proc Natl Acad Sci USA.* (2014) 111:13187–92. doi: 10.1073/pnas.1407616111
5. Pasquevich KA, Estein SM, Garcia Samartino C, Zwerdling A, Coria LM, Barrionuevo P, et al. Immunization with recombinant Brucella species outer membrane protein Omp16 or Omp19 in adjuvant induces specific $CD4^+$ and $CD8^+$ T cells as well as systemic and oral protection against *Brucella abortus* infection. *Infect Immun.* (2009) 77:436–45. doi: 10.1128/IAI.00123-09

6. Pasquevich KA, Ibanez AE, Coria LM, Garcia Samartino C, Estein SM, Zwerdling A, et al. An oral vaccine based on U-Omp19 induces protection against *B. abortus* mucosal challenge by inducing an adaptive IL-17 immune response in mice. *PLoS ONE.* (2011) 6:e16203. doi: 10.1371/journal.pone.0016203
7. Tibor A, Decelle B, Letesson JJ. Outer membrane proteins Omp10, Omp16, and Omp19 of *Brucella* spp. are lipoproteins. *Infect Immun.* (1999) 67:4960–2.
8. Ibanez E, Coria LM, Carabajal MV, Delpino MV, Risso GS, Cobiello PG, et al. A bacterial protease inhibitor protects antigens delivered in oral vaccines from digestion while triggering specific mucosal immune responses. *J Control Release.* (2015) 220 (Pt A):18–28. doi: 10.1016/j.jconrel.2015.10.011
9. Coria LM, Ibanez AE, Tkach M, Sabbione F, Bruno L, Carabajal MV, et al. A *Brucella* spp. protease inhibitor limits antigen lysosomal proteolysis, increases cross-presentation, and enhances $CD8^+$ T cell responses. *J Immunol.* (2016) 196:4014–29. doi: 10.4049/jimmunol.1501188
10. Moreno E. Retrospective and prospective perspectives on zoonotic brucellosis. *Front Microbiol.* (2014) 5:213. doi: 10.3389/fmicb.2014.00213
11. Pappas G, Papadimitriou P, Akritidis N, Christou L, Tsianos EV. The new global map of human brucellosis. *Lancet Infect Dis.* (2006) 6:91–9. doi: 10.1016/S1473-3099(06)70382-6
12. Chomel B, DeBess EE, Mangiamele DM, Reilly KF, Farver TB, Sun RK, et al. Changing trends in the epidemiology of human brucellosis in California from 1973 to 1992: a shift toward foodborne transmission. *J Infect Dis.* (1994) 170:1216–23. doi: 10.1093/infdis/170.5.1216
13. Garcell HG, Garcia EG, Pueyo PV, Martin IR, Arias AV, Alfonso Serrano RN. Outbreaks of brucellosis related to the consumption of unpasteurized camel milk. *J Infect Public Health.* (2016) 9:523–7. doi: 10.1016/j.jiph.2015.12.006
14. Rhodes HM, Williams DN, Hansen GT. Invasive human brucellosis infection in travelers to and immigrants from the Horn of Africa related to the consumption of raw camel milk. *Travel Med Infect Dis.* (2016) 14:255–60. doi: 10.1016/j.tmaid.2016.03.013
15. Leong KN, Chow TS, Wong PS, Hamzah SH, Ahmad N, Ch'ng CC. Outbreak of human brucellosis from consumption of raw goats' milk in Penang, Malaysia. *Am J Trop Med Hyg.* (2015) 93:539–41. doi: 10.4269/ajtmh.15-0246
16. Yoo JR, Heo ST, Lee KH, Kim YR, Yoo SJ. Foodborne outbreak of human brucellosis caused by ingested raw materials of fetal calf on Jeju Island. *Am J Trop Med Hyg.* (2015) 92:267–9. doi: 10.4269/ajtmh.14-0399
17. Sangari FJ, Seoane A, Rodriguez MC, Aguero J, Garcia Lobo JM. Characterization of the urease operon of *Brucella abortus* and assessment of its role in virulence of the bacterium. *Infect Immun.* (2007) 75:774–80. doi: 10.1128/IAI.01244-06
18. Delpino MV, Marchesini MI, Estein SM, Comerci DJ, Cassataro J, Fossati CA, et al. A bile salt hydrolase of *Brucella abortus* contributes to the establishment of a successful infection through the oral route in mice. *Infect Immun.* (2007) 75:299–305. doi: 10.1128/IAI.00952-06
19. von Bargen K, Gorvel JP, Salcedo SP. Internal affairs: investigating the *Brucella* intracellular lifestyle. *FEMS Microbiol Rev.* (2012) 36:533–62. doi: 10.1111/j.1574-6976.2012.00334.x
20. Salvo Romero E, Alonso Cotoner C, Pardo Camacho C, Casado Bedmar M, Vicario M. The intestinal barrier function and its involvement in digestive disease. *Rev Esp Enferm Dig.* (2015) 107:686–96. doi: 10.17235/reed.2015.3846/2015
21. Czibener C, Ugalde JE. Identification of a unique gene cluster of *Brucella* spp. that mediates adhesion to host cells. *Microbes Infect.* (2012) 14:79–85. doi: 10.1016/j.micinf.2011.08.012
22. Herrmann K, Bukata L, Melli L, Marchesini MI, Caramelo J J, Comerci DJ. Identification and characterization of a high-affinity choline uptake system of *Brucella abortus. J Bacteriol.* (2013) 195:493–501. doi: 10.1128/JB.01929-12
23. Schafer A, Tauch A, Jager W, Kalinowski J, Thierbach G, Puhler A. Small mobilizable multi-purpose cloning vectors derived from the *Escherichia coli* plasmids pK18 and pK19: selection of defined deletions in the chromosome of *Corynebacterium glutamicum. Gene.* (1994) 145:69–73. doi: 10.1016/0378-1119(94)90324-7
24. de Wergifosse P, Lintermans P, Limet JN, Cloeckaert A. Cloning and nucleotide sequence of the gene coding for the major 25-kilodalton outer membrane protein of *Brucella abortus. J Bacteriol.* (1995) 177:1911–4. doi: 10.1128/jb.177.7.1911-1914.1995
25. Goel D, Bhatnagar R. Intradermal immunization with outer membrane protein 25 protects Balb/c mice from virulent *B. abortus* 544. *Mol Immunol.* (2012) 51:159–68. doi: 10.1016/j.molimm.2012.02.126
26. Paixao TA, Roux CM, den Hartigh AB, Sankaran-Walters S, Dandekar S, Santos RL, et al. Establishment of systemic *Brucella melitensis* infection through the digestive tract requires urease, the type IV secretion system, and lipopolysaccharide O antigen. *Infect Immun.* (2009) 77:4197–208. doi: 10.1128/IAI.00417-09
27. von Bargen K, Gagnaire A, Arce-Gorvel V, de Bovis B, Baudimont F, Chasson L, et al. Cervical lymph nodes as a selective niche for brucella during oral infections. *PLoS ONE.* (2014) 10:e0121790. doi: 10.1371/journal.pone.0121790
28. Brown PJ, de Pedro MA, Kysela DT, Van der Henst C, Kim J, De Bolle X, et al. Polar growth in the Alphaproteobacterial order Rhizobiales. *Proc Natl Acad Sci USA.* (2012) 109:1697–701. doi: 10.1073/pnas.1114476109
29. Cloeckaert A, de Wergifosse P, Dubray G, Limet JN. Identification of seven surface-exposed Brucella outer membrane proteins by use of monoclonal antibodies: immunogold labeling for electron microscopy and enzyme-linked immunosorbent assay. *Infect Immun.* (1990) 58:3980–7.
30. Domian J, Quon KC, Shapiro L. Cell type-specific phosphorylation and proteolysis of a transcriptional regulator controls the G1-to-S transition in a bacterial cell cycle. *Cell.* (1997) 90:415–24. doi: 10.1016/S0092-8674(00)80502-4
31. Hayat S, Peters C, Shu N, Tsirigos KD, Elofsson A. Inclusion of dyad-repeat pattern improves topology prediction of transmembrane beta-barrel proteins. *Bioinformatics.* (2016) 32:1571–3. doi: 10.1093/bioinformatics/btw025
32. Tsirigos D, Elofsson A, Bagos PG. PRED-TMBB2: improved topology prediction and detection of beta-barrel outer membrane proteins. *Bioinformatics.* (2016) 32:i665–71. doi: 10.1093/bioinformatics/btw444
33. Tessaro SV, Forbes LB. Experimental *Brucella abortus* infection in wolves. *J Wildl Dis.* (2004) 40:60–5. doi: 10.7589/0090-3558-40.1.60
34. Rossetti CA, Drake KL, Siddavatam P, Lawhon SD, Nunes JE, Gull T, et al. Systems biology analysis of *Brucella* infected Peyer's patch reveals rapid invasion with modest transient perturbations of the host transcriptome. *PLoS ONE.* (2013) 8:e81719. doi: 10.1371/journal.pone.0081719
35. Nakato G, Hase K, Suzuki M, Kimura M, Ato M, Hanazato M, et al. Cutting Edge: *Brucella abortus* exploits a cellular prion protein on intestinal M cells as an invasive receptor. *J Immunol.* (2012) 189:1540–4. doi: 10.4049/jimmunol.1103332
36. Tibor A, Wansard V, Bielartz V, Delrue R, M., Danese I, Michel P, et al. Effect of omp10 or omp19 deletion on *Brucella abortus* outer membrane properties and virulence in mice. *Infect Immun.* (2002) 70:5540–6. doi: 10.1128/IAI.70.10.5540-5546.2002
37. de Souza Filho JA, de Paulo Martins V, Campos PC, Alves-Silva J, Santos NV, de Oliveira FS, et al. Mutant *Brucella abortus* membrane fusogenic protein induces protection against challenge infection in mice. *Infect Immun.* (2015) 83:1458–64. doi: 10.1128/IAI.02790-14
38. Turroni F, Foroni E, O'Connell Motherway M, Bottacini F, Giubellini V, Zomer A, et al. Characterization of the serpin-encoding gene of *Bifidobacterium breve* 210B. *Appl Environ Microbiol.* (2010) 76:3206–19. doi: 10.1128/AEM.02938-09
39. Shiga Y, Yamagata H, Tsukagoshi N, Udaka S. BbrPI, an extracellular proteinase inhibitor of Bacillus brevis, protects cells from the attack of exogenous proteinase. *Biosci Biotechnol Biochem.* (1995) 59:2348–50. doi: 10.1271/bbb.59.2348
40. Mkaouar H, Akermi N, Mariaule V, Boudebbouze S, Gaci N, Szukala F, et al. Siropins, novel serine protease inhibitors from gut microbiota acting on human proteases involved in inflammatory bowel diseases. *Microb Cell Fact.* (2016) 15:201. doi: 10.1186/s12934-016-0596-2
41. Ivanov D, Emonet C, Foata F, Affolter M, Delley M, Fisseha M, et al. A serpin from the gut bacterium Bifidobacterium longum inhibits eukaryotic elastase-like serine proteases. *J Biol Chem.* (2006) 281:17246–52. doi: 10.1074/jbc.M601678200
42. Farouk A. Antibacterial activity of proteolytic enzymes. *Int J Pharmaceut.* (1982) 12:295–8. doi: 10.1016/0378-5173(82)90100-4
43. Felsenfeld O, Gyr K. Action of some pancreatic enzymes on *Vibrio cholerae. Med Microbiol Immunol.* (1977) 163:53–60. doi: 10.1007/BF02126709

44. Deghelt M, Mullier C, Sternon JF, Francis N, Laloux G, Dotreppe D, et al. G1-arrested newborn cells are the predominant infectious form of the pathogen *Brucella abortus*. *Nat Commun.* (2014) 5:4366. doi: 10.1038/ncomms5366
45. De Nisco NJ, Abo RP, Wu CM, Penterman J, Walker GC. Global analysis of cell cycle gene expression of the legume symbiont Sinorhizobium meliloti. *Proc Natl Acad Sci USA.* (2014) 111:3217–24. doi: 10.1073/pnas.1400421111
46. Jenal U. The role of proteolysis in the *Caulobacter crescentus* cell cycle and development. *Res Microbiol.* (2009) 160:687–95. doi: 10.1016/j.resmic.2009.09.006
47. Francis N, Poncin K, Fioravanti A, Vassen V, Willemart K, Ong TA, et al. CtrA controls cell division and outer membrane composition of the pathogen *Brucella abortus*. *Mol Microbiol.* (2017) 103:780–97. doi: 10.1111/mmi.13589
48. Belaaouaj A, Kim KS, Shapiro SD. Degradation of outer membrane protein A in *Escherichia coli* killing by neutrophil elastase. *Science.* (2000) 289:1185–8. doi: 10.1126/science.289.5482.1185
49. Hirche TO, Benabid R, Deslee G, Gangloff S, Achilefu S, Guenounou M, et al. Neutrophil elastase mediates innate host protection against *Pseudomonas aeruginosa*. *J Immunol.* (2008) 181:4945–54. doi: 10.4049/jimmunol.181.7.4945
50. Verstreate DR, Creasy MT, Caveney NT, Baldwin CL, Blab MW, Winter AJ. Outer membrane proteins of *Brucella abortus*: isolation and characterization. *Infect Immun.* (1982) 35:979–89.
51. Goolab S, Roth RL, van Heerden H, Crampton MC. Analyzing the molecular mechanism of lipoprotein localization in *Brucella*. *Front Microbiol.* (2015) 6:1189. doi: 10.3389/fmicb.2015.01189
52. Starr T, Ng TW, Wehrly TD, Knodler LA, Celli J. Brucella intracellular replication requires trafficking through the late endosomal/lysosomal compartment. *Traffic.* (2008) 9:678–94. doi: 10.1111/j.1600-0854.2008.00718.x

11

CD8^{+} T-Cell Response to HIV Infection in the Era of Antiretroviral Therapy

Federico Perdomo-Celis[1], *Natalia A. Taborda*[1,2] *and Maria T. Rugeles*[1*]

[1] *Grupo Inmunovirología, Facultad de Medicina, Universidad de Antioquia, Medellín, Colombia,* [2] *Grupo de Investigaciones Biomédicas Uniremington, Programa de Medicina, Facultad de Ciencias de la Salud, Corporación Universitaria Remington, Medellín, Colombia*

Correspondence:
Maria T. Rugeles
maria.rugeles@udea.edu.co

Although the combined antiretroviral therapy (cART) has decreased the deaths associated with the immune deficiency acquired syndrome (AIDS), non-AIDS conditions have emerged as an important cause of morbidity and mortality in HIV-infected patients under suppressive cART. Since these conditions are associated with a persistent inflammatory and immune activation state, major efforts are currently made to improve the immune reconstitution. CD8^{+} T-cells are critical in the natural and cART-induced control of viral replication; however, CD8^{+} T-cells are highly affected by the persistent immune activation and exhaustion state driven by the increased antigenic and inflammatory burden during HIV infection, inducing phenotypic and functional alterations, and hampering their antiviral response. Several CD8^{+} T-cell subsets, such as interleukin-17-producing and follicular CXCR5^{+} CD8^{+} T-cells, could play a particular role during HIV infection by promoting the gut barrier integrity, and exerting viral control in lymphoid follicles, respectively. Here, we discuss the role of CD8^{+} T-cells and some of their subpopulations during HIV infection in the context of cART-induced viral suppression, focusing on current challenges and alternatives for reaching complete reconstitution of CD8^{+} T-cells antiviral function. We also address the potential usefulness of CD8^{+} T-cell features to identify patients who will reach immune reconstitution or have a higher risk for developing non-AIDS conditions. Finally, we examine the therapeutic potential of CD8^{+} T-cells for HIV cure strategies.

Keywords: CD8^{+} T-cell, HIV, antiretroviral therapy, IL-17, exhaustion, CXCR5

EPIDEMIOLOGY OF HIV INFECTION AND IMPACT OF ANTIRETROVIRAL THERAPY

The human immunodeficiency virus type-1 (HIV) infection remains an important public health problem, particularly in developing countries. As a result of the long-term subclinical presentation of this infection, a high rate of shortfall at diagnosis is evidenced worldwide, and almost half of the HIV-infected patients are not aware of their HIV status (1). Therefore, most of the available data on HIV epidemiology is based on estimates, particularly in resource-limited settings (2). This issue dramatically affects public health policies; representing a major barrier for HIV global control. Thus, according to UNAIDS 2017 data, at the end of 2016, 36.7 million people lived with HIV, and of these, 17.8 million were women, and 2.1 million were children. The problem is increasing, as the global annual number of new HIV infections is 1.8 million, and deaths associated with the acquired immune deficiency syndrome (AIDS) reach 1 million.

The most important advance in the clinical management of HIV infection was the development of antiretroviral drugs and their therapeutic combination to suppress systemic viral load. Indeed, the combined antiretroviral therapy (cART), i.e., combination of three or more antiretroviral drugs, generally including at least two drugs of different mechanisms of action (1), has been effective in decreasing the deaths associated with AIDS. According to UNAIDS 2017 estimates, global AIDS-related deaths declined in 48% between 2005 and 2016, with near to eight million deaths prevented since the introduction of the therapy in 1995. Moreover, the decrease in the viral load by cART and consequent lower transmission risk, has led to the reduction of 16% of new HIV infections between 2010 and 2016. In addition, pre-exposure and post-exposure prophylaxis are recommended in some countries for prevention of HIV infection (3). Thus, cART constitutes a critical strategy for the control of HIV-associated morbidity and mortality, as well as a transmission prevention approach.

The World Health Organization (WHO) and Centers for Disease Control and Prevention (CDC) recommends the initiation of cART as soon as possible after diagnosis, resulting in improved viral control and prevention of AIDS conditions (available at https://www.who.int/hiv/topics/treatment/en/ and https://aidsinfo.nih.gov/guidelines). However, guidelines for management HIV-infected patients in some Latin American countries, such as Colombia, have clearly defined indications for initiation of cART, based on $CD4^+$ T-cell counts and viral load (4). Importantly, from the total diagnosed patients in Colombia, 89.9% received at least one dose of antiretroviral drugs, although the number of patients receiving continuous therapy and with viral suppression (plasma or serum viral load <20 copies RNA/mL) only reached 66.6% of treated patients. This reflects the poor health system that is not able to sustain antiretroviral supply, in addition to problems with therapy adherence; these problems might be common in other Latin American countries. Overall, the strategies to increase the rate of diagnosis and the rapid initiation and maintenance of cART, will help to achieve the 90-90-90 target for HIV-infected patients (2).

CURRENT CHALLENGES OF THE ANTIRETROVIRAL THERAPY

In addition to important issues in prevention, screening, and diagnosis of HIV-infection, the treatment of diagnosed patients has faced several challenges and pitfalls. These issues can be divided as following: (i) operative, related to coverage, adherence, and adequate monitoring of therapy; (ii) virological, related to generation of viral resistance to antiretroviral drugs, and (iii) immunological, related to immune reconstitution failure. Operative challenges include those associated with the lack of the required financial resources for implementing integral HIV programs; inadequate stocks of antiretroviral drugs; limited health system infrastructures, low acceptance of cART initiation and long-term adherence with absence of proven methods to ensure treatment adherence and an adequate follow-up. The complexity of cART regimens and the side effects of antiretroviral drugs are also a major complaint in HIV-infected patients. Moreover, the persistent stigma associated with HIV infection limits the timely detection of cases and early initiation of cART (5). The **second** type of cART challenge is the antiretroviral drugs resistance, which is the most frequent type of therapy failure, inducing a change in the first-line cART scheme (6). Drug resistance results from the high rate of viral mutations, enhanced by a poor cART adherence, pharmacokinetics limitations, inadequate dosing or drug interactions (7). In addition, a weak monitoring and limited indicators for antiretroviral drugs resistance reduce the rate of successful cART (8). Finally, partial immune reconstitution by cART is a major concern in the setting of viral suppression. It has recently attracted more attention, as it has been associated with increased non-AIDS conditions and related mortality, despite the reduction in AIDS-related deaths (9). Indeed, non-AIDS conditions, such as cardiovascular disease or stroke, are responsible for around 42% of deaths among HIV-infected patients with viral suppression induced by cART. Moreover, the mortality rate in these individuals is higher than in the general population, even excluding the AIDS-related conditions (10, 11).

Importantly, the success of cART in reducing AIDS-related deaths and increasing the life expectancy of HIV-infected patients, has resulted in a high number of patients over 50 years living with HIV (available at https://www.cdc.gov/hiv/group/age/olderamericans/index.html). Thus, the presence of concomitant diseases, such as metabolic or cardiovascular pathologies, and their respective medications, influence the choice of antiretroviral drugs for cART regimens, and increase the risk of side effects due to drug interactions (12).

$CD8^+$ T-CELLS, EFFECTOR FUNCTIONS, AND SUBPOPULATIONS

Activation and Differentiation of $CD8^+$ T-Cells

$CD8^+$ T-cells are part of the adaptive immune system, playing a critical role for protection against foreign organisms and malignancies (13). The activation of naïve $CD8^+$ T-cells requires three signals, provided by antigen-presenting cells (APC). Initially, there is the recognition of the antigen by the T-cell receptor (TCR); in the case of $CD8^+$ T-cells, the peptides are 8–10 amino acids in length and are presented by major histocompatibility complex (MHC) class I molecules. Second, costimulatory signals are required, such as the binding of CD80 or CD86 from the APC to the CD28 molecule expressed by the $CD8^+$ T-cell, and finally an alarm signal produced in response to pathogens, such as IL-12 and type I interferon (IFN), among others (14, 15).

After activation, $CD8^+$ T-cells undergo clonal expansion, generating a large pool of effector cells. These cells exhibit high effector functions, such as the expression of cytokines, cytotoxic molecules and a high capacity for degranulation (16–19). Additionally, at this point, effector $CD8^+$ T-cells acquire the ability to migrate to peripheral tissues (20). After clonal expansion, effector cells suffer massive apoptosis, in a period known as contraction phase. Finally, the remaining antigen-specific $CD8^+$ T-cells constitute the pool of memory cells, which decrease their effector profile, remaining in a quiescent state expecting a new antigenic challenge. This period, which can last the whole life of the individual, is known as the memory phase (21). Several $CD8^+$ T-cells differentiation models propose that memory cells can differentiate into effector cells once they are exposed to activation signals, acquiring a high capacity for cytokine production and cytotoxic potential (22).

$CD8^+$ T-Cells Effector Mechanisms

$CD8^+$ T-cell effector mechanisms can be classified in lytic (cytotoxicity) and non-lytic (cytokine production) (**Figure 1**). These effector functions are primarily regulated by the balance between the T-bet, Eomes, and Runx families of transcription factors (23–26). Indeed, these transcription factors not only bind to DNA sequences of effector molecules such as granzyme B and IFN-γ, but also cooperate with chromatin remodeling proteins to regulate chromatin accessibility of key genes in activated $CD8^+$ T-cells (27). The cytotoxic capacity of $CD8^+$ T-cells depends on the content of their lytic granules and their degranulation capacity (28, 29). Lytic granules are secretory lysosomes containing effector molecules, such as granzymes and perforin (30). The core of the granule is surrounded by a lipid bilayer containing lysosome-associated membrane glycoproteins (LAMP), including LAMP-1 (CD107a), LAMP-2 (CD107b), and LAMP-3 (CD63) (31). During the degranulation process, the granule membrane is fused with the plasma membrane of the activated $CD8^+$ T-cell, and the content of the granule is released into the immunological synapse between the $CD8^+$ T-cell and the target cell (29). Of note, LAMP molecules are not found on the surface of resting $CD8^+$ T-cells. Therefore, the evaluation of the surface expression of CD107a/b allows to identify the degranulation of $CD8^+$ T-cells (28, 29). In addition, lytic granules also contain the membrane pore-forming protein granulysin (32), the proteoglycan matrix protein serglycin (33), the perforin inhibitor calreticulin (34), and the lysosomal enzymes cathepsins (35). Moreover, apoptosis-inducing Fas ligand (CD95L) is stored in specialized secretory lysosomes of $CD8^+$ T-cells and the degranulation process controls its expression at the cell surface (36).

Perforin and granzymes are the most abundant proteins within the lytic granules of $CD8^+$ T-cells and cooperate for inducing death of target cells (37). Apparently, granzymes work in a perforin-dependent manner, since initial studies in mast cell lines, the presence of perforin was required for granzyme B-induced death of target cells (38). Thus, the pore formation by perforin facilitates the entry of granzymes into target cells (39). However, granzymes could be internalized by endocytosis, after binding to the mannose-6-phosphate receptor in target cells (40). Molecular effector mechanisms can vary among granzyme subtypes, inducing apoptosis through caspase-dependent and independent mechanisms (41). Once in the cytosol of target cells, granzymes cleave the BH3-interacting domain death agonist (BID) and pro-caspase 3 (42, 43). Truncated BID alters the mitochondrial membrane, inducing the release of pro-apoptotic factors such as cytochrome C, involved in the formation of the apoptosome (44), and endonuclease G, which causes DNA fragmentation (45). In addition, active caspase 3 also induces endonuclease and protease activation, causing degradation of cellular DNA and cytoskeletal proteins (46).

Cytokines secreted by $CD8^+$ T-cells include IFN-γ, TNF-α, and IL-2, important for promoting antiviral, inflammatory responses, and T-cell survival and proliferation, respectively (47). Additionally, $CD8^+$ T-cells secrete the β-chemokines macrophage inflammatory protein (MIP)-1α (CCL3), MIP-1β (CCL4), and regulated upon activation, normal T-cell expressed and secreted (RANTES; CCL5). These chemokines bind to the receptors CCR1, CCR3, CCR4, and CCR5, some of them, previously characterized as HIV co-receptors (48); therefore they play an important role in this infection by blocking viral binding and entry into target cells (49, 50).

$CD8^+$ T-Cell Subpopulations

Several $CD8^+$ T-cell subsets have been described, based on the expression of the differentiation markers CD45RA, CD45RO, CCR7, CD62L, CD27, and CD28, among others. The most extended classification divides them into naïve, central memory, effector memory, and terminal effector cells; each of them has different effector capacities, particularly evaluated by the expression of granzymes, perforin, IFN-γ, the degranulation ability, and *in vitro* cytotoxicity [**Table 1**; (18, 51)]. The lowest functional capacity is observed for naïve $CD8^+$ T-cells, which have low expression of effector molecules, reduced degranulation capacity and low *in vitro* cytotoxicity. Central memory cells have a low/intermediate cytotoxic potential, given their low basal expression of granzymes and perforin, which confers them a limited immediate *in vitro* cytotoxicity. However, these cells can degranulate and express *de novo* effector molecules after polyclonal or antigen-specific stimulation (22, 52). Finally, effector memory and terminal effector cells are characterized by a high cytotoxic capacity (**Table 1**).

Of note, the distribution of $CD8^+$ T-cell subsets and their effector machinery also vary according to the body tissues and compartments, with effector $CD8^+$ T-cells mainly located in blood and inflamed tissues, and naïve and central memory cells primarily found in secondary lymphoid organs (**Table 1**). Particularly, their transcriptional program determines this cell distribution and effector function. Thus, $CD8^+$ T-cells in lymphoid tissues, as well as in gastrointestinal mucosa, from healthy individuals, have a lower expression of perforin and granzyme B compared with blood cells, which is associated with a low expression of T-bet in these tissues (53–55). Interestingly, $CD8^+$ T-cells in lymphoid tissues are poised to upregulate cytotoxic molecules and rapidly exert effector functions, similar

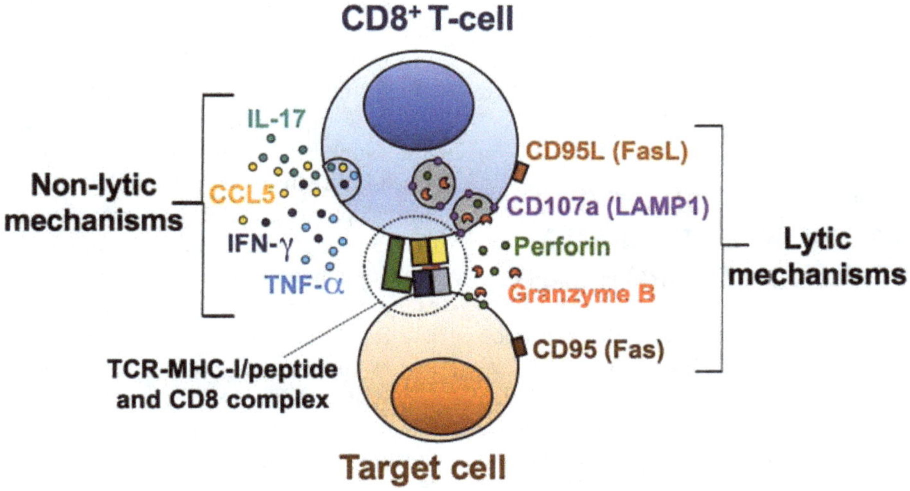

FIGURE 1 | Lytic and non-lytic effector mechanisms of CD8$^+$ T-cells. CD8$^+$ T-cells are activated after recognition of an MHC-I/peptide complex, which binds to the TCR and CD8 molecules. The cytotoxic potential of CD8$^+$ T-cells is determined by the expression of cytotoxic molecules granzyme B and perforin, and a coordinated degranulation process, which can be evaluated by the cell membrane expression of CD107a (LAMP1). Receptor-mediated cell death via CD95L/CD95 interaction is also a lytic mechanism of CD8$^+$ T-cells. Activated CD8$^+$ T-cells can also produce cytokines such as IFN-γ, TNF-α, and IL-17, and the β-chemokine CCL5, which exert a variety of antiviral, inflammatory, and regulatory functions.

TABLE 1 | Effector capacity of CD8$^+$ T-cells according to their differentiation stage.

Cell subset	Phenotype	Degranulation (CD107a/b expression)	Cytotoxic molecules expression (granzymes and/or perforin)	*In vitro* cytotoxicity	*De novo* synthesis of granzymes and/or perforin*	IFN-γ production*	Main location
Naïve	CD45RA$^+$ CD45RO$^-$ CCR7$^+$ CD62L$^+$ CD28$^+$ CD27$^+$ CD57$^-$	–	–	–	–	–	Secondary lymphoid tissues
Central memory	CD45RA$^-$ CD45RO$^+$ CCR7$^+$ CD62L$^+$ CD28$^+$ CD27$^+$ CD57$^-$	++	++	++	++	+++	Secondary lymphoid tissues
Effector memory	CD45RA$^-$ CD45RO$^+$ CCR7$^-$ CD62L$^-$ CD28$^{+/-}$CD27$^{+/-}$CD57$^{-/+}$	+++	+++	+++	+	+++	Blood and inflamed tissues
Terminal effector	CD45RA$^+$ CD45RO$^-$ CCR7$^-$ CD62L$^-$ CD28$^-$ CD27$^-$ CD57$^+$	+++	+++	+++	+	+++	Blood and inflamed tissues

After 5 h stimulation.

to long-lived memory CD8$^+$ T-cells (22). However, they also upregulate trafficking markers such as CXCR3 to egress from lymphoid tissues (53). Moreover, compared with blood cells, memory CD8$^+$ T-cells from tonsil, lymph nodes, and spleen exhibit higher tissue residency markers such as CD69, CD103, and CD49a, but lower expression of T-bet, eomes, perforin, and granzyme B. Therefore, cells from blood and tissue compartment form distinct phenotypic and functional clusters (56).

According to the cytokines they produce, several subpopulations of CD8$^+$ T-cells have been described. Similar to CD4$^+$ T-cells, IFN-γ-producing, and IL-5/IL-13-producing CD8$^+$ T-cells are designated as Tc1 and Tc2 cells, respectively (57). Regulatory CD8$^+$ T-cell subsets have also been described (58). Moreover, IL-17-producing CD8$^+$ T-cells (Tc17) can be induced by polarizing cytokines such as Transforming Growth Factor (TGF)-β1 and IL-6 (59). This population is characterized by the expression of the C-type lectin receptor CD161 (60), the transcription factor retinoic acid receptor-related orphan nuclear receptor (ROR)-γt (61), and its main localization is the intestinal tract (62–64). Importantly, the IL-17 cytokine family is constituted by six proteins that share homology (IL-17A through IL-17F) (65). The most widely studied is IL-17A (here referred as IL-17), and pro-inflammatory and immunomodulatory effects have been described (66). In the context of HIV infection, this cytokine has attracted attention due to its beneficial effects in the gut mucosa, such as the promotion of the conformation of tight junctions in epithelial cells (67), secretion of antimicrobial peptides (68), as well as recruitment of immune cells to sites of mucosal injury (69). In this sense, Tc17 cells could promote gut homeostasis, exerting a protective mechanism during HIV infection. Finally, similar to CD4$^+$ T-cells, follicular CXCR5-expressing CD8$^+$ T-cells have been characterized (70), and their role during HIV infection is examined below.

PROGRESSIVE DYSFUNCTION OF CD8$^+$ T-CELLS DURING HIV INFECTION AND POOR RECONSTITUTION DESPITE cART

CD8$^+$ T-cells are important in the control of HIV replication (71), as evidenced by: (i) emergence of HIV-specific CD8$^+$ T-cells coinciding with the decrease of viremia in acutely infected patients (72); (ii) a potent HIV-specific CD8$^+$ T cell response contribute to the reduction of the pool of HIV-infected cells and the HIV reservoir (73); (iii) increase in viral load in SIV-infected macaques after CD8$^+$ T-cell depletion (74, 75); (iii) associations between the frequency and/or functional capacity of HIV-specific CD8$^+$ T-cells and limited viral replication and/or disease non-progression in HIV-infected patients (76, 77); (iv) appearance of viral escape mutations to evade the immune pressure of HIV-specific CD8$^+$ T-cells (78); (v) requirement of CD8$^+$ T-cells for maintaining therapy-induced viral suppression in SIV-infected macaques (79). In fact, some CD8$^+$ T-cells features have been proposed as correlate of protection in HIV-infected patients (80).

While HIV-specific CD8$^+$ T-cells control the virus during acute HIV/SIV infection, their cytotoxic potential dramatically decreases along with disease progression and are no longer capable of exerting an appropriate antiviral response (81, 82). Certainly, CD8$^+$ T-cells suffer important alterations in their frequency, differentiation, and activation profile, undergoing immune exhaustion, and progressive dysfunction (24, 83–87). Compared with seronegative individuals, the total pool of circulating CD8$^+$ T-cells is persistently increased in untreated HIV-infected patients (88), with higher frequency of memory subsets and reduction of naïve cells (89, 90). In addition, patients exhibit higher expression of the activation markers HLA-DR, CD38, and Ki-67 (91), and immune exhaustion markers such as programmed death (PD)-1 and T-cell immunoglobulin and mucin-domain containing-3 (TIM-3) (92). Remarkably, the HLA-DR$^+$ CD38$^+$ Ki-67$^+$ PD-1$^+$ phenotype in CD8$^+$ T-cells characterizes the effector phase after acute viral infections or vaccination, which is associated with disease control (16, 93–96). Nonetheless, the expression of these molecules during chronic HIV infection is accompanied by the impairment of CD8$^+$ T-cell lytic and non-lytic mechanisms (24, 83, 97), as well as the proliferative ability and survival (98–100). Specific subpopulations, such as Tc17 cells, are decreased in gut mucosa and blood during HIV/SIV infections (101–103). Importantly, these alterations are observed in HIV-specific CD8$^+$ T-cells (76, 104), as well as cells specific for other pathogens, such as cytomegalovirus (CMV), Epstein-Barr virus, influenza virus, and adenovirus (105, 106). Taking into account that HIV-specific cells constitute <20% of the total CD8$^+$ T-cell population (107, 108), these data reflect the massive bystander activation that CD8$^+$ T-cells undergo during HIV infection.

Considering that a large size of viral burden is a product of infected cells in lymph nodes and gastrointestinal mucosa (109), and there is a low distribution of antiretroviral drugs to these compartments (110), an effective CD8$^+$ T-cell response in these tissues is required to control viral replication and the reservoir size. Nonetheless, the cytolytic activity of lymph node CD8$^+$ T-cells is reduced in chronically HIV-infected patients (both untreated and on cART) compared with seronegative controls (53). Furthermore, lymph node and rectal HIV-specific CD8$^+$ T-cells have lower expression of granzyme B and perforin, as well as T-bet, compared with blood cells (53, 55). Thus, while there is a regulated cytolytic function in CD8$^+$ T-cells in lymphoid tissues and gut mucosa, there is apparently a poorer cytotoxic response in HIV-infected patients. Intriguingly, HIV controllers maintain low viral load in the absence of therapy and despite this low cytotoxic potential of CD8$^+$ T-cells in lymphoid tissues (53, 111). Thus, it is possible that non-lytic mechanisms and a polyfunctional response, including IFN-γ, TNF-α, and MIP-1β production, as well as degranulation, are critical in the control of HIV infection in lymphoid and gastrointestinal tissues (111, 112).

Along with the suppression of viral load and the increase in the CD4$^+$ T-cell counts, cART induces improvement of some of the CD8$^+$ T-cell alterations found in HIV-infected patients (113–115), whereas treatment discontinuation causes the increase of CD8$^+$ T-cell activation and dysfunction (116, 117). However, compared with seronegative individuals, cART does not fully reconstitute the CD8$^+$ T-cell counts (88, 118), the proportions of memory subsets, the levels of activation and exhaustion markers (91, 118–121), and their functional capacity (24, 122). In addition, the loss of Tc17 cells and CD161-expressing CD8$^+$ T-cells is not restored in HIV-infected patients under suppressive cART (101, 102, 120). Interestingly, in seronegative individuals, HLA-DR$^+$ CD38$^+$ cells constitute the main IL-17-producing subset among CD8$^+$ T-cells (120), consistent with an effector memory profile of HLA-DR-expressing CD8$^+$ T-cells (123). However, this subset is decreased in HIV-infected patients on cART (120). Remarkably, early initiation of cART is associated with improved reconstitution of CD8$^+$ T-cell counts and activation levels (124, 125), whereas a long treatment is required for improvement of some CD8$^+$ T-cell phenotypic and functional disturbances (120, 123).

It is important to mention that the decrease in antigen load with ART induces a decline in the frequency of circulating HIV-specific CD8$^+$ T-cells (108, 115, 126, 127), with subsequent increases after treatment interruption or failure (108, 127, 128). Changes in the frequencies of circulating CMV-specific CD8$^+$ T-cells are also observed in patients with treatment interruption (108, 115, 127). HIV-specific CD8$^+$ T-cells are maintained in lymph nodes (128) and exert potent antiviral responses in *ex vivo* assays (129), but are not able to suppress viral replication in the absence of therapy. This issue represents a major challenge in the setting of supervised treatment interruptions strategies in the search of HIV cure strategies (130). Certainly, memory virus-specific CD8$^+$ T-cells respond to the changes in antigen load and the inflammatory milieu during cART, actively migrating within body compartments and possibly modulating their effector response.

CAUSES OF CD8$^+$ T-CELL DYSFUNCTION DURING HIV INFECTION

Three factors are major determinants of CD8$^+$ T-cell dysfunction during chronic infections (131): persistent antigen, negative costimulation, and chronic inflammation. In addition, the loss of CD4$^+$ T-cell help enhances CD8$^+$ T-cell dysfunction during HIV infection (132), whereas cell-intrinsic defects may also contribute to this pathogenic process (133). Remarkably, even in the context of cART-induced viral suppression, the three major determinants of CD8$^+$ T-cells dysfunction are present, since there is a residual HIV replication and microbial burden that maintain a persistent antigen load (110, 134, 135), induce continuous expression of inhibitory receptors (131), and the secretion of inflammatory mediators (136–138).

Persistent Antigen and Chronic Inflammation

Chronic immune activation is a hallmark of HIV infection (139), and it is associated with phenotypic and functional changes of immune cell populations (140), impairment of antiviral mechanisms (141), increase in the number of target cells (142), CD4$^+$ T-cell regenerative failure (143, 144), and risk of organ damage (145). HIV-associated immune activation is explained by the persistent viral replication and reactivation of HIV reservoirs, recurrence of co-infections, loss of the integrity of the gut mucosa, and increased systemic levels of pro-inflammatory cytokines [such as IL-6, IL-1β, and tumor necrosis factor (TNF)-α], among other factors (139). Of note, the maintenance of low immune activation levels characterizes non-pathogenic simian immunodeficiency virus (SIV) infection in natural hosts despite sustained viral replication (146). Moreover, the levels of immune activation predict the magnitude of CD4$^+$ T-cell depletion better than viral loads in HIV-infected patients (91, 147), and are associated with disease progression, the development of AIDS-defining and non-AIDS conditions, and mortality (148–150).

Tissue reservoirs (i.e., tissues containing cells with integrated HIV) promote a persistent antigenic burden during HIV infection, even during cART. In a macaque model of SIV infection, the primary reservoir sites of infection were lymphoid tissues (~98% of total RNA$^+$ cells), including lymph nodes, spleen, and gut-associated lymphoid tissues (GALT) (109). Other tissues, such as brain, kidney, heart or lung, individually contributed to <1% of RNA$^+$ cells (109). Similarly HIV tissue reservoirs are predominant in GALT (151), and lymph nodes (152). In lymphoid follicles, CD4$^+$ T-cells, particularly of the CXCR5$^+$ follicular subset, exhibit high levels of infection (153), and free virions are captured by follicular dendritic cells (154). Remarkably, although cART decreases the HIV reservoir size in lymph nodes, HIV RNA and DNA can still be detected after years of therapy (152, 155), whereas there is minimal cART-induced change in HIV DNA in gut tissues (109). Thus, viral reservoirs constitute an important source of persistent antigen, even during cART.

The loss of the integrity of the gut mucosa is also responsible for a high antigenic burden that consequently drives immune dysfunction (156). Mechanistically, this process can be viewed as follows (**Figure 2A**):

1. Alteration in the gut mucosa: during HIV/SIV infection, it is induced by the decrease of mucosal IL-17/IL-22-producing cells (157, 158), loss of gut junctional complexes (159, 160), changes in the microbiota composition (161), and persistence of HIV reservoirs in GALT (151).
2. Microbial translocation: Gut barrier disruption allows the passage of microbial products from the intestinal lumen to the lamina propria and systemic circulation (162).
3. Activation of immune cells by microbial-associated molecular patterns (MAPS) via pathogen-recognition receptors (PRRs): innate immune cells are activated by microbial components via PRRs, such as Toll-like receptors (TLR) (163, 164). Importantly, in chronic inflammatory settings (165, 166), as well as during HIV infection (167), CD4$^+$, and CD8$^+$ T-cells may upregulate TLR-2, 3, 4, 7, and 9 expression (167, 168), and human T-cells can respond *in vitro* to several MAPS (168, 169). In the case of CD4$^+$ T-cells, this TLR-mediated activation renders them more susceptible to HIV replication (170) and apoptosis (169), whereas in the case of CD8$^+$ T cells, TLR engagement lowers the activation threshold (171), which can be deleterious in a chronic setting. Thus, T-cell exposure to TLR agonists may directly contribute to increased T-cell activation during chronic HIV infection.
4. Cytokine secretion and immune cells activation and dysfunction: IL-1β, IL-18, IL-6, TNF-α, and type-I IFN induced by PRRs ligation promote the activation of innate and adaptive immune cells (172, 173). Moreover, cytokines such as IL-15 and IL-12 are an important signal for bystander activation of CD8$^+$ T-cells, particularly memory subsets (105).

Negative Costimulation

As previously mentioned, CD8$^+$ T-cells from HIV-infected patients exhibit increased expression of inhibitory receptors such as PD-1, TIM-3, lymphocyte Activation Gene-3 (LAG-3), CD160, and 2B4 (85, 120, 174). Overall, these receptors interfere with TCR signaling by competing with costimulatory ligands, modulating intracellular pathways, or inducing inhibitory molecules in T-cells; these mechanisms decrease the response of antigen-specific cells to cognate stimulation (175). Expression of inhibitory receptors, particularly PD-1, is also associated with a reduced functional capacity of total CD8$^+$ T-cells after polyclonal stimulation, such as lower degranulation capacity, with consequent decreased release of the cytotoxic molecules granzyme B and perforin (123), and a lower proportion of IL-17-producing cells [(120); **Figure 2A**]. Moreover, activated/exhausted CD8$^+$ T-cells present higher susceptibility to apoptosis (104, 176, 177), as in the case of Tc17 cells, which are highly activated and exhausted during HIV infection and are susceptible to activation-induced cell death (102, 178). Finally, cell-intrinsic defects, such as an impaired signaling machinery (133), and an altered transcriptional, epigenetic, and metabolic profile may also account for the observed dysfunction in activated/exhausted CD8$^+$ T-cells during HIV infection (24, 179, 180).

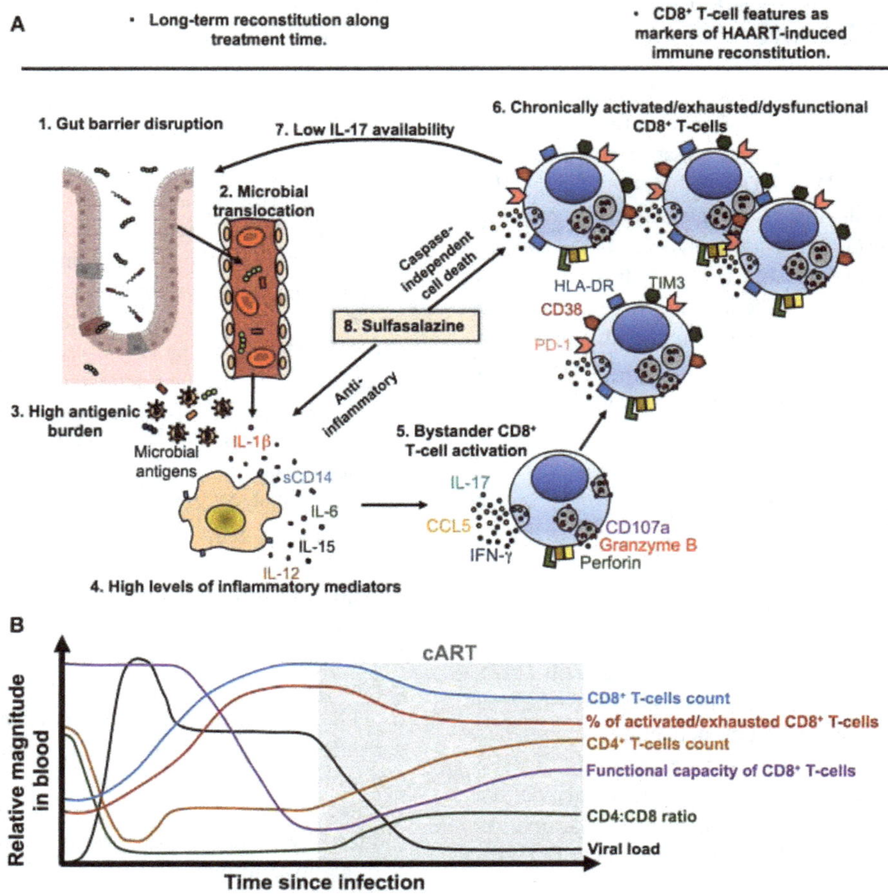

FIGURE 2 | Model of CD8+ T-cell activation, exhaustion and dysfunction during treated HIV infection. **(A)** During chronic HIV, and despite cART-induced viral suppression, gut barrier disruption (1) causes the passage of microbial products to systemic circulation (microbial translocation, 2), contributing to a high antigenic burden together with residual HIV replication and ongoing co-infections (3). Microbial products and other antigens activate innate immune cells such as monocytes/macrophages, which activate and release soluble CD14 (sCD14) and inflammatory cytokines such as IL-1β, IL-6, IL-15, and IL-12 (4). Particularly, IL-15 and IL-12 induce bystander activation of CD8+ T-cells (5), which in early stages of disease may exhibit potent cytotoxic capacity and cytokine production. Nonetheless, chronic bystander stimulation induces exhaustion and dysfunction of CD8+ T-cells (6), which have an increased expression of HLA-DR, CD38, PD-1 and TIM3, and lower degranulation capacity and IL-17 secretion, among other alterations. The low secretion of IL-17 causes a low availability of this cytokine and its beneficial effects on gut mucosa, worsening the gut barrier disruption (7). In this setting, sulfasalazine could be a therapeutic approach to target the inflammatory environment and activated/dysfunctional CD8+ T-cells, through the inhibition of inflammatory cytokine secretion and induction of caspase-independent cell death (8). **(B)** Model of the dynamic of viral load, CD4+ T-cells count, CD8+ T-cells count, CD4:CD8 ratio, the frequency of activated/exhausted CD8+ T-cells and their functional capacity in HIV-infected patients before and after ART beginning. Of note, the viral load is efficiently suppressed and the CD4+ T-cells count are recovered after treatment beginning, but the CD8+ T-cells features remain disturbed despite therapy.

POTENTIAL IMMUNOMODULATORY STRATEGIES FOR IMPROVING CD8+ T-CELLS IMMUNE RECONSTITUTION DURING ANTIRETROVIRAL THERAPY

cART Intensification

Some studies indicate that the intensification of the cART with HIV integrase inhibitors, such as raltegrevir promotes the normalization of the level of activation of CD8+ T-cells (181, 182). Indeed, according with their mechanism of action, integrase inhibitors decrease the levels of proviral DNA (182–185), impacting in the reservoir size and the consequent antigenic burden and immune activation. The effect of raltegravir intensification of cART is also evidenced by the decrease in the levels of the coagulation marker D-dimer (184).

Anti-inflammatory Agents

Since chronic immune activation and systemic inflammation are important determinants of HIV-associated morbidity and mortality, some anti-inflammatory drugs have been explored in the setting of HIV infection, including acetylsalicylic acid, statins, and hydroxychloroquine [reviewed in (186)]. Among them, the treatment with the statins atorvastatin or rosuvastatin in the presence of cART has shown a reduction in the levels of HLA-DR/CD38 and/or PD-1-expressing CD8+ T-cells compared with placebo controls (187–189). We also explored the effect of sulfasalazine (SSZ) on the reconstitution of CD8$^+$ T-cells functional capacity, focused on IL-17 production (120). Sulfasalazine molecule combines the antibiotic sulphapyridine with the anti-inflammatory drug 5-aminosalicylic acid, and has been used in the treatment of chronic inflammatory diseases (190). Previous reports indicated that SSZ not only inhibits macrophage activation and secretion of TNF-α (191, 192), but also induces apoptosis of activated—and possibly dysfunctional—T-cells (193). Certainly, *in vitro* analyses with cells derived from HIV-infected patients on cART, showed that SSZ induces caspase-independent cell death of CD8$^+$ T-cells co-expressing HLA-DR and CD38 (120), possibly through the mitochondrio-nuclear translocation of the apoptosis- inducing factor (AIF), that induces DNA fragmentation (193). Moreover, SSZ decreased the levels of LPS-induced IL-1β. These mechanisms were associated with an increase in the proportion of Tc17 cells in HIV-infected patients [(120); **Figure 2A**]. Interestingly, clinical observations from Colombian health care programs for HIV indicate that SSZ improves the symptoms of HIV-infected patients suffering wasting syndrome. This effect could be related with the abnormal T-cell activation in this group of individuals (194), that is targeted by SSZ. Thus, the use of SSZ and/or other anti-inflammatory drugs could be considered for managing patients with poor response to cART or with advance/progressive disease; large clinical studies that address its usefulness are needed.

Cytokines

Due to the high relevance of Tc17 cells in the context of HIV infection, previous studies have evaluated different strategies to reconstitute this population, as well as mucosa-associated invariant T (MAIT) cells, which are an important IL-17-producing CD161^{hi} CD8$^+$ subset. The administration of IL-7, a member of the γ-common chain family of cytokines, to HIV-infected patients on cART increases the frequency and number of circulating MAIT cells (195). *In vitro*, IL-7 also promotes the cytotoxic capacity and cytokine production of MAIT cells (196). This approach could be relevant in the clinical setting to limit the deterioration of the gut barrier, most likely preventing microbial co-infections. Another member of the γ-common chain, IL-21, promotes the survival, expansion, and cytotoxic responses of antigen-specific CD8$^+$ T-cells (197–199). Accordingly, the administration of IL-21 to SIV-infected rhesus macaques increased the expression of cytotoxic molecules and polyfunctional CD8$^+$ T-cells, compared with untreated controls (200). A functionally-related cytokine, IL-15, also increased the levels of granzyme B$^+$ and perforin$^+$ CD8$^+$ T-cells after administration (in the form of complex between IL-15 and IL-15 receptor α) in uninfected and SHIV-infected rhesus macaques, both in cells from peripheral blood, lymph nodes, and mucosa (201). Interestingly, IL-15 treatment also promoted the migration of cytotoxic CD8$^+$ T-cells to lymphoid follicles (201), whereas administration of an IL-15 superagonist to SIV-infected macaques induced this effect through the induction of the expression of the follicle-homing chemokine receptor CXCR5 in CD8$^+$ T-cells (202). Thus, γ-common chain cytokines are potentially useful as immunotherapies for promoting CD8$^+$ T-cells function HIV-infected patients, and clinical studies are required to evaluate their effectiveness.

Checkpoint Therapy

Checkpoint therapy (i.e., blockade of the aforementioned inhibitory receptors or their ligands) may constitute an important strategy to improve CD8$^+$ T-cell function in HIV-infected patients on cART. Certainly, *in vitro* blockade of PD-1 or its ligands PD-L1/L2 promotes HIV or SIV-specific CD8$^+$ T-cells function and proliferative capacity (83, 203). Similarly, evidence in macaque models of SIV infection indicates that anti-PD-1 antibody therapy increases the frequencies of SIV-specific CD8$^+$ T-cells in blood and gut, with improved polyfunctional capacity and proliferative potential; this effect is associated with significant reductions in viral load and increased survival of infected macaques (204). Interestingly, PD-1 blockade also promotes the response of CD8$^+$ T-cells against gut-resident pathogens, as well as contribute to reduce gut epithelial damage, microbial translocation, and immune activation (205). Moreover, the administration of anti-PD-1 antibody to rhesus macaques prior initiation of cART enhanced the antiviral function of CD8$^+$ T-cells, whereas promoted the expansion of CXCR5$^+$ perforin$^+$ granzyme B$^+$ CD8$^+$ T-cells after cART interruption, resulting in a better control of viremia (206). Interestingly, the CXCR5$^+$ subset is the main CD8$^+$ T-cell population responding to PD-1 blockade (207), which would be important in the context of HIV infection due to the role of follicles as tissue reservoirs (discussed below). Another effect of PD-1 axis blockade would be the reversal of HIV latency (208), that could contribute to recognition and elimination of infected cells by functionally improved HIV-specific CD8$^+$ T-cells. In line with this evidence, a phase I clinical trial of an anti-PD-L1 antibody in 8 HIV-infected patients on cART showed that the frequency of Gag-specific CD8$^+$ T-cells expressing IFN-γ or CD107a increased from baseline to day 28 post-treatment, although there was no statistical significance, most likely due to high inter-individual variability. There were no changes in the CD4$^+$ T-cell counts or CD4:CD8 ratio (209). Importantly, an overall safety has been shown for the anti-PD-L1 or anti-PD1 antibody therapy, even in patients with concomitant malignancies (209, 210). Together, these studies indicate that PD-1 axis blockade could improve the antiviral function of CD8$^+$ T-cells during HIV infection, along with other beneficial effects on the levels of microbial translocation, immune activation and viral reservoirs.

CD8$^+$ T-CELLS AS CORRELATES OF IMMUNE RECONSTITUTION DURING ANTIRETROVIRAL THERAPY

A large body of evidence indicate that monitoring CD4$^+$ T-cell counts, and viral load is informative of the effectiveness of cART-induced viral suppression in HIV-infected patients. Typically, CD4$^+$ T-cells increase rapidly in the first weeks of treatment, followed by a more gradual increase, depending on the level of nadir CD4$^+$ T-cells or the naïve subpopulation at the time of treatment initiation (211–215). Moreover, HIV-infected patients who maintain viral suppression and had CD4$^+$ T-cells ≥300 cells/μL are unlikely to experience counts <200 cells/μL (threshold for opportunistic infection risk), suggesting that routine CD4$^+$ T-cells monitoring may be unnecessary in some scenarios (216). Certainly, undetectable viral load or CD4$^+$ T-cell counts do not reflect the immunological alterations that are present in treated HIV-infected patients. In contrast, the persistently high CD8$^+$ T-cell counts and low CD4:CD8 ratio are indicative of partial immune reconstitution in treated HIV-infected patients, and, due to their accessibility in low-income settings and predictive power of adverse clinical outcomes (88, 217, 218), could be useful tools for immune monitoring of these individuals. Moreover, in HIV-infected patients under long-term suppressive cART (more than 25 months) there is a recovery in the proportion of CD107a$^+$ and IL-17$^+$ CD8$^+$ T-cells, reaching similar levels to those seen in seronegative individuals (120, 123). These findings suggest a potential usefulness of these CD8$^+$ T-cell functional markers to predict immune reconstitution in HIV-infected patients on cART, in addition to others currently used such as the CD8$^+$ T-cell counts and the CD4:CD8 ratio (88, 217, 218).

In summary, cART-induced immune reconstitution is a long-term and incomplete process. After treatment initiation, viral load is rapidly controlled and CD4$^+$ T-cell counts are progressively recovered. However, CD8$^+$ T-cell counts remain increased despite cART, along with a low CD4:CD8 ratio (**Figure 2B**). Moreover, the frequency of activated/exhausted CD8$^+$ T-cells do not completely return to basal levels, and some grade of dysfunction remains in several CD8$^+$ T-cell subsets (**Figure 2B**). The improvement of cART effectiveness may require the combination of strategies such as an early beginning of therapy, rigorous clinical monitoring, the use of reliable biomarkers and possibly the use of immunomodulatory therapies.

CXCR5$^+$ CD8$^+$ T-CELLS AND THEIR ROLE DURING HIV INFECTION

Another subpopulation of CD8$^+$ T-cells that is relevant in the setting of HIV infection is that expressing CXCR5, since they could be a potential therapeutic cell-based strategy to eradicate HIV in follicles (219), an important body viral reservoir (153, 220). CXCR5-expressing CD8$^+$ T-cells follow a particular dynamic during HIV/SIV infection. A common observation across studies is the increase in the proportion of CXCR5$^+$ CD8$^+$ T-cells in lymphoid follicles in HIV-infected patients, compared with seronegative controls (70, 221–223). A similar accumulation of follicular CXCR5$^+$ CD8$^+$ T-cells has been observed in SIV-infected macaques (224, 225). This accumulation is associated with the inflammatory/immune activation environment within follicles and increased levels of the CXCR5-ligand CXCL13 in HIV-infected patients, but not with the levels of viral replication or antigens, both during HIV (222) and SIV infection (225). Moreover, CXCR5$^+$ CD8$^+$ T-cells could also migrate within lymph nodes in response to CXCL10, which is ligand of CXCR3, as has been observed in SIV-infected macaques (224). Interestingly, CXCR5$^+$ CD4$^+$ T-cells also accumulate during chronic HIV infection (153, 223, 226), whereas this process is also driven by the local inflammation in SIV-infected macaques (227). Accordingly, increased immune activation and inflammatory cytokines secretion is present in lymph nodes from chronically HIV-infected patients (228). Interestingly, lymphotoxin α and β, and TNF are required for the expression of CXCL13 by murine follicular stromal cells (229), CXCL13 is expressed in chronic inflammation (230), and is a marker of chronic inflammation in HIV-infected patients, even during cART (231). Thus, the antigen burden in lymphoid tissues, both by infected CD4$^+$ T-cells or virion-bearing follicular dendritic cells, may induce an inflammatory environment that in turn promote the production of CXCL13, contributing to the accumulation of CXCR5$^+$ CD8$^+$ T-cells.

Importantly, ART does not decrease the frequency of CXCR5$^+$ CD8$^+$ T-cells in human lymph nodes (222), which is in agreement with the low drug distribution to these tissues and consequent unchanged inflammatory environment, in comparison with blood (110). In addition, the compromise in follicles architecture during HIV infection may also be responsible for the increased passage of CD8$^+$ T-cells and other cell types to these compartments (232).

On the other hand, circulating CXCR5-expressing CD8$^+$ T-cells, which exhibit a transitional memory phenotype, are decreased in untreated HIV-infected patients compared with seronegative controls, but are maintained in patients under suppressive cART (233). Interestingly, the decrease in CXCR5$^+$ CCR7$^-$ CD8$^+$ T-cells is associated with the increase in CXCR5$^-$ CCR7$^-$ cells, which are most likely an effector memory population. Moreover, the frequency of CXCR5^{hi} CCR7$^{-/lo}$ CD8$^+$ T-cells is inversely correlated with the level of systemic HIV replication in untreated HIV-infected patients, particularly in elite controllers (233). Strikingly, while similar correlations between the number of circulating human CXCR5$^+$ CD8$^+$ T-cells and systemic viral load have been reported (221), comparable associations were obtained between the frequencies of lymph node-confined memory CXCR5$^+$ CD8$^+$ T-cells and systemic viral load in HIV controllers patients (53). Thus, immune activation and local inflammation, but not viral replication, are apparently major drivers of CXCR5$^+$ CD8$^+$ T-cells (and CXCR5$^+$ CD4$^+$ T-cells) accumulation in lymphoid follicles during chronic HIV/SIV infection (**Figure 3**). Once in the lymphoid follicles, antigen-specific CXCR5$^+$ CD8$^+$ T-cells could partially eliminate infected cells, being reflected in lower local and systemic viral load, as has been observed in SIV-infected macaques (234). In fact, a role of this subpopulation in the control of HIV (70, 221) and SIV (225, 235) replication has been proposed, their antiviral function in follicles could be an important mechanism of disease protection, and its frequency could be as useful correlate of limited viral replication. If the systemic viral load, immune activation and/or tissue inflammation decrease, these cells could egress from the follicles, enter systemic circulation and search for other lymphoid follicles or tissues (**Figure 3**). However, it is yet unclear which other factors may

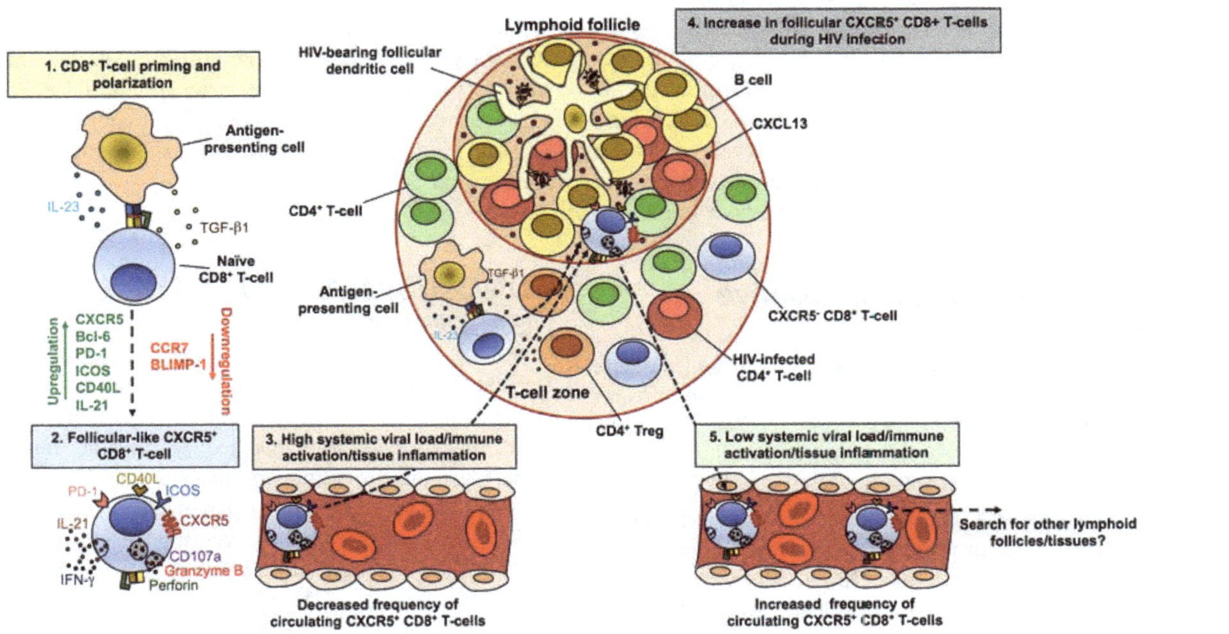

FIGURE 3 | Model of the dynamics of CXCR5+ CD8+ T-cells during HIV infection. CD8+ T-cells are polarized to a follicular-like CXCR5+ profile after priming by an antigen-presenting cell that secrete TGF-β1 and IL-23 (1). These cytokines induce the up-regulation of CXCR5, Bcl-6, PD-1, ICOS, CD40L and IL-21, with down-regulation of CCR7 and BLIMP-1 (2). In circulation or peripheral tissues, follicular-like CXCR5+ CD8+ T-cells also exhibit a cytotoxic potential and production of IFN-γ. During chronic HIV infection and in the setting of high viral load and consequent increased immune activation and tissue inflammation, there is an accumulation of CXCR5+ CD8+ T-cells in lymphoid follicles, in response to CXCL13 (4). The high levels of TGF-β1 produced by antigen-presenting cells or regulatory T cells (Treg), may also induce the differentiation and accumulation of CXCR5+ CD8+ T-cells. Once in the follicles, CXCR5+ CD8+ T-cells exert an antiviral effect, which can be reflected in lower viral replication and the subsequent decrease in the immune activation/tissue inflammation and the egress of this subset from follicles. In circulation, CXCR5+ CD8+ T-cells possibly search for other lymphoid follicles or peripheral tissues (5).

influence the induction of CXCR5 and follicle migration of CD8+ T-cells.

In order to explore the differentiation conditions of human CXCR5+ CD8+ T-cells, we evaluated the effect of TGF-β1, IL-23, and IL-12, which promote the differentiation of human follicular CD4+ T-cells (236) and induce the expression of CXCR5 in non-human primate CD8+ T-cells (234). *In vitro*, TGF-β1 plus IL-23 (in the presence of TCR stimulation) induced the expression of CXCR5 in purified CD8+ T-cells from healthy individuals, as well as a follicular-like phenotypic and transcriptional profile, such as the up-regulation of PD-1, inducible T-cell costimulatory (ICOS), CD40L and *BCL6*, and the down-regulation of CCR7 and *PRDM1* (Perdomo-Celis F, In press). These data suggest that, *in vivo*, TGF-β1 and IL-23 may be polarizing factors for follicular-like CXCR5+ CD8+ T-cells, which could then migrate to lymphoid follicles for exerting immune surveillance (**Figure 2**). Considering the increased levels of regulatory T cells (Treg)-derived TGF-β1 in lymphoid tissues during HIV infection (237), there could be an appropriate environment for the differentiation and accumulation of follicular-like CXCR5+ CD8+ T-cells (**Figure 3**). Importantly, the induction of the expression of CXCR5 in CD8+ T-cells through cytokine stimulation or genetic engineering may be a useful strategy for improving the migration of these cells to lymphoid follicles and boost follicular antiviral responses that help to eradicate viral reservoirs in these structures (202, 238, 239).

CD8+ T-CELL-BASED STRATEGIES TO TREAT OR CURE HIV INFECTION

Current strategies for CD8+ T-cell-based strategies to treat or cure HIV infection are based on stimulating pre-existing and/or inducing *de novo* HIV-specific immune responses through vaccine therapies or redirecting HIV-specific CD8+ T-cells and improving their function and persistence after adoptive transfer. The latter adoptive transfer strategies can be divided in (i) Expansion of HIV-specific CD8+ T-cells; (ii) Artificial CD8+ TCR; (iii) Chimeric antigen receptors (CAR); (iv) Selection of CD8+ T-cells with long-term persistence; (v) Induction of HIV-specific CD8+ T-cells from virus-naïve donor cells. Of note, these strategies may also be accompanied by the aforementioned immunomodulatory approaches, in order to reach a global reconstitution of the CD8+ T-cell response, as well as with latency-reversing agents, to induce the reactivation of viral reservoir (240), particularly in the case of patients receiving cART.

CD8+ T-Cell-Based Vaccines

Several HIV vaccine candidates have been focused on the induction of CD8+ T-cell responses in order to control viremia, i.e., as a therapeutic approach. They range from whole attenuated virus, vector viruses containing HIV proteins, DNA plasmids, and HIV peptides [reviewed in (241)]. Importantly, immunization should be performed with multiple selected peptides based on conserved regions of HIV proteins, which induce subdominant but effective CD8$^+$ T-cell responses, and are restricted by the most common HLA alleles in a specific population (242, 243). Nonetheless, in general, a low and transient reduction of viral load has been observed with most therapeutic vaccines (241), indicating that a combination of this and other approaches is required for a relevant impact on disease progression.

HIV-Specific CD8$^+$ T-Cells Adoptive Transfer

First reports including small cohorts of HIV-infected patients (some of them receiving cART) demonstrated that the infusion of autologous CD8$^+$ T-cells enriched for HIV-specific cells targeting several viral proteins (expanded *ex vivo* through polyclonal stimulation), transiently decreased plasma viremia or productively infected cells, and increased CD4$^+$ T-cell counts (244, 245). Nonetheless, in other studies, a rapid apoptosis of adoptively transferred HIV-specific CD8$^+$ T-cells was associated with failure in the reduction of viral load (246). Moreover, transfer of HIV-specific CD8$^+$ T-cells induced selection of escape mutant HIV variants, which was associated with rise in viral load and decrease of CD4$^+$ T-cells (247). More recently, other approaches based on infusion of CD8$^+$ T-cells specific for multiple HIV antigens (248) demonstrated efficacy in the control of autologous reservoir virus (249). Similarly, CD8$^+$ T-cells transduced with vectors expressing a TCR targeting the relevant HIV epitope SL9 in Gag protein, showed lysis capacity and reduced infectious cells *in vivo* in SCID mice (250), as well as functional capacity in cells derived from cART-receiving patients (251). However, engineered TCR may have recognition of self-epitopes, resulting in severe reactions such as cardiac toxicity (252), which limits the use of this approach. The use of CAR CD8$^+$ T-cells may overcome the problems of viral escape, HIV-induced HLA downregulation, and immune exhaustion (253). First-generation CAR T-cells containing the extracellular domain of human CD4 linked to the CD3ζ chain (CD4ζ) showed prolonged survival and trafficking to gut mucosa, although did not change viral load in HIV-infected patients (254). More recently, the CD4ζ CAR was re-engineered to express the 4-1BB costimulatory domain, inducing a more potent HIV suppressing capacity *in vitro* and *in vivo* in a humanized mouse model (255). CAR T-cells have also been designed with expression of single-chain variable fragments of broadly neutralizing antibodies (256), or carbohydrate-recognition domain of C-type lectin, both targeting gp120 (257). Another approach to improve the survival of adoptively transferred HIV-specific CD8$^+$ T-cells is to select those with a long-term memory profile. Accordingly, *ex vivo* expanded HIV-specific CD28$^+$ CD8$^+$ T-cells survived for at least 84 days after infusion in cART-receiving patients and maintained central memory characteristics (258). Finally, functional HIV-specific CD8$^+$ T-cells can be generated from HIV-negative donors through priming with peptide-pulsed dendritic cells, followed by polyclonal expansion. This approach could be useful in the setting of hematopoietic stem cell transplantation in HIV-infected patients to recover or improve the virus-specific CD8$^+$ T-cell response (259).

In summary, these studies demonstrate the potential of CD8$^+$ T-cell-based therapeutic strategies for HIV treatment or cure strategies. More importantly, combination of different strategies, such as vaccine induction of virus-specific CD8$^+$ T-cells and subsequent adoptive transfer, could limit viral replication and/or rebound after cART interruption, as recently evidenced in a macaque model (260).

CONCLUSIONS AND FUTURE PERSPECTIVES

Despite intense research on HIV, there is no preventing vaccine and cure available for this infection. In fact, a high incidence is still reported worldwide, underlying the importance of providing an optimal cART and health care management to HIV-infected patients, not only for improving their quality of life and preventing several co-morbidities, but also for breaking the chain of transmission. Thus, the characterization of HIV-infected patients under suppressive cART is required to understand the benefits, pitfalls, and challenges of cART, to identify novel immunomodulatory targets, and to elucidate potential strategies for reaching a functional or sterilizing cure for this infection. Despite complete suppression of viral load and reconstitution of CD4$^+$ T-cells, HIV-infected patients exhibit increased systemic inflammation levels and a compromised CD8$^+$ T-cells response, characterized by high activation/exhaustion and impaired lytic and non-lytic mechanisms. Some of the phenotypic and/or functional CD8$^+$ T-cell features could be used in the clinical setting to identify those patients reaching immune reconstitution during continuous suppressive cART. Some of the CD8$^+$ T-cell alterations, such as low IL-17 production, could be targeted by immunomodulatory drugs. Finally, follicular CXCR5$^+$ CD8$^+$ T-cells could be a therapeutic weapon for targeting viral reservoirs in lymphoid follicles, along with other CD8$^+$ T-cell-based strategies.

AUTHOR CONTRIBUTIONS

FP-C, NT, and MR reviewed the literature and wrote the manuscript.

ACKNOWLEDGMENTS

We thank Dr. Juan C. Zapata for critically reviewing this manuscript. Thanks to Angela Betancur for her administrative support.

REFERENCES

1. WHO Guidelines Approved by the Guidelines Review Committee. *Consolidated Guidelines on the Use of Antiretroviral Drugs for Treating and Preventing HIV Infection: Recommendations for a Public Health Approach.* Geneva: World Health OrganizationCopyright (c) World Health Organization (2013).
2. Levi J, Raymond A, Pozniak A, Vernazza P, Kohler P, Hill A. Can the UNAIDS 90-90-90 target be achieved? A systematic analysis of national HIV treatment cascades. *BMJ Glob Heal.* (2016) 1:e000010. doi: 10.1136/bmjgh-2015-000010
3. Saag MS, Benson CA, Gandhi RT, Hoy JF, Landovitz RJ, Mugavero MJ, et al. Antiretroviral drugs for treatment and prevention of HIV infection in adults: 2018 recommendations of the International Antiviral Society-USA Panel. *JAMA.* (2018) 320:379–96. doi: 10.1001/jama.2018.8431
4. Ministerio de Salud y Protección Social, Fondo de Población de las Naciones Unidas - UNFPA. *Guía de Práctica Clínica Basada en la Evidencia Científica Para la Atención de la Infección por VIH/Sida en Adolescentes (con 13 años o más de edad) y Adultos.* (2014)
5. Bigna JJR, Plottel CS, Koulla-Shiro S. Challenges in initiating antiretroviral therapy for all HIV-infected people regardless of CD4 cell count. *Infect Dis Poverty.* (2016) 5:85. doi: 10.1186/s40249-016-0179-9
6. DHHS Panel on Antiretroviral Guidelines for Adults and Adolescents. *Guidelines for the Use of Antiretroviral Agents in Adults and Adolescents With HIV.* Washington, DC: Department of Health and Human Services (2018).
7. Tang MW, Shafer RW. HIV-1 antiretroviral resistance: scientific principles and clinical applications. *Drugs.* (2012) 72:e1–25. doi: 10.2165/11633630-000000000-00000
8. Aldous JL, Haubrich RH. Defining treatment failure in resource-rich settings. *Curr Opin HIV AIDS.* (2009) 4:459–66. doi: 10.1097/COH.0b013e328331dea5
9. Wilson EMP, Sereti I. Immune restoration after antiretroviral therapy: the pitfalls of hasty or incomplete repairs. *Immunol Rev.* (2013) 254:343–54. doi: 10.1111/imr.12064
10. Croxford S, Kitching A, Desai S, Kall M, Edelstein M, Skingsley A, et al. Mortality and causes of death in people diagnosed with HIV in the era of highly active antiretroviral therapy compared with the general population: an analysis of a national observational cohort. *Lancet Public Heal.* (2017) 2:e35–46. doi: 10.1016/S2468-2667(16)30020-2
11. Antiretroviral Therapy Cohort Collaboration. Causes of death in HIV-1-infected patients treated with antiretroviral therapy, 1996-2006: collaborative analysis of 13 HIV cohort studies. *Clin Infect Dis.* (2010) 50:1387–1396. doi: 10.1086/652283
12. Hughes CA, Tseng A, Cooper R. Managing drug interactions in HIV-infected adults with comorbid illness. *CMAJ.* (2015) 187:36–43. doi: 10.1503/cmaj.131626
13. Zhang N, Bevan MJ. CD8(+) T cells: foot soldiers of the immune system. *Immunity.* (2011) 35:161–8. doi: 10.1016/j.immuni.2011.07.010
14. Curtsinger JM, Johnson CM, Mescher MF. CD8 T cell clonal expansion and development of effector function require prolonged exposure to antigen, costimulation, and signal 3 cytokine. *J Immunol.* (2003) 171:5165–71. doi: 10.4049/jimmunol.171.10.5165
15. Curtsinger JM, Valenzuela JO, Agarwal P, Lins D, Mescher MF. Cutting edge: type I IFNs provide a third signal to CD8 T cells to stimulate clonal expansion and differentiation. *J Immunol.* (2005) 174:4465–9. doi: 10.4049/jimmunol.174.8.4465
16. Miller JD, van der Most RG, Akondy RS, Glidewell JT, Albott S, Masopust D, et al. Human effector and memory $CD8^+$ T cell responses to smallpox and yellow fever vaccines. *Immunity.* (2008) 28:710–22. doi: 10.1016/j.immuni.2008.02.020
17. Hamann D, Baars PA, Rep MHG, Hooibrink B, Kerkhof-Garde SR, Klein MR, et al. Phenotypic and functional separation of memory and effector human $CD8^+$ T cells. *J Exp Med.* (1997) 186:1407–18. doi: 10.1016/S0165-2478(97)85793-8
18. Wolint P, Betts MR, Koup RA, Oxenius A. Immediate cytotoxicity but not degranulation distinguishes effector and memory subsets of $CD8^+$ T cells. *J Exp Med.* (2004) 199:925–36. doi: 10.1084/jem.200 31799
19. Bachmann MF, Barner M, Viola A, Kopf M. Distinct kinetics of cytokine production and cytolysis in effector and memory T cells after viral infection. *Eur J Immunol.* (1999) 29:291–9. doi: 10.1002/(SICI)1521-4141(199901)29:01<291::AID-IMMU291>;3.0.CO;2-K
20. Weninger W, Manjunath N, Von Andrian UH. Migration and differentiation of $CD8^+$ T cells. *Immunol Rev.* (2002) 186:221–3. doi: 10.1034/j.1600-065X.2002.18618.x
21. Wherry EJ, Ahmed R. Memory CD8 T-cell differentiation during viral infection. *J Virol.* (2004) 78:5535–45. doi: 10.1128/JVI.78.11.5535-5545.2004
22. Akondy RS, Fitch M, Edupuganti S, Yang S, Kissick HT, Li KW, et al. Origin and differentiation of human memory CD8 T cells after vaccination. *Nature.* (2017) 552:362–367. doi: 10.1038/nature24633
23. Paley MA, Kroy DC, Odorizzi PM, Johnnidis JB, Dolfi DV, Barnett BE, et al. Progenitor and terminal subsets of $CD8^+$ T cells cooperate to contain chronic viral infection. *Science.* (2012) 338:1220–5. doi: 10.1126/science.1229620
24. Buggert M, Tauriainen J, Yamamoto T, Frederiksen J, Ivarsson MA, Michaëlsson J, et al. T-bet and eomes are differentially linked to the exhausted phenotype of $CD8^-$ T cells in HIV infection. *PLoS Pathog.* (2014) 10:e1004251. doi: 10.1371/journal.ppat.1004251
25. McLane LM, Banerjee PP, Cosma GL, Makedonas G, Wherry EJ, Orange JS, et al. Differential localization of T-bet and eomes in CD8 T cell memory populations. *J Immunol.* (2013) 190:3207–15. doi: 10.4049/jimmunol.1201556
26. Cruz-Guilloty F, Pipkin ME, Djuretic IM, Levanon D, Lotem J, Lichtenheld MG, et al. Runx3 and T-box proteins cooperate to establish the transcriptional program of effector CTLs. *J Exp Med.* (2009) 206:51 LP—59. doi: 10.1084/jem.20081242
27. van der Veeken J, Zhong Y, Sharma R, Mazutis L, Dao P, Pe'er D, et al. Natural genetic variation reveals key features of epigenetic and transcriptional memory in virus-specific CD8 T cells. *Immunity.* (2019) 50:1202–17.e7. doi: 10.1016/j.immuni.2019.03.031
28. Betts MR, Brenchley JM, Price DA, De Rosa SC, Douek DC, Roederer M, et al. Sensitive and viable identification of antigen-specific $CD8^+$ T cells by a flow cytometric assay for degranulation. *J Immunol Methods.* (2003) 281:65–78. doi: 10.1016/S0022-1759(03)00265-5
29. Betts MR, Koup RA. Detection of T-cell degranulation: CD107a and b. *Methods Cell Biol.* (2004) 75:497–512. doi: 10.1016/S0091-679X(04)75020-7
30. Peters PJ. Cytotoxic T lymphocyte granules are secretory lysosomes, containing both perforin and granzymes. *J Exp Med.* (1991) 173:1099–109. doi: 10.1084/jem.173.5.1099
31. Fukuda M. Lysosomal membrane glycoproteins: structure, biosynthesis, and intracellular trafficking. *J Biol Chem.* (1991) 266:21327–30.
32. Stenger S, Hanson DA, Teitelbaum R, Dewan P, Niazi KR, Froelich CJ, et al. An antimicrobial activity of cytolytic T cells mediated by granulysin. *Science.* (1998) 282:121–5. doi: 10.1126/science.282.5386.121
33. Metkar SS, Wang B, Aguilar-Santelises M, Raja SM, Uhlin-Hansen L, Podack E, et al. Cytotoxic cell granule-mediated apoptosis: perforin delivers granzyme b-serglycin complexes into target cells without plasma membrane pore formation. *Immunity.* (2002) doi: 10.1016/S1074-7613(02)00286-8
34. Dupuis M, Schaerer E, Krause KH, Tschopp J. The calcium-binding protein calreticulin is a major constituent of lytic granules in cytolytic T lymphocytes. *J Exp Med.* (1993) 16:417–28. doi: 10.1084/jem.177.1.1
35. Balaji KN, Schaschke N, Machleidt W, Catalfamo M, Henkart PA. Surface cathepsin B protects cytotoxic lymphocytes from self-destruction after degranulation. *J Exp Med.* (2002) 196:493–503. doi: 10.1084/jem.20011836
36. Bossi G, Griffiths GM. Degranulation plays an essential part in regulating cell surface expression of Fas ligand in T cells and natural killer cells. *Nat Med.* (1999) 5:90–6. doi: 10.1038/4779
37. Lieberman J. The ABCs of granule-mediated cytotoxicity: new weapons in the arsenal. *Nat Rev Immunol.* (2003) 3:361–70. doi: 10.1038/nri1083
38. Shiver JW, Henkart PA. A noncytotoxic mast cell tumor line exhibits potent IgE-dependent cytotoxicity after transfection with the cytolysin/perforin gene. *Cell.* (1991) 64:1175–81. doi: 10.1016/0092-8674(91)90272-Z
39. Lopez JA, Susanto O, Jenkins MR, Lukoyanova N, Sutton VR, Law RHP, et al. Perforin forms transient pores on the target cell plasma membrane to facilitate rapid access of granzymes during killer cell attack. *Blood.* (2013) doi: 10.1182/blood-2012-07-446146

40. Motyka B, Korbutt G, Pinkoski MJ, Heibein JA, Caputo A, Hobman M, et al. Mannose 6-phosphate/insulin-like growth factor II receptor is a death receptor for granzyme B during cytotoxic T cell-induced apoptosis. *Cell.* (2000) 103:491–500. doi: 10.1016/S0092-8674(00)00140-9
41. Lord SJ, Rajotte RV, Korbutt GS, Bleackley RC. Granzyme B: a natural born killer. *Immunol Rev.* (2003) 193:31–8. doi: 10.1034/j.1600-065X.2003.00044.x
42. Barry M, Heibein JA, Pinkoski MJ, Lee SF, Moyer RW, Green DR, et al. Granzyme B short-circuits the need for caspase 8 activity during granule-mediated cytotoxic T-lymphocyte killing by directly cleaving Bid. *Mol Cell Biol.* (2000) 20:3781–94. doi: 10.1128/MCB.20.11.3781-3794.2000
43. Atkinson EA, Barry M, Darmon AJ, Shostak I, Turner PC, Moyer RW, et al. Cytotoxic T lymphocyte-assisted suicide: caspase 3 activation is primarily the result of the direct action of granzyme B. *J Biol Chem.* (1998) 273:21261–6. doi: 10.1074/jbc.273.33.21261
44. Zou H, Li Y, Liu X, Wang X. An APAf-1. cytochrome C multimeric complex is a functional apoptosome that activates procaspase-9. *J Biol Chem.* (1999) 274:11549–56. doi: 10.1074/jbc.274.17.11549
45. Li LY, Luo X, Wang X. Endonuclease G is an apoptotic DNase when released from mitochondria. *Nature.* (2001) 412:95–9. doi: 10.1038/35083620
46. Elmore S. Apoptosis: a review of programmed cell death. *Toxicol Pathol.* (2007) 35:495–516. doi: 10.1080/01926230701320337
47. Gulzar N, Copeland K. CD8$^+$ T-cells: function and response to HIV infection. *Curr HIV Res.* (2004) 2:23–37. doi: 10.2174/1570162043485077
48. Choe H, Farzan M, Sun Y, Sullivan N, Rollins B, Ponath PD, et al. The β-chemokine receptors CCR3 and CCR5 facilitate infection by primary HIV-1 isolates. *Cell.* (1996) 85:1135–48. doi: 10.1016/S0092-8674(00)81313-6
49. Saunders KO, Ward-Caviness C, Schutte RJ, Freel SA, Overman RG, Thielman NM, et al. Secretion of MIP-1β and MIP-1α by CD8$^+$ T-lymphocytes correlates with HIV-1 inhibition independent of coreceptor usage. *Cell Immunol.* (2011) 266:154–64. doi: 10.1016/j.cellimm.2010.09.011
50. Cocchi F, DeVico AL, Garzino-Demo A, Arya SK, Gallo RC, Lusso P. Identification of RANTES, MIP-1α, and MIP-1β as the major HIV-suppressive factors produced by CD8$^+$ T cells. *Science.* (1995) 27:1811–5. doi: 10.1126/science.270.5243.1811
51. Romero P, Zippelius A, Kurth I, Pittet MJ, Touvrey C, Iancu EM, et al. Four functionally distinct populations of human effector-memory CD8$^+$ T lymphocytes. *J Immunol.* (2007) 178:4112–9. doi: 10.4049/jimmunol.178.7.4112
52. Abdelsamed HA, Moustaki A, Fan Y, Dogra P, Ghoneim HE, Zebley CC, et al. Human memory CD8 T cell effector potential is epigenetically preserved during *in vivo* homeostasis. *J Exp Med.* (2017) 214:1593–606 doi: 10.1084/jem.20161760
53. Reuter MA, Del Rio Estrada PM, Buggert M, Petrovas C, Ferrando-Martinez S, Nguyen S, et al. HIV-specific CD8$^+$ T cells exhibit reduced and differentially regulated cytolytic activity in lymphoid tissue. *Cell Rep.* (2017) 21:3458–70. doi: 10.1016/j.celrep.2017.11.075
54. Kiniry BE, Ganesh A, Critchfield JW, Hunt PW, Hecht FM, Somsouk M, et al. Predominance of weakly cytotoxic, T-bet(Low)Eomes(Neg) CD8(+) T-cells in human gastrointestinal mucosa: implications for HIV infection. *Mucosal Immunol.* (2017) 10:1008–20. doi: 10.1038/mi.2016.100
55. Kiniry BE, Hunt PW, Hecht FM, Somsouk M, Deeks SG, Shacklett BL. Differential expression of CD8(+) T cell cytotoxic effector molecules in blood and gastrointestinal mucosa in HIV-1 infection. *J Immunol.* (2018) 200:1876–88. doi: 10.4049/jimmunol.1701532
56. Buggert M, Nguyen S, Salgado-Montes de Oca G, Bengsch B, Darko S, Ransier A, et al. Identification and characterization of HIV-specific resident memory CD8(+) T cells in human lymphoid tissue. *Sci Immunol.* (2018) 3:eaar4526. doi: 10.1126/sciimmunol.aar4526
57. Mittrücker HW, Visekruna A, Huber M. Heterogeneity in the differentiation and function of CD8$^+$ T cells. *Arch Immunol Ther Exp.* (2014) 62:449–58. doi: 10.1007/s00005-014-0293-y
58. Yu Y, Ma X, Gong R, Zhu J, Wei L, Yao J. Recent advances in CD8(+) regulatory T cell research. *Oncol Lett.* (2018) 15:8187–94. doi: 10.3892/ol.2018.8378
59. Srenathan U, Steel K, Taams LS. IL-17+ CD8$^+$ T cells: differentiation, phenotype and role in inflammatory disease. *Immunol Lett.* (2016) 178:20–6. doi: 10.1016/j.imlet.2016.05.001
60. Billerbeck E, Kang Y-H, Walker L, Lockstone H, Grafmueller S, Fleming V, et al. Analysis of CD161 expression on human CD8$^+$ T cells defines a distinct functional subset with tissue-homing properties. *Proc Natl Acad Sci USA.* (2010) 107:3006–11. doi: 10.1073/pnas.0914839107
61. Huber M, Heink S, Grothe H, Guralnik A, Reinhard K, Elflein K, et al. Th17-like developmental process leads to CD8$^+$Tc17 cells with reduced cytotoxic activity. *Eur J Immunol.* (2009) 39:1716–25. doi: 10.1002/eji.200939412
62. Maggi L, Santarlasci V, Capone M, Peired A, Frosali F, Crome SQ, et al. CD161 is a marker of all human IL-17-producing T-cell subsets and is induced by RORC. *Eur J Immunol.* (2010) 40:2174–81. doi: 10.1002/eji.200940257
63. Kondo T, Takata H, Matsuki F, Takiguchi M. Cutting edge: phenotypic characterization and differentiation of human CD8$^+$ T cells producing IL-17. *J Immunol.* (2009) 182:1794–8. doi: 10.4049/jimmunol.0801347
64. Fergusson JR, Hühn MH, Swadling L, Walker LJ, Kurioka A, Llibre A, et al. CD161int CD8$^+$ T cells: a novel population of highly functional, memory CD8$^+$ T cells enriched within the gut. *Mucosal Immunol.* (2016) 9:401–13. doi: 10.1038/mi.2015.69
65. Iwakura Y, Ishigame H, Saijo S, Nakae S. Functional specialization of interleukin-17 family members. *Immunity.* (2011) 34:149–62. doi: 10.1016/j.immuni.2011.02.012
66. Veldhoen M. Interleukin 17 is a chief orchestrator of immunity. *Nat Immunol.* (2017) 18:612–21. doi: 10.1038/ni.3742
67. Lee JS, Tato CM, Joyce-Shaikh B, Gulan F, Cayatte C, Chen Y, et al. Interleukin-23-independent IL-17 production regulates intestinal epithelial permeability. *Immunity.* (2015) 43:727–38. doi: 10.1016/j.immuni.2015.09.003
68. Liang SC, Tan X-Y, Luxenberg DP, Karim R, Dunussi-Joannopoulos K, Collins M, et al. Interleukin (IL)-22 and IL-17 are coexpressed by Th17 cells and cooperatively enhance expression of antimicrobial peptides. *J Exp Med.* (2006) 203:2271–9. doi: 10.1084/jem.20061308
69. Miyamoto M, Prause O, Sjostrand M, Laan M, Lotvall J, Linden A. Endogenous IL-17 as a mediator of neutrophil recruitment caused by endotoxin exposure in mouse airways. *J Immunol.* (2003) 170:4665–72. doi: 10.4049/jimmunol.170.9.4665
70. Leong YA, Chen Y, Ong HS, Wu D, Man K, Deleage C, et al. CXCR5+ follicular cytotoxic T cells control viral infection in B cell follicles. *Nat Immunol.* (2016) 17:1187–96. doi: 10.1038/ni.3543
71. McBrien JB, Kumar NA, Silvestri G. Mechanisms of CD8$^+$ T cell-mediated suppression of HIV/SIV replication. *Eur J Immunol.* (2018) 48:898–914. doi: 10.1002/eji.201747172
72. Borrow P, Lewicki H, Hahn BH, Shaw GM, Oldstone MB. Virus-specific CD8$^+$ cytotoxic T-lymphocyte activity associated with control of viremia in primary human immunodeficiency virus type 1 infection. *J Virol.* (1994) 68:6103–10.
73. Takata H, Buranapraditkun S, Kessing C, Fletcher JLK, Muir R, Tardif V, et al. Delayed differentiation of potent effector CD8$^+$ T cells reducing viremia and reservoir seeding in acute HIV infection. *Sci Transl Med.* (2017) 9:eaag1809. doi: 10.1126/scitranslmed.aag1809
74. Jin X, Bauer DE, Tuttleton SE, Lewin S, Gettie A, Blanchard J, et al. Dramatic rise in plasma viremia after CD8(+) T cell depletion in simian immunodeficiency virus-infected macaques. *J Exp Med.* (1999) 189:991–8. doi: 10.1084/jem.189.6.991
75. Schmitz JE, Kuroda MJ, Santra S, Sasseville VG, Simon MA, Lifton MA, et al. Control of viremia in simian immunodeficiency virus infection by CD8$^+$ lymphocytes. *Science.* (1999) 283:857–60.
76. Saez-Cirion A, Lacabaratz C, Lambotte O, Versmisse P, Urrutia A, Boufassa F, et al. HIV controllers exhibit potent CD8 T cell capacity to suppress HIV infection *ex vivo* and peculiar cytotoxic T lymphocyte activation phenotype. *Proc Natl Acad Sci USA.* (2007) 104:6776–81. doi: 10.1073/pnas.0611244104
77. Betts MR, Nason MC, West SM, De Rosa SC, Migueles SA, Abraham J, et al. HIV nonprogressors preferentially maintain highly functional HIV-specific CD8$^+$ T cells. *Blood.* (2006) 107:4781–89. doi: 10.1182/blood-2005-12-4818
78. Borrow P, Lewicki H, Wei X, Horwitz MS, Peffer N, Meyers H, et al. Antiviral pressure exerted by HIV-1-specific cytotoxic T lymphocytes (CTLs) during primary infection demonstrated by rapid selection of CTL escape virus. *Nat Med.* (1997) 3:205–11. doi: 10.1038/nm0297-205

79. Cartwright EK, Spicer L, Smith SA, Lee D, Fast R, Paganini S, et al. $CD8^+$ lymphocytes are required for maintaining viral suppression in SIV-infected macaques treated with short-term antiretroviral therapy. *Immunity.* (2016) 45:656–68. doi: 10.1016/j.immuni.2016.08.018
80. Makedonas G, Betts MR. Living in a house of cards: re-evaluating $CD8^+$ T-cell immune correlates against HIV. *Immunol Rev.* (2011) 239:109–24. doi: 10.1111/j.1600-065X.2010.00968.x
81. Roberts ER, Carnathan DG, Li H, Shaw GM, Silvestri G, Betts MR. Collapse of cytolytic potential in SIV-specific $CD8^+$ T cells following acute siv infection in rhesus macaques. *PLoS Pathog.* (2016) 12:e1006135. doi: 10.1371/journal.ppat.1006135
82. Demers KR, Makedonas G, Buggert M, Eller MA, Ratcliffe SJ, Goonetilleke N, et al. Temporal dynamics of $CD8^+$ T cell effector responses during primary HIV infection. *PLoS Pathog.* (2016) 12:e1005805. doi: 10.1371/journal.ppat.1005805
83. Day CL, Kaufmann DE, Kiepiela P, Brown JA, Moodley ES, Reddy S, et al. PD-1 expression on HIV-specific T cells is associated with T-cell exhaustion and disease progression. *Nature.* (2006) 443:350–4. doi: 10.1038/nature05115
84. Appay V, Papagno L, Spina CA, Hansasuta P, King A, Jones L, et al. Dynamics of T cell responses in HIV infection. *J Immunol.* (2002) 168:3660–6. doi: 10.4049/jimmunol.168.7.3660
85. Champagne P, Ogg GS, King AS, Knabenhans C, Ellefsen K, Nobile M, et al. Skewed maturation of memory HIV-specific CD8 T lymphocytes. *Nature.* (2001) 410:106–11. doi: 10.1038/35065118
86. Hoffmann M, Pantazis N, Martin GE, Hickling S, Hurst J, Meyerowitz J, et al. Exhaustion of activated CD8 T cells predicts disease progression in primary HIV-1 infection. *PLoS Pathog.* (2016) 12:1–19. doi: 10.1371/journal.ppat.1005661
87. Papagno L, Spina CA, Marchant A, Salio M, Rufer N, Little S, et al. Immune activation and $CD8^+$ T-cell differentiation towards senescence in HIV-1 infection. *PLoS Biol.* (2004) 2:e20. doi: 10.1371/journal.pbio.0020020
88. Helleberg M, Kronborg G, Ullum H, Ryder LP, Obel N, Gerstoft J. Course and clinical significance of $CD8^+$ T-cell counts in a large cohort of HIV-infected individuals. *J Infect Dis.* (2015) 211:1726–34. doi: 10.1093/infdis/jiu669
89. Roederer M, Dubs JG, Anderson MT, Raju PA, Herzenberg LA, Herzenberg LA. CD8 naive T cell counts decrease progressively in HIV-infected adults. *J Clin Invest.* (1995) 95:2061–6. doi: 10.1172/JCI117892
90. Chen G, Shankar P, Lange C, Valdez H, Skolnik PR, Wu L, et al. CD8 T cells specific for human immunodeficiency virus, Epstein-Barr virus, and cytomegalovirus lack molecules for homing to lymphoid sites of infection. *Blood.* (2001) 98:156–64. doi: 10.1182/blood.V98.1.156
91. Hunt PW, Martin JN, Sinclair E, Bredt B, Hagos E, Lampiris H, et al. T cell activation is associated with lower CD4+ T cell gains in human immunodeficiency virus-infected patients with sustained viral suppression during antiretroviral therapy. *J Infect Dis.* (2003) 187:1534–43. doi: 10.1086/374786
92. Kuchroo VK, Anderson AC, Petrovas C. Coinhibitory receptors and CD8 T cell exhaustion in chronic infections. *Curr Opin HIV AIDS.* (2014) 9:439–45. doi: 10.1097/COH.0000000000000088
93. Lindgren T, Ahlm C, Mohamed N, Evander M, Ljunggren H-G, Bjorkstrom NK. Longitudinal analysis of the human T cell response during acute hantavirus infection. *J Virol.* (2011) 85:10252–60. doi: 10.1128/JVI.05548-11
94. McElroy AK, Akondy RS, Harmon JR, Ellebedy AH, Cannon D, Klena JD, et al. A case of human lassa virus infection with robust acute T-cell activation and long-term virus-specific T-cell responses. *J Infect Dis.* (2017) 215:1862–72. doi: 10.1093/infdis/jix201
95. Chandele A, Sewatanon J, Gunisetty S, Singla M, Onlamoon N, Akondy RS, et al. Characterization of human CD8 T cell responses in dengue virus-infected patients from India. *J Virol.* (2016) 90:11259–78. doi: 10.1128/JVI.01424-16
96. Akondy RS, Monson ND, Miller JD, Edupuganti S, Teuwen D, Wu H, et al. The yellow fever virus vaccine induces a broad and polyfunctional human memory $CD8^+$ T cell response. *J Immunol.* (2009) 183:7919–30. doi: 10.4049/jimmunol.0803903
97. Peretz Y, He Z, Shi Y, Yassine-Diab B, Goulet JP, Bordi R, et al. CD160 and PD-1 co-expression on HIV-specific CD8 T cells defines a subset with advanced dysfunction. *PLoS Pathog.* (2012) 8:e1002840. doi: 10.1371/journal.ppat.1002840
98. Lichterfeld M, Kaufmann DE, Yu XG, Mui SK, Addo MM, Johnston MN, et al. Loss of HIV-1–specific $CD8^+$ T cell proliferation after acute HIV-1 infection and restoration by vaccine-induced HIV-1–specific $CD4^+$ T cells. *J Exp Med.* (2004) 200:701–12 doi: 10.1084/jem.20041270
99. Day CL, Kiepiela P, Leslie AJ, van der Stok M, Nair K, Ismail N, et al. Proliferative capacity of epitope-specific CD8 T-cell responses is inversely related to viral load in chronic human immunodeficiency virus type 1 infection. *J Virol.* (2007) 81:434–8. doi: 10.1128/JVI.01754-06
100. Yan J, Sabbaj S, Bansal A, Amatya N, Shacka JJ, Goepfert PA, et al. HIV-specific $CD8^+$ T cells from elite controllers are primed for survival. *J Virol.* (2013) 87:5170–81. doi: 10.1128/JVI.02379-12
101. Gaardbo JC, Hartling HJ, Thorsteinsson K, Ullum H, Nielsen SD. CD3+CD8+CD161high Tc17 cells are depleted in HIV-infection. *AIDS.* (2013) 27:659–62. doi: 10.1097/QAD.0b013e32835b8cb3
102. Cosgrove C, Ussher JE, Rauch A, Gärtner K, Kurioka A, Hühn MH, et al. Early and nonreversible decrease of CD161++/MAIT cells in HIV infection. *Blood.* (2013) 121:951–61. doi: 10.1182/blood-2012-06-436436
103. Nigam P, Kwa S, Velu V, Amara RR. Loss of IL-17-producing CD8 T cells during late chronic stage of pathogenic simian immunodeficiency virus infection. *J Immunol.* (2011) 186:745–53. doi: 10.4049/jimmunol.1002807
104. Hua S, Lécuroux C, Sáez-Cirión A, Pancino G, Girault I, Versmisse P, et al. Potential role for HIV-specific CD38-/HLA-DR+ CD8+ T cells in viral suppression and cytotoxicity in HIV controllers. *PLoS ONE.* (2014) 9:2–11. doi: 10.1186/1471-2334-14-S2-P64
105. Bastidas S, Graw F, Smith MZ, Kuster H, Gunthard HF, Oxenius A. CD8+ T cells are activated in an antigen-independent manner in HIV-infected individuals. *J Immunol.* (2014) 192:1732–44. doi: 10.4049/jimmunol.1302027
106. Doisne J-M, Urrutia A, Lacabaratz-Porret C, Goujard C, Meyer L, Chaix M-L, et al. CD8+ T cells specific for EBV, cytomegalovirus, and influenza virus are activated during primary HIV infection. *J Immunol.* (2004) 173:2410–8. doi: 10.4049/jimmunol.173 4.2410
107. Betts MR, Ambrozak DR, Douek DC, Bonhoeffer S, Brenchley JM, Casazza JP, et al. Analysis of total human immunodeficiency virus (HIV)-specific CD4+ and CD8+ T-cell responses: relationship to viral load in untreated HIV infection. *J Virol.* (2001) 75:11983–91. doi: 10.1128/JVI.75.24.11983-11991.2001
108. Casazza JP, Betts MR, Picker LJ, Koup RA. Decay kinetics of human immunodeficiency virus-specific CD8? T cells in peripheral blood after initiation of highly active antiretroviral therapy. *J Virol.* (2001) 75:6508–16. doi: 10.1128/JVI.75.14.6508-6516.2001
109. Estes JD, Kityo C, Ssali F, Swainson L, Makamdop KN, Del Prete GQ, et al. Defining total-body AIDS-virus burden with implications for curative strategies. *Nat Med.* (2017) 23:1271–6. doi: 10.1038/nm.4411
110. Fletcher CV, Staskus K, Wietgrefe SW, Rothenberger M, Reilly C, Chipman JG, et al. Persistent HIV-1 replication is associated with lower antiretroviral drug concentrations in lymphatic tissues. *Proc Natl Acad Sci USA.* (2014) 111:2307–12. doi: 10.1073/pnas.1318249111
111. Ferre AL, Hunt PW, Critchfield JW, Young DH, Morris MM, Garcia JC, et al. Mucosal immune responses to HIV-1 in elite controllers: a potential correlate of immune control. *Blood.* (2009) 113:3978–89. doi: 10.1182/blood-2008-10-182709
112. Critchfield JW, Young DH, Hayes TL, Braun JV, Garcia JC, Pollard RB, et al. Magnitude and complexity of rectal mucosa HIV-1-specific CD8+ T-cell responses during chronic infection reflect clinical status. *PLoS ONE.* (2008) 3:e3577. doi: 10.1371/journal.pone.0003577
113. Rehr M, Cahenzli J, Haas A, Price DA, Gostick E, Huber M, et al. Emergence of polyfunctional CD8+ T cells after prolonged suppression of human immunodeficiency virus replication by antiretroviral therapy. *J Virol.* (2008) 82:3391–404. doi: 10.1128/JVI.02383-07
114. Streeck H, Brumme ZL, Anastario M, Cohen KW, Jolin JS, Meier A, et al. Antigen load and viral sequence diversification determine the functional profile of HIV-1-specific CD8+ T cells. *PLoS Med.* (2008) 5:e100. doi: 10.1371/journal.pmed.0050100
115. Rinaldo CRJ, Huang XL, Fan Z, Margolick JB, Borowski L, Hoji A, et al. Anti-human immunodeficiency virus type 1 (HIV-1) CD8(+) T-lymphocyte reactivity during combination antiretroviral therapy in HIV-1-infected patients with advanced immunodeficiency. *J Virol.* (2000) 74:4127–38. doi: 10.1128/JVI.74.9.4127-4138.2000

116. Garcia F, Plana M, Vidal C, Cruceta A, O'Brien WA, Pantaleo G, et al. Dynamics of viral load rebound and immunological changes after stopping effective antiretroviral therapy. *AIDS.* (1999) 13:F79–86. doi: 10.1097/00002030-199907300-00002
117. Serwanga J, Mugaba S, Betty A, Pimego E, Walker S, Munderi P, et al. CD8 T-cell responses before and after structured treatment interruption in ugandan adults who initiated ART with CD4 T cells <200 cell/muL: the DART trial STI substudy. *AIDS Res Treat.* (2011) 2011:875028. doi: 10.1155/2011/875028
118. Tanko RF, Soares AP, Masson L, Garrett NJ, Samsunder N, Abdool Karim Q, et al. Residual T cell activation and skewed CD8+ T cell memory differentiation despite antiretroviral therapy-induced HIV suppression. *Clin Immunol.* (2018) 195:127–38. doi: 10.1016/j.clim.2018.06.001
119. Trautmann L, Janbazian L, Chomont N, Said EA, Gimmig S, Bessette B, et al. Upregulation of PD-1 expression on HIV-specific CD8+ T cells leads to reversible immune dysfunction. *Nat Med.* (2006) 12:1198–202. doi: 10.1038/nm1106-1329b
120. Perdomo-Celis F, Feria MG, Taborda NA, Rugeles MT. A low frequency of IL-17-producing CD8+ T-cells is associated with persistent immune activation in people living with HIV despite HAART-induced viral suppression. *Front Immunol.* (2018) 9:2502. doi: 10.3389/fimmu.2018.02502
121. Migueles SA, Weeks KA, Nou E, Berkley AM, Rood JE, Osborne CM, et al. Defective human immunodeficiency virus-specific CD8+ T-cell polyfunctionality, proliferation, and cytotoxicity are not restored by antiretroviral therapy. *J Virol.* (2009) 83:11876–89. doi: 10.1128/JVI.01153-09
122. Kelleher AD, Sewell WA, Cooper DA. Effect of protease therapy on cytokine secretion by peripheral blood mononuclear cells (PBMC) from HIV-infected subjects. *Clin Exp Immunol.* (1999) 115:147–52. doi: 10.1046/j.1365-2249.1999.00761.x
123. Perdomo-Celis F, Velilla PA, Taborda NA, Rugeles MT. An altered cytotoxic program of CD8+ T-cells in HIV-infected patients despite HAART-induced viral suppression. *PLoS ONE.* (2019) 14:e0210540. doi: 10.1371/journal.pone.0210540
124. Cao W, Mehraj V, Trottier B, Baril JG, Leblanc R, Lebouche B, et al. Early initiation rather than prolonged duration of antiretroviral therapy in hiv infection contributes to the normalization of CD8 T-cell counts. *Clin Infect Dis.* (2016) 62:250–7. doi: 10.1093/cid/civ809
125. Jenabian MA, El-Far M, Vyboh K, Kema I, Costiniuk CT, Thomas R, et al. Immunosuppressive tryptophan catabolism and gut mucosal dysfunction following early HIV infection. *J Infect Dis.* 212:355–66. doi: 10.1093/infdis/jiv037
126. Ogg GS, Jin X, Bonhoeffer S, Moss P, Nowak MA, Monard S, et al. Decay kinetics of human immunodeficiency virus-specific effector cytotoxic T lymphocytes after combination antiretroviral therapy. *J Virol.* (1999) 73:797–800.
127. Mollet L, Li TS, Samri A, Tournay C, Tubiana R, Calvez V, et al. Dynamics of HIV-specific CD8+ T lymphocytes with changes in viral load.The RESTIM and COMET Study Groups. *J Immunol.* (2000) 165:1692–704. doi: 10.4049/jimmunol.165.3.1692
128. Altfeld M, Van Lunzen J, Frahm N, Yu XG, Schneider C, Eldridge RL, et al. Expansion of pre-existing, lymph node-localized CD8+ T cells during supervised treatment interruptions in chronic HIV-1 infection. *J Clin Invest.* (2002) 109:837–43. doi: 10.1172/JCI14789
129. Killian MS, Roop J, Ng S, Hecht FM, Levy JA. CD8+ cell anti-HIV activity rapidly increases upon discontinuation of early antiretroviral therapy. *J Clin Immunol.* (2009) 29:311–8. doi: 10.1007/s10875-009-9275-y
130. Kaufmann DE, Lichterfeld M, Altfeld M, Addo MM, Johnston MN, Lee PK, et al. Limited durability of viral control following treated acute HIV infection. *PLoS Med.* (2004) 1:e36. doi: 10.1371/journal.pmed.00 10036
131. McLane LM, Abdel-Hakeem MS, Wherry EJ. CD8 T cell exhaustion during chronic viral infection and cancer. *Annu Rev Immunol.* (2019) 37:457–95. doi: 10.1146/annurev-immunol-041015-05 5318
132. Chevalier MF, Julg B, Pyo A, Flanders M, Ranasinghe S, Soghoian DZ, et al. HIV-1-specific interleukin-21+ CD4+ T cell responses contribute to durable viral control through the modulation of HIV-specific CD8+ T cell function. *J Virol.* (2011) 85:733–41. doi: 10.1128/JVI.02 030-10
133. Schweneker M, Favre D, Martin JN, Deeks SG, Joseph M, McCune JM. HIV-induced changes in T cell signaling pathways. *J Immunol.* (2008) 180:6490–500. doi: 10.4049/jimmunol.180.10.6490
134. Dornadula G, Zhang H, VanUitert B, Stern J, Livornese LJ, Ingerman MJ, et al. Residual HIV-1 RNA in blood plasma of patients taking suppressive highly active antiretroviral therapy. *JAMA.* (1999) 282:1627–32. doi: 10.1001/jama.282.17.1627
135. Ouedraogo DE, Makinson A, Vendrell JP, Casanova ML, Nagot N, Cezar R, et al. Pivotal role of HIV and EBV replication in the long-term persistence of monoclonal gammopathy in patients on antiretroviral therapy. *Blood.* (2013) 122:3030–3. doi: 10.1182/blood-2012-12-470393
136. Kuller LH, Tracy R, Belloso W, De Wit S, Drummond F, Lane HC, et al. Inflammatory and coagulation biomarkers and mortality in patients with HIV infection. *PLoS Med.* (2008) 5:e203. doi: 10.1371/journal.pmed.0050203
137. Baker JV, Neuhaus J, Duprez D, Kuller LH, Tracy R, Belloso WH, et al. Changes in inflammatory and coagulation biomarkers: a randomized comparison of immediate versus deferred antiretroviral therapy in patients with HIV infection. *J Acquir Immune Defic Syndr.* (2011) 56:36–43. doi: 10.1097/QAI.0b013e3181f7f61a
138. Neuhaus J, Jacobs DR Jr, Baker JV, Calmy A, Duprez D, La Rosa A, et al. Markers of inflammation, coagulation, and renal function are elevated in adults with HIV infection. *J Infect Dis.* (2010) 201:1788–95. doi: 10.1086/652749
139. Paiardini M, Müller-Trutwin M. HIV-associated chronic immune activation. *Immunol Rev.* (2013) 254:78–101. doi: 10.1111/imr.12079
140. Kestens L, Vanham G, Gigase P, Young G, Hannet I, Vanlangendonck F, et al. Expression of activation antigens, HLA-DR and CD38, on CD8 lymphocytes during HIV-1 infection. *AIDS.* (1992) 6:793–7. doi: 10.1097/00002030-199208000-00004
141. Boasso A, Shearer GM, Chougnet C. Immune dysregulation in human immunodeficiency virus infection: know it, fix it, prevent it? *J Intern Med.* (2009) 265:78–96. doi: 10.1111/j.1365-2796.2008.02043.x
142. Biancotto A, Iglehart SJ, Vanpouille C, Condack CE, Lisco A, Ruecker E, et al. HIV-1-induced activation of CD4+T cells creates new targets for HIV-1 infection in human lymphoid tissue *ex vivo*. *Blood.* (2008) 111:699–704. doi: 10.1182/blood-2007-05-088435
143. Schacker TW, Brenchley JM, Beilman GJ, Reilly C, Pambuccian SE, Taylor J, et al. Lymphatic tissue fibrosis is associated with reduced numbers of naïve CD4+ T cells in human immunodeficiency virus type 1 infection. *Clin Vaccine Immunol.* (2006) 13:556–60. doi: 10.1128/CVI.13.5.556-560.2006
144. Douek DC, Betts MR, Hill BJ, Little SJ, Lempicki R, Metcalf JA, et al. Evidence for increased T cell turnover and decreased thymic output in HIV infection. *J Immunol.* (2001) 167:6663–8. doi: 10.4049/jimmunol.167.11.6663
145. Moroni M, Antinori S. HIV and direct damage of organs: disease spectrum before and during the highly active antiretroviral therapy era. *AIDS.* (2003) 17 (Suppl 1):S51–64. doi: 10.1097/00002030-200304001-00008
146. Chahroudi A, Bosinger SE, Vanderford TH, Paiardini M, Silvestri G. Natural SIV hosts: showing AIDS the door. *Science.* (2012) 335:1188–93. doi: 10.1126/science.1217550
147. Goicoechea M, Smith D, Liu L. Determinants of CD4+ T cell recovery during suppressive antiretroviral therapy: association of immune activation, T cell maturation markers, and cellular HIV-1 DNA. *J Infect.* (2006) 194:29–37. doi: 10.1086/504718
148. Sandler NG, Wand H, Roque A, Law M, Nason MC, Nixon DE, et al. Plasma levels of soluble CD14 independently predict mortality in HIV infection. *J Infect Dis.* (2011) 203:780–90. doi: 10.1093/infdis/jiq118
149. Hunt PW, Sinclair E, Rodriguez B, Shive C, Clagett B, Funderburg N, et al. Gut epithelial barrier dysfunction and innate immune activation predict mortality in treated HIV infection. *J Infect Dis.* (2014) 210:1228–38. doi: 10.1093/infdis/jiu238
150. Cheru LT, Park EA, Saylor CF, Burdo TH, Fitch KV, Looby S, et al. I-FABP is higher in people with chronic hiv than elite controllers, related to sugar and fatty acid intake and inversely related to body fat in people with HIV. *Open forum Infect Dis.* (2018) 5:ofy288. doi: 10.1093/ofid/ofy288

151. Chun T-W, Nickle DC, Justement JS, Meyers JH, Roby G, Hallahan CW, et al. Persistence of HIV in gut-associated lymphoid tissue despite long-term antiretroviral therapy. *J Infect Dis.* (2008) 197:714–20. doi: 10.1086/527324
152. Wong JK, Gunthard HF, Havlir DV, Zhang ZQ, Haase AT, Ignacio CC, et al. Reduction of HIV-1 in blood and lymph nodes following potent antiretroviral therapy and the virologic correlates of treatment failure. *Proc Natl Acad Sci USA.* (1997) 94:12574–9. doi: 10.1073/pnas.94.23.12574
153. Perreau M, Savoye A-L, De Crignis E, Corpataux J-M, Cubas R, Haddad EK, et al. Follicular helper T cells serve as the major CD4 T cell compartment for HIV-1 infection, replication, and production. *J Exp Med.* (2013) 216:143–56. doi: 10.1084/jem.20121932
154. Spiegel H, Herbst H, Niedobitek G, Foss HD, Stein H. Follicular dendritic cells are a major reservoir for human immunodeficiency virus type 1 in lymphoid tissues facilitating infection of CD4+ T-helper cells. *Am J Pathol.* (1992) 140:15–22.
155. Gunthard HF, Havlir DV, Fiscus S, Zhang ZQ, Eron J, Mellors J, et al. Residual human immunodeficiency virus (HIV) Type 1 RNA and DNA in lymph nodes and HIV RNA in genital secretions and in cerebrospinal fluid after suppression of viremia for 2 years. *J Infect Dis.* (2001) 183:1318–27. doi: 10.1086/319864
156. Brenchley JM, Douek DC. HIV infection and the gastrointestinal immune system. *Mucosal Immunol.* (2008) 1:23–30. doi: 10.1038/sj.mi.2007.1750001
157. Klatt NR, Estes JD, Sun X, Ortiz AM, Barber JS, Harris LD, et al. Loss of mucosal CD103 DCs and IL-17 and IL-22 lymphocytes is associated with mucosal damage in SIV infection. *Mucosal Immunol.* (2012) 5:646–57. doi: 10.1038/mi.2012.38
158. Ryan ES, Micci L, Fromentin R, Paganini S, McGary CS, Easley K, et al. Loss of function of intestinal IL-17 and IL-22 producing cells contributes to inflammation and viral persistence in SIV-infected rhesus macaques. *PLoS Pathog.* (2016) 12:e1005412. doi: 10.1371/journal.ppat.1005412
159. Estes JD, Harris LD, Klatt NR, Tabb B, Pittaluga S, Paiardini M, et al. Damaged intestinal epithelial integrity linked to microbial translocation in pathogenic simian immunodeficiency virus infections. *PLoS Pathog.* (2010) 6:e1001052. doi: 10.1371/journal.ppat.1001052
160. Chung CY, Alden SL, Funderburg NT, Fu P, Levine AD. Progressive proximal-to-distal reduction in expression of the tight junction complex in colonic epithelium of virally-suppressed HIV+ individuals. *PLoS Pathog.* (2014) 10:e1004198. doi: 10.1371/journal.ppat.1004198
161. Dinh DM, Volpe GE, Duffalo C, Bhalchandra S, Tai AK, Kane AV, et al. Intestinal Microbiota, microbial translocation, and systemic inflammation in chronic HIV infection. *J Infect Dis.* (2015) 211:19–27. doi: 10.1093/infdis/jiu409
162. Sandler NG, Douek DC. Microbial translocation in HIV infection: causes, consequences and treatment opportunities. *Nat Rev Microbiol.* (2012) 10:655–66. doi: 10.1038/nrmicro2848
163. Lore K, Betts MR, Brenchley JM, Kuruppu J, Khojasteh S, Perfetto S, et al. Toll-like receptor ligands modulate dendritic cells to augment cytomegalovirus- and HIV-1-specific T cell responses. *J Immunol.* (2003) 171:4320–8. doi: 10.4049/jimmunol.171.8.4320
164. Svard J, Paquin-Proulx D, Buggert M, Noyan K, Barqasho B, Sonnerborg A, et al. Role of translocated bacterial flagellin in monocyte activation among individuals with chronic HIV-1 infection. *Clin Immunol.* (2015) 161:180–9. doi: 10.1016/j.clim.2015.08.018
165. Hammond T, Lee S, Watson MW, Flexman JP, Cheng W, Fernandez S, et al. Toll-like receptor (TLR) expression on CD4+ and CD8+ T-cells in patients chronically infected with hepatitis C virus. *Cell Immunol.* (2010) 264:150–5. doi: 10.1016/j.cellimm.2010.06.001
166. Tripathy A, Khanna S, Padhan P, Smita S, Raghav S, Gupta B. Direct recognition of LPS drive TLR4 expressing CD8(+) T cell activation in patients with rheumatoid arthritis. *Sci Rep.* (2017) 7:933. doi: 10.1038/s41598-017-01033-7
167. Miller Sanders C, Cruse JM, Lewis RE. Toll-like receptor and chemokine receptor expression in HIV-infected T lymphocyte subsets. *Exp Mol Pathol.* (2010) 88:26–31. doi: 10.1016/j.yexmp.2009.09.006
168. Song Y, Zhuang Y, Zhai S, Huang D, Zhang Y, Kang W, et al. Increased expression of TLR7 in CD8(+) T cells leads to TLR7-mediated activation and accessory cell-dependent IFN-gamma production in HIV type 1 infection. *AIDS Res Hum Retroviruses.* (2009) 25:1287–95. doi: 10.1089/aid.2008.0303
169. Funderburg N, Luciano AA, Jiang W, Rodriguez B, Sieg SF, Lederman MM. Toll-like receptor ligands induce human T cell activation and death, a model for HIV pathogenesis. *PLoS ONE.* (2008) 3:e1915. doi: 10.1371/journal.pone.0001915
170. Thibault S, Tardif MR, Barat C, Tremblay MJ. TLR2 signaling renders quiescent naive and memory CD4+ T cells more susceptible to productive infection with X4 and R5 HIV-type 1. *J Immunol.* (2007) 179:4357–66. doi: 10.4049/jimmunol.179.7.4357
171. Mercier BC, Cottalorda A, Coupet C-A, Marvel J, Bonnefoy-Berard N. TLR2 engagement on CD8 T cells enables generation of functional memory cells in response to a suboptimal TCR signal. *J Immunol.* (2009) 182:1860–7. doi: 10.4049/jimmunol.0801167
172. Brenchley JM, Price DA, Schacker TW, Asher TE, Silvestri G, Rao S, et al. Microbial translocation is a cause of systemic immune activation in chronic HIV infection. *Nat Med.* (2006) 12:1365–71. doi: 10.1038/nm1511
173. Stacey AR, Norris PJ, Qin L, Haygreen EA, Taylor E, Heitman J, et al. Induction of a striking systemic cytokine cascade prior to peak viremia in acute human immunodeficiency virus type 1 infection, in contrast to more modest and delayed responses in acute hepatitis B and C virus infections. *J Virol.* (2009) 83:3719–33. doi: 10.1128/JVI.01844-08
174. Yamamoto T, Price DA, Casazza JP, Ferrari G, Nason M, Chattopadhyay PK, et al. Surface expression patterns of negative regulatory molecules identify determinants of virus-specific CD8+ T-cell exhaustion in HIV infection. *Blood.* (2011) 117:4805–15. doi: 10.1182/blood-2010-11-317297
175. Wherry EJ, Kurachi M. Molecular and cellular insights into T cell exhaustion. *Nat Rev Immunol.* (2015) 15:486–99. doi: 10.1038/nri3862
176. Chun T-W, Justement JS, Sanford C, Hallahan CW, Planta MA, Loutfy M, et al. Relationship between the frequency of HIV-specific CD8+ T cells and the level of CD38+CD8+ T cells in untreated HIV-infected individuals. *Proc Natl Acad Sci USA.* (2004) 101:2464–9. doi: 10.1073/pnas.0307328101
177. Petrovas C, Casazza JP, Brenchley JM, Price DA, Gostick E, Adams WC, et al. PD-1 is a regulator of virus-specific CD8+ T cell survival in HIV infection. *J Exp Med.* (2006) 203:2281–92. doi: 10.1084/jem.20061496
178. Leeansyah E, Ganesh A, Quigley MF, Sönnerborg A, Andersson J, Hunt PW, et al. Activation, exhaustion, and persistent decline of the antimicrobial MR1-restricted MAIT-cell population in chronic HIV-1 infection. *Blood.* (2013) 121:1124–35. doi: 10.1182/blood-2012-07-445429
179. Sen DR, Kaminski J, Barnitz RA, Kurachi M, Gerdemann U, Yates KB, et al. The epigenetic landscape of T cell exhaustion. *Science.* (2016) 354:1165–9. doi: 10.1126/science.aae0491
180. Bengsch B, Johnson AL, Kurachi M, Odorizzi PM, Pauken KE, Attanasio J, et al. Bioenergetic insufficiencies due to metabolic alterations regulated by the inhibitory receptor PD-1 are an early driver of CD8+ T cell exhaustion. *Immunity.* (2016) 45:358–73. doi: 10.1016/j.immuni.2016.07.008
181. Llibre JM, Buzon MJ, Massanella M, Esteve A, Dahl V, Puertas MC, et al. Treatment intensification with raltegravir in subjects with sustained HIV-1 viraemia suppression: a randomized 48-week study. *Antivir Ther.* (2012) 17:355–64. doi: 10.3851/IMP1917
182. Buzón JM, Massanella M, Llibre JM, Esteve A, Dahl V, Puertas MC, et al. HIV-1 replication and immune dynamics are affected by raltegravir intensification of HAART-suppressed subjects. *Nat Med.* (2010) 16:460–5. doi: 10.1038/nm.2111
183. Nicastri E, Tommasi C, Abbate I, Bonora S, Tempestilli M, Bellagamba R, et al. Effect of raltegravir on the total and unintegrated proviral HIV DNA during raltegravir-based HAART. *Antivir Ther.* (2011) 16:797–803. doi: 10.3851/IMP1833
184. Hatano H, Strain MC, Scherzer R, Bacchetti P, Wentworth D, Hoh R, et al. Increase in 2-long terminal repeat circles and decrease in D-dimer after raltegravir intensification in patients with treated HIV Infection: a randomized, placebo-controlled trial. *J Infect Dis.* (2013) 208:1436–42. doi: 10.1093/infdis/jit453
185. Arponen S, Benito J, Lozano S, Blanco F, Garrido C, De Mendoza C. More pronounced effect of integrase inhibitor Raltegravir on proviral DNA reduction that other antiretroviral drugs in patients achieving undetectable viremia. In: *15TH Conference on Retroviruses and Opportunistic Infections # 796.* Boston, MA (2008)

186. Bandera A, Colella E, Rizzardini G, Gori A, Clerici M. Strategies to limit immune-activation in HIV patients. *Expert Rev Anti Infect Ther.* (2017) 15:43–54. doi: 10.1080/14787210.2017.1250624
187. Nakanjako D, Ssinabulya I, Nabatanzi R, Bayigga L, Kiragga A, Joloba M, et al. Atorvastatin reduces T-cell activation and exhaustion among HIV-infected cART-treated suboptimal immune responders in Uganda: a randomised crossover placebo-controlled trial. *Trop Med Int Health.* (2015) 20:380–90. doi: 10.1111/tmi.12442
188. Ganesan A, Crum-Cianflone N, Higgins J, Qin J, Rehm C, Metcalf J, et al. High dose atorvastatin decreases cellular markers of immune activation without affecting HIV-1 RNA levels: results of a double-blind randomized placebo controlled clinical trial. *J Infect Dis.* (2011) 203:756–64. doi: 10.1093/infdis/jiq115
189. Funderburg NT, Jiang Y, Debanne SM, Labbato D, Juchnowski S, Ferrari B, et al. Rosuvastatin reduces vascular inflammation and T-cell and monocyte activation in HIV-infected subjects on antiretroviral therapy. *J Acquir Immune Defic Syndr.* (2015) 68:396–404. doi: 10.1097/QAI.0000000000000478
190. Plosker GL, Croom KF. Sulfasalazine: a review of its use in the management of rheumatoid arthritis. *Drugs.* (2005) 65:1825–49. doi: 10.2165/00003495-200565130-00008
191. Szabo C, Haskó G, Szabó C, Németh ZH, Deitch EA. Sulphasalazine inhibits macrophage activation: inhibitory effects on inducible nitric oxide synthase expression, interleukin-12 production and major histocompatibility complex II expression. *Immunology.* (2001) 103:473-8. doi: 10.1046/j.1365-2567.2001.01272.x
192. Rodenburg RJT, Ganga A, Van Lent PLEM, Van De Putte LBA, Van Venrooij WJ. The antiinflammatory drug sulfasalazine inhibits tumor necrosis factor alpha expression in macrophages by inducing apoptosis. *Arthritis Rheum.* (2000) 43:1941–50. doi: 10.1002/1529-0131(200009)43:9<1941::AID-ANR4>3.0.CO;2-O
193. Liptay S, Bachem M, Häcker G, Adler G, Debatin KM, Schmid RM. Inhibition of nuclear factor kappa B and induction of apoptosis in T-lymphocytes by sulfasalazine. *Br J Pharmacol.* (1999) 128:1361–9. doi: 10.1038/sj.bjp.0702937
194. Schneider T, Ullrich R, Bergs C, Schmidt W, Riecken EO, Zeitz M. Abnormalities in subset distribution, activation, and differentiation of T cells isolated from large intestine biopsies in HIV infection. The Berlin Diarrhoea/Wasting Syndrome Study Group. *Clin Exp Immunol.* (1994) 95:430–5.
195. Sortino O, Richards E, Dias J, Leeansyah E, Sandberg JK, Sereti I. IL-7 treatment supports CD8+ mucosa-associated invariant T-cell restoration in HIV-1-infected patients on antiretroviral therapy. *AIDS.* (2018) 32:825–8. doi: 10.1097/QAD.0000000000001760
196. Leeansyah E, Svärd J, Dias J, Buggert M, Nyström J, Quigley MF, et al. Arming of MAIT cell cytolytic antimicrobial activity is induced by IL-7 and defective in HIV-1 infection. *PLoS Pathog.* (2015) 11:e1005072. doi: 10.1371/journal.ppat.1005072
197. Li Y, Bleakley M, Yee C. IL-21 influences the frequency, phenotype, and affinity of the antigen-specific CD8 T cell response. *J Immunol.* (2005) 175:2261–9. doi: 10.4049/jimmunol.175.4.2261
198. Novy P, Huang X, Leonard WJ, Yang Y. Intrinsic IL-21 signaling is critical for CD8 T cell survival and memory formation in response to vaccinia viral infection. *J Immunol.* (2011) 186:2729–38. doi: 10.4049/jimmunol.1003009
199. White L, Krishnan S, Strbo N, Liu H, Kolber MA, Lichtenheld MG, et al. Differential effects of IL-21 and IL-15 on perforin expression, lysosomal degranulation, and proliferation in CD8 T cells of patients with human immunodeficiency virus-1 (HIV). *Blood.* (2007) 109:3873–80. doi: 10.1182/blood-2006-09-045278
200. Pallikkuth S, Rogers K, Villinger F, Dosterii M, Vaccari M, Franchini G, et al. Interleukin-21 administration to rhesus macaques chronically infected with simian immunodeficiency virus increases cytotoxic effector molecules in T cells and NK cells and enhances B cell function without increasing immune activation or viral replication. *Vaccine.* (2011) 29:9229–38. doi: 10.1016/j.vaccine.2011.09.118
201. Watson DC, Moysi E, Valentin A, Bergamaschi C, Devasundaram S, Fortis SP, et al. Treatment with native heterodimeric IL-15 increases cytotoxic lymphocytes and reduces SHIV RNA in lymph nodes. *PLoS Pathog.* (2018) 14:e1006902. doi: 10.1371/journal.ppat.1006902
202. Webb GM, Li S, Mwakalundwa G, Folkvord JM, Greene JM, Reed JS, et al. The human IL-15 superagonist ALT-803 directs SIV-specific CD8+ T cells into B-cell follicles. *Blood Adv.* (2018) 2:76–84. doi: 10.1182/bloodadvances.2017012971
203. Velu V, Kannanganat S, Ibegbu C, Chennareddi L, Villinger F, Freeman GJ, et al. Elevated expression levels of inhibitory receptor programmed death 1 on simian immunodeficiency virus-specific CD8 T cells during chronic infection but not after vaccination. *J Virol.* (2007) 81:5819–28. doi: 10.1128/JVI.00024-07
204. Velu V, Titanji K, Zhu B, Husain S, Pladevega A, Lai L, et al. Enhancing SIV-specific immunity *in vivo* by PD-1 blockade. *Nature.* (2009) 458:206–10. doi: 10.1038/nature07662
205. Dyavar Shetty R, Velu V, Titanji K, Bosinger SE, Freeman GJ, Silvestri G, et al. PD-1 blockade during chronic SIV infection reduces hyperimmune activation and microbial translocation in rhesus macaques. *J Clin Invest.* (2012) 122:1712–6. doi: 10.1172/JCI60612
206. Mylvaganam GH, Chea LS, Tharp GK, Hicks S, Velu V, Iyer SS, et al. Combination anti-PD-1 and antiretroviral therapy provides therapeutic benefit against SIV. *JCI Insight.* (2018) 3:122940. doi: 10.1172/jci.insight.122940
207. Im SJ, Hashimoto M, Gerner MY, Lee J, Kissick HT, Burger MC, et al. Defining CD8+T cells that provide the proliferative burst after PD-1 therapy. *Nature.* (2016) 537:417–21. doi: 10.1038/nature19330
208. Fromentin R, DaFonseca S, Costiniuk CT, El-Far M, Procopio FA, Hecht FM, et al. PD-1 blockade potentiates HIV latency reversal *ex vivo* in CD4 + T cells from ART-suppressed individuals. *Nat Commun.* (2019) 10:814. doi: 10.1038/s41467-019-08798-7
209. Gay CL, Bosch RJ, Ritz J, Hataye JM, Aga E, Tressler RL, et al. Clinical trial of the anti-PD-L1 antibody BMS-936559 in HIV-1 infected participants on suppressive antiretroviral therapy. *J Infect Dis.* (2017) 215:1725–33. doi: 10.1093/infdis/jix191
210. Ostios-Garcia L, Faig J, Leonardi GC, Adeni AE, Subegdjo SJ, Lydon CA, et al. Safety and efficacy of PD-1 inhibitors among HIV-positive patients with non-small cell lung cancer. *J Thorac Oncol.* (2018) 13:1037–42. doi: 10.1016/j.jtho.2018.03.031
211. Pakker NG, Kroon EDMB, Roos MTL, Otto SA, Hall D, Wit FWNM, et al. Immune restoration does not invariably occur following long-term HIV-1 suppression during antiretroviral therapy. *AIDS.* (1999) 13:203–12. doi: 10.1097/00002030-199902040-00008
212. Notermans DW, Pakker NG, Hamann D, Foudraine NA, Kauffmann RH, Meenhorst PL, et al. Immune reconstitution after 2 years of successful potent antiretroviral therapy in previously untreated human immunodeficiency virus type 1-infected adults. *J Infect Dis.* (1999) 180:1050–6. doi: 10.1086/315013
213. Lok JJ, Bosch RJ, Benson CA, Collier AC, Robbins GK, Shafer RW, et al. Long-term increase in CD4+ T-cell counts during combination antiretroviral therapy for HIV-1 infection. *AIDS.* (2010) 24:1867–76. doi: 10.1097/QAD.0b013e32833adbcf
214. Negredo E, Massanella M, Puig J, Perez-Alvarez N, Gallego-Escuredo JM, Villarroya J, et al. Nadir CD4 T cell count as predictor and high CD4 T cell intrinsic apoptosis as final mechanism of poor CD4 T cell recovery in virologically suppressed HIV-infected patients: clinical implications. *Clin Infect Dis.* (2010) 50:1300–8. doi: 10.1086/651689
215. Robbins GK, Spritzler JG, Chan ES, Asmuth DM, Gandhi RT, Rodriguez BA, et al. Incomplete reconstitution of T cell subsets on combination antiretroviral therapy in the AIDS clinical trials group protocol 384. *Clin Infect Dis.* (2009) 48:350–61. doi: 10.1086/595888
216. Gale HB, Gitterman SR, Hoffman HJ, Gordin FM, Benator DA, Labriola AM, et al. Is frequent CD4+ T-lymphocyte count monitoring necessary for persons with counts >=300 cells/muL and HIV-1 suppression? *Clin Infect Dis.* (2013) 56:1340–3. doi: 10.1093/cid/cit004
217. Serrano-Villar S, Sainz T, Lee SA, Hunt PW, Sinclair E, Shacklett BL, et al. HIV-infected individuals with low CD4/CD8 ratio despite effective antiretroviral therapy exhibit altered T cell subsets, heightened CD8+ T cell

activation, and increased risk of non-AIDS morbidity and mortality. *PLoS Pathog.* (2014) 10:e1004078. doi: 10.1371/journal.ppat.1004078
218. Serrano-Villar S, Pérez-Elías MJ, Dronda F, Casado JL, Moreno A, Royuela A, et al. Increased risk of serious non-AIDS-related events in HIV-infected subjects on antiretroviral therapy associated with a low CD4/CD8 ratio. *PLoS ONE.* (2014) 9:e85798. doi: 10.1371/journal.pone.0085798
219. Perdomo-Celis F, Taborda NA, Rugeles MT. Follicular CD8+ T cells: origin, function and importance during HIV infection. *Front Immunol.* (2017) 8:1241. doi: 10.3389/fimmu.2017.01241
220. Banga R, Procopio FA, Noto A, Pollakis G, Cavassini M, Ohmiti K, et al. PD-1+ and follicular helper T cells are responsible for persistent HIV-1 transcription in treated aviremic individuals. *Nat Med.* (2016) 22:754–61. doi: 10.1038/nm.4113
221. He R, Ye L. Follicular CXCR5-expressing CD8+ T-cells curtail chronic viral infection. *Nature.* (2016) 537:412–6. doi: 10.1038/nature19317
222. Petrovas C, Ferrando-Martinez S, Gerner MY, Casazza JP, Pegu A, Deleage C, et al. H I V Follicular CD8 T cells accumulate in HIV infection and can kill infected cells *in vitro* via bispecific antibodies. *Sci Transl Med.* (2017) 9:eaag2285. doi: 10.1126/scitranslmed.aag2285
223. Moysi E, Pallikkuth S, De Armas LR, Gonzalez LE, Ambrozak D, George V, et al. Altered immune cell follicular dynamics in HIV infection following influenza vaccination. *J Clin Invest.* (2018) 128:3171–85. doi: 10.1172/JCI99884
224. Ferrando-Martinez S, Moysi E, Pegu A, Andrews S, Makamdop KN, Ambrozak D, et al. Accumulation of follicular CD8+T cells in pathogenic SIV infection. *J Clin Invest.* (2018) 128:2089–103. doi: 10.1172/JCI96207
225. Rahman MA, McKinnon KM, Karpova TS, Ball DA, Venzon DJ, Fan W, et al. Associations of simian immunodeficiency virus (SIV)-specific follicular CD8 + T cells with other follicular T cells suggest complex contributions to SIV viremia control. *J Immunol.* (2018) 200:2714–26. doi: 10.4049/jimmunol.1701403
226. Lindqvist M, van Lunzen J, Soghoian DZ, Kuhl BD, Ranasinghe S, Kranias G, et al. Expansion of HIV-specific T follicular helper cells in chronic HIV infection. *J Clin Invest.* (2012) 122:3271–80. doi: 10.1172/JCI64314
227. Petrovas C, Yamamoto T, Gerner MY, Boswell KL, Wloka K, Smith EC, et al. CD4 T follicular helper cell dynamics during SIV infection. *J Clin Invest.* (2012) 122:3281–94. doi: 10.1172/JCI63039
228. Biancotto A, Grivel JC, Iglehart SJ, Vanpouille C, Lisco A, Sieg SF, et al. Abnormal activation and cytokine spectra in lymph nodes of people chronically infected with HIV-1. *Blood.* (2007) 109:4272–9. doi: 10.1182/blood-2006-11-055764
229. Ngo VN, Korner H, Gunn MD, Schmidt KN, Riminton DS, Cooper MD, et al. Lymphotoxin alpha/beta and tumor necrosis factor are required for stromal cell expression of homing chemokines in B and T cell areas of the spleen. *J Exp Med.* (1999) 189:403–12. doi: 10.1084/jem.189.2.403
230. Hjelmstrom P, Fjell J, Nakagawa T, Sacca R, Cuff CA, Ruddle NH. Lymphoid tissue homing chemokines are expressed in chronic inflammation. *Am J Pathol.* (2000) 156:1133–8. doi: 10.1016/S0002-9440(10)64981-4
231. Mehraj V, Ramendra R, Isnard S, Dupuy FP, Lebouché B, Costiniuk C, et al. CXCL13 as a biomarker of immune activation during early and chronic HIV infection. *Front Immunol.* (2019) 10:289. doi: 10.3389/fimmu.2019.00289
232. Wood GS. The immunohistology of lymph nodes in HIV infection: a review. *Prog AIDS Pathol.* (1990) 2:25–32.
233. Perdomo-Celis F, Taborda NA, Rugeles MT. Circulating CXCR5-expressing CD8+T-cells are major producers of IL-21 and associate with limited HIV replication. *J Acquir Immune Defic Syndr.* (2018) 78:473–82. doi: 10.1097/QAI.0000000000001700
234. Mylvaganam GH, Rios D, Abdelaal HM, Iyer S, Tharp G, Mavinger M, et al. Dynamics of SIV-specific CXCR5+ CD8 T cells during chronic SIV infection. *Proc Natl Acad Sci USA.* (2017) 114:1976–81. doi: 10.1073/pnas.1621418114
235. Li S, Folkvord JM, Rakasz EG, Abdelaal HM, Wagstaff RK, Kovacs KJ, et al. Simian immunodeficiency virus-producing cells in follicles are partially suppressed by CD8 + cells *in vivo.* *J Virol.* (2016) 90:11168–80. doi: 10.1128/JVI.01332-16
236. Schmitt N, Liu Y, Bentebibel SE, Munagala I, Bourdery L, Venuprasad K, et al. The cytokine TGF-beta co-opts signaling via STAT3-STAT4 to promote the differentiation of human TFH cells. *Nat Immunol.* (2014) 15:856–65. doi: 10.1038/ni.2947
237. Nilsson J, Boasso A, Velilla PA, Zhang R, Vaccari M, Franchini G, et al. HIV-1-driven regulatory T-cell accumulation in lymphoid tissues is associated with disease progression in HIV/AIDS. *Blood.* (2006) 108:3808–17. doi: 10.1182/blood-2006-05-021576
238. Ayala VI, Deleage C, Trivett MT, Jain S, Coren LV, Breed MW, et al. CXCR5-dependent entry of CD8 T cells into rhesus macaque B-cell follicles achieved through T-cell engineering. *J Virol.* (2017) 91:e02507–16. doi: 10.1128/JVI.02507-16
239. Haran KP, Hajduczki A, Pampusch MS, Mwakalundwa G, Vargas-Inchaustegui DA, Rakasz EG, et al. Simian immunodeficiency virus (SIV)-specific chimeric antigen receptor-T cells engineered to target B cell follicles and suppress SIV replication. *Front Immunol.* (2018) 9:492. doi: 10.3389/fimmu.2018.00492
240. Chomont N, Okoye AA, Favre D, Trautmann L. Wake me up before you go: a strategy to reduce the latent HIV reservoir. *AIDS.* (2018) 32:293–8. doi: 10.1097/QAD.0000000000001695
241. Pantaleo G, Levy Y. Therapeutic vaccines and immunological intervention in HIV infection: a paradigm change. *Curr Opin HIV AIDS.* (2016) 11:576–84. doi: 10.1097/COH.0000000000000324
242. Karlsson I, Kloverpris H, Jensen KJ, Stryhn A, Buus S, Karlsson A, et al. Identification of conserved subdominant HIV Type 1 CD8(+) T Cell epitopes restricted within common HLA Supertypes for therapeutic HIV Type 1 vaccines. *AIDS Res Hum Retroviruses.* (2012) 28:1434–43. doi: 10.1089/aid.2012.0081
243. Borthwick N, Ahmed T, Ondondo B, Hayes P, Rose A, Ebrahimsa U, et al. Vaccine-elicited human T cells recognizing conserved protein regions inhibit HIV-1. *Mol Ther.* (2014) 22:464–75. doi: 10.1038/mt.2013.248
244. Lieberman J, Skolnik PR, Parkerson GR III, Fabry JA, Landry B, Bethel J, et al. Safety of autologous, *ex vivo*-expanded human immunodeficiency virus (HIV)-specific cytotoxic T-lymphocyte infusion in HIV-infected patients. *Blood.* (1997) 90:2196–206.
245. Brodie SJ, Lewinsohn DA, Patterson BK, Jiyamapa D, Krieger J, Corey L, et al. *In vivo* migration and function of transferred HIV-1-specific cytotoxic T cells. *Nat Med.* (1999) 5:34–41. doi: 10.1038/4716
246. Tan R, Xu X, Ogg GS, Hansasuta P, Dong T, Rostron T, et al. Rapid death of adoptively transferred T cells in acquired immunodeficiency syndrome. *Blood.* (1999) 93:1506–10.
247. Koenig S, Conley AJ, Brewah YA, Jones GM, Leath S, Boots LJ, et al. Transfer of HIV-1-specific cytotoxic T lymphocytes to an AIDS patient leads to selection for mutant HIV variants and subsequent disease progression. *Nat Med.* (1995) 1:330–6. doi: 10.1038/nm0495-330
248. Lam S, Sung J, Cruz C, Castillo-Caro P, Ngo M, Garrido C, et al. Broadly-specific cytotoxic T cells targeting multiple HIV antigens are expanded from HIV+ patients: implications for immunotherapy. *Mol Ther.* (2015) 23:387–95. doi: 10.1038/mt.2014.207
249. Sung JA, Lam S, Garrido C, Archin N, Rooney CM, Bollard CM, et al. Expanded cytotoxic T-cell lymphocytes target the latent HIV reservoir. *J Infect Dis.* (2015) 212:258–63. doi: 10.1093/infdis/jiv022
250. Joseph A, Zheng JH, Follenzi A, Dilorenzo T, Sango K, Hyman J, et al. Lentiviral vectors encoding human immunodeficiency virus type 1 (HIV-1)-specific T-cell receptor genes efficiently convert peripheral blood CD8 T lymphocytes into cytotoxic T lymphocytes with potent *in vitro* and *in vivo* HIV-1-specific inhibitory activity. *J Virol.* (2008) 82:3078–89. doi: 10.1128/JVI.01812-07
251. Mummert C, Hofmann C, Huckelhoven AG, Bergmann S, Mueller-Schmucker SM, Harrer EG, et al. T-cell receptor transfer for boosting HIV-1-specific T-cell immunity in HIV-1-infected patients. *AIDS.* (2016) 30:2149–58. doi: 10.1097/QAD.0000000000001176
252. Linette GP, Stadtmauer EA, Maus MV, Rapoport AP, Levine BL, Emery L, et al. Cardiovascular toxicity and titin cross-reactivity of affinity-enhanced T cells in myeloma and melanoma. *Blood.* (2013) 122:863–71. doi: 10.1182/blood-2013-03-490565
253. Maldini CR, Ellis GI, Riley JL. CAR T cells for infection, autoimmunity and allotransplantation. *Nat Rev Immunol.* (2018) 18:605–16. doi: 10.1038/s41577-018-0042-2

254. Mitsuyasu RT, Anton PA, Deeks SG, Scadden DT, Connick E, Downs MT, et al. Prolonged survival and tissue trafficking following adoptive transfer of CD4zeta gene-modified autologous CD4(+) and CD8(+) T cells in human immunodeficiency virus-infected subjects. *Blood.* (2000) 96:785–93.

255. Leibman RS, Richardson MW, Ellebrecht CT, Maldini CR, Glover JA, Secreto AJ, et al. Supraphysiologic control over HIV-1 replication mediated by CD8 T cells expressing a re-engineered CD4-based chimeric antigen receptor. *PLoS Pathog.* (2017) 13:e1006613. doi: 10.1371/journal.ppat.1006613

256. Liu B, Zou F, Lu L, Chen C, He D, Zhang X, et al. Chimeric antigen receptor T cells guided by the single-chain Fv of a broadly neutralizing antibody specifically and effectively eradicate virus reactivated from latency in CD4+ T lymphocytes isolated from HIV-1-infected individuals receiving suppressive C. *J Virol.* (2016) 90:9712–24. doi: 10.1128/JVI.00852-16

257. Ghanem MH, Bolivar-Wagers S, Dey B, Hajduczki A, Vargas-Inchaustegui DA, Danielson DT, et al. Bispecific chimeric antigen receptors targeting the CD4 binding site and high-mannose Glycans of gp120 optimized for anti-human immunodeficiency virus potency and breadth with minimal immunogenicity. *Cytotherapy.* (2018) 20:407–19. doi: 10.1016/j.jcyt.2017.11.001

258. Chapuis AG, Casper C, Kuntz S, Zhu J, Tjernlund A, Diem K, et al. HIV-specific CD8+ T cells from HIV+ individuals receiving HAART can be expanded *ex vivo* to augment systemic and mucosal immunity *in vivo*. *Blood.* (2011) 117:5391–402. doi: 10.1182/blood-2010-11-32 0226

259. Patel S, Lam S, Cruz CR, Wright K, Cochran C, Ambinder RF, et al. Functionally active HIV-specific T cells that target gag and Nef can be expanded from virus-naive donors and target a range of viral epitopes: implications for a cure strategy after allogeneic hematopoietic stem cell transplantation. *Biol Blood Marrow Transplant.* (2016) 22:536–41. doi: 10.1016/j.bbmt.2015.12.007

260. Fan J, Liang H, Ji X, Wang S, Xue J, Li D, et al. CTL-mediated immunotherapy can suppress SHIV rebound in ART-free macaques. *Nat Commun.* (2019) 10:2257. doi: 10.1038/s41467-019-09725-6

12

Candida spp. Determination and Th1/Th2 Mixed Cytokine Profile in Oral Samples from HIV+ Patients with Chronic Periodontitis

Sarah M. Lomeli-Martinez[1,2], Eulogio Valentin-Goméz[3,4], Juan J. Varela-Hernández[5], Monserrat Alvarez-Zavala[6], Karina Sanchez-Reyes[6], Moises Ramos-Solano[6], Rodolfo I. Cabrera-Silva[6], Victor M. Ramirez-Anguiano[7], Manuel A. Lomeli-Martinez[1], Silvia Y. Martinez-Salazar[5], Luz A. González-Hernández[6,8] and Jaime F. Andrade-Villanueva[6,8]**

[1] Department of Wellbeing and Sustainable Development, Centro Universitario del Norte, University of Guadalajara, Colotlán, Mexico, [2] Biological and Agricultural Sciences Ph.D. Program, Centro Universitario de la Ciénega, University of Guadalajara, Ocotlán, Mexico, [3] GMCA Research Unit, Department of Microbiology and Ecology, University of Valencia, Valencia, Spain, [4] Severe Infection Group, Health Research Institute "La Fe," Valencia, Spain, [5] Department of Medical and Life Sciences, Centro Universitario de la Ciénega, University of Guadalajara, Ocotlán, Mexico, [6] HIV and Immunodeficiencies Research Institute, Clinical Medicine Department, Centro Universitario de Ciencias de la Salud-University of Guadalajara, Guadalajara, Mexico, [7] Department of Integrated Dentistry Clinics, Centro Universitario de Ciencias de la Salud, University of Guadalajara, Guadalajara, Mexico, [8] HIV Unit Department, University Hospital "Fray Antonio Alcalde," University of Guadalajara, Guadalajara, Mexico

***Correspondence:**
Luz A. González-Hernández
luceroga08@gmail.com
Jaime F. Andrade-Villanueva
drjandradev@gmail.com

Background: Chronic periodontitis (CP), caused by bacteria and fungi, appears in up to 66% of HIV-patients. The impact and association of HIV-treatment (HAART) and *Candida* itself has not been properly evaluated in the development and progression of CP. The immunopathogenesis is characterized by CD4$^+$ T-cells activation and the balance between the T-helper 1 (Th1) and T-helper 2 (Th2) or a mixed cytokine profile. Currently, the associated causes of an immune response in HIV-patients with CP is controversial. Our aims were the determination of *Candida* spp. and cytokine profile in oral samples from HIV-positive patients with CP, considering the CD4$^+$ T cells levels and HAART use.

Methods: From 500 HIV-positive patients evaluated, 228 patients were enrolled. Patients were separated in groups: (A) $n = 53$ ($\leq$200 CD4$^+$ T-cells on HAART); (B) $n = 57$ ($\leq$200 CD4$^+$ T-cells without HAART); (C) $n = 50$ (>200 CD4$^+$ T-cells without HAART); (D) $n = 68$ (>200 CD4$^+$ T-cells on HAART). *Candida* spp. were isolated from the oral biofilm and crevicular fluid in CHROMagar and confirmed by endpoint PCR. Cytokine levels were measured by beads-based immunoassay in saliva by flow cytometry.

Results: 147 patients (64.5%) were positive to *Candida spp*. and 204 strains were isolated; 138 (67.6%) were *C. albicans* and the remaining *C. non-albicans* species (*C. glabrata*>*C. tropicalis*>*C. krusei*>*C. dubliniensis)*. In this study, CHROMagar showed good sensitivity (95%) but poor specificity (68%); since of the 152 samples identified as *C. albicans*, only 131 were confirmed by PCR; from the 10 samples identified as *C. glabrata*, only six were confirmed. Finally, of the 42 samples detected as *C. tropicalis*, only five were confirmed. When evaluating *Candida* spp. presence, group A and D had higher isolation, while group B had the highest species diversity. Whereas, group C had a significant reduction of *Candida* spp. Despite the presence of *Candida* and HAART, we found a Th1/Th2 hybrid profile in the saliva of patients with low CD4$^+$ T-cell count (group A).

Conclusion: Abundance and diversity of the *Candida* spp. detected in HIV-patients with CP could be related to HAART and low CD4$^+$ T-cells levels. Also, the immunosuppression might promote a local Th1/Th2 hybrid cytokine profile.

Keywords: ***Candida*** **spp, chronic periodontitis, HIV, HAART, cytokines**

INTRODUCTION

In HIV positive (HIV+) patients, periodontitis represents one of the first opportunistic pathologies that manifest in the oral cavity, appearing in up to 66% of these patients (1). Periodontitis is a disease caused by both Gram-positive and negative bacteria and oral fungi. It is characterized by inflammation in the gum and adjacent tissues, which causes the destruction of teeth structural supports (2, 3). The mechanisms of damage include both the direct tissue damage caused by the bacterial products of the dental biofilm and the indirect damage produced by the bacterial induction of host inflammatory and immune response (2–5). The immunopathogenesis of periodontitis is orchestrated by the innate and adaptive immune response, mainly through the activation of CD4$^+$ T cells and the balance between the T helper 1 (Th1) and T helper 2 (Th2) subtypes or a mixed cytokine profile (5, 6). Th1 signature cytokines are interleukin-2 (IL-2) and Interferon-gamma (IFN-γ), while Th2 cells secrete their signature cytokine interleukin 4 (IL-4) plus interleukin 5 (IL-5) and interleukin 10 (IL-10). It is well-known, that oral response against fungi in HIV negative (HIV-) subjects is orchestrated by a Th17 profile, this cytokine profile promote inflammation through the induction of a Th1 cytokine profile (inflammatory), recruitment of neutrophils, and production of reactive oxygen species such as nitrogen oxide (NO). This oral microenvironment is produced by infiltrating immune cells that are stimulated by the presence of opportunistic microorganisms and commensal bacteria that are part of the subgingival biofilm. This proinflammatory microenvironment (IL-1β, IFN- γ, IL-6, NO) is associated to bone loss, and the induction of a Th2 profile is a compensatory mechanism that controls the inflammation and promotes immune homeostasis (7).

Since HIV infection is characterized by the depletion of CD4$^+$ T cells and several changes in the whole cellular and humoral immune response that could lead to an immunodeficient state, which may allow subgingival colonization by different pathogens, HIV+ patients exhibit more oral manifestations that HIV- subjects (8). One of such pathogens is *Candida*, which can aggregate jointly with other bacteria to the subgingival biofilm and attach to the epithelial cells of patients with periodontal disease (8–10). *C. albicans* is the most frequent species identified in patients with periodontal disease. However, other species have also been found like *C. tropicalis*, *C. glabrata*, *C. krusei*, and *C. guilliermondii* (8, 10, 11). Also, it has been suggested that *Candida* spp. play a role in both the pathogenesis and the severity of periodontal disease (11–13). These last aspects gather importance in HIV+ patients. Both the local and systemic effects of the periodontal disease and the chronic immune activation associated with a co-infection are crucial factors in AIDS severity and progression. Furthermore, periodontal bacteria favor Epstein-Barr virus and Kaposi's sarcoma-associated herpesvirus reactivation (14).

It has been reported that CD4$^+$ T cells count >200 cells/μL increase the probability to acquire oral manifestations such as oropharyngeal candidiasis (OPC) (15, 16). A possible explanation to this susceptibility is by the depletion of Th17 (particularly in the gut) and an increase of a Th2 profile in the mucosa of HIV+ patients, as both factors are associated with susceptibility to mucosal candidiasis (7, 17, 18). In OPC, CD8$^+$ T cells are recruited to the mucosa in response to Candida infection, promoting a proinflammatory microenvironment characterized by a Th1 cytokine profile (19). This compensatory response in OPC is reflected in a Th1/Th2 cytokine profile, however, the establishment of a similar immune profile has not been described in CP.

In our knowledge, HIV+ patients with CP have been studied without considering *Candida* infection, nor the clinical conditions of the patients, such as CD4$^+$ T cell count and HAART. In addition, they do not evaluate if CD4$^+$ T cell count or HAART could modify the cytokine environment or promote atypical *Candida* spp. colonization in the mouth. Several studies analyzed the role of *Candida* spp. in mucosal infection in HIV+ patients, however, most of them are focused in OPC, while this comorbidity has been studied microbiologically and immunologically, other infections driven by *Candida* spp. such as CP, remain poorly known. We hypothesized that *Candida* spp. colonization in HIV+ patients with CP is associated with a Th1/Th2 profile independently of the immune state and the presence of HAART, however, these two last factors are related to the diversity of *Candida* spp.

Our aims were the determination of *Candida* spp. and cytokine profile in oral samples from HIV+ patients with CP, considering the CD4$^+$ T cells levels and HAART use.

MATERIALS AND METHODS

Study Population

We performed a cross-sectional (observational) study including 500 HIV+ patients with untreated CP in the last 3 months. HIV patients were recruited from the HIV clinic of the tertiary care university hospital "Antiguo Hospital Civil de Guadalajara—Fray Antonio Alcalde" (a 1,000-bed teaching hospital in Western Mexico) from February to September 2017. Non-inclusion criteria were pregnancy, breastfeeding, no sign of CP, oral candidiasis, and use of dental prostheses. This study was carried out in accordance with the recommendations of the Declaration of Helsinki, World Medical Association with written informed consent from all subjects. The protocol was approved by the ethics committee in research of the "Antiguo Hospital Civil de Guadalajara—Fray Antonio Alcalde" with registry number 020/16 (20). All subjects gave written informed consent in accordance with the Declaration of Helsinki.

The sample size was calculated using a finite population proportion formula based on the prevalence previously reported (21). Detailed sociodemographic, immunological, and health-related information were obtained during the scheduled medical visit.

Selected patients were grouped as follows: Group (A) patients with $CD4^+ \leq 200$ cells/μL on HAART; Group (B) patients with $CD4^+ \leq 200$ cells/μL without HAART; Group (C) patients with $CD4^+ > 200$ cells/μL without HAART; and Group (D) patients with $CD4^+ > 200$ cells/μL on HAART.

Periodontal Evaluation

The periodontal evaluation was performed by a periodontist with a North Carolina periodontal probe number 12 (Hu-Friedy). This analysis evaluated the mesiobuccal, buccal, distobuccal, mesiolingual, lingual, and distolingual site of each tooth (except the third molars). In each site: sounding depth, Clinical Attachment Level (CAL) and bleeding on probing were evaluated. Periodontitis diagnosis was established according to the Disease Control/American Association of Periodontology Classification (22), which considers the CAL scale.

Sample Collection

Crevicular fluid and subgingival biofilm were obtained from the most severe site in each oral quadrant at the base of the periodontal pocket. The crevicular fluid was obtained by introducing filter paper for 60 s. Subgingival biofilm was obtained with a sterile Gracey curette (Hu-Friedy). For *Candida* spp. identification, crevicular fluid, and subgingival biofilm were collected in thioglycolate medium (BD) tubes. Non-stimulated saliva samples were collected in a clean 2 mL amber tubes and stored at −70°C. All samples were collected before noon after periodontal evaluation.

Candida spp. Detection by CHROMagar®

Crevicular fluid and subgingival biofilm were streak-plated in CHROMagar Candida® medium, incubated at 36°C for 48 h. Identification was carried out by colorimetric changes as specified by the manufacturer's instructions. All CHROMagar were analyzed by a certified microbiologist.

Endpoint PCR From Yeast Colonies

Endpoint PCR was performed in yeast colonies as previously described (https://openwetware.org/wiki/Smolke:Protocols/Yeast_Colony_PCR). Briefly, primary *Candida* spp. acquired from the CHROMagar were re-cultured overnight in yeast 1% extract, 2% peptone, and 2% dextrose (YPD) medium. Yeast colonies were harvested with a sterile pipette tip and resuspended in 3 μL of freshly made NaOH (20 mM). Cells were lysed and incubated at 95°C for 10 min. The 3 μL were used as molds for the PCR reaction, which was performed in a total volume of 25 μL. PCR mix was made with 5 mM dNTPs, 15 mM $MgCl_2$, and Taq polymerase following the manufacturer's instruction (MyTaq™ DNA Polymerase Kit, Bioline). Three percent of DMSO was added to improve reaction as previously described (23) and 10 mM of primers specific for every species (**Table 1**).

TABLE 1 | Primer sets used for *Candida* spp. PCR detection.

***Candida*spp.**	**Primer set**	**References**
C. albicans	INT1 5′ AAGTATTTGGGAGAAGGGAAAGGG 3′	(24)
	INT2 5′ AAAATGGGCATTAAGGAAAAGAGC 3′	
C. tropicalis	CTf 5′ TGATAGTTAGGAAAGATCAGGTG 3′	(24)
	CTr 5′ CACACACATGGGATATGTT 3′	
C. glabrata	CGf 5′ ACATATGTTTGCTGAAAAGGC 3′	(24)
	CGr 5′ AGAAGTCCTGAACACTAAGAAAAAGT 3′	
C. parapsilosis	CPf 5′ AGGGATTGCCAATATGCCCA 3′	(24)
	CPr 5′ GTGACATTGTGTAGATCCTTGG 3′	

Endpoint PCR was performed in a MiniCycler MJ Research thermal cycler. PCR program was as follows: 5 min of denaturalization at 95°C, 30 cycles of 30 s at 94°C (denaturalization), 30 s at 50°C (hybridization), and 30 s at 72°C (elongation). Afterward, a final elongation at 72°C for 10 min was performed (24).

Electrophoresis

DNA fragments from the PCR reaction were separated in 2% agarose gel (CONDA Micro and Molecular Biology®) prepared with TAE buffer (Tris-acetate 40 mM, pH 8.5; EDTA 0.05 mM). Ten microliter of Red Safe® (iNtRON) were added. Photographs were taken with a UVITEC transilluminator.

Cytokine Determination

Saliva samples were centrifuged at 1,000 g for 10 min, the supernatant was recollected and used for the assay. LEGENDplex Human T Helper Cytokine Th1/Th2 Panel kit (BioLegend) was used for cytokines detection. The evaluated cytokines were: IL-2, IL-4, IL-5, IL-6, IL-10, IL-13, IFN-γ, and Tumor Necrosis Factor-alpha (TNF-α). The assay was performed following manufacturer recommendations. Samples were read using the NxT Attune flow cytometer (Applied Bioscience) and analyzed with the LEGENDplex v8 Software (BioLegend).

Statistical Analysis

Data were analyzed using Statistical Package for the Social Scientist (SPSS) version 23 (IBM) and GraphPad Prism 6 software. Medians and interquartile ranges (IQR) or means and standard deviations (SD) were reported depending on data distribution. Sociodemographic and *Candida* spp. presence data were compared with either Student's *t*-test, Fisher exact, or Chi-square, according to the variable analyzed; binary linear regression analysis was performed to estimate the association

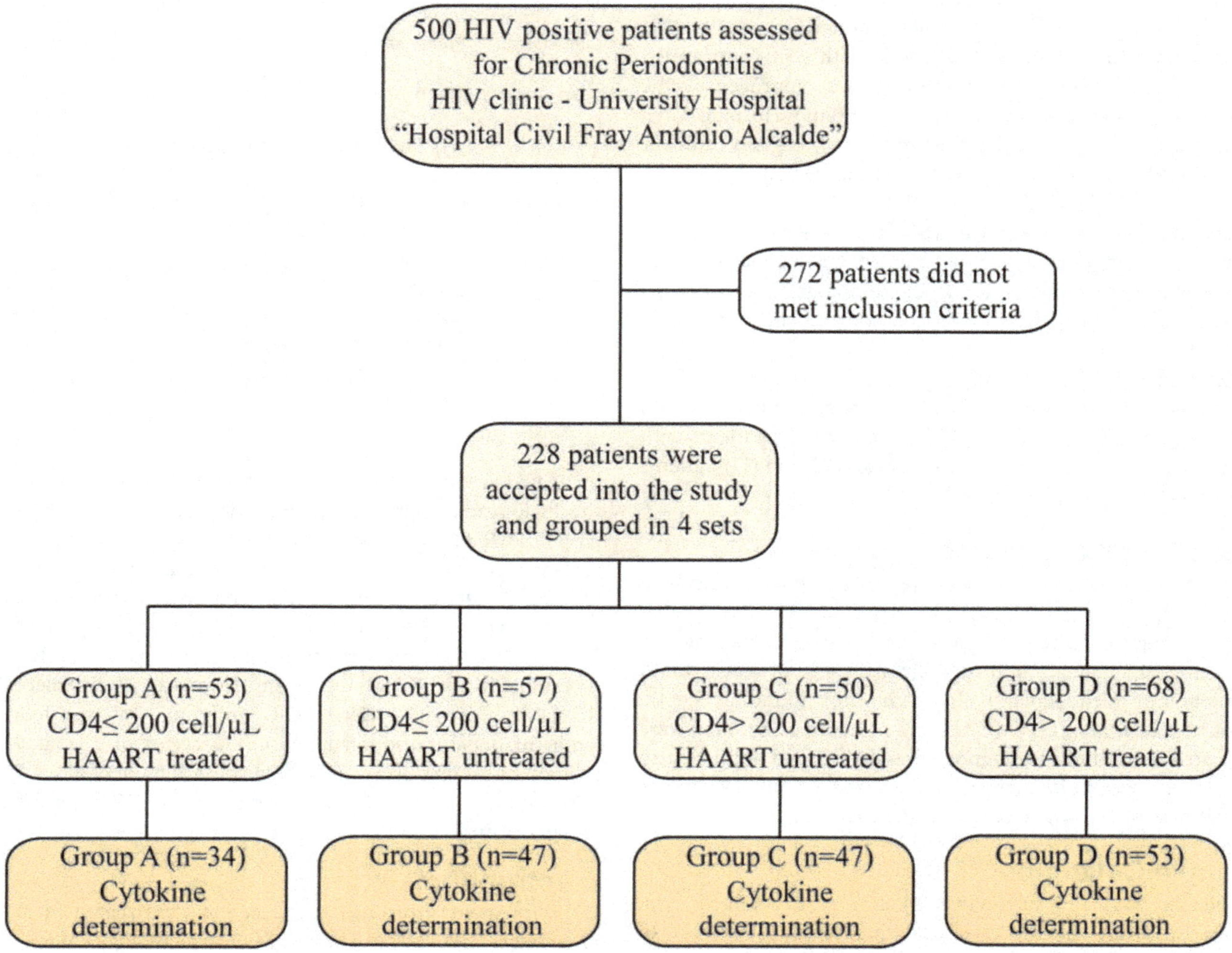

FIGURE 1 | Flowchart of patient recruitment and distribution. Two hundred twenty-eight patients were selected after exclusion criteria and separated into four groups. Due to low quality in saliva samples, we were not able to determine the cytokines profile in the samples from all patients included in this study.

of candida presence, considering the following variables: use of HAART, age, gender, level of $CD4^+$ T cells (> or ≤200 cells/μL), tobacco, alcohol, and drug use; and Cohen's kappa coefficient (κ) was reported. The cytokines differences between the different groups were estimated using the Kruskal-Wallis test with Dunn's Multiple Comparison test. Shapiro-Wilks normality test was significant, so the data distribution was considered non-Gaussian. p-values < 0.05 were considered significant.

RESULTS

Group Study Characteristics

Periodontal evaluation was performed in 500 HIV+ volunteer patients. After assessing the selection criteria, 228 patients were included in the study. Next, patients were divided into different groups: 53 patients were assigned to Group A, 57 patients to Group B, 50 patients to Group C, and 68 patients to Group D (**Figure 1**).

Cytokine determination in saliva was performed only in 34 from Group A, 47 from Group B, 47 from Group C, and 53 from Group D; this due to lack of enough sample or samples that were blood-stained. It was observed a significant difference among age, $CD4^+$ T cells count, CD4/CD8 ratio, viral load, duration of HAART, and grades of severity according to the CAL scale. Regarding age, the group with the older patients was group D (43 ± 11 years; $p = 0.05$). Patients with ≤200 $CD4^+$ T cells had a median of 17 months under HAART compared to the 38 months among patients with >200 $CD4^+$ T cells ($p = 0.0001$). Furthermore, this last group also had an undetectable viral load ($p = 0.0001$). In addition, group B—with ≤200 CD4 $^+$ T cells- presented less "mild" cases and more "severe" cases, according to the CAL classification, when compared against group C—with >200 $CD4^+$ T cells-, both groups without HAART ($p = 0.05$).

In respect to gender, the majority of our patients were men (4:1). Because in group B there was only one woman, a significant difference was found but this statistic finding should

TABLE 2 | Sociodemographic characteristics including all patients.

	Group A $n = 53$	Group B $n = 57$	Group C $n = 50$	Group D $n = 68$	*p*-value*
Age (years)	37.3 ± 9	36.9 ± 8	37 ± 12	42.6 ± 11	0.05
Mean (SD)					
Gender					0.05#
Female	10 (19%)	1 (2%)	11 (22%)	15 (22%)	
Male	43 (81%)	56 (98%)	39 (78%)	53 (78%)	
Tobacco use:					ns
Yes	34 (64%)	38 (67%)	31 (62%)	47 (69%)	
No	19 (36%)	19 (33%)	19 (38%)	21 (31%)	
Drugs use:					ns
Yes	34 (64%)	31 (54%)	24 (48%)	41 (60%)	
No	19 (36%)	26 (46%)	26 (52%)	27 (40%)	
Alcohol use:					ns
Yes	40 (76%)	41 (72%)	38 (76%)	53 (78%)	
No	13 (24%)	16 (28%)	12 (24%)	15 (22%)	
Diabetes:					ns
Present	2 (4%)	4 (7%)	2 (4%)	4 (6%)	
Absent	51 (96%)	53 (93%)	48 (96%)	64 (94%)	
$CD4^+$ (cells/mL)	41	38	366	503	0.0001
Median (IQR)	(11–109)	(19–89)	(264–552)	(354–697)	
CD4/CD8 ratio	0.1	0.11	0.42	0.54	0.0001
Median (IQR)	(0.05–0.17)	(0.05–0.16)	(0.25–0.67)	(0.40–0.77)	
Viral load (copies/mL)	31,400	149,000	30,600	38	0.0001
Median (IQR)	(428–297,250)	(57,800–411,436)	(183–77,750)	(20–78)	
Type of HAART:					ns
No medication	–	100%	100%	–	
PI-based	19 (36%)	–	–	23 (34%)	
NNRT-based	18 (34%)	–	–	33 (48%)	
INI-based	7 (13%)	–	–	4 (6%)	
Other	9 (17%)	–	–	8 (12%)	
Duration in treatment (months)	17 (6–23)	–	–	38 (24–104)	0.0001
CAL classification:					
Mild	7 (13.2%)	7 (12.2%)	13 (26%)	12 (17.6%)	0.05
Moderate	15 (28.3%)	14 (24.5%)	17 (34%)	24 (35.2%)	ns
Severe	31 (58.4%)	36 (63.1%)	20 (40%)	32 (47%)	0.05

**Fisher's exact test, Chi-squared test, ANOVA, Kruskal-Wallis, and Mann-Whitney U-tests. #Statistical significance was found only with Group B because it only had one female patient; however, between the rest of the groups, there were no statistical differences; SD, standard deviation; IQR, interquartile range; ns, no significance. Group A: ≤200 $CD4^+$ on HAART; group B: ≤200 $CD4^+$ without HAART; group C: >200 $CD4^+$ without HAART; group D: >200 $CD4^+$ on HAART.*

be considered with caution. We did not find differences among the four groups in terms of the habits of smoking, drinking or drug use, but is important to emphasize that more than 62% of patients used tobacco, that is already considered as a risk factor for CP. Besides, diabetes was absent in more than 93% in all groups, that is relevant considering that it is another known risk factor for CP and was absent in the majority of our patients (25). The treatment scheme in the groups under HAART was based mainly in non-nucleoside reverse transcriptase inhibitors (NNRT), followed by protease inhibitors (PI), and integrase inhibitors; nonetheless, there were no differences statistically significant between the groups. Complete sociodemographic data is described in **Table 2**.

After the logistic regression analysis, we found a significantly association with the presence of *Candida* spp. with levels ≤200 cells/μL of $CD4^+$ T cells (OR: 3.59 CI 95% 1.89–6.80; $p = 0.0001$), the use of PIs (OR: 2.67 CI 95% 1.13–6.29; $p = 0.025$) and NNTRIs (OR: 2.99 CI 95% 1.37–6.49; $p = 0.006$; $\kappa = 0.408$).

Candida spp. Varies Between Groups and Identification Methods

HIV infection is associated with an increased colonization rate by *Candida* spp. as well as the development of other diseases, such as periodontal disease. Our first goal was to identify the *Candida* spp. present in the different groups of HIV+ patients with periodontal disease.

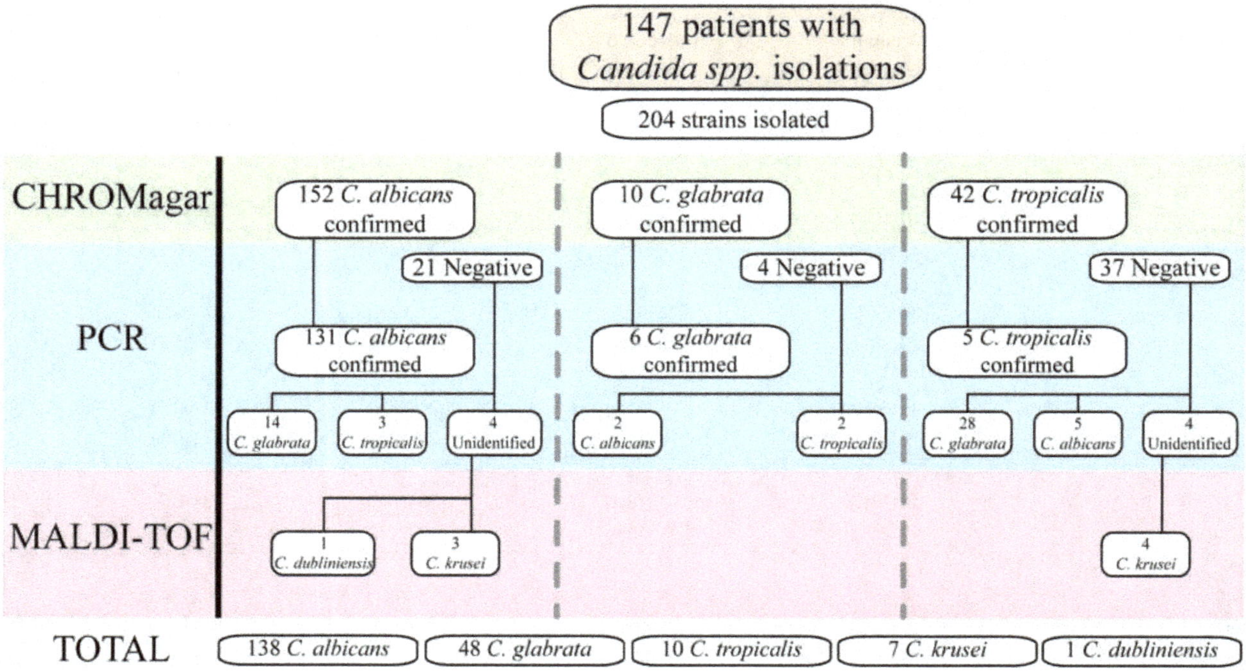

FIGURE 2 | *Candida* spp. identification by methods. All samples were cultivated first in CHROMagar for initial identification. Afterward, all identified *Candida* spp. by traditional microbiologic methods were evaluated by PCR technique to confirm the species. If the PCR for the specific species found in CHROMagar was negative, further PCRs were made for other *Candida* spp. Any *Candida* spp. that was not confirmed by PCR, due to lack of the primers specific for that species, were identified through MALDI-TOF technique.

From the 228 patients included in the study, 147 (64.5%) were positive to *Candida* spp. In total 204 strains were isolated, of which 138 (67.6%) were *C. albicans,* and the remaining 66 (32.4%) had *C. non-albicans* species. The identified *non-albicans* species were: 48 (23.6%) *C. glabrata*, 10 (4.9%) *C. tropicalis*, 7 (3.4%) *C. krusei*, and 1 (0.5%) *C. dubliniensis.*

In 145 (71.1%) of the total isolated strains, only one type of *Candida* was isolated, while the remaining 59 isolated strains (28.9%) more than one type of *Candida* were isolated. The most common combinations were: *C. albicans* + *C. glabrata* (19.6%), *C. albicans* + *C. krusei* (4.9%), *C. glabrata* + *C. tropicalis* (2%), and *C. albicans* + *C. glabrata* + *C. tropicalis* (1.5%). When comparing all combinations between the study groups, Group C had significantly fewer combinations in comparison with Group D ($p = 0.011$). The distribution of *Candida* spp. strains separated by groups are shown in the **Supplementary Table 1**.

Identification of Candida Species With Different Methods

When carrying out this study, it was necessary to use different methods of identification for *Candida* spp., including conventional methods as well as molecular techniques. At the beginning, with streak-plating technique by CHROMagar, *C. albicans, C. glabrata,* and *C. tropicalis* were identified in 152, 10, and 42 samples; respectively. However, of the 152 *C. albicans* identified, molecular confirmation was positive in 131 of these samples. Therefore, PCR for the other *Candida* species was performed in the remaining 21 samples; 14 of these samples were positive for *C. glabrata,* and 3 for *C. tropicalis.* The last four samples were not identified by PCR. From the 10 samples identified as *C. glabrata*, six were confirmed by molecular techniques. The remaining four samples were tested by PCR for the other *Candida* species, two were identified as *C. albicans* and the others as *C. tropicalis.* The last 42 samples were detected as *C. tropicalis*, but only five were confirmed by PCR. In the other 37 samples, 28 were identified as *C. glabrata,* and five as *C. albicans.* Again, four samples were not identified to any *Candida* spp. by PCR.

The eight samples that were negative in all PCRs were sent to "La Fe" Hospital in Valencia, Spain. *Candida* spp. was detected through matrix-assisted laser desorption/ionization time-of-flight mass spectrometry (MALDI-TOF MS). From the four samples detected as *C. albicans* by streak-plating technique, one was identified as *C. dubliniensis* and the remaining as *C. krusei.* The four samples detected as *C. tropicalis* by plating were confirmed as *C. krusei* by MALDI-TOF MS. A summary is provided in **Figure 2**.

With this information, we compared the accuracy of CHROMagar Candida medium to identify *Candida* spp. with streak-plating technique against PCR; results are shown in **Table 3**.

Candida spp. and Colonization Varies Depending on $CD4^+$ T Cells Count and HAART

In the course of HIV infection, the rate of Candida infection is inversely related to the $CD4^+$ T cells count. When evaluating

TABLE 3 | Capacity of *Candida* spp. identification with CHROMagar Candida Medium.

Marker	Value	95% confidence interval
Sensibility	95%	89.8–97.9%
Specificity	68%	55.6–79.1%
Positive likelihood ratio	2.98	2.09–4.26
Negative likelihood ratio	0.07	0.04–0.16
Positive predictive value	86%	81.4–89.9%
Negative predictive value	87%	75.4–93.1%
Accuracy	86%	80.8–90.7%

TABLE 4 | Patients with presence of *Candida* spp. in each group.

	Group A $n = 53$ (%)	Group B $n = 57$ (%)	Group C $n = 50$ (%)	Group D $n = 68$ (%)	*p*-value
***Candida* spp.**	**36 (68)**	**45 (78)**	**13 (26)**	**51 (75)**	A vs. C[a]*** B vs. C[a]*** D vs. C[a]***
C. albicans	26 (49)	27 (47)	11 (22)	29 (43)	A vs. C[a]** B vs. C[a]** D vs. C[a]*
C. glabrata	9 (17)	11 (19)	2 (4)	15 (22)	B vs. C[b]* D vs. C[b]**
C. tropicalis	0 (0)	4 (7)	0 (0)	5 (7)	ns
C. krusei	1 (2)	2 (3)	0 (0)	2 (3)	ns
C. dubliniensis	0 (0)	1 (2)	0 (0)	0 (0)	n/a

*Groups were compared between each other for overall Candida infection and for each individual Candida spp. detected. Total Candida identification is shown with their percentage (round up) for every group. Statistically significant p-values are shown. For C. dubliniensis, the statistical comparison was not performed because only one group had this species (n/a). As not every patient in each group had Candida, the amount of Candida spp. detected and total patient per group differs. [a]Chi-squared test; [b]Fisher's exact test; *$p < 0.05$; **$p < 0.01$; ***$p < 0.001$; ns, no statistical significance.*

Candida spp. between the groups, *C. albicans* and *C. glabrata* were identified in all of them; *C. krusei* was detected in Groups A, B, and D; *C. tropicalis* in Group B and D, while *C. dubliniensis* was present exclusively in Group B.

When analyzing the number of patients with *Candida* in each group, we found a significant reduction of *Candida* spp. in the Group C in comparison with the other groups ($p \leq 0.001$ vs. A, B, D). As well, *C. albicans* was significantly diminished in Group C ($p < 0.01$ vs. A and B; $p < 0.05$ vs. D). For patients with *C. glabrata*, Group C had also a significant decrease in comparison with B and D ($p < 0.05$ and $p < 0.01$, respectively). Data are shown in **Table 4**.

Th1/Th2 Mixed Cytokines Profile in the Saliva Is Mainly Promoted by Low CD4$^+$ T Cell Count

Saliva samples from HIV+ patients with CP and *Candida* spp. growth were analyzed to evaluate if CD4$^+$ T cell count or HAART modifies the local Th1 and Th2 related cytokine expression. With respect to Th1-related cytokines, IFN-γ was significantly higher in group A and B in relation to group D; the levels of TNF-α in group A were significantly higher against group D, and significantly higher to group B for IL-2. Finally, group B had significantly more IL-6 in comparison with group C and D.

Regarding Th2 signature cytokines, group A had a significant increase of IL-5 in comparison with group B and D; whilst both groups with low CD4$^+$ T cell count (A and B) had a significant increase of IL-10 and IL-4 respect to group D. Group A was also significant with group C for IL-4. When comparing cytokine expression in each group, there was no difference for IL-13 (**Table 5**; **Figure S1**). We were able to observe a mixed increase of some Th1 and Th2 cytokines, although a major predisposition for a Th2 profile was found. Interestingly, the groups with more levels of cytokines overall are the ones with low CD4$^+$ T cell count.

DISCUSSION

This study is one of the few studies that measure CP in different groups considering the CD4$^+$ T cell count and HAART. Because other studies divided their groups differently to ours, we separate and regroup our data as required to better compare our results with the literature.

In this study, patients with CP and CD4$^+$ T cells $\leq$200 cells/μL had a major prevalence of *Candida* infection (73.7%) than the one reported in previous studies (11–13, 26). In addition, the number of patients, in this study, colonized with *C. albicans* (40.8%), *C. tropicalis* (3.9%), and *C. krusei* (2.2%) is less than the ones found previously (11, 26). However, similar results to ours were found by another group (27). Furthermore, we found a higher amount of *C. glabrata* colonization (16.2%) in comparison with the literature (11, 26–28).

Regarding the distribution of *Candida* spp. isolation, *C. albicans* (67.7%), *C. glabrata* (23.5%), and *C. krusei* (3.4%) had a major distribution than the one reported (13, 29, 30). On the other hand, the distribution that we detected for *C. tropicalis* (4.9%) was lower than previous papers (13, 29, 30). Like previous studies, we identified *C. dubliniensis* in one of the patients (0.5%) (26, 29, 30). This is the first study in Mexico that identifies *Candida dubliniensis* in HIV+ patients with CP; it was previously reported in USA (31) and this could increase the relevance of screening this species in Mexican populations with CP.

In this study, we required to use several techniques for *Candida* spp. identification. Currently, several authors have considered the use of CHROMagar Candida medium as a diagnostic test directly from the oral cavity (27, 28, 32). Taking advantage that we used this technique, we evaluated the CHROMagar effectiveness as a diagnosis technique. Since CHROMagar is a presumptive test, we confirmed our results with endpoint PCR and found a sensibility of 95%, a specificity of 68%, and an accuracy of 86% for CHROMagar. These results differ from the studies that suggest a sensibility and a specificity of 99% (33, 34). These discrepancies could be explained by the different saliva sampling techniques used: isotopes method (28, 30, 35), mouthwash method (11), filter papers method (12, 36); or the identification technique performed: biochemistry

TABLE 5 | Cytokine levels in saliva samples from HIV+ patients per group.

Cytokine median ± IQR (pg/mL)	Group A	Group B	Group C	Group D	*p-value*
Th1 PROFILE					
IFN-γ	11.79 (7.10–25.21)	7.89 (6.63–23.39)	7.07 (6.0–17.23)	7.07 (3.31–8.23)	A vs. D***
					B vs. D*
TNF-α	5.35 (5.05–9.54)	5.05 (4.03–8.77)	5.05 (4.57–7.54)	5.05 (1.98–5.25)	A vs. D**
IL-2	15.18 (15.18–19.65)	15.18 (4.84–15.18)	15.18 (4.84–16.47)	15.18 (4.84–16.32)	A vs. B*
IL-6	19.03 (4.26–59.96)	40.79 (5.09–145)	4.83 (2.43–28.91)	4.82 (3.37–5.37)	B vs. D***
					B vs. C**
Th2 PROFILE					
IL-4	15.65 (5.79–33.63)	9.9 (5.17–36.85)	5.75 (2.27–13.75)	5.17 (2.13–9.89)	A vs. D**
					A vs. C*
					B vs. D**
IL-5	4.08 (4.08–10.39)	4.08 (2.98–4.08)	4.08 (2.98–4.08)	4.08 (2.98–4.08)	A vs. D**
					A vs. B*
IL-10	2.89 (2.83–11.22)	4.17 (2.83–13.53)	2.83 (2.39–4.25)	2.83 (2.27–2.87)	A vs. D*
					B vs. D**
IL-13	13.48 (12.47–17.81)	12.47 (5.49–17.81)	13.08 (5.45–23.68)	8.43 (3.81–15.16)	ns

*Measurements of Th1 and Th2 profile's cytokines levels in all groups. All values are reported in pg/mL. Median and interquartile range (IQR) are shown. Kruskal-Wallis test was performed to evaluate differences. The p-values with statistical significance are reported as follows: *p < 0.5; **p < 0.01; ***p < 0.001; ns, no statistical significance.*

tests (11, 28, 30), chromogenic medium (12, 28, 36) PCR (29) or MALDI-TOF MS (27). Therefore, an acquisition technique should be standardized when CHROMagar is used. Nonetheless, considering our results we suggest that CHROMagar Candida Medium requires a confirmatory technique, such as PCR, to ensure the results, especially for *Candida non-albicans species*, as recommended by other authors (24, 29, 32).

It is known, that the interaction of various *Candida* spp. with bacteria from the dental plaque promotes bacterial colonization and proliferation in the periodontal pockets. This contributes to the progression of periodontal disease (8). We isolated in 71.1% of the patients a single *Candida* spp.; and two or more *Candida* spp. in 28.9% of our patients. During the periodontal evaluation, the most severe patients were the ones with two or more *Candida* spp. (CAL $\geq$5 mm). Also, we detected an increase distribution of the *C. albicans* + *C. glabrata* coinfection (19.6%) in comparison with other studies (26, 29). Our results suggest that a transition to coinfection with multiple *Candida* spp. is a factor that facilitates CP and increases severity. Clark et al. (29), did a study with HIV+ Mexican patients without a periodontal evaluation and through a different acquisition technique (mouthwash) and they found in 94.1% of their patients a single *Candida* spp. and two or more species in 6.5% of them. Furthermore, the most frequent *Candida non-albicans* species that we found was *C. glabrata* (23.6%) in comparison with Clark et al. (29), which found *C. tropicalis*. In this sense, the differences found between our study and Clark et al. (29) study could be related to potential geographical environmental factors; it has already been proposed that environmental factors could have importance in the type of *Candida* spp. in oral colonization, factors that could be relevant when we compared our results with the literature (37).

The use of HAART and the immune reconstitution have been associated with a significant reduction of viral load and opportunistic infections, including oral manifestations like oral hairy leukoplakia, Kaposi's sarcoma and oral candidiasis (10, 21). However, it remains controversial the effect of HAART in incidence and severity of the atypical periodontal diseases, such as linear gingival erythema, necrotizing periodontitis and CP (10, 21, 38, 39); the latter, probably caused by the known effect of HAART over the salivary flow (hyposalivation, xerostomia, or dysgeusia), which modifies the oral microbiota and facilitates *Candida* spp. colonization (40, 41); yet other studies could not find a correlation between *Candida* colonization and HAART usage (29, 30, 42, 43). In this sense, we evaluated if the presence of HAART affected the amount of *Candida* colonization in CP. We detected that groups with HAART, especially with the use of PIs and NNRTIs, had a significant increase of *Candida* colonization. Interestingly, we also found an increase in diversity. Therefore, we suggest that a secondary effect of HAART is the promotion of oral dysbiosis.

Concerning $CD4^+$ T cell count, the groups with $CD4^+$ T cells count $\leq$200 cells/μL had a significant increase of *Candida* spp. colonization in comparison with the groups with $CD4^+$ T cell count >200 cells/μL (OR: 3.59; $p = 0.0001$). This finding is consistent with the literature (11, 44). In summary, $CD4^+$ T cell count in HIV+ patients play a major role in the subgingival colonization of *Candida* spp. in CP. It has been reported that during periodontal disease the expression of $CD4^+$, $CXCR5^+$, and $CCR5^+$ is increased (45, 46); the latter has also been reported increased in smokers (47). This overexpression facilitates the entry of HIV virions through dendritic cells (DC) and macrophages, which are the prevalent cells in the oral mucosa; this could cause major cell death, local inflammation, and promotion for pathogen colonization like *Candida*. On average, 66% of HIV+ patients in our study are current smokers, it seems that this continues to be an important factor for the

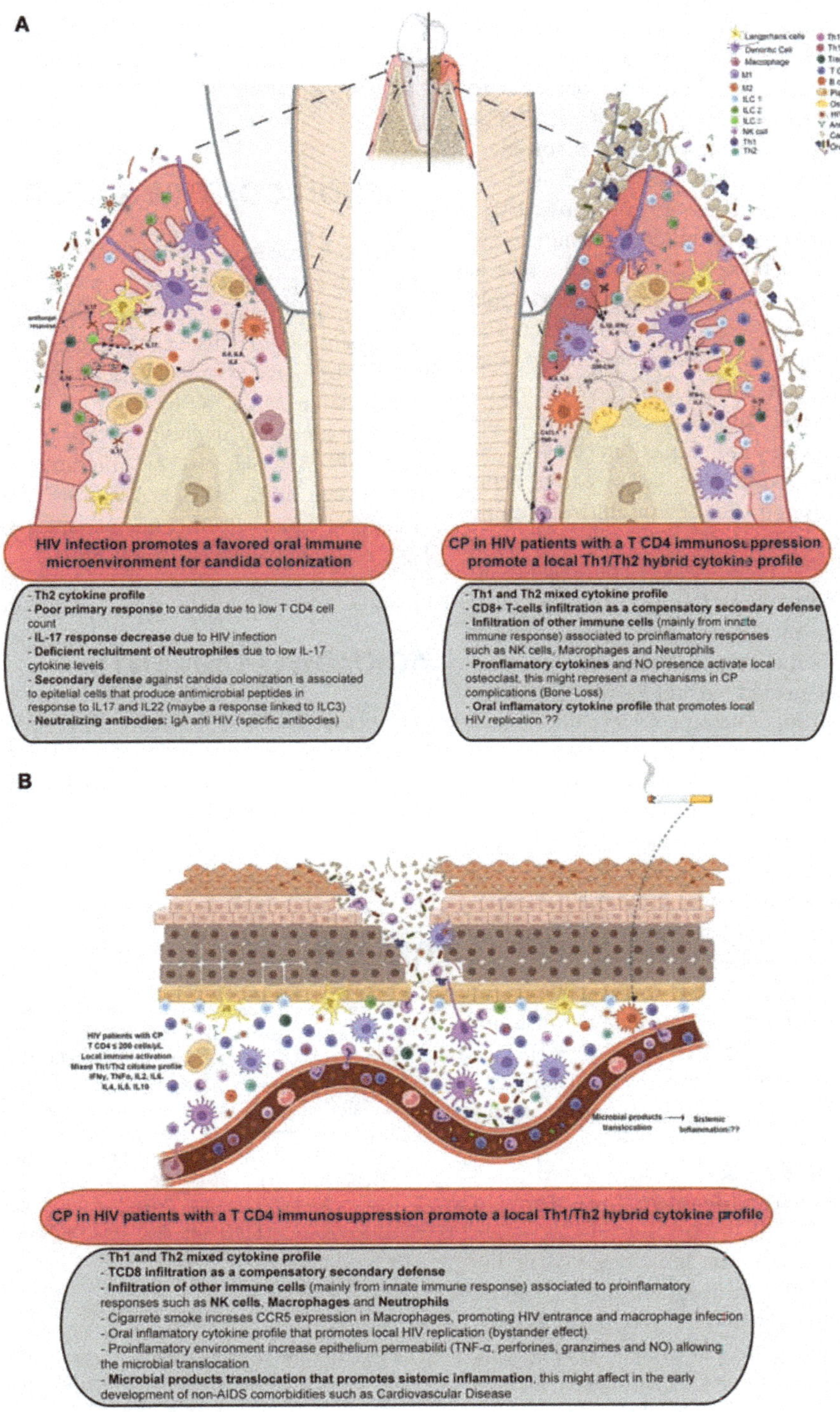

FIGURE 3 | Proposal of the immune response in HIV patients with CP. **(A)** Suggests the progression to CP in the oral cavity while **(B)** shows a proposal for the involvement of CP in the systemic inflammation environment of HIV patients. Created with BioRender.

development of periodontal disease, but in our study, it was not shown that tobacco influenced *Candida* colonization.

Lastly, we assessed the local cytokine environment occurring in HIV+ patients with CP. For this, we analyzed saliva samples and found that the patients had a mixed cytokine profile. Similar results have been found previously in the literature, however, the cytokine diversity has varied within the studies (17, 18, 48, 49). This could be attributed to discrepancies in selection criteria within the studies and the period of the disease -acute or chronic-. In addition, we saw that the most increase of cytokines occurred in the groups with low $CD4^+$ T cell count. A plausible theory for this finding is that cytokine production could be innate-mediated. DC and macrophages could be the main cells producing cytokine as they have been observed to remain prevalent in oral mucosa during periodontal disease (45, 46). Although, other types of cells could be involved in the cytokine environment, such as innate lymphoid cells (ILC) and natural killer (NK) cells. Li and Reeves (50) showed that ILC are increased and activated in oral mucosa during simian immunodeficiency viral infection, these cells can produce several cytokines and we consider that the innate immune system should be studied further in CP, as well as evaluating the role of ILC and NK cells in human's oral cavity. As we previously mentioned, HIV+ patients have a dominant Th2 cytokine environment, irrespective of periodontal disease status (18), since the immune response against *Candida* spp. requires a plethora of immune cells (mainly $CD8^+$ T cells); the presence of a Th1 cytokine profile seems to be essential in the development of a resolutive immune response in CP. It is unknown, whether the Th2 cytokines present in the Th2/Th1 profile remains as a consequence in the oral immune microenvironment by the HIV infection, or if they are a secondary immune reactivation in order to establish a homeostatic mechanism. Something that we did observe is that the Th1/Th2 profile is present in all groups colonized with one or more *Candida* spp., despite their clinical, and demographic differences.

Though it has been reported that smoking promotes a Th1/Th2 cytokine profile in the saliva of HIV+ patients with OPC (51), in our study this factor did not have a major impact in the establishment of the mixed cytokine profile, since the majority of our study population presented a Th1/Th2 cytokine profile yet only 40% of them reported smoking habits. We considered that the shift in the local immune response from a Th2 to a Th1/Th2 profile is linked directly to the presence of *Candida* spp. (regardless of colonization), this data is consistent with the previous cytokine profile reported in OPC (17). In a non-HIV context, the progression of CP evolves from Th1/Th2 to Th1/Th17 profile (52, 53). Unfortunately, in our study we did not evaluate the Th17 profile. Whether these results are an early phase, which will further develop into a Th1/Th17 cytokine profile remains unknown and an interesting question to be answered in future studies.

With these findings and what it has been reported in the literature (7), we proposed a potential diagram of the immune physiopathology of CP in patients with HIV (**Figure 3**). Briefly, the loss of Th17 cytokines and increased presence of the Th2 profile, facilitate the oral colonization with pathogens such as *Candida* spp. This colonization activates local innate immune cells -DC, macrophages, ILC, NK cells, and others- which secrete Th1 cytokines, promoting the presence of a Th1/Th2 profile, and also secreting chemoattractant (TNF-α, CXCL1, and GM-CSF), that allows neutrophils recruitment and increase their survivability (54). At the same time, the release of ROS elements promotes bone resorption by activated osteoclasts (55). This local immune behavior is strengthened by smoking habit that increases the CCR5 expression, which facilitates local HIV entrance to DC and macrophages, promoting an onset of a "trojan horse" effect and a major local inflammation. Altogether, this damage promotes the destruction of the teeth architecture and facilitates the translocation of microbial products that could be enhancing a systemic inflammation.

AUTHOR CONTRIBUTIONS

SL-M performed the recruitment of patients, their periodontal evaluations, saliva acquisition, and original draft. SL-M, LG-H, VR-A, and ML-M helped with the diagnosis, evaluation, and assessment for inclusion or exclusion of patients for this paper. SL-M, EV-G, and JV-H performed PCRs and Candida identification. MA-Z, KS-R, MR-S, and RC-S performed cytokine determination and analysis. SL-M, JV-H, EV-G, RC-S, MA-Z, KS-R, MR-S, LG-H, and JA-V literature search, writing, review, and editing. SL-M, RC-S, MA-Z, KS-R, and MR-S developed the tables and figures for this manuscript. EV-G, SM-S, LG-H, and JA-V acquired the funds for this project.

ACKNOWLEDGMENTS

We thank GMCA Research Unit (University of Valencia, Spain) and Severe Infection Group (Health Research Institute La Fe, Valencia, Spain) for their technical support in Candida identification.

REFERENCES

1. Groenewegen H, Bierman WFW, Delli K, Dijkstra PU, Nesse W, Vissink A, et al. Severe periodontitis is more common in HIV- infected patients. *J Infect.* (2018) 78:171–7. doi: 10.1016/j.jinf.2018.11.008
2. Artega Chirinos F, Quiñónez B, Prado J, Florido R. Enfermedades periodontales asociadas a la infección del virus de inmunodeficiencia adquirida, reporte de lesiones orales y corporales. *Rev ADM.* (2008) LXV:322–6. Available online at: https://www.medigraphic.com/pdfs/adm/od-2008/od086h.pdf
3. Gonçalves LS, Gonçalves BML, Fontes TV. Periodontal disease in HIV-infected adults in the HAART era: clinical, immunological, and microbiological aspects. *Arch Oral Biol.* (2013) 58:1385–96. doi: 10.1016/j.archoralbio.2013.05.002
4. Agbelusi GA, Eweka OM, Umeizudike KA, Okoh M. Oral manifestations of HIV. In: *Current Perspectives in HIV Infection.* InTech (2013). Available oline at: http://www.intechopen.com/books/current-perspectives-in-hiv-infection/oral-manifestations-of-hiv doi: 10.5772/52941
5. Silva N, Abusleme L, Bravo D, Dutzan N, Garcia-Sesnich J, Vernal R, et al. Host response mechanisms in periodontal diseases. *J Appl Oral Sci.* (2015) 23:329–55. doi: 10.1590/1678-775720140259
6. Ohlrich E, Cullinan M, Seymour G. The immunopathogenesis of periodontal disease. *Aust Dent J.* (2009) 54:S2–10. doi: 10.1111/j.1834-7819.2009.01139.x
7. Heron SE, Elahi S. HIV infection and compromised mucosal immunity: oral manifestations and systemic inflammation. *Front Immunol.* (2017) 8:241. doi: 10.3389/fimmu.2017.00241
8. Sardi JCO, Duque C, Mariano FS, Peixoto ITA, Höfling JF, Gonçalves RB. *Candida* spp. in periodontal disease: a brief review. *J Oral Sci.* (2010) 52:177–85. doi: 10.2334/josnusd.52.177

9. Murray PA. Periodontal diseases in patients infected by human immunodeficiency virus. *Periodontol 2000.* (1994) 6:50–67. doi: 10.1111/j.1600-0757.1994.tb00026.x
10. Mataftsi M, Skoura L, Sakellari D. HIV infection and periodontal diseases: an overview of the post-HAART era. *Oral Dis.* (2011) 17:13–25. doi: 10.1111/j.1601-0825.2010.01727.x
11. Lourenço AG, Ribeiro AERA, Nakao C, Motta ACF, Antonio LGL, Machado AA, et al. Oral *Candida* spp carriage and periodontal diseases in HIV-infected patients in Ribeirão Preto, Brazil. *Rev Inst Med Trop Sao Paulo.* (2017) 59:e29. doi: 10.1590/s1678-9946201759029
12. Gaetti-Jardim Júnior E, Nakano V, Wahasugui TC, Cabral FC, Gamba R, Avila-Campos MJ. Occurrence of yeasts, enterococci and other enteric bacteria in subgingival biofilm of HIV-positive patients with chronic gingivitis and necrotizing periodontitis. *Braz J Microbiol.* (2008) 39:257–61. doi: 10.1590/S1517-83822008000200011
13. Junqueira JC, Vilela SFG, Rossoni RD, Barbosa JO, Costa ACBP, Rasteiro VMC, et al. Oral colonization by yeasts in HIV-positive patients in Brazil. *Rev Inst Med Trop Sao Paulo.* (2012) 54:17–24. doi: 10.1590/S0036-46652012000100004
14. Imai K, Ochiai K. Role of histone modification on transcriptional regulation and HIV-1 gene expression: possible mechanisms of periodontal diseases in AIDS progression. *J Oral Sci.* (2011) 53:1–13. doi: 10.2334/josnusd.53.1
15. Adeshnee MNHW. HIV-Associated oral lesions in HIV-seropositive patients at an HIV treatment clinic in South Africa. *J AIDS Clin Res.* (2015) 6:422. doi: 10.4172/2155-6113.1000422
16. Bodhade AS, Ganvir SM, Hazarey VK. Oral manifestations of HIV infection and their correlation with CD4 count. *J Oral Sci.* (2011) 53:203–11. doi: 10.2334/josnusd.53.203
17. Leigh JE, Steele C, Wormley FL, Luo W, Clark RA, Gallaher W, et al. Th1/Th2 cytokine expression in saliva of HIV-positive and HIV-negative individuals: a pilot study in HIV-positive individuals with oropharyngeal candidiasis. *J Acquir Immune Defic Syndr Hum Retrovirol.* (1998) 19:373–80. doi: 10.1097/00042560-199812010-00008
18. Vastardis S, Leigh JE, Wozniak K, Yukna R, Fidel PL. Influence of periodontal disease on Th1/Th2-type cytokines in saliva of HIV-positive individuals. *Oral Microbiol Immunol.* (2003) 18:88–91. doi: 10.1034/j.1399-302X.2003.00045.x
19. Leigh JE, McNulty KM, Fidel PL. Characterization of the immune status of CD8+ T cells in oral lesions of human immunodeficiency virus-infected persons with oropharyngeal Candidiasis. *Clin Vaccine Immunol.* (2006) 13:678–83. doi: 10.1128/CVI.00015-06
20. World Medical Association. World medical association declaration of Helsinki. *JAMA.* (2013) 310:2191–4. doi: 10.1001/jama.2013.281053
21. Kroidl A, Schaeben A, Oette M, Wettstein M, Herfordt A, Häussinger D. Prevalence of oral lesions and periodontal diseases in HIV-infected patients on antiretroviral therapy. *Eur J Med Res.* (2005) 10:448–53. Available online at: https://daignet.de/site-content/die-daig/fachorgan/archiv/2005/ejomr-2005-vol.10/448.pdf
22. Armitage GC. Development of a classification system for periodontal diseases and conditions. *Ann Periodontol.* (1999) 4:1–6. doi: 10.1902/annals.1999.4.1.1
23. Chakrabarti R, Schutt CE. The enhancement of PCR amplification by low molecular weight amides. *Nucleic Acids Res.* (2001) 29:2377–81. doi: 10.1093/nar/29.11.2377
24. Martínez JMG, Gómez EV, Pemán J, Cantón E, García MG, del Castillo Agudo L. Identification of pathogenic yeast species by polymerase chain reaction amplification of the RPS0 gene intron fragment. *J Appl Microbiol.* (2010) 108:1917–27. doi: 10.1111/j.1365-2672.2009.04595.x
25. Gupta N, Gupta ND, Garg S, Goyal L, Gupta A, Khan S, et al. The effect of type 2 diabetes mellitus and smoking on periodontal parameters and salivary matrix metalloproteinase-8 levels. *J Oral Sci.* (2016) 58:156–63. doi: 10.2334/josnusd.58.1
26. Campisi G, Pizzo G, Milici ME, Mancuso S, Margiotta V. Candidal carriage in the oral cavity of human immunodeficiency virus–infected subjects. *Oral Surg Oral Med Oral Pathol Oral Radiol.* (2002) 93:281–6. doi: 10.1067/moe.2002.120804
27. Mushi MF, Mtemisika CI, Bader O, Bii C, Mirambo MM, Groß U, et al. High oral carriage of non- albicans *Candida* spp. among HIV-infected individuals. *Int J Infect Dis.* (2016) 49:185–8. doi: 10.1016/j.ijid.2016.07.001
28. Jabra-Rizk MA, Ferreira SMS, Sabet M, Falkler WA, Merz WG, Meiller TF. Recovery of Candida dubliniensis and other yeasts from human immunodeficiency virus-associated periodontal lesions. *J Clin Microbiol.* (2001) 39:4520–2. doi: 10.1128/JCM.39.12.4520-4522.2001
29. Clark-Ordóñez I, Callejas-Negrete OA, Aréchiga-Carvajal ET, Mouriño-Pérez RR. Candida species diversity and antifungal susceptibility patterns in oral samples of HIV/AIDS patients in Baja California, Mexico. *Med Mycol.* (2017) 55:myw069. doi: 10.1093/mmy/myw069
30. Costa CR, Cohen AJ, Fernandes OFL, Miranda KC, Passos XS, Souza LKH, et al. Asymptomatic oral carriage of Candida species in HIV-infected patients in the highly active antiretroviral therapy era. *Rev Inst Med Trop Sao Paulo.* (2006) 48:257–61. doi: 10.1590/S0036-46652006000500004
31. Kirkpatrick WR, Revankar SG, Mcatee RK, Lopez-Ribot JL, Fothergill AW, McCarthy DI, et al. Detection of Candida dubliniensis in oropharyngeal samples from human immunodeficiency virus-infected patients in North America by primary CHROMagar candida screening and susceptibility testing of isolates. *J Clin Microbiol.* (1998) 36:3007–12.
32. Hulimane S, Maluvadi-Krishnappa R, Mulki S, Rai H, Dayakar A, Kabbinahalli M. Speciation of Candida using CHROMagar in cases with oral epithelial dysplasia and squamous cell carcinoma. *J Clin Exp Dent.* (2018) 10:e657–e660. doi: 10.4317/jced.54737
33. Nadeem SG, Hakim ST, Kazmi SU. Use of CHROMagar Candida for the presumptive identification of Candida species directly from clinical specimens in resource-limited settings. *Libyan J Med.* (2010) 5:2144. doi: 10.3402/ljm.v5i0.2144
34. Nayak S, Kavitha B, Sriram G, Saraswathi T, Sivapathasundharam B, Dorothy A. Comparative study of Candida by conventional and CHROMagar method in non-denture and denture wearers by oral rinse technique. *Indian J Dent Res.* (2012) 23:490–7. doi: 10.4103/0970-9290.104956
35. Ribeiro Ribeiro AL, de Alencar Menezes TO, de Melo Alves-Junior S, de Menezes SAF, Marques-da-Silva SH, Rosário Vallinoto AC. Oral carriage of Candida species in HIV-infected patients during highly active antiretroviral therapy (HAART) in Belém, Brazil. *Oral Surg Oral Med Oral Pathol Oral Radiol.* (2015) 120:29–33. doi: 10.1016/j.oooo.2015.03.008
36. Canabarro A, Valle C, Farias MR, Santos FB, Lazera M, Wanke B. Association of subgingival colonization of Candida albicans and other yeasts with severity of chronic periodontitis. *J Periodontal Res.* (2013) 48:428–32. doi: 10.1111/jre.12022
37. Hannula J, Dogan B, Slots J, Okte E, Asikainen S. Subgingival strains of Candida albicans in relation to geographical origin and occurrence of periodontal pathogenic bacteria. *Oral Microbiol Immunol.* (2001) 16:113–8. doi: 10.1034/j.1399-302x 2001.016002113.x
38. Yin MT, Dobkin JF, Grbic JT. Epidemiology, pathogenesis, and management of human immunodeficiency virus infection in patients with periodontal disease. *Periodontol.* (2007) 44:55–81. doi: 10.1111/j.1600-0757.2007.00205.x
39. Ryder MI. An update on HIV and periodontal disease. *J Periodontol.* (2002) 73:1071–8. doi: 10.1902/jop.2002.73.9.1071
40. Shinozaki S, Moriyama M, Hayashida J-N, Tanaka A, Maehara T, Ieda S, et al. Close association between oral Candida species and oral mucosal disorders in patients with xerostomia. *Oral Dis.* (2012) 18:667–72. doi: 10.1111/j.1601-0825.2012.01923.x
41. López-Verdín S, Andrade-Villanueva J, Zamora-Perez AL, Bologna-Molina R, Cervantes-Cabrera JJ, Molina-Frechero N. Differences in salivary flow level, xerostomia, and flavor alteration in mexican HIV patients who did or did not receive antiretroviral therapy. *AIDS Res Treat.* (2013) 2013:613278. doi: 10.1155/2013/613278
42. Cannon RD, Chaffin WL. Oral colonization by *Candida albicans*. *Crit Rev Oral Biol Med.* (1999) 10:359–83. doi: 10.1177/10454411990100030701
43. Margiotta V, Campisi G, Mancuso S. Plasma HIV-1 RNA and route of transmission in oral candidiasis and oral hairy leukoplakia. *Oral Dis.* (2008) 6:194–5. doi: 10.1111/j.1601-0825.2000.tb00333.x
44. Delgado ACD, de Jesus Pedro R, Aoki FH, Resende MR, Trabasso P, Colombo AL, et al. Clinical and microbiological assessment of patients with a long-term diagnosis of human immunodeficiency virus infection and Candida oral colonization. *Clin Microbiol Infect.* (2009) 15:364–71. doi: 10.1111/j.1469-0691.2009.02707.x

45. Cutler CW, Jotwani R. Oral mucosal expression of HIV-1 receptors, co-receptors, and α-defensins: tableau of resistance or susceptibility to HIV infection? *Adv Dent Res.* (2006) 19:49–51. doi: 10.1177/154407370601900110
46. Kweon M-N. Sublingual mucosa: a new vaccination route for systemic and mucosal immunity. *Cytokine.* (2011) 54:1–5. doi: 10.1016/j.cyto.2010.12.014
47. Cornwell WD, Kim V, Fan X, Vega ME, Ramsey FV, Criner GJ, et al. Activation and polarization of circulating monocytes in severe chronic obstructive pulmonary disease. *BMC Pulm Med.* (2018) 18:101. doi: 10.1186/s12890-018-0664-y
48. Takeichi O, Haber J, Kawai T, Smith DJ, Moro I, Taubman MA. Cytokine Profiles of T-lymphocytes from gingival tissues with pathological pocketing. *J Dent Res.* (2000) 79:1548–55. doi: 10.1177/00220345000790080401
49. Berglundh T, Liljenberg B, Lindhe J. Some cytokine profiles of T-helper cells in lesions of advanced periodontitis. *J Clin Periodontol.* (2002) 29:705–9. doi: 10.1034/j.1600-051X.2002.290807.x
50. Li H, Reeves RK. Functional perturbation of classical natural killer and innate lymphoid cells in the oral mucosa during SIV infection. *Front Immunol.* (2013) 3:417. doi: 10.3389/fimmu.2012.00417
51. Slavinsky J, Myers T, Swoboda RK, Leigh JE, Hager S, Fidel PL. Th1/Th2 cytokine profiles in saliva of HIV-positive smokers with oropharyngeal candidiasis. *Oral Microbiol Immunol.* (2002) 17:38–43. doi: 10.1046/j.0902-0055.2001.00080.x
52. Dezerega A, Maggiolo S, Garrido M, Dutzan N. The TH17 vs. TREG imbalance in the pathogenesis of periodontitis: new approach for dichotomy TH1 vs. TH2. *Rev Clínica Periodoncia, Implantol y Rehabil Oral.* (2008) 1:70–2. doi: 10.1016/S0718-5391(08)70012-0
53. Gaffen SL, Hajishengallis G. A new inflammatory cytokine on the block: re-thinking periodontal disease and the Th1/Th2 paradigm in the context of Th17 cells and IL-17. *J Dent Res.* (2008) 87:817–28. doi: 10.1177/154405910808700908
54. Prame Kumar K, Nicholls AJ, Wong CHY. Partners in crime: neutrophils and monocytes/macrophages in inflammation and disease. *Cell Tissue Res.* (2018) 371:551–65. doi: 10.1007/s00441-017-2753-2
55. Herrera BS, Martins-Porto R, Maia-Dantas A, Campi P, Spolidorio LC, Costa SKP, et al. iNOS-derived nitric oxide stimulates osteoclast activity and alveolar bone loss in ligature-induced periodontitis in rats. *J Periodontol.* (2011) 82:1608–15. doi: 10.1902/jop.2011.100768

13

Dengue Virus Serotype 2 and its Non-Structural Proteins 2A and 2B Activate NLRP3 Inflammasome

*Gaurav Shrivastava[1†], Giovani Visoso-Carvajal[1], Julio Garcia-Cordero[1], Moisés Leon-Juarez[2], Bibiana Chavez-Munguia[3], Tomas Lopez[4], Porfirio Nava[5], Nicolás Villegas-Sepulveda[1] and Leticia Cedillo-Barron[1]**

[1] Departmento de Biomedicina Molecular Centro de Investigación y Estudios Avanzados-Instituto Politécnico Nacional, Mexico City, Mexico, [2] Departamento de Inmunobioquímica, Instituto Nacional de Perinatología, Mexico City, Mexico, [3] Departamento de Infectomica y Biologia Molecular, Centro de Investigación y Estudios Avanzados-Instituto Politécnico Nacional, Mexico City, Mexico, [4] Departamento de Genética del Desarrollo y Fisiología Molecular, Instituto de Biotecnología, UNAM Cuernavaca, Cuernavaca, Mexico, [5] Departamento de Fisiologia, Biofisica y Neurociencias, Cinvestav Zacatenco, Mexico City, Mexico

***Correspondence:**
Leticia Cedillo-Barron
lcedillo@cinvestav.mx

†Present address:
Gaurav Shrivastava,
Laboratory of Malaria and Vector Research, National Institute of Allergy and Infectious Diseases (NIAID), National Institutes of Health (NIH), Rockville, MD, United States

Dengue is the most prevalent and rapidly transmitted mosquito-borne viral disease of humans. One of the fundamental innate immune responses to viral infections includes the processing and release of pro-inflammatory cytokines such as interleukin (IL-1β and IL-18) through the activation of inflammasome. Dengue virus stimulates the Nod-like receptor (NLRP3-specific inflammasome), however, the specific mechanism(s) by which dengue virus activates the NLRP3 inflammasome is unknown. In this study, we investigated the activation of the NLRP3 inflammasome in endothelial cells (HMEC-1) following dengue virus infection. Our results showed that dengue infection as well as the NS2A and NS2B protein expression increase the NLRP3 inflammasome activation, and further apoptosis-associated speck-like protein containing caspase recruitment domain (ASC) oligomerization, and IL-1β secretion through caspase-1 activation. Specifically, we have demonstrated that NS2A and NS2B, two proteins of dengue virus that behave as putative viroporins, were sufficient to stimulate the NLRP3 inflammasome complex in lipopolysaccharide (LPS)-primed endothelial cells. In summary, our observations provide insight into the dengue-induced inflammatory response mechanism and highlight the importance of DENV-2 NS2A and NS2B proteins in activation of the NLRP3 inflammasome during dengue virus infection.

Keywords: dengue, inflammasome, non-structural proteins NS2A and NS2B, viroporins, IL-1β, NLRP3, Caspase-1

INTRODUCTION

Dengue Virus (DENV) is a positive-sense single-stranded RNA virus from the Flaviviridae family. Dengue is caused by any of the four serotypes DENV-1 to DENV-4. It is transmitted to humans by female mosquitoes of the genus, *Aedes* (1, 2). The infection results in a broad spectrum of illness ranging from subclinical and mild self-limiting to severe dengue fever (DF) (2, 3). Severe dengue is associated with a secondary infection with a heterologous serotype (1, 3), and is characterized by immune dysfunction that can progress to life-threatening hypovolemic shock due to hemorrhage and leakage of vascular fluid. During severe infection, a massive and aberrant production of cytokines called a "cytokine storm" contributes to its deadly pathology (4). For example, the interleukin IL-1β plays a crucial role in the cytokine storm during dengue infection (5, 6). It is an extremely potent cytokine that is regulated and induced by dengue-infected macrophages and monocytes (6–8). Further, most dengue virus-infected patients present with fever, which is the most common symptom caused by the endogenous pyrogen molecule (EP). Additionally, the pro-inflammatory cytokine IL-1β has been shown to play a crucial role in increasing the deregulation of hemostasis and thrombosis during DENV infection (4, 6, 9). A dual pathway is required for the production of IL-1β, the priming signal, to stimulate the transcription and synthesis of pro-IL-1β, which must undergo post-translational cleavage to mature IL-1β by activated caspase-1. Caspase-1 activation is regulated by a second independent stimulus such as the "inflammasome," a multi-protein complex assembled upon activation (10).

Pathogen recognition receptors (PPRs) include several nucleotide-binding domain leucine rich repeat-containing proteins (NLRPs) and other innate immune receptors, such as AIM2, which show different specificities toward pathogen- and danger-associated molecular patterns (10). During viral infections, NLRP3, binds to caspase-1 through the adaptor molecule, ASC containing a caspase recruitment domain, to assemble the inflammasome (11). The NLRP3 inflammasome responds to many stimuli from viral components, such as ATP and reactive oxygen species (ROS). Evaluation of macrophages infected with dengue virus has revealed that C-type lectin 5A (CLEC5A) plays a crucial role in dengue virus-induced NLRP3 activation (12).

Increased amounts of IL-1β have been observed in dengue virus patients (4) and several viral proteins have been linked to this process. It is also demonstrated that platelets from dengue-infected patients contribute to increased vascular permeability during infection by the synthesis and release of IL-1β (13). Spleen Tyrosine Kinase (Syk) augments IL-1β induction during antibody-enhanced dengue virus infection in primary human monocytes, however caspase-1 and NLRP3 are required for the maturation of pro-IL-1β during antibody-dependent enhancement (7). Altogether, these observations indicated that inflammasome activation might play a critical role in the pathogenesis of DENV infection. However, the molecular mechanisms through which DENV-2 provides secondary signals that activate the inflammasome are still elusive.

Several reports have confirmed the role of viroporins in inflammasome activation during viral infections (14). These molecules participate in several steps of the life cycle and are usually associated with the pathogenesis of viral infections. Viroporins are small, hydrophobic, transmembrane proteins that cause changes in the cellular permeability by forming hydrophilic pores in host cellular membranes, and disturb balance among the corresponding intracellular ions (e.g., Na^+, K^+, Ca^{++}, Cl^-, and H^+). The ion concentration changes induced by those proteins often activates innate immune responses aimed to counter the viral infection (15–17). Interestingly, several viroporins from different viruses have been shown to activate the NLRP3 inflammasome by disrupting the Ca^{++} balance, including Rotavirus NSP4 (18), HCV p7 (19), EMCV 2B (20), Agnoprotein (21), polio 2BC (22), Influenza PB1-F2 (23), and coxsackievirus 2B (24). Calcium levels are disturbed in two ways; primarily, free cytosolic Ca^{++} are elevated through the release of Ca^{++} from the endoplasmic reticulum, Golgi complex, mitochondria, and lysosomes and secondly, influx of extracellular Ca^{++} via plasma membrane channels or Ca^{++} pump disturbance (25).

Among the dengue virus non-structural proteins (NS1, NS2A, NS2B, NS3, NS4A, NS4B, and NS5), DENV NS2B has been reported to participate in replication, as a co-factor of viral protease and degradation of cGAS (26). In addition, DENV protease complex NS2B3 has been shown to partially cleave mitochondrial fusion proteins i.e., Mfn1 and Mfn2 resulting in the inhibition of mitochondrial fusion. Also, DENV induces cytopathic effects through destabilizing the interferon response and facilitating mitochondrial membrane potential (MMP) disruption (27). In our lab, two non-structural proteins (NSP) DENV-2 NS2B and DENV-2 NS2A have been demonstrated to behave as viroporins. Both molecules permeabilize different membrane models by forming membrane channels, as well as self-oligomerize and participate in a range of viral functions (28, 29). Furthermore, DENV NS2A a 22–25 kDa hydrophobic transmembrane protein plays a critical role in the virus life cycle by modulating the replication, viral assembly, and viral release probably by inhibiting the interferon and JAK-STAT pathways (30–32). DENV NS2A hydrophobic regions have demonstrated to have strong interactions with several Eukariothic model membrane systems (33). Although several studies have provided some clues regarding the role of different molecules of DENV that trigger the inflammatory process (34, 35), the mechanism of NLRP3 activation is not fully understood. In the current study, we have attempted to shed more light on the role of the putative viroporins NS2B and NS2A in the regulation of inflammasome activation. Initially, we demonstrated that macrovascular endothelial cells (HMEC-1) infected with DENV-2 activate the NLRP3 inflammasome, followed by ASC oligomerization, activation of caspase-1 and secretion of IL-1β. We further investigated whether this phenomenon is conserved in other cell lines such HepG2 and THP-1 cells. Finally, we have evaluated whether the viroporin-like proteins, NS2A, and NS2B, which induce changes in membrane permeability (29), are able to trigger the activation of the inflammasome. Thus, we found that the expression of recombinant NS2A-GFP and NS2B-GFP in the ER and mitochondria of HMEC-1 cells, significant increases the expression of NLRP3, ASC oligomerization, caspase-1 activation, and IL-1β secretion in the cell supernatant after priming with LPS. Furthermore, using a genetic knockout strain (ASC gene) and also pharmacological agents (NLRP3 inhibitor or caspase-1 inhibitor), we demonstrated that IL-1β release during DENV infection relays mainly in the assembly of the NLRP3 inflammasome and the activation of Caspase-1. Finally, we suggest that NS2A may be involved in intracellular Ca^{++} homeostasis and/or mitochondrial disruption, thereby boosting the activation of the NLRP3 inflammasome that leads to the overproduction of IL-1β. In summary, our observations unravel the mechanism by which dengue virus activates the NLRP3 inflammasome and emphasize the activity of viroporins in inducing NLRP3 inflammasome activation.

TABLE 1 | List of Antibodies.

Antibody list			
Host	**Target**	**Brand**	**No cat.**
Mouse	αGolgi 97	Thermo Fisher	A-21270
Rabbit	αNS3	Genetex	GTX124252
Rabbit	αGM130	Abcam	ab-52649
Rabbit	αCalnexin	Abcam	ab232433
Mouse	αTOM22	Abcam	ab-57523
Mouse	αNLRP3	Adipogen	AG-20B-0014-C100
Rat	αNS5	LCB	(38)*
Rabbit	αGAPDH	Genetex	GTX100118
Rabbit	αASC	Adipogen	AG-25B-0006
Rabbit	αCasp-1	Abcam	ab-108362
Goat	αMouse HRP	Invitrogen	626520
Goat	αRabbit HRP	Invitrogen	656120
Goat	αMouse Alexa 486	Invitrogen	A11001
Goat	αRabbit Cy3	Invitrogen	A10521
Goat	αRat HRP	Invitrogen	629520
Goat	αRat FITC	Thermo Fisher	31629

MATERIALS AND METHODS

Cell Culture and DENV Serotype 2

HMEC-1 (HMEC line 1; Centers for Disease Control, Atlanta, GA, USA) were grown at 37°C under 5% CO_2 in MCDB131 medium (Gibco/Life Technologies, Carlsbad, CA, USA) supplemented with 10% fetal bovine serum, 1 mg/mL hydrocortisone (Sigma Aldrich, St. Louis, MO, USA), 10 ng/mL epidermal growth factor (Gibco), 100 U penicillin, and 100 mg/mL streptomycin. Cells were detached by treatment with 1,000 U/mL trypsin and 0.5 mM EDTA. Mosquito C6/36 cells derived from *Aedes albopictus* were grown in MEM supplemented with 10% fetal bovine Serum (FBS) (Gibco Carlsbad, CA) at 34°C. The DENV-2 with high nucleotide sequence homology to the New Guinea strain; (36) was obtained from a clinical isolate from a 1997 DF patient from the Mexican east coast. The stock preparation and titration have been described previously (37). The virus stock was prepared by infecting a C6/36 cell monolayer in 75 cm^2 tissue culture flasks at 75–85% confluence. When the infected monolayer showed cytopathic effects, the cells supernatant were homogenized and diluted in a 40% polyethylene glycol solution in 2 M NaCl (Sigma-Aldrich St. Louis, MO) and incubated at 4°C overnight. The suspension was centrifuged at 6,000 rpm for 1 h, and then the virus stock in the bottom was resuspended in 1/15 of the total volume with a glycine buffer (Tris 50 mM, Glycine 200 mM, NaCl 100 mM and EDTA 1 mM) and 1/30 of the total volume of FBS. The virus was homogenized, aliquoted and frozen at −70°C until use.

Antibodies

The **Table 1** describe all the antibodies used during this work.

Plasmid Construction

The full length cDNAs encoding the NS2A and NS2B proteins of DENV-2 were cloned in the eukaryotic expression vector pEGFPN1 (Clontech). Briefly, the cDNAs encoding NS2A and NS2B were obtained by reverse transcription and PCR (by using specific oligonucleotides) of total RNA extracted from DENV-2 infected C6/36 cells with Trizol (Gibco, USA) according the manufacturer instructions. Both NS2A and NS2B amplicons and the plasmid pEGFPN1 were digested simultaneously with the restriction enzymes XhoI and HindIII (New England Biolabs), and then ligated in frame with GFP. The plasmid constructs pNS2A-GFP and pNS2B-GFP were verified by DNA sequencing. Further, the bulk production of plasmids were obtained by using endotoxin free Maxiprep kit (Qiagen, USA).

SDS-PAGE and Immunoblotting

Protein samples were resolved by SDS-PAGE using 12 or 15 % gels for 80 min at 100 V (Mini-Protean Cell; Amersham Biosciences, Piscataway, NJ, USA) and then electro transferred (120 V for 2 h) onto nitrocellulose membranes (Hybond ECL; GE Healthcare, Little Chalfont, UK). Membranes were blocked and then incubated with the appropriate primary antibody, followed by the appropriate horseradish peroxidase (HRP)-conjugated secondary antibody (1:3,000) in PBS-Tween-20. After further washing with PBS-Tween-20, the membranes were developed with western lightning enhanced chemiluminescence reagent (Pearce, Rockford, IL, USA). The membranes were stripped if necessary. All the antibodies used in this work are presented in **Table 1**.

Mitochondrial Membrane Potential Assay

HMEC-1 cells were seeded at 1 × 10^5 per well in a 6 well-plate and transiently transfected with plasmids i.e., GFP, NS2A-GFP, NS2B-GFP. After 36 h post-transfection, HMEC-1 cells were treated with 175 mM with Tetramethyl rodhamine Methyl Ester Perchlorate (TMRE Waltham, Massachusetts, USA) in MCDB base medium and incubate for 30 min at 37°C. Then TMRE solution was discarded and the cells were washed. Cells were detached and washed with 2 times with PBS 1X, and cells pellets resuspended in 0.2% BSA in 1X PBS. Mitochondria membrane potential was analyzed in the flow-cytometry at 488 nm.

Quantification of IL-1β Production

LPS-primed HMEC-1 cells were grown in 24 well-plates, transfected as described earlier and incubated at 5% CO_2 and 37°C overnight. Further, cell supernatants were harvested at the indicated times post-transfection and analyzed for the presence of IL-1β using an enzyme-linked immunosorbent assay (Human IL-1β ELISA Kit II BD biosciences San Jose CA, USA) according to the manufacturer's instructions, and the concentration of IL-1β of the unknown samples and controls was determined from a standard curve. Samples producing signals higher than that of the highest standard (250 pg/ml) were diluted and re-analyzed. Each sample was run in triplicate and the assay were repeated for at least three times. The absorbance was read at 450 nm within 30 min of stopping reaction.

Transmission Electron Microscopy Analysis

The HMEC-1 cells were grown overnight in a 25 cm^2 tissue culture flasks (Corning, New York, USA). Then, cells were mock-infected or infected with DENV-2 at 5 MOIs for 48 h. Further, the samples were fixed with 2.5% of glutaraldehyde in 0.1 M Sodium cacodylate buffer (pH 7.2) for 1 h at room temperature (RT), and post-fixed with 1% osmium tetroxide for 1 h at RT. The samples were dehydrated through an ethanol gradient and propylene oxide, and then were embedded in Polybed epoxy resins and polymerized at 60°C for 24 h. Finally, 70 nm thin sections were stained with uranyl acetate and citrate and then the preparations were analyzed by using a Jeol JEM-1011 transmission electron microscope (JeolLtd.,Tokyo, Japan).

Transfection and Immunofluorescence

HMEC-1 cells were trypsinized and resuspended in MCDB131 medium. Cells were then seeded on glass coverslips (1 × 10^5 cells/ mL). After 24 h, the culture medium was removed, and the monolayers were washed and transfected. Briefly,HMEC-1 cells were grown at 50% confluence in a 6-well-plate, the medium was removed, and the cells were exposed to the transfection complex with different constructed plasmids [1 μg of DNA and 1 μl of Lipofectamine 2000 reagent (Invitrogen Life Technologies) mixed in 100 μl of serum-free Opti-MEM] for 4.5 h at 37°C. Then the cells were cultured in complete medium. At different times post-tranfections, the cells were fixed with 4% paraformaldehyde (Sigma-Aldrich, St. Louis, MO, USA) in PBS for 20 min at room temperature, permeabilized with a solution of PBS supplemented with 0.1% Triton-X100 and blocked with 10% normal goat serum. The cell monolayer was incubated for 60 min with primary antibodies. Further, glass cover slip was washed and the following fluorochrome-conjugated secondary antibodies were added. Irrelevant isotype antibody was used as a negative control. Nuclei were labeled with DAPI (1 μg/ml) in PBS for 10 min, and the slides were mounted with VECTASHIELD (Vector Labs, Burlingame, CA, USA). The images were captured with a confocal microscope (Leica SP2, Barcelona, Spain).

Knockout of ASC by CRISPR-CAS9 Technology

The knockout was performed according to the protocol (37). lentiCRISPR v2 was a gift from Feng Zhang (Addgene plasmid # 52961; http://n2t.net/addgene:52961; RRID:Addgene_52961). Briefly, to clone the specific guide RNA specific to the vector, 5 μg of the lentiviral CRISPR plasmid (lentiCRISPRv2) was digested with BsmBI for 30 min at 37°C. In parallel, guide RNA was phosphorylated and annealed with each pair of oligos. The reaction mixture contained 1 μl Oligo Forward (100 μM), 1 μl Oligo Reverse (100 μM), 1 μl of 10X T4 Ligation Buffer (NEB), 6.5 μl dd H_2O, 0.5 μl T4 PNK (NEB M0201S). Briefly, the phosphorylation/annealing reactions of the guide RNA were performed at 37°C for 30 min, 95°C for 5 min and then ramped down to 25°C at the rate of 5°C/min. The annealed oligos were diluted at a 1:200. The ligation reaction was incubated at room temperature for 10 min. Later, 1.5 μl ligated vector DNA was mixed with 20 μl competent Stbl3 bacterial cells, and incubated on ice for 30 min. After incubation, the cells were heat-shocked at 42°C for 45 s and more tubes were placed on ice for 2 min. SOC media (50 μl) was added and the bacteria were cultured at 37°C for 60 min on a shaker. Cultured bacteria were plated on LB-Agar plates and analyzed by colony PCR using the forward primer from the vector plasmid and the reverse primer from the reverse guide RNA (S-1). The amplified DNA was analyzed in 2% agarose gel and the expected band size (125 bp) was observed. Further, HEK 293T (3 × 10^6) cells were plated and then transfected with 4 μg of pLentiCRISPR v2 encoding sgRNA against GFP (control) or human ASC and packaging plasmids pVSVg and psPAX2 (1 μg each). After 6 h of transfection, 10 mL growth medium (cDMEM with 20% FBS) was replaced. Viral supernatants were collected after 48 and 72 h of transfection, concentrated by centrifugation at 20,000 × g for 2 h and was used to transduce the HMEC-1 cells in the presence of polybrene (2 μg/ml) in the 6-well plate containing HMEC-1 media. The plates were centrifuged for 45 min at 2,000 × g at 37°C, followed incubation at 37°C under 5% CO_2 in MCDB131. After 12 h (overnight incubation), cells were tripsinized, washed and transferred to a 75 cm^2 tissue culture flask with HMEC-1 media containing puromycin (1 μg/mL). The cells were checked every 3 days and the puromycin-containing medium was changed. Surviving populations derived in this manner were propagated and expanded for 6 weeks before cryopreserving stock cultures. The expression of wild type and ASC KO HMEC-1 was verified by western blotting with Anti-ASC antibody.

RESULTS

Dengue Virus Infection Activates the NLRP3 Inflammasome in HMEC-1 Cells

Considering the major function of endothelial cells during the infection with dengue virus, we wanted to evaluate whether DENV is capable of triggering the immune response mediated by the inflammasome in HMEC-1 cells. We initially characterized the inflammasome activation induced by DENV-2, in different cell lines such as HepG2, THP-1 (**Figures S1**, **S2**), and our experimental model HMEC-1 cells. Cell lysates from DENV-2 infected (5 MOI) HMEC-1 and mock-infected (UV treated DENV-2) cells were western blotted for caspase 1. As shown in **Figure S1A**, DENV-2 infection induced and increased the cleavage of caspase-1, when compared with mock-infected cells. LPS/ATP stimuli was used as a positive control. Moreover, DENV-2 infection was confirmed by western blotting DENV-2 NS3 protein in THP-1 cells (**Figure S2A**) and by western blotting and imaging (immunofluorescence) DENV-2 NS5 protein in HMEC-1 cells (**Figure 1A** and **Figure S1B**).

Likewise, to determine whether DENV-2 activates the NLRP3 inflammasome, cell lysates from DENV-2 infected HMEC-1 cells were analyzed by western blot at different infection times using specific anti-NLRP3 antibody. During DENV-2 infection. Changes in the NLRP3 expression were observed at the late phase (36 and 48 h) pos-DENV-2 infection, in contrast to HMEC-1 untreated and mock-infected cell controls, shown low expression

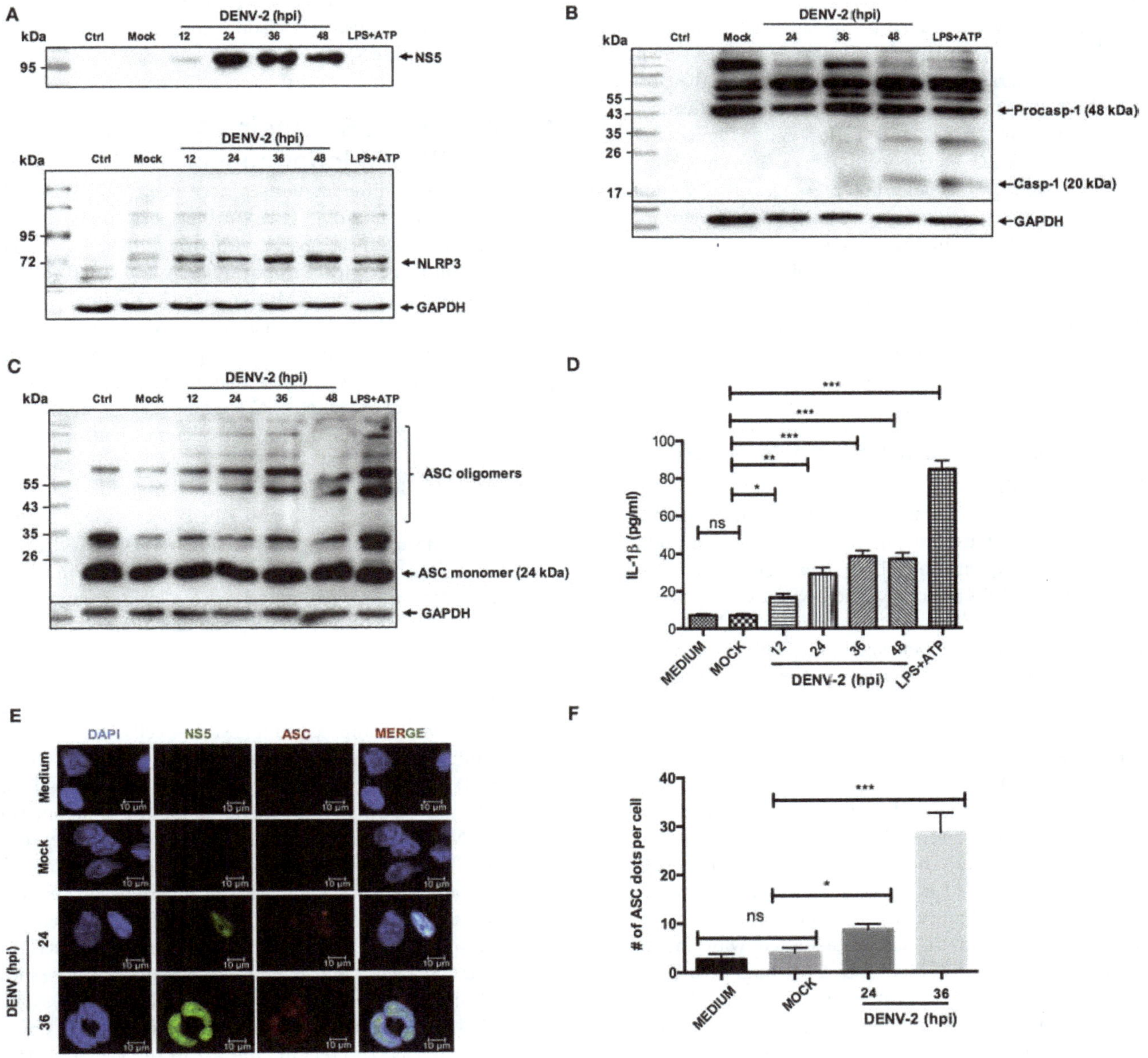

FIGURE 1 | NLRP3 inflammasome activation by DENV-2. HMEC-1 were infected with DENV-2 (5 MOI) at different time points, mock-infected or treated with LPS (1 μg/mL) and ATP (5 mM) as a positive control. Cell lysates were analyzed by western blot using an anti-NLRP3 antibody (1:500) **(A)**, an anti-NS5 antibody (1:100) **(B)**, an anti-caspase-1 antibody (1:1,000) **(C)**, or an anti-ASC antibody (1:1,000) **(D)**. HMEC-1 were infected with DENV-2 (5 MOI) at different time points, mock-infected or treated with LPS (1 μg/mL) for 6 h followed by ATP (5 mM) for 45 min as a positive control, and cell-free supernatants were collected at 12, 24, 36, and 48 h post-infection and analyzed for IL-1β by ELISA **(E)**, HMEC-1 were infected with DENV-2 (5 MOI) at 24 and 36 h or mock-infected. Cells were stained with anti-NS5 (green) and anti-ASC (red) and analyzed by confocal microscopy. Mock-treated cells were also examined. Nuclei were visualized by staining with DAPI **(F)**. The number (#) of ASC puncta per cell was counted by confocal microscopy. ASC puncta was calculated from a total of 20 cells. Data are representative of at least three independent experiments, and indicate the mean ± S.D. **(E,F)**. $^{*}P < 0.05$, $^{**}P < 0.01$, and $^{***}P < 0.001$. ns, non significant.

of NLRP3. In the positive control, the HMEC-1 cells treated with LPS (1 μg/mL) (LPS -O111:B4, sigma Aldrich) (signal 1) for 6 h, and ATP for 45 min (signal 2), to induce the assembly of the inflammasome complex, a high expression of NLRP3 was observed (**Figure 1A**). Western blot analysis showed the activated caspase 1 (~20 kDa) at 24 h post-infection, and a more prominent band was observed at 48 h post-infection with DENV-2 (**Figure 1B**). To analyze the oligomerization of the ASC adapter protein, western blot analysis was conducted on the cell lysates infected with DENV-2 at 24, 36, and 48 h post-infection, and cells treated with LPS and ATP. No oligomerization of ASC was observed in mock-infected HMEC-1 cells, however prominent oligomerization of ASC was observed after 12, 24, 36, and 48 h post-infection with DENV-2, along with the positive control (LPS + ATP) (**Figure 1C**). As expected, a significant increase of IL-1β was detected in the supernatant of DENV-2-infected cells at 36 and 48 h post-infection, in contrast with mock-infected cell supernatant (**Figure 1D**). Similar to the observed with HMEC-1, DENV-2 triggered caspase-1 activation and IL-1β secretion in HepG2 and THP-1 cells (**Figures S2B–E**). Furthermore, HMEC-1 cells were DENV-2 or mock-infected at different time points and the presence of ASC punctate structures, which serve as a marker of the "inflammasome complex," were found in the cells infected with DENV-2 at 36 h, in contrast to mock-infected cells (**Figure 1E**). The number of ASC puncta structures per cell was calculated for total 20 cells (**Figure 1F**). Taken together, these results demonstrate that DENV-2 induces activation of the NLRP3 inflammasome in HepG2, THP1, and HMEC-1 cells.

Expression and Localization of NS2A in HMEC-1 Cells

To fully characterize the subcellular localization of DENV-2 NS2A and evaluate its role in inflammasome activation, the NS2A (657 bp) sequence of DENV-2 was cloned as an eGFP-fused protein (eGFPN1 vector). The pNS2A-GFP, pNS2B-GFP, and pGFPN1 plasmids were transfected into HMEC-1 cells and analyzed by western blot and immunofluorescence assays at different times (24 and 48 h) to determine the subcellular localization of DENV-2 NS2A. The expression of NS2A-GFP, was observed in the perinuclear space in HMEC-1, demonstrating its functional expression in the cytoplasmic region (**Figure 2A**). In addition, NS2A-GFP and NS2B-GFP and GFP transfected cells were lysed, and analyzed by western blot using anti-GFP antibody. Clear bands were observed in the transfected cells with DENV constructs. The molecular weight for NS2A-GFP (48 kDa) and NS2B (43 kDa) were as expected according to the fusion protein (**Figure 2B**). Additionaly a sharp 27-kDa band was observed in the cells transfected with the NS2A-GFP and NS2B-GFP (in this case, GFP might be produced as a result of leaky translation scanning in the frame fused transcript) as well as in the parental vector GFP (as expected). Using different organelle markers for ER, Golgi apparatus, and mitochondria, we observed that NS2A exhibited significant overlap with calnexin A, which is a transmembrane protein that resides in the ER membrane, indicating that NS2A partially localizes to the ER network. Further, NS2A co-localized with mitochondria (MitoTracker) and Tom22, an outer mitochondrial membrane protein. In contrast, NS2A did not co-localize with the Golgi apparatus marker (GOLGI) (**Figure 2C**). Hence, our co-localization studies indicated that the NS2A protein localizes to both the ER and mitochondria organelles with Pearson's coefficient values of 0.79 and 0.81, respectively (**Figure 2D**). The Pearson's coefficients between NS2A and the different markers analyzed were calculated as average values from 20 individual cells. It is important to demonstrate that the NS2A-GFP and NS2B-GFP behave as the viral proteins in the context of DENV infection. Thus, we evaluated the localization of NS2B protein by infecting and transfecting cells simultaneously to corroborate the localization of NS2B. We observed the same localization pattern of NS2B during DENV-2 infection as well as during transfection of NS2B-GFP tag. Thus, GFP tag does not modify the localization of the NS2B (**Figure S3**).

NS2A and NS2B Proteins Are Sufficient to Trigger NLRP3 Inflammasome

Viroporins from different viruses have been demonstrated to activate the inflammasome (14). Furthermore, we have shown that NS2A and NS2B behave as viroporins, thus, we evaluated the ability of dengue virus viroporin NS2A and NS2B to trigger inflammasome activation. HMEC-1 cells were primed with LPS (O111:B4, sigma Aldrich) (signal 1) followed by transfection with GFP-tagged plasmids expressing dengue NS2A, NS2B, proteins. Western blot analysis demonstrated higher protein levels of NLRP3 expression, ASC oligomerization, and caspase-1 activation in LPS-primed HMEC-1 cells transiently expressing NS2A or NS2B but not in HMEC-1 cells transfected with NS3, and NS2B-NS3 with the parental plasmid (eGFPN1). We also found that NS2A and NS2B expression triggered Caspase-1 cleavage in HepG2 cells (**Figure S1C**). ATP (5 mM) stimulation was used as a positive control for an NLRP3 inflammasome inducer (**Figures 3A–C**). Cell free supernatants were collected at 36 h post-transfection and the presence of IL-1β was analyzed using an enzyme-linked immunosorbent assay (ELISA). As expected, significant IL-1β was released from LPS-primed HMEC-1 cells transfected with pNS2A-GFP or pNS2B-GFP vectors when compared with HMEC-1 cells transfected with pNS3-GFP, pNS2B-NS3-GFP or the parental vector (peGFPN1) (**Figure 3D**). This data strongly suggested a direct involvement of NS2A and NS2B in the activation of the inflammasome complex (NLRP3, ASC, Caspase-1) and the subsequently release of IL-1β. To support the above results, we also examined the oligomerization of ASC as a marker of inflammasome complex activation by NS2A and NS2B. To do this, HMEC-1 cells were primed with LPS for 6 h followed by transfection with peGFPN1-plasmid or GFP tagged NS2A and NS2B plasmid. We have shown that ASC punctate structures were formed in the cytoplasm of HMEC-1 cells transfected with the plasmid expressing the NS2A-GFP and NS2B-GFP, in contrast to the cells transfected with peGFPN1 (**Figure 3E**). As a positive control, HMEC-1 cells were re-treated with ATP for 45 min to observe the presence of ASC punctate structures. The number of ASC per cell was counted and demonstrated the role of DENV-2 NS2A and NS2B in inflammasome activation (**Figure 3F**). We also examined the intracellular localization of NLRP3. In agreement with previous reports (39), stimulation of LPS-primed cells with HMEC-1 induced NLRP3 expression in the cytosol. Upon cell transfection with dengue NS2A-GFP after 36 h, NLRP3 was redistributed to the perinuclear region or cytoplasmic granular structures, which are considered a hallmark of NLRP3 activation, in contrast to resting or control cells transfected only with GFP. We also shown that NLRP3 was co-localized with NS2A-GFP in HMEC-1 cells, in contrast to either GFP or NS2B-GFP (not shown). About 60% of cells expressing the NS2A-GFP showed very strong co-localization with NLRP3, very as a 0.8427 (>0.5) Pearson's coefficient was observed (**Figures 3G,H**). Together,

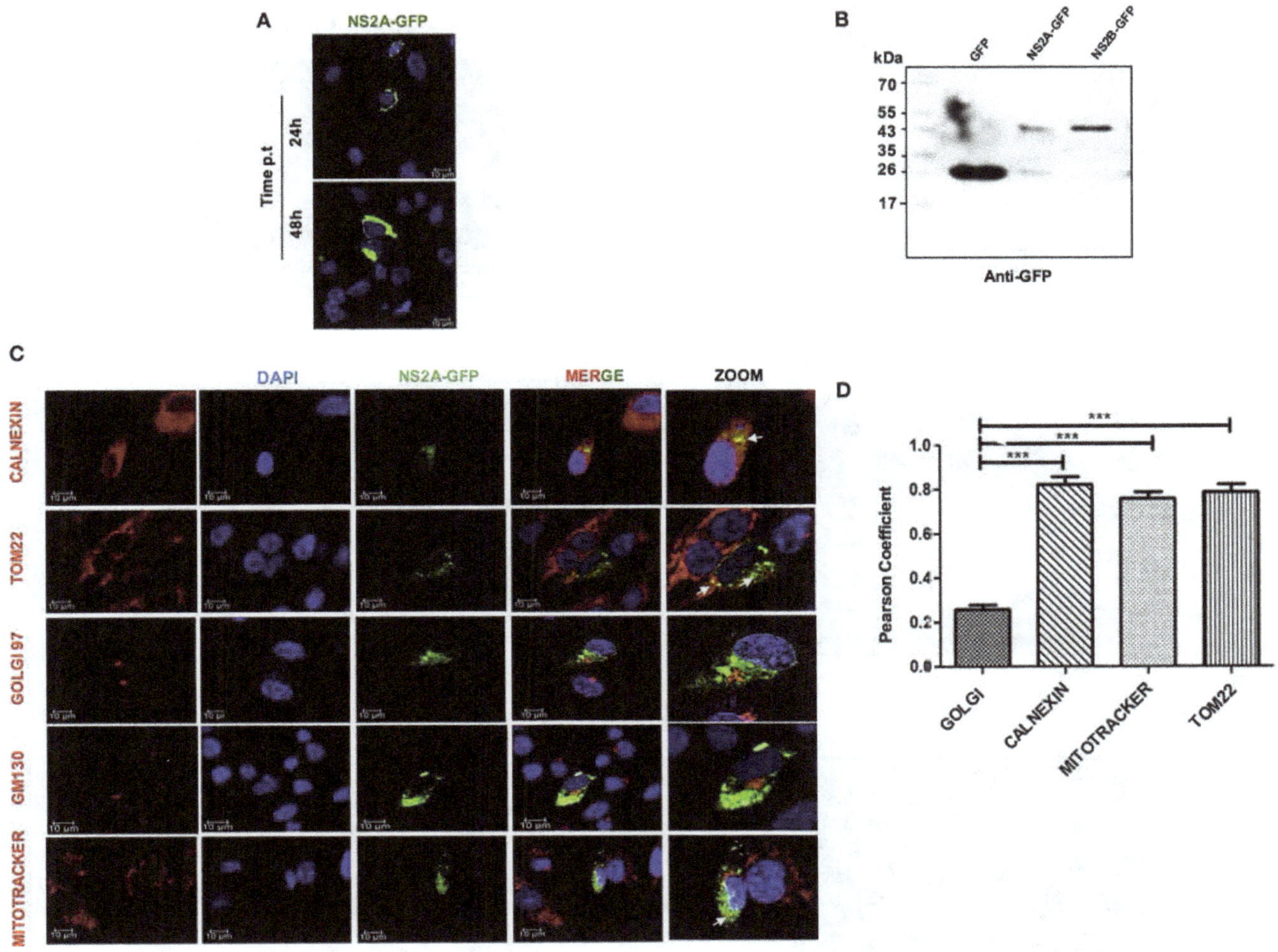

FIGURE 2 | Expression and localization of NS2A protein in HMEC-1 cells. **(A)** HMEC-1 cells were transiently transfected with plasmids coding for NS2A-GFP and analyzed at 24 and 48 h. Cells were fixed and analyzed by confocal microscopy **(B)**. HMEC-1 cells were transiently transfected with the plasmids coding for GFP and the NS2A-GFP protein and cell lysates were analyzed by western blot using an anti-GFP antibody (1:1,000). Lane 1: molecular weight (MW), Lane 2: pEGFPN1 transfected lysate, Lane 3: pNS2A-GFP transfected cell lysate showing band of GFP (27 kDa) as well as NS2A-GFP (48 kDa) and NS2B-GFP (43 kDa) **(C)**. To evaluate the localization of the NS2A protein, HMEC-1 cells were transfected with a plasmid encoding GFP-tagged DENV-2 NS2A and stained with either anti-calnexin (ER Marker; red), anti-GM (Golgi marker; red), MitoTracker (mitochondrial marker; red) or TOM22 (mitochondrial outer membrane marker, red) and observed with a confocal microscope 24 h after transfection **(D)**. Pearson's Coefficient of the NS2A-GFP localization in different membrane organelles. $^{***}P < 0.001$.

these data provide evidence that the expression of dengue virus viroporins, NS2A, and NS2B are sufficient to activate the NLRP3 inflammasome.

Confirmation of a NS2A and NS2B Effect on Inflammasome Activation by CRISPR-CAS9

Next, to confirm the effect of NS2A and NS2B in the activation of NLRP3 inflammasome, the ASC gene was knocked out in HMEC-1 cells using a lenti-CRISPRv2-ASC viral particle. ASC guide RNA was cloned in a lenti-CRISPRv2 vector and the confirmation of cloned lenti-CRISPRv2-ASC was obtained with colony-PCR using appropriate primers that showed the positive clone as 125 bp by agarose gel electrophoresis (**Figure S4B**). In addition to ASC, NLRP3 and CASP-1 guide RNA were also cloned into the lentiCRISPRv2 plasmid (**Figure S4A**). To confirm the ASC knockout, HMEC-1 transduced cell lysates were analyzed by western blot; a complete ASC gene knockout was observed, and a lack of ASC was confirmed in HMEC-1 transduced cells (**Figure 4A**). Then, $ASC^{-/-}$ HMEC-1 cells were selected to analyze inflammasome activation due to NS2A and NS2B. To do this, $ASC^{-/-}$ HMEC-1 cells or WT HMEC-1 cells were primed with 1 μg/mL LPS for 6 h and then transfected with peEGFPN, pNS2A-GFP, and pNS2B-GFP for 36 h. As a positive control, cells were primed with 2 μg/mL LPS for 6 h followed by 5 mM ATP for 45 min. Lysates were analyzed by western blot and demonstrated caspase-1 activation due to the presence of NS2A and ATP in WT HMEC-1 cells in contrast to $ASC^{-/-}$ HMEC-1 cells (**Figure 4B**). Cell supernatants were also analyzed for IL-1β secretion, which was absent in $ASC^{-/-}$ HMEC-1 cells, in contrast to WT HMEC-1. A similar result was observed for ATP.

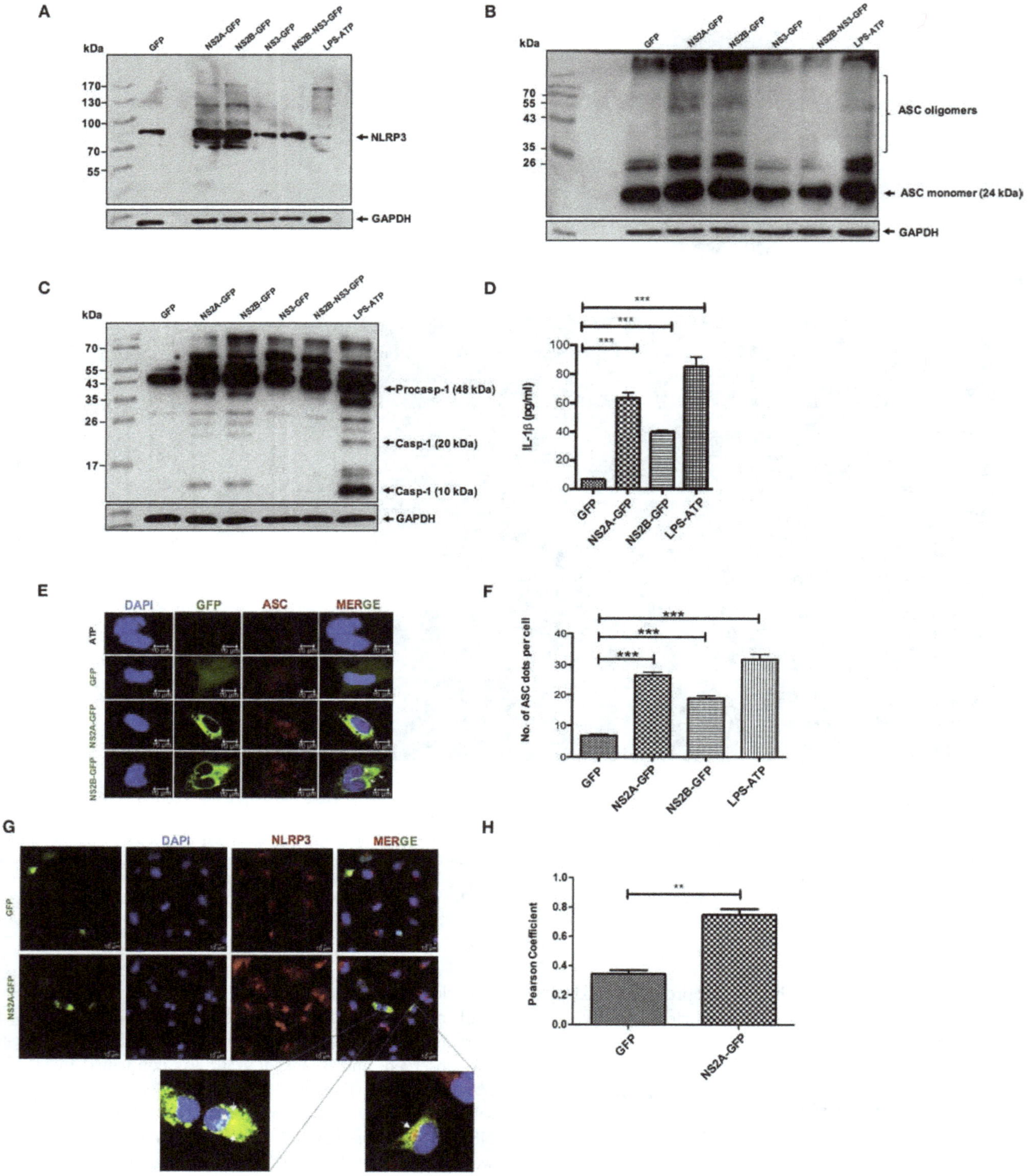

FIGURE 3 | NLRP3 inflammasome activation by DENV-2 viroporin, NS2A, and NS2B. HMEC-1 cells were transfected with the expression plasmid encoding GFP-tagged DENV-2 NS2A, NS2B, or the pEGFPN1 empty vector for 36 h or treated with LPS (1 μg/mL) for 6 h followed by ATP (5 mM) for 45 min as a positive control. Cell lysates were analyzed by western blot using **(A)** an anti-NLRP3 antibody (1:500), **(B)** an anti-ASC antibody (1:1,000), and **(C)** an anti-caspase-1 antibody (1:1,000). **(D)** HMEC-1 cells were transfected with the expression plasmid encoding GFP-tagged DENV-2 NS2A, NS2B, or the pEGFPN1 empty vector for 36 h or treated with LPS (1 μg/mL) for 6 h followed by ATP (5 mM) for 45 min as a positive control, and the cell free supernatant was analyzed for IL-1β by ELISA. **(E)** HMEC-1

(Continued)

FIGURE 3 | cells were transfected with expression plasmids encoding GFP-tagged DENV-2 NS2A, NS2B, or the pEGFPN1 parental vector for 36 h or treated with LPS (1 μg/mL) for 6 h followed by ATP (5 mM) for 45 min as a positive control, and the cells were stained with anti-ASC (Red) and analyzed by a confocal microscope. **(F)** The number (#) of ASC puncta per cell was counted by confocal microscopy. ASC puncta was calculated from a total of 20 cells. **(G)** HMEC-1 cells were transfected with pNS2A-GFP, or the pEGFPN1 empty vector for 36 h and the cells were stained with anti-NLRP3 (1:200) (Red) and analyzed by a confocal microscope. Nuclei were visualized by staining with DAPI. **(H)** Pearson's Coefficient of the NS2A-GFP or GFP co-localization with NLRP3. Data are representative of at least three independent experiments, and indicate the mean ± S.D. **(D,F,H)**. $^{**}P < 0.01$ and $^{***}P < 0.001$.

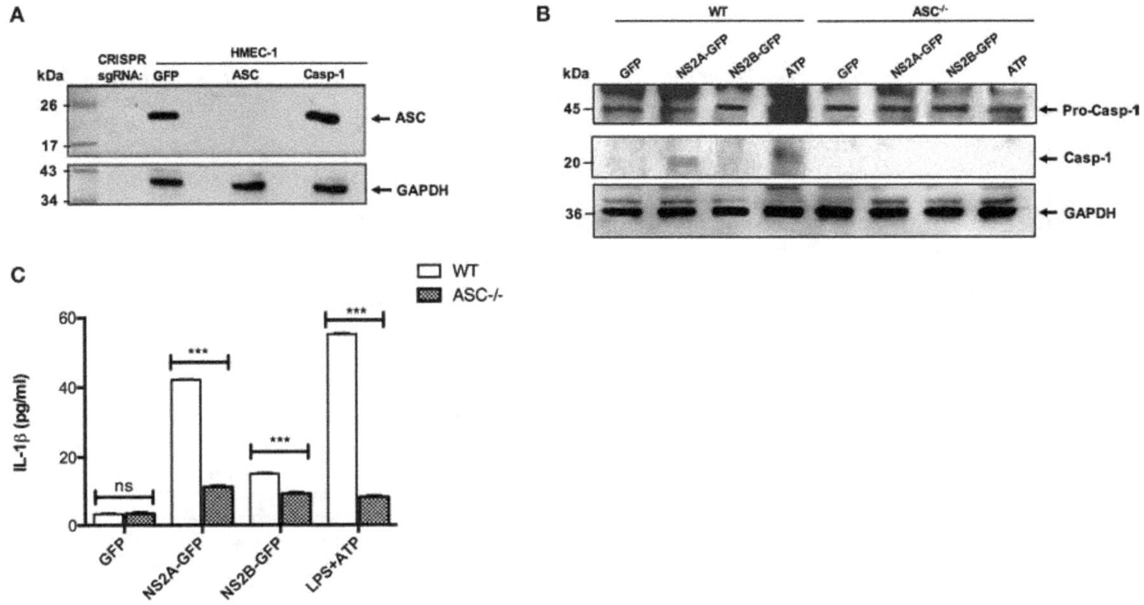

FIGURE 4 | Confirmation of inflammasome activation by viroporin via CRISPR-CAS 9. **(A)** HMEC-1 lysates expressing lentiCRISPRv2-GFP/Caspase/ASC were resolved by western blot. The primary antibody against ASC was used at a 1:1,000 dilution. HRP-anti rabbit was used as the secondary antibody (1:5,000). **(B)** $ASC^{-/-}$ HMEC-1 cells and WT HMEC-1 cells were primed with LPS 1 μg/mL for 6 h, followed by transfection with GFP, NS2A-GFP, and NS2B-GFP for 36 h. Positive control cells were primed with LPS 1 μg/mL for 6 h, followed by 5 mM ATP for 45 min. Lysates were analyzed using western blot. Caspase-1 primary antibody was used at a 1:1,000 dilution. HRP-anti rabbit was used as the secondary antibody (1:5,000). **(C)** HMEC-1 cells (WT or $ASC^{-/-}$) were transfected with the expression plasmid encoding DENV-2 NS2A-GFP, NS2B-GFP or the pEGFPN1 parental vector for 36 h or treated with LPS (1 μg/mL) for 6 h followed by ATP (5 mM) for 45 min as a positive control, and the cell free supernatant was analyzed for IL-1β by ELISA. $^{***}P < 0.001$.

This result confirmed the effects of NS2A on caspase-1 activation and the subsequent inflammasome assembly (**Figure 4C**).

NS2A and NS2B Mediated Inflammasome Activation Was Dependent on NLRP3 and Caspase-1

Further, we examined whether IL-1β release was dependent on the NLRP3 inflammasome activation induced by DENV viral proteins (NS2A, NS2B). We found the absence of caspase-1 activation in the presence of glyburide (NLRP3 inhibitor) in extracts from cells transfected with pNS2B-GFP and a significant reduction in cells transfected with pNS2A-GFP. However, activation of caspase-1 was observed in non-treated cells due to pNS2A-GFP or pNS2B-GFP (**Figure 5A**). Similarly, IL-1β secretion was reduced in the presence of the NLRP3 inhibitor, suggesting that NS2A and NS2B activate caspase-1 and promote secretion of IL-1β, are dependent on NLRP3 (**Figure 5B**). Studies also suggested the existence of other pathways through which IL-1β is secreted (40, 41). Therefore, to determine whether secretion of IL-1β was dependent on caspase-1, HMEC-1 cells were treated with YVAD (a caspase-1 inhibitor) for 1 h prior to transfection with the pNS2A-GFP and pNS2B-GFP plasmids. After 36 h post-transfection, a reduced secretion of IL-1β in the presence of the caspase-1 inhibitor (YVAD) was observed, suggesting that NS2A and NS2B-dependent secretion of IL-1β requires caspase-1 activation (**Figure 5C**). As a positive control, ATP was used; however, the NLRP3 inhibitor had low effect on caspase 1 activation, as observed by western blot, while IL-1β secretion was reduced up to 50 %, as observed by ELISA. However, in the presence of the caspase-1 inhibitor, secretion of IL-1β was reduced by 50% due to ATP. These observations suggested that activation of the inflammasome, and subsequently, secretion of IL-1β in the cell supernatant by dengue virus viroporins NS2A and NS2B were specific to NLRP3 and Caspase-1.

Regulation of Ca^{++} Might Impair Inflammasome Activation

NS2A and NS2B proteins are mainly localized at the endoplasmic reticulum (ER) (33, 42). We therefore investigated whether the activation of NLRP3 involved the release of Ca^{++} from organelles. To this end, we analyzed if a cell-permeable

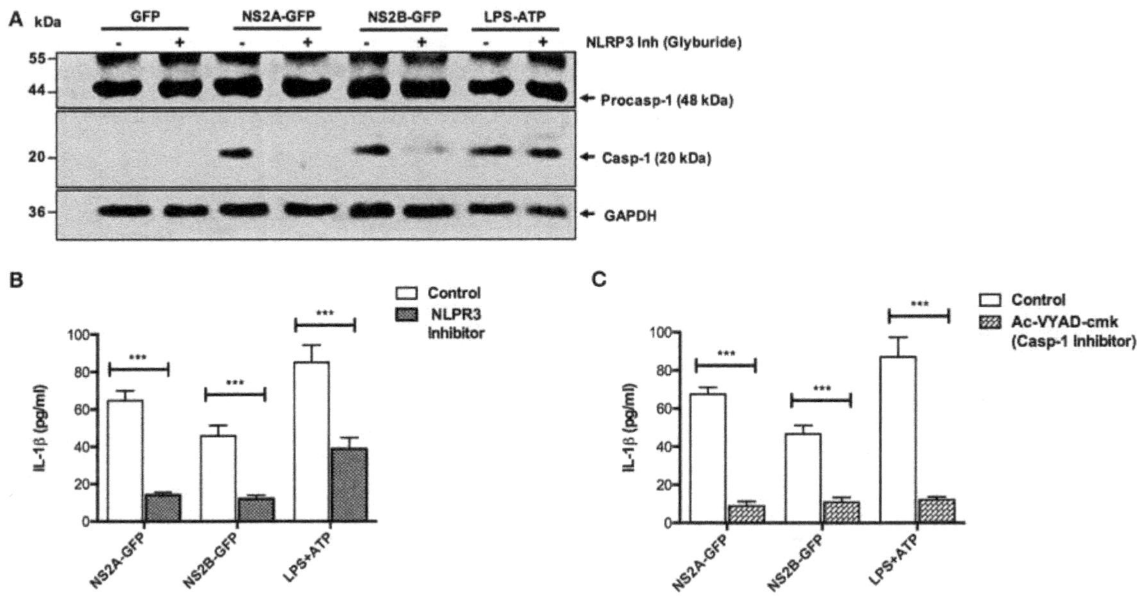

FIGURE 5 | NLRP3 and caspase-1 specific activation of the inflammasome by NS2A and NS2B. HMEC-1 cells were transfected with expression plasmids encoding NS2A-GFP, NS2B-GFP or the pEGFPN1 empty vector for 36 h or treated with LPS (1 μg/mL) for 6 hrs followed by ATP (5 mM) for 1 h as a positive control, in the presence or absence of Glyburide (200 μM). **(A)** The cell lysates were analyzed by western blot using an anti-Caspase 1 antibody (1:1,000), and **(B)** the cell free supernatant was analyzed for IL-1β by ELISA. **(C)** HMEC-1 cells were transfected with expression plasmids encoding NS2A-GFP, NS2B-GFP or the pEGFPN1 empty vector for 36 h or treated with LPS (1 μg/mL) for 6 h followed by ATP (5 mM) for 45 min as a positive control, in the presence or absence of AcVYAD-cmk (50 μM), and the cell free supernatant was analyzed for IL-1β by ELISA. Data are representative of at least three independent experiments and indicate the mean ± S.D. **(B,C)**. ***$P < 0.001$.

Ca^{++}chelator BAPTA-AM inhibit inflammasome activation induced by NS2A-GFP, NS2B-GFP. We found that cells treated with the Ca^{++} chelator significantly decreased caspase-1 activation due to DENV-2 NS2A, NS2B, and ATP (**Figure 6A**). Furthermore, treatment of HMEC-1 with BAPTA-AM significantly blocked IL-1β secretion by DENV-2 NS2A (**Figure 6B**). These results suggest that DENV viroporins may induce Ca^{++} flux in the cytoplasm from intracellular storages, which activate the NLRP3 inflammasome.

ROS Generation Is Required for DENV-2, NS2A Driven NLRP3 Inflammasome

Several viral proteins including viroporins induce membrane permeability, ionic imbalance and can disrupt mitochondria functions (43, 44). Therefore, we investigated if DENV-2 infection affects the mitochondria in HMEC-1 cells. As shown in **Figure 7A** elongated mitochondria were detected in infected HMEC-1 when compared to uninfected HMEC-1 cells which exhibit a typical mitochondria ultrastructural morphology (Mt) (**Figure 7A**). In addition, as expected from our previous results NS2A over-expression induced changes in the mitochondrial morphology, those mithocondria appearing as fragmented, longed entities or with perinuclear localization, in contrast to the typical elongated healthy mitochondria (**Figure 7B**). To further analyze the effects of DENV-2 viroporin on the mitochondria, we evaluated whether DENV viroporins could change the mitochondrial membrane potential ($\Delta\Psi$m). We found that the flow cytometric distribution of the fluorescence intensity of the $\Delta\Psi$m indicator in HMEC-1 transfected with pNS2A-GFP decreased membrane potential and fail to sequester TMRE approximately 1.84-fold compared to that in HMEC-1 cells transfected with pEGFPN1 (**Figure 7C**). NS2B-transfected HMEC-1 cells showed only a minor effect in mitochondrial membrane potential compared to HMEC-1 cells transfected with pEGFPN1 (**Figures 7C,D**). These data suggest that NS2A induce changes in mitochondrial integrity and polarized the mitochondrial membrane potential ($\Delta\Psi$m).

Additionally, mitochondria are reported to play a crucial role in the activation of the NLRP3 inflammasome (45–47). Specifically, mitochondrial ROS has found to be important in fueling NLRP3 inflammasome activation (48, 49). Therefore, we tested the effect of Mito-TEMPO, a scavenger specific for mitochondrial ROS (50, 51), in the activation of the NLRP3 inflammasome due to DENV-2 viroporins. Treatment with the antioxidant Mito-TEMPO had inhibitory effects on the secretion of IL-1β in HMEC-1 transfected with DENV-2 pNS2A-GFP and pNS2B-GFP, as well as on the response to ATP (**Figure 7E**). Thus, our data strongly suggest that the generation of ROS during DENV-2 viroporin expression might act as a stress signal for inflammasome activation, which in turn is crucial for IL-1β production.

DISCUSSION

The main finding of our present study is that DENV-2, a positive-strand RNA virus, triggers NLRP3 inflammasome–mediated

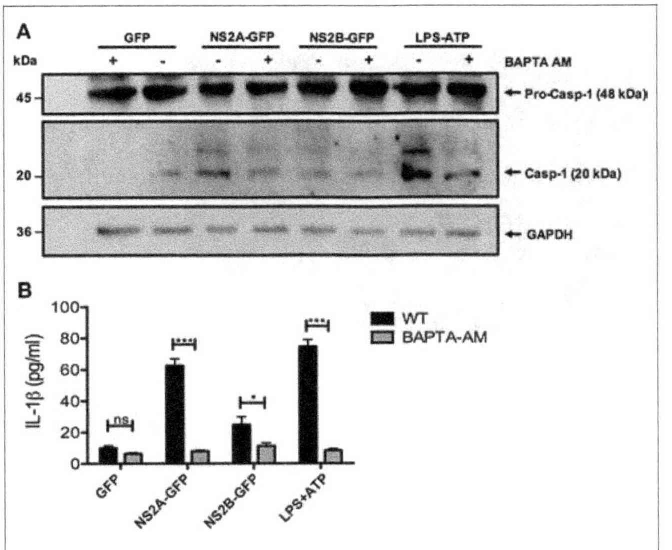

FIGURE 6 | Requirement of increased intracellular Ca^{++} concentration for NLRP3 inflammasome activation by NS2A and NS2B. HMEC-1 cells were transfected with plasmids encoding NS2A-GFP, NS2B-GFP, or the pEGFPN1 empty vector for 36 h or treated with LPS (1 µg/mL) for 6 hrs followed by ATP (5 mM) for 45 min as a positive control, in the presence or absence of BAPTA-AM (10 µM). **(A)** The cell lysates were analyzed by western blot using an anti-caspase-1 antibody (1:1,000), and **(B)** the cell free supernatants were analyzed for IL-1β by ELISA. Data are representative of at least three independent experiments, and indicate the mean ± S.D. **(B)**. $^{*}P < 0.05$ and $^{***}P < 0.001$. ns, non significant.

IL-1β production through the expression of the virus-encoded NS2A, NS2B proteins. Our data reveal the physiopathologic relevance of the NLRP3 inflammasome during DENV-2 infection, which may provide therapeutic targets along these pathways for novel anti-DENV-2 treatment.

Endogenous pyrogens (Ex: IL-1β) is induced during dengue virus infection causes fever, a primary symptom of the disease (4). IL-1β processing and release is regulated by caspase-1 through the activation of an inflammasome complex (10). Although dengue virus pathogenesis is not fully elucidated, recent evidence support the central role of pro-inflammatory cytokines in endothelial activation and plasma leakage during DENV-2 infection (4, 6, 52). In this study, we found that DENV-2 triggered NLRP3 activation in endothelial cells (HMEC-1). Microvascular endothelial cells are regarded as the permissive target of DENV-2 (53) and we have demonstrated that DENV-2 is able to activate the inflammasome complex by NLRP3 expression, ASC oligomerization, and caspase-1 activation, following IL-1β secretion in the cell supernatant. These data are in agreement with a recent study that demonstrate NLRP3 inflammasome activation in DENV-2-infected macrophages in cultures and in platelets (12, 13). In addition, a study reported the increased expression of caspase-1 in DENV-2-infected cultured cells (54).

Several studies have reported NLRP3 and RIG-I inflammasome-induced caspase-1 activation during RNA virus infections (55–58). An array of RNA viruses have also been shown to induce IL-1β production through the NLRP3 inflammasome (59). Flaviviruses, including the West Nile virus, swine fever virus (CSFV), Japanese encephalitis virus, and hepatitis C virus, have been shown to assemble the NLRP3 inflammasome and promote IL-1β production during infection (60–63). Our results clearly demonstrated that DENV-2 was able to activate the NLRP3 inflammasome on its own, without the prerequisite for priming the cells with another pathogen associated molecular pattern (PAMP), which was previously shown to be necessary for other viruses, such as encephalomyocarditis virus and stomatitis vesicular virus (VSV) (63). A wide range of stimuli have been reported to activate the NLRP3 inflammasome, including bacterial components, environment irritants, endogenous danger signals from damaged cells, and other viruses (64, 65). Three mechanisms for NLRP3 inflammasome activation have been suggested so far. First, according to the "ion channel model," high concentrations of extracellular ATP can induce K+ efflux through the P2X7 ATP-gated ion channel, by forming cell membrane pannexin-1 pores, and further facilitating the influx of PAMPs and damage-associated molecular patterns (DAMPs), which trigger NLRP3 activation (66). The second model is the "lysosomal rupture model," in which large crystals and environmental irritants are phagocytosed and induce the release of cathepsin B by lysosome rupture. Released cathepsin B further activates NLRP3 (67). The third model is "mitochondrial ROS," in which damaged mitochondria produce a large amount of ROS that stimulates NLRP3 inflammasome activation (68, 69). Although a recent study on macrophages and platelets have shown the importance of the Syk-coupled C-type lectin CLEC5A and RIP kinases during DENV-2-induced NLRP3 inflammasome activation (12, 13), no direct role of dengue proteins in the activation of inflammasomes have been reported.

We recently reported that dengue virus NS2B and NS2A proteins behave as viroporins (28, 29). Therefore, we investigated the mechanism by which the proposed dengue virus like-viroporins (NS2A & NS2B) activate the NLRP3 inflammasome, as several viroporins of RNA viruses have been reported to activate the NLRP3 inflammasome (14). Our results showed a clear activation of the NLRP3 inflammasome by both the DENV-2 NS2B and NS2A proteins.

Several viruses encode viroporins that increase the permeability of host cellular, endoplasmic, and mitochondrial membranes, facilitating virus entry and exit mechanisms. The increased ion concentration helps viral replication and transcription. Increased ion concentration (Na^{+}, K^{+}, Ca^{++}) by viroporins trigger NLRP3 inflammasome activation (14). Using the DENV-2 viroporins, NS2A and NS2B GFP fused-proteins, we have shown that DENV-2 NS2A and NS2B were able to activate the NLRP3 inflammasome complex following IL-1β secretion in the cell supernatant. Furthermore, NS2A was shown to colocalize with NLRP3. Recently, it has been demonstrated that DENV-2 envelope protein domain III and M proteins also trigger NLRP3 activation (34, 35). Furthermore, studies have reported that some RNA viruses (Chikungunya and Zika) activate the AIM2-specific inflammasome (70, 71). Since several DNA viruses have been reported to be sensed by AIM2, the mechanism by which AIM2 senses RNA viruses remains unknown. Here, we demonstrated

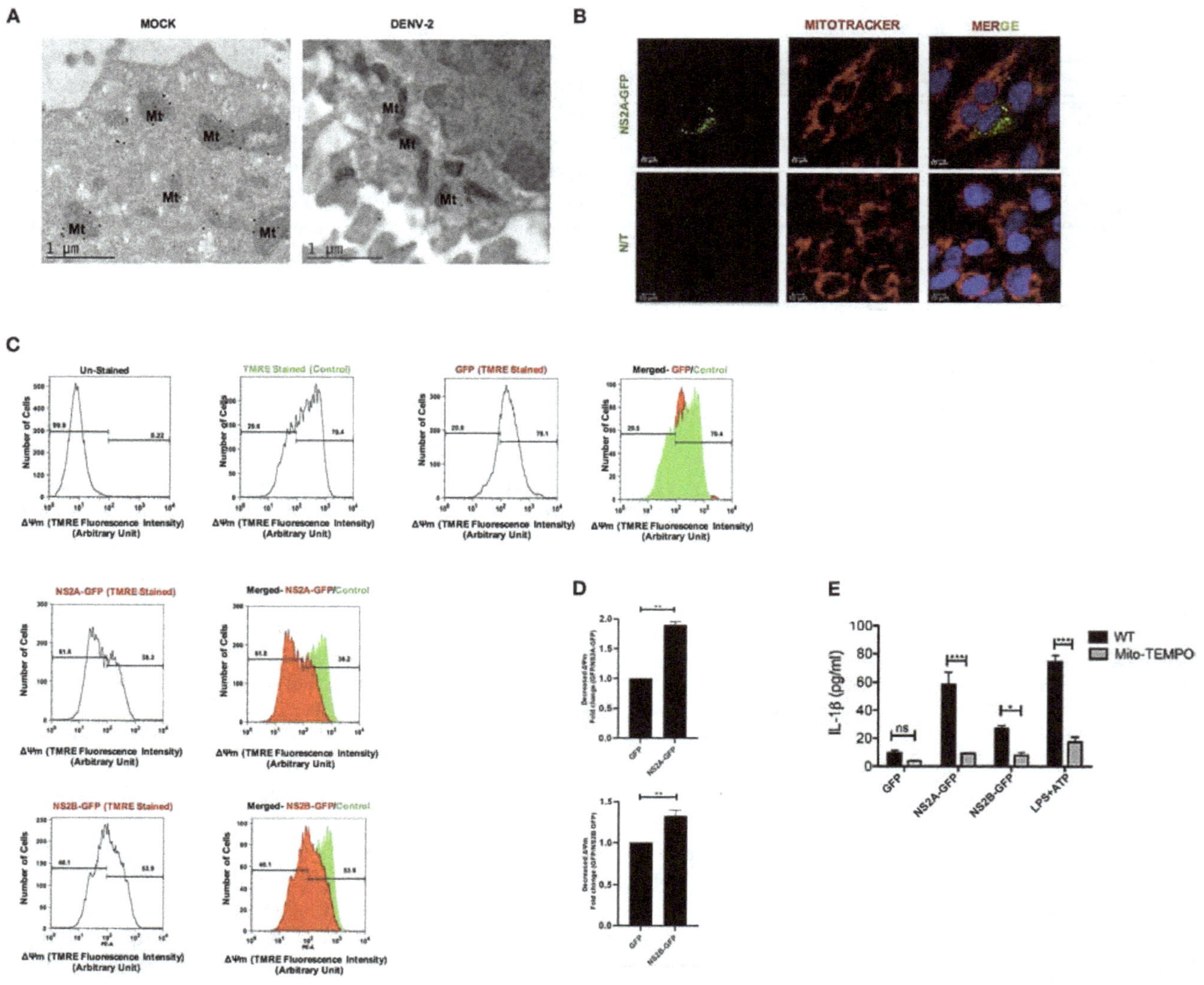

FIGURE 7 | DENV-2 viroporin induce the NLRP3 inflammasome through the mitochondria. **(A)** Ultra-thing sections (TME) images (70 nm) of resin-embedded HMEC-1 cells, stained with uranyl acetate. Ultrastructural analysis of non-infected and DENV-2 infected HMEC-1 cells show their typical structure of mitochondria (Mt), captured by Jeol JEM-1011 transmission electron microscope (JeolLtd.,Tokyo, Japan). **(B)** To evaluate the localization of the NS2A protein within mitochondria, HMEC-1 cells were transfected with pNS2A-GFP for 36 h, stained with Mito Tracker (mitochondrial marker; red) and analyzed by confocal microscopy. **(C,D)** Mitochondrial membrane potential was detected in HMEC-1 cells transfected with plasmids encoding NS2A-GFP, NS2B-GFP, or the pEGFPN1 parental plasmid for 36 h and stained with TMRE (175 mM) for 30 min and analyzed using flow cytometry at 488 nm (excitation peak-595 nm, emission-575 nm). **(E)** HMEC-1 cells were transfected with expression plasmids encoding NS2A-GFP, NS2B-GFP, or the pEGFPN1 empty vector for 36 h, treated with LPS (1 µg/mL) for 6 h followed by ATP (5 mM) for 45 min as a positive control, in the presence or absence of Mito-TEMPO (10 µM), and the cell free supernatant was analyzed for IL-1β by ELISA. Data are representative of at least three independent experiments and indicate the mean ± S.D. $^{*}P < 0.05$, $^{**}P < 0.01$, and $^{***}P < 0.001$. ns, non significant.

that IL-1β secretion by NS2A and NS2B was specific to NLRP3 and caspase-1.

In platelets, inflammasome induction by Dengue virus is dependent on ROS production in the mitochondria (13). We observed that IL-1β production induced by both NS2A and NS2B was dependent on ROS; one hypothesis is that the expression of these proteins in mitochondria could be part of the mechanism. Induction of IL-1β secretion has two components; since the secretion was inhibited by both Mito-TEMPO and BAPTA-AM, these suggest that both Ca^{++} and ROS production are necessary for IL-1β secretion. Alternatively, one of these events induces the other. In this sense, it was reported that ATP can activate the inflammasome by inducing Ca^{++} that triggers mitochondrial ROS production (72); it has already been reported that viroporins regulate NLRP3 activation through calcium mobilization (25). These studies support our results.

In summary, the current study shows that DENV-2 infection triggers inflammasome and high level of IL-1β in HMEC-1 as well as in THP-1, HepG2 via NLRP3 inflammasome activation. We also oberved that the maturation and secretion of IL-1β during DENV-2 infection is mediated by NLRP3 inflammasome. DENV-2 NS2A and NS2B protein were found to facilitate the assembly of the NLRP3 inflammasome complex and lead to caspase-1 activation and IL-1β secretion through calcium mobilization or by disrupting mitochondria potential and by inducing ROS production. Further research is required for an in-depth understanding the role of these viroporins in the regulation of innate immunity. These results reveal a novel mechanism for the DENV-2-mediated inflammatory response, which may provide therapeutic targets along these pathways for novel strategies to treat DENV-2 associated disease.

AUTHOR CONTRIBUTIONS

GS and GV-C performed research, analyzed data, and wrote the paper. JG-C, GV-C, ML-J, and BC-M performed research, analyzed the data, and prepared the images. GS, GV-C, JG-C, BC-M, ML-J, TL, PN, NV-S, and LC-B conceived, designed, conducted the research, interpreted data, and wrote the paper.

ACKNOWLEDGMENTS

We thank the microscope and cytometry facility team of the CINVESTAV. We thank Raul Bonilla for excellent technical assistance. GS and GV-C are fellow holders from the National Council for Science and Technology (CONACYT) Mexico. Additionally, JG-C, ML-J, PN, TL, NV-S, and LC-B are members of the National System of Researchers, SNI.

SUPPLEMENTARY MATERIAL

Figure S1 | DENV-2 and NS2A, NS2B tagged with GFP activate NLRP3 inflammasome in HepG2 cells. Cells were infected with DENV-2 at (5 MOI), mock infected or treated with LPS (1 μg/mL) for 6 hrs followed by ATP (5 mM) for 45 min as a positive control. **(A)** Cell lysates were analyzed by western blot using an anti-caspase-1 antibody (1:1,000) and anti-NS5 antibody (1:100); **(B)** HMEC-1 were infected with DENV-2 (5 MOI) for 36 h or treated with medium. Immunofluorescence with double staining was performed in HMEC-1 using anti-NS5 antibody (1:100) and anti-NLRP3 antibody (1:500) **(C)** HepG2 cells were transfected with either parental plasmid eGFPN1, pNS2A-GFP, pNS2B-GFP, or treated with LPS (1 μg/mL) for 6 h followed by ATP (5 mM) for 1 h as a positive control. At 36 h post-tranfection, cell lysates were analyzed for western blot with anti-caspase-1 antibody (1:1,000). ←Expression of NLRP3.

Figure S2 | THP1 cells infected wit DENV 2 trigger the NLRP3 inflammasome activation. THP-1 cells grown in RPMI 1640 medium supplemented with 10% FBS in a 37°C incubator with 5% CO_2 were differentiated for 1 days with 100nM phorbol-12-myristate-13-acetate (PMA), followed by DENV-2 infection at 5 MOIs or mock infected. At 24 and 48 h cell lysates and supernatants were obtained. **(A)** Infection was detected by western blot with anti-NS3 dengue antibody (Genetex USA). **(B)** Western blot of the same lysates were analyzed with Pro-Caspase 1, and GAPDH. **(C)** Caspasa and IL-1β. **(D)** Inflammasome Assay monitor released caspase-1 in culture medium. THP-1 cells grown in RPMI 1640 medium supplemented with 10% FBS in a 37°C incubator with 5% CO_2 were differentiated for 1 days with 100 nM phorbol-12-myristate-13-acetate (PMA), followed by infected with either Mock or DENV-2 (5 MOIs for 2 h). After the 24 and 48 h post-infection half of the culture medium (50 μl/well) was transferred to a second plate, 50 μl/well of Caspase-Glo® 1 Reagent or Caspase-Glo® 1 YVAD-CHO Reagent was added and luminescence was recorded using a GloMax® Multi+ Detection System as directed in the GloMax® Multi+ Detection System with Instinct® Software Technical Manual #TM340. For cells, 100 μl/well of reagent was added directly to 100μl/well of cultured cells. **(E)** THP-1 cells grown in RPMI 1640 medium supplemented with 10% FBS in a 37°C incubator with 5% CO_2 were differentiated for 1 days with 100 nM phorbol-12-myristate-13-acetate (PMA), followed by infected with either Mock or DENV-2 (5 MOIs for 2 h). After the 24 and 48 h post-infection, supernatants were collected and IL-1β was checked using R&D IL-1β Elisa kit. ns, non significant, $^{***}P < 0.001$.

Figure S3 | The expression of NS2B in infected HMEC-1 cells has the same distribution as transfected pNS2B-GFP. **(A)** HMEC-1 cells were infected with DENV-2 at 5 MOI. 24 and 48 h post-infection, the cells were fixed and stained with anti-NS2B polyclonal antibody (RED) and then analyzed by confocal microscopy **(B)** To evaluate the distribution of NS2B, HMEC-1 cells were infected with DENV-2 at 5 MOI for 24 h, further the same cells were transiently transfected with plasmid coding for NS2B-GFP and analyzed at 24 h post-transfection. Cells were fixed with 4 % paraformaldehyde and stained with anti-NS2B polyclonal antibody (RED) and analyzed by confocal microscopy.

Figure S4 | Confirmation of guide RNA cloning in LentiCRISPR plasmid. **(A)** Guide RNA specific to NLRP3, ASC and Caspase-1 were cloned in LentiCRISPRv2 plasmid, according to protocol. Clones were transformed in STBL3 bacteria and Colony PCR of transformed clones, specific to lenti-CRISPRv2 (NLRP3, Caspase-1, ASC), was performed. Bands corresponding to 125 bp showed positive clones for the respective Guide RNA. Amplified PCR were resolved using 0.8% agarose gel. **(B)** Sequence of guide RNA used.

REFERENCES

1. Schmidt AC. Response to dengue fever–the good, the bad, and the ugly? *N Engl J Med.* (2010) 363:484–7. doi: 10.1056/NEJMcibr1005904
2. World Health Organization. Dengue: guidelines for diagnosis, treatment, prevention, and control. *Spec Program Res Train Trop Dis.* World Health Organization (2009) 147. Available online at: https://apps.who.int/iris/
3. Vaughn DW, Green S, Kalayanarooj S, Innis BL, Nimmannitya S, Suntayakorn S, et al. Dengue in the early febrile phase: viremia and antibody responses. *J Infect Dis.* (1997) 176:322–330. doi: 10.1086/514048
4. Bozza FA, Cruz OG, Zagne SMO, Azeredo EL, Nogueira RMR, Assis EF, et al. Multiplex cytokine profile from dengue patients: MIP-1beta and IFN-gamma as predictive factors for severity. *BMC Infect Dis.* (2008) 8:86. doi: 10.1186/1471-2334-8-86
5. Malavige GN, Ogg GS. Pathogenesis of vascular leak in dengue virus infection. *Immunology.* (2017) 51:261–9. doi: 10.1111/imm.12748
6. Suharti C, Van Gorp ECM, Setiati TE, Dolmans WMV, Djokomoeljanto RJ, Hack CE, et al. The role of cytokines in activation of coagulation and fibrinolysis in dengue shock syndrome. *Thromb Haemost.* (2002) 87:42–46. doi: 10.1055/s-0037-1612941
7. Callaway JB, Smith SA, McKinnon KP, de Silva AM, Crowe JE Jr, Ting JP. Spleen Tyrosine Kinase (Syk) mediates IL-1β induction by primary human monocytes during antibody-enhanced dengue virus infection. *J Biol Chem.* (2015) 290:17306–20. doi: 10.1074/jbc.M115.664136

8. Houghton-Trivino N, Martin K, Giaya K, Rodriguez JA, Bosch I, Castellanos JE. [Comparison of the transcriptional profiles of patients with dengue fever and dengue hemorrhagic fever reveals differences in the immune response and clues in immunopathogenesis. *Biomedica.* (2010) 30:587–97. doi: 10.7705/biomedica.v30i4.297
9. Jaiyen Y, Masrinoul P, Kalayanarooj S, Pulmanausahakul R, Ubol S. Characteristics of dengue virus-infected peripheral blood mononuclear cell death that correlates with the severity of illness. *Microbiol Immunol.* (2009) 53:442–50. doi: 10.1111/j.1348-0421.2009.00148.x
10. Davis BK, Wen H, Ting JP-Y. The inflammasome NLRs in immunity, inflammation, and associated diseases. *Annu Rev Immunol.* (2011) 29:707–35. doi: 10.1146/annurev-immunol-031210-101405
11. Lamkanfi M, Dixit VM. Modulation of inflammasome pathways by bacterial and viral pathogens. *J Immunol.* (2011) 187:597–602. doi: 10.4049/jimmunol.1100229
12. Wu MF, Chen ST, Yang AH, Lin WW, Lin YL, Chen NJ et al. CLEC5A is critical for dengue virus-induced inflammasome activation in human macrophages. *Blood.* (2013) 121:95–106. doi: 10.1182/blood-2012-05-430090
13. Hottz ED, Lopes JF, Freitas C, Valls-de-Souza R, Oliveira MF, Bozza MT et al. Platelets mediate increased endothelium permeability in dengue through NLRP3-inflammasome activation. *Blood.* (2013) 122:3405–14. doi: 10.1182/blood-2013-05-504449
14. Guo HC, Jin Y, Zhi XY, Yan D, Sun SQ. NLRP3 inflammasome activation by viroporins of animal viruses. *Viruses.* (2015) 7:3380–91. doi: 10.3390/v7072777
15. Sze CW, Tan YJ. Viral membrane channels: role and function in the virus life cycle. *Viruses.* (2015) 7:3261–84. doi: 10.3390/v7062771
16. Luis Nieva J, Carrasco L. Viroporins: structures and functions beyond cell membrane permeabilization. *Viruses.* (2015) 7:5169–71. doi: 10.3390/v7102866
17. Nieto-Torres JL, Verdiá-Báguena C, Castaño-Rodriguez C, Aguilella VM, Enjuanes L. Relevance of viroporin ion channel activity on viral replication and pathogenesis. *Viruses.* (2015) 7:3552–73. doi: 10.3390/v7072786
18. Hyser JM, Collinson-Pautz MR, Utama B, Estes MK. Rotavirus disrupts calcium homeostasis by NSP4 viroporin activity. *mBio.* (2010) 1:e00265-10. doi: 10.1128/mBio.00265-10
19. Griffin SD, Beales LP, Clarke DS, Worsfold O, Evans SD, Jaeger J, et al. The p7 protein of hepatitis C virus forms an ion channel that is blocked by the antiviral drug, Amantadine. *FEBS Lett.* (2003) 535:34–8. doi: 10.1016/S0014-5793(02)03851-6
20. Ito M, Yanagi Y, Ichinohe T. Encephalomyocarditis virus viroporin 2B activates NLRP3 inflammasome. *PLoS Pathog.* (2012) 8:e1002857. doi: 10.1371/journal.ppat.1002857
21. Suzuki T, Orba Y, Okada Y, Sunden Y, Kimura T, Tanaka S, et al. The human polyoma JC virus agnoprotein acts as a viroporin. *PLoS Pathog.* (2010) 6:e1000801. doi: 10.1371/journal.ppat.1000801
22. Aldabe R, Irurzun A, Carrasco L. Poliovirus protein 2BC increases cytosolic free calcium concentrations. *J Virol.* (1997) 71:6214–7. doi: 10.1128/JVI.71.8.6214-6217.1997
23. Henkel M, Mitzner D, Henklein P, Meyer-Almes FJ, Moroni A, Difrancesco ML, et al. The proapoptotic influenza A virus protein PB1-F2 forms a nonselective ion channel. *PLoS ONE.* (2010) 5:e11112. doi: 10.1371/journal.pone.0011112
24. Van Kuppeveld FJM, Hoenderop JGJ, Smeets RLL, Willems PHGM, Dijkman HBPM, Galama JMD, et al. Coxsackievirus protein 2B modifies endoplasmic reticulum membrane and plasma membrane permeability and facilitates virus release. *EMBO J.* (1997) 16:3519–32. doi: 10.1093/emboj/16.12.3519
25. Hyser JM, Estes MK. Pathophysiological Consequences of Calcium-Conducting Viroporins. *Annu Rev Virol.* (2015) 2:473–96. doi: 10.1146/annurev-virology-100114-054846
26. Aguirre S, Luthra P, Sanchez-Aparicio MT, Maestre AM, Patel J, Lamothe F, et al. Dengue virus NS2B protein targets cGAS for degradation and prevents mitochondrial DNA sensing during infection. *Nat Microbiol.* (2017) 2:17037. doi: 10.1038/nmicrobiol.2017.37
27. Yu CY, Liang JJ, Li JK, Lee YL, Chang BL, Su CI, et al. Dengue virus impairs mitochondrial fusion by cleaving mitofusins. *PLoS Pathog.* (2015) 11:e1005350. doi: 10.1371/journal.ppat.1005350
28. León-Juárez M, Martínez-Castillo M, Shrivastava G, García-Cordero J, Villegas-Sepulveda N, Mondragón-Castelán M, et al. Recombinant Dengue virus protein NS2B alters membrane permeability in different membrane models. *Virol J.* (2016) 13:1. doi: 10.1186/s12985-015-0456-4
29. Shrivastava G, García-Cordero J, León-Juárez M, Oza G, Tapia-Ramírez J, Villegas-Sepulveda N, et al. NS2A comprises a putative viroporin of Dengue virus 2. *Virulence.* (2017) 8:1450–6. doi: 10.1080/21505594.2017.1356540
30. Leung JY, Pijlman GP, Kondratieva N, Hyde J, Mackenzie JM, Khromykh AA. Role of nonstructural protein NS2A in flavivirus assembly. *J Virol.* (2008) 82:4731–41. doi: 10.1128/JVI.00002-08
31. Xie X, Gayen S, Kang C, Yuan Z, Shi PY. Membrane topology and function of dengue virus NS2A protein. *J Virol.* (2013) 87:4609–22. doi: 10.1128/JVI.02424-12
32. Xie X, Zou J, Puttikhunt C, Yuan Z, Shi PY. Two distinct sets of NS2A molecules are responsible for dengue virus RNA synthesis and virion assembly. *J Virol.* (2015) 89:1298–313. doi: 10.1128/JVI.02882-14
33. Nemésio H, Villalaín J. Membrane interacting regions of Dengue virus NS2A protein. *J Phys Chem B.* (2014) 118:10142–55. doi: 10.1021/jp504911r
34. Khan RA, Afroz S, Minhas G, Battu S, Khan N. Dengue virus envelope protein domain III induces pro-inflammatory signature and triggers activation of inflammasome. *Cytokine.* (2019) 123:154780. doi: 10.1016/j.cyto.2019.154780
35. Pan P, Zhang Q, Liu W, Wang W, Lao Z, Zhang W, et al. Dengue virus M protein promotes NLRP3 inflammasome activation to induce vascular leakage in mice. *J Virol.* (2019) 93:e00996-19. doi: 10.1128/JVI.00996-19
36. Gruenberg A, Woo WS, Biedrzycka A, Wright PJ. Partial nucleotide sequence and deduced amino acid sequence of the structural proteins of dengue virus type 2, New Guinea C and PUO-218 strains. *J Gen Virol.* (1988) 69:1391–8. doi: 10.1099/0022-1317-69-6-1391
37. García Cordero J, León Juárez M, González-Y-Merchand JA, Cedillo Barrón L, Gutiérrez Castañeda B. Caveolin-1 in lipid rafts interacts with dengue virus NS3 during polyprotein processing and replication in HMEC-1 cells. *PLoS ONE.* (2014) 9:e90704. doi: 10.1371/journal.pone.0090704
38. García-Cordero J, Carrillo-Halfon S, León-Juárez M, Romero-Ramírez H, Valenzuela-León P, López-González M, et al. Generation and characterization of a rat monoclonal antibody against the RNA polymerase protein from Dengue Virus-2. *Immunol Invest.* (2014) 43:28–40. doi: 10.3109/08820139.2013.833622
39. Bauernfeind FG, Horvath G, Stutz A, Alnemri ES, MacDonald K, Speert D, et al. Cutting edge: NF-kappaB activating pattern recognition and cytokine receptors license NLRP3 inflammasome activation by regulating NLRP3 expression. *J Immunol.* (2009) 183:787–91. doi: 10.4049/jimmunol.0901363
40. Lopez-Castejon G, Brough D. Understanding the mechanism of IL-1β secretion. *Cytokine Growth Factor Rev.* (2011) 22:189–95. doi: 10.1016/j.cytogfr.2011.10.001
41. Eder C. Mechanisms of interleukin-1beta release. *Immunobiology.* (2009) 214:543–53. doi: 10.1016/j.imbio.2008.11.007
42. Welsch S, Miller S, Romero-Brey I, Merz A, Bleck CK, Walther P, et al. Composition and three-dimensional architecture of the dengue virus replication and assembly sites. *Cell Host Microbe.* (2009) 5:365–75. doi: 10.1016/j.chom.2009.03.007
43. Madan V, Castelló A, Carrasco L. Viroporins from RNA viruses induce caspase-dependent apoptosis. *Cell Microbiol.* (2008) 10:437–51. doi: 10.1111/j.1462-5822.2007.01057.x
44. Anand SK, Tikoo SK. Viruses as modulators of mitochondrial functions. *Adv Virol. (*2013):738–94. doi: 10.1155/2013/738794
45. Zhou R, Yazdi AS, Menu P, Tschopp J. A role for mitochondria in NLRP3 inflammasome activation. *Nature.* (2011) 469:221–5. doi: 10.1038/nature09663
46. Shimada K, Crother TR, Karlin J, Dagvadorj J, Chiba N, Chen S, et al. Oxidized mitochondrial DNAactivates the NLRP3 inflammasome during apoptosis. *Immunity.* (2012) 36:401–14. doi: 10.1016/j.immuni.2012.01.009
47. Nakahira K, Haspel JA, Rathinam VA, Lee SJ, Dolinay T, Lam HC, et al. Autophagy proteins regulate innate immune responses by inhibiting the release of mitochondrial DNA mediated by the NALP3 inflammasome. *Nat Immunol.* (2011) 12:222–30. doi: 10.1038/ni.1980
48. Heid ME, Keyel PA, Kamga C, Shiva S, Watkins SC, Salter RD. Mitochondrial reactive oxygen species induces NLRP3-dependent lysosomal

damage and inflammasome activation. *J Immunol.* (2013) 191:5230–8. doi: 10.4049/jimmunol.1301490
49. Sorbara MT, Girardin SE. Mitochondrial ROS fuel the inflammasome. *Cell Res.* (2011) 21:558–60. doi: 10.1038/cr.2011.20
50. Trnka J, Blaikie FH, Logan A, Smith RA, Murphy MP. Antioxidant properties of MitoTEMPOL and its hydroxylamine. *Free Radic Res.* (2009) 43:4–12. doi: 10.1080/10715760802582183
51. Dikalova AE, Bikineyeva AT, Budzyn K, Nazarewicz RR, McCann L, Lewis W, et al. Therapeutic targeting of mitochondrial superoxide in hypertension. *Circ Res.* (2010) 107:106–16. doi: 10.1161/CIRCRESAHA.109.214601
52. Pang T, Cardosa MJ, Guzman MG. Of cascades and perfect storms: the immunopathogenesis of dengue haemorrhagic fever-dengue shock syndrome (DHF/DSS). *Immunol Cell Biol.* (2007) 85:43–45. doi: 10.1038/sj.icb.7100008
53. Talavera D, Castillo AM, Dominguez MC, Gutierrez AE, Meza I. IL8 release, tight junction and cytoskeleton dynamic reorganization conducive to permeability increase are induced by dengue virus infection of microvascular endothelial monolayers. *J Gen Virol.* (2004) 85(Pt 7):1801–13. doi: 10.1099/vir.0.19652-0
54. Nasirudeen AM, Liu DX. Gene expression profiling by microarray analysis reveals an important role for caspase-1 in dengue virus-induced p53-mediated apoptosis. *J Med Virol.* (2009) 81:1069–81. doi: 10.1002/jmv.21486
55. Wang X, Jiang W, Yan Y, Gong T, Han J, Tian Z, et al. RNA viruses promote activation of the NLRP3 inflammasome through a RIP1-RIP3-DRP1 signaling pathway. *Nat Immunol.* (2014) 15:1126–33. doi: 10.1038/ni.3015
56. Takeuchi O, Akira S. MDA5/RIG-I and virus recognition. *Curr Opin Immunol.* (2008) 20:17–22. doi: 10.1016/j.coi.2008.01.002
57. Kell AM, Gale M Jr. RIG-I in RNA virus recognition. *Virology.* (2015) 479–80:110–21. doi: 10.1016/j.virol.2015.02.017
58. Jacobs SR, Damania B. NLRs, inflammasomes, and viral infection. *J Leukoc Biol.* (2012) 92:469–77. doi: 10.1189/jlb.0312132
59. Chen IY, Ichinohe T. Response of host inflammasomes to viral infection. *Trends Microbiol.* (2015) 23:55–63. doi: 10.1016/j.tim.2014.09.007
60. Kaushik DK, Gupta M, Kumawat KL, Basu A. NLRP3 inflammasome: key mediator of neuroinflammation in murine Japanese encephalitis. *PLoS ONE.* (2012) 7:e32270. doi: 10.1371/journal.pone.0032270
61. Negash AA, Ramos HJ, Crochet N, Lau DT, Doehle B, Papic N et al. IL-1β production through the NLRP3 inflammasome by hepatic macrophages links hepatitis C virus infection with liver inflammation and disease. *PLoS Pathog.* (2013) 9:e1003330. doi: 10.1371/journal.ppat.1003330
62. Ramos HJ, Lanteri MC, Blahnik G, Negash A, Suthar MS, Brassil MM, et al. IL-1beta signaling promotes CNS-intrinsic immune control of West Nile virus infection. *PLoS Pathog.* (2012)8:e1003039. doi: 10.1371/journal.ppat.1003039
63. Fan S, Yuan J, Deng S, Chen Y, Xie B, Wu K, et al. Activation of interleukin-1β release by the classical swine fever virus is dependent on the NLRP3 inflammasome, which affects virus growth in monocytes. *Front Cell Infect Microbiol.* (2018) 8:225. doi: 10.3389/fcimb.2018.00225
64. Rathinam VA, Fitzgerald KA. Inflammasome complexes: emerging mechanisms and effector functions. *Cell.* (2016) 165:792–800. doi: 10.1016/j.cell.2016.03.046
65. He Y, Hara H, Núñez G. Mechanism and regulation of NLRP3 inflammasome activation. *Trends Biochem Sci.* (2016) 41:1012–21. doi: 10.1016/j.tibs.2016.09.002
66. Kanneganti TD, Lamkanfi M, Kim YG, Chen G, Park JH, Franchi L, et al. Pannexin-1-mediated recognition of bacterial molecules activates the cryopyrin inflammasome independent of Toll-like receptor signaling. *Immunity.* (2007) 26:433–43. doi: 10.1016/j.immuni.2007.03.008
67. Hornung V, Bauernfeind F, Halle A, Samstad EO, Kono H, Rock KL, et al. Silica crystals and aluminum salts activate the NALP3 inflammasome through phagosomal destabilization. *Nat Immunol.* (2008) 9:847–56. doi: 10.1038/ni.1631
68. Cruz CM, Rinna A, Forman HJ, Ventura AL, Persechini PM, Ojcius DM. ATP activates a reactive oxygen species-dependent oxidative stress response and secretion of proinflammatory cytokines in macrophages. *J Biol Chem.* (2007) 282:2871–9. doi: 10.1074/jbc.M608083200
69. Zhou R, Tardivel A, Thorens B, Choi I, Tschopp J. Thioredoxin-interacting protein links oxidative stress to inflammasome activation. *Nat Immunol.* (2010) 11:136–40. doi: 10.1038/ni.1831
70. Ekchariyawat P, Hamel R, Bernard E, Wichit S, Surasombatpattana P, Talignani L, et al. Inflammasome signaling pathways exert antiviral effect against Chikungunya virus in human dermal fibroblasts. *Infect Genet Evol.* (2015) 32:401–8. doi: 10.1016/j.meegid.2015.03.025
71. Hamel R, Dejarnac O, Wichit S, Ekchariyawat P, Neyret A, Luplertlop N, et al. Biology of zika virus infection in human skin cells. *J Virol.* (2015) 89:8880–96. doi: 10.1128/JVI.00354-15
72. Murakami T, Ockinger J, Yu J, Byles V, McColl A, Hofer AM, et al. Critical role for calcium mobilization in activation of the NLRP3 inflammasome. *Proc Natl Acad Sci U S A.* (2012) 109:11282–7. doi: 10.1073/pnas.1117765109

14

E6/E7 and E6* from HPV16 and HPV18 Upregulate IL-6 Expression Independently of p53 in Keratinocytes

*Cristina Artaza-Irigaray[1], Andrea Molina-Pineda[1,2], Adriana Aguilar-Lemarroy[1], Pablo Ortiz-Lazareno[1], Laura P. Limón-Toledo[3], Ana L. Pereira-Suárez[4], Wendoline Rojo-Contreras[5] and Luis F. Jave-Suárez[1]**

[1] Centro de Investigación Biomédica de Occidente, Instituto Mexicano del Seguro Social, Guadalajara, Mexico, [2] Programa de Doctorado en Ciencias Biomédicas, Centro Universitario de Ciencias de la Salud, Universidad de Guadalajara, Guadalajara, Mexico, [3] Centro Médico Nacional de Occidente, Instituto Mexicano del Seguro Social, Hospital de Ginecología y Obstetricia, Guadalajara, Mexico, [4] Departamento de Fisiología, Centro Universitario de Ciencias de la Salud, Universidad de Guadalajara, Guadalajara, Mexico, [5] Instituto Mexicano del Seguro Social, Hospital General Regional 110, Guadalajara, Mexico

***Correspondence:**
Luis F. Jave-Suárez
lfjave@yahoo.com

Keratinocyte infection with high-risk human papillomavirus genotypes has been linked to cancer development. In cervix, the alpha HPV16 and HPV18 have been reported as the mayor causative agents of cervical cancer. Oncogenic progression and chronic inflammation are closely related processes, with IL-6 as one of the main pro-inflammatory cytokines involved. However, there are limited studies about the regulation of IL-6 by low and high risk HPVs and the HPV proteins implicated in this modulation. In this work, we report the overexpression of IL-6 in HPV infected cervical cancer derived cell lines (HeLa and SiHa) compared to non-tumorigenic keratinocytes (HaCaT), and in Cervical Intraepithelial Neoplasia grade 1 HPV16 and HPV18 positive cervical samples compared to HPV negative samples without lesions. Moreover, we generated HaCaT keratinocytes that express E5, E6, and E7 from high risk (16 or 18) or low risk (62 and 84) HPVs. E5 proteins do not modify IL-6 expression, while E7 modestly increase it. Interestingly, E6 proteins in HaCaT cells upregulate IL-6 mRNA expression and protein secretion. Indeed, in HaCaT cells that express high risk HPV16E6 or HPV18E6 proteins, only the truncated E6* isoforms were expressed, showing the stronger IL-6 overexpression, while in HaCaT cells that express low risk HPV62 and HPV84 full length E6 proteins, IL-6 was also upregulated but not so drastically. Since HaCaT cells have a mutated p53 form that is not degraded by the introduction of E6 or E6/E7, it seems that E6/E7 regulate IL-6 by an additional mechanism independent of p53. In addition, basal keratinocytes showed a strong expression of IL-6R using immunohistochemistry, suggesting an autocrine mechanism over proliferative cells. Altogether, IL-6 cytokine expression in keratinocytes is upregulated by E6 and E7 proteins from HPVs 16, 18, 62, and 84, especially by high risk HPV16 and HPV18 E6*, which may contribute to promote a pro-inflammatory and highly proliferative microenvironment that can persist over time and lead to cervical tumorigenesis.

Keywords: IL-6, E6*, cervical cancer, chronic inflammation, human papillomavirus, HPV16, HPV18

INTRODUCTION

Human Papillomaviruses (HPVs) are small non-encapsulated dsDNA viruses that show tropism for squamous epithelium therefore causing cutaneous or mucosal infections. Most HPV infections persist asymptomatically during all the lifetime; however, some of them can have clinical presentations from benign to malignant growth (1). Over 200 HPV genotypes have been identified and classified in taxonomic categories based on nucleotide sequence comparisons, genome organization, biology, and pathogenicity (2). *Alpha*, *Beta*, *Gamma*, *Mu*, and *Nu* genera hold all the HPVs described to date, and principally, the *Alpha* genus harbors all oncogenic HPVs associated to anogenital cancers (1). This subset of viruses has been extensively studied and they are referred to as high-risk HPVs (HR-HPVs) to distinguish them from the rest of HPV types, the low-risk HPVs (LR-HPVs), that commonly cause only benign epithelial lesions (3).

Cervical Cancer (CC) is the fourth leading cause of cancer deaths in women worldwide, and the second most frequent cancer in Mexico (4). HR-HPV persistent infection is the main etiological factor for CC development and HPV16 and HPV18 are the major HPV types associated to cervical carcinogenesis worldwide being therefore the best studied HPVs (5). Meantime, HPV62 and HPV84, considered as non-carcinogenic HPVs, are often found in cervical samples of Mexican women with different grades of lesions, but never in single infection in CC samples (6, 7). HR-HPV oncoproteins E5, E6, and E7 are the primary viral factors responsible for initiation and progression of CC. E6 and E7 proteins disrupt p53 and Rb functions, respectively, a crucial event for the cellular transformation, but additional important cellular targets have also been identified. Alterations on many cellular pathways lead to the overcoming of negative growth regulation by host cell proteins and to genomic instability which finally results in malignant progression (8). The comparison of HR-HPVs oncoproteins against their non-oncogenic LR-HPV counterparts has revealed that the limited activities of the LR-HPV proteins, like their inability to degrade Rb and p53, may have allowed these low risk viruses to send fewer distress signals and therefore to better coexist with their host cell (9, 10).

HPV gene transcription is controlled by two main promoters whose activation is regulated by the differentiation state of the infected cell. This results in the synthesis of polycistronic mRNAs, which are further regulated by alternative splicing processes (11). Alternative splicing within E6-E7 ORFs has been exclusively observed in HR-HPVs, not in LR-HPVs (12). When no splicing occurs within E6 ORF, full length E6 (fl-E6) protein is expressed, while E7 protein can be transcribed from mRNAs with or without splicing of E6. Moreover, for the splicing process in HPV16 E6-E7 mRNA, the spliceosome recognizes a donor splice site within E6 ORF and one of the different acceptor sites located in the early mRNA, leading to different shorter E6 mRNA transcripts called E6*, mainly E6*I (also called E6*) and E6*II, being E6*I the most abundant spliced E6 (13). Regarding HPV18, it appears to transcribe only one short E6 isoform, the E6*I (14).

On the other hand, an important player during the carcinogenic process is interleukin-6 (IL-6), a pleiotropic cytokine mainly reported as a pro-inflammatory molecule. IL-6 leads to inhibition of apoptosis in cells during inflammation through the activation of JAK-STAT signaling pathways after its binding to IL-6 receptor (IL-6R); however, as these pathways maintain cells progressing toward neoplastic growth, inflammation, and cancer are two closely related processes (15, 16). IL-6 is highly up-regulated in many cancers and is considered as a crucial cytokine during tumorigenesis. Therapeutic strategies targeting the IL-6 pathway are in development for cancers and inflammatory diseases. Regarding CC, high microenvironmental IL-6 levels promote angiogenesis and CC development (17). Also, IL-6 expression is higher in CC tissue compared to non-tumorigenic adjacent tissue and this overexpression is correlated with tumor size and poor prognosis (18). Furthermore, it has been reported that overexpression of IL-6 enhances the tumorigenic activity of basal cell carcinoma cells by inhibiting apoptosis and promoting angiogenesis (19). An interesting study on cytokine expression in HPV immortalized epithelial cells showed that in human keratinocytes immortalized with E6 and E7 genes from carcinogenic alpha HPV16 and beta HPV38, IL-6 mRNA expression and protein secretion was higher than in control cells (20), suggesting that the presence of E6/E7 from carcinogenic HPVs increases IL-6 expression. Interestingly, the target proteins of the high risk E6 and E7, p53, and Rb, regulate the expression of IL-6 negatively, raising the question whether degradation of those proteins are the main mechanisms of IL-6 induction by high risk HPVs. As we mention before low risk HPVs are unable to induce p53 and Rb degradation.

Therefore, the aim of this work was to evaluate the influence of HR HPVs 16 and 18 and LR HPVs 62 and 84 viral E6, E7, and E5 proteins on IL-6 expression in keratinocytes and whether this influence is mediated through p53.

MATERIALS AND METHODS

Cell Culture and Cell Line

HaCaT, HeLa (HPV18+) and SiHa (HPV16+), Lenti-X 293T cells were cultivated in Dulbecco's Modified Eagle Medium (DMEM) with L-glutamine (584 mg/L), sodium pyruvate (110 mg/L), penicillin (100 U/ml), streptomycin (100 µg/ml), 10% Fetal Bovine Serum (FBS) and specific concentrations of D-glucose for each cell line (4.5 g/L for HaCaT and Lenti-X 293T cells, and 1 g/L for HeLa and SiHa cells) (Gibco, Thermo Fisher Scientific, Waltham, MA). Lenti-X 293T cells were grown in medium supplemented with Tet-Free FBS (Clontech, Mountain View, CA). hTERT-scrambled and hTERT-crisp53 (primary human keratinocytes immortalized with hTERT and then silenced for p53 with Crispr/Cas9 system) were cultivated as previously described and Feeder layer was prepared by treating NIH 3T3 cells with Mytomycin C (0.5 mg/ml) for 2 h (21).

Abbreviations: CC, cervical cancer; CIN1, Cervical Intraepithelial Neoplasia grade 1; HR-HPV, High-Risk Human Papillomavirus; LR-HPV, Low-Risk Human Papillomavirus; fl-E6, full length E6; IL-6R, IL-6 receptor.

Cloning of E5, E6, and E7 From HPV16, 18, 62, or 84

E5, E6, and E7 Open Reading Frames (ORFs) from HPV16, 18, 62 or 84 were amplified by PCR from genomic DNA (gDNA) extracted from cervical biopsies of women infected with those viruses with primers described in **Table S1**. PCR experiments were done using *Expand High Fidelity PCR System kit* (Sigma-Aldrich, Toluca, Mexico), PCR products were separated by agarose gel electrophoresis and the bands of interest were purified with *Wizard SV Gel and PCR Clean-Up System kit* (Promega, Madison, WI). Each PCR product was first cloned in the pGEM-T Easy vector (Promega). For HPV18E5, a synthetic DNA fragment flanked with EcoRI restriction sites (gBlock) was constructed using the sequence of HPV18E5 as template (*Integrated DNA Technologies*, Coralville, IA) and cloned into the pGEM-T Easy vector. Then, the ORFs of E5, E6, and E7 were subcloned in the expression vector pLVX-Puro (Clontech) using EcoRI enzyme for restriction, Antarctic Alkaline Phosphatase for vector dephosphorylation and T4 DNA ligase for ligation (New England Biolabs, Ipswich, MA), following the provider instructions. Cloned genes were sequenced using *BigDye® Terminator Cycle Sequencing kit* (Applied Biosystems, Thermo Fisher Scientific) and *ABI PRISM 310 Genetic Analyzer*. The obtained sequences were aligned with reference sequences reported in the NCBI by using the *CLC MainWorkbench7.0* software (Qiagen Bioinformatics, Redwood City, CA). Plasmids obtained on this way were pLVX-16E5, pLVX-16E6, pLVX-16E7, pLVX-18E5, pLVX-18E6, pLVX-18E7, pLVX-62E5, pLVX-62E6, pLVX-62E7, pLVX-84E5, pLVX-84E6, and pLVX-84E7. These plasmids were further used to produce lentiviral particles.

Production of Lentiviral Particles Carrying Viral Genes and Infection of HaCaT Cells

Lenti-X 293T cells were transfected with each of the 12 pLVX expression vectors and the pLVX-Puro empty vector using the *Lenti-X HTX Packaging System* (Clontech) and Lipofectamine 2000 transfection reagent (Thermo Fisher Scientific). Cell supernatants were collected following the *Lenti-X Lentiviral Expression System* (Clontech) instructions and the presence of lentivirus was confirmed with *Lenti-X GoStix™* (Clontech). HaCaT cells were individually infected with the lentiviral particles containing each viral gene and selected with 0.5 μg/ml of Puromycin antibiotic for approximately 2 weeks until control cells (HaCaT cells without any infection) were death. The transduced HaCaT cells HaCaT-pLVX, HaCaT-16E5, HaCaT-16E6, HaCaT-16E7, HaCaT-18E5, HaCaT-18E6, HaCaT-18E7, HaCaT-62E5, HaCaT-62E6, HaCaT-62E7, HaCaT-84E5, HaCaT-84E6, and HaCaT-84E7 were grown in the same conditions as the parental HaCaT cell line.

Quantitative PCR Analysis

RNA was extracted with *RNeasy Plus Mini Kit* (Qiagen, Cat. No. 74136) or *All Prep DNA/RNA Mini kit* (Qiagen, Germantown, MD) and cDNA was obtained with *Transcriptor First Strand cDNA Synthesis Kit* (Roche, Pleasanton, CA) or *Revert Aid H Minus First Strand cDNA Synthesis Kit* (Thermo Fisher Scientific) following the manufacturers' instructions. Quantitative PCR (qPCR) was performed using the *LightCycler 2.0* platform (Roche) and the *LightCycler FastStart DNA Master plus SYBR Green I Kit* (Roche). In addition, the *Agilent Technologies Stratagene Mx3005P* equipment (Serial No. DE10901331) and the *MESA GREEN qPCR MasterMix Plus for SYBR Assay* (Eurogentec, Liege, Belgium) were used. β-actin, GAPDH, RPLP0 and RPL32 were used as reference genes. The results were analyzed with *Light Cycler Software 4.1* or the *MxPro qPCR Software*. E5, E6, and E7 qPCR products were visualized in 2% agarose gels. Primers used to amplify HPV16 E6/E6* were the following: Fwd ACTGCAATGTTTCAGGACCCA and Rev TCAGGACACAGTGGCTTTT, the product size was 343 bp for fl-E6 and 161 bp for E6*. All additional primer pairs used in this work are described in **Table S1**.

Western Blot and ELISA Test

For protein detection by western blot, 50 μg of protein were separated in a polyacrylamide *Mini-PROTEAN TGX Gel* (Bio-Rad, Hercules, CA) and transferred to a PVDF membrane by semi-dry transfer using the *iBlot Dry Blotting System* (Thermo Fisher Scientific). The membrane was blocked for 1 h at 37°C with *PBS Odyssey Blocking Buffer* (Li-COR Biosciences, Lincoln, NE). Then, primary antibody was added and the membrane was incubated overnight at 4°C: Anti-p53 mouse monoclonal IgG2a (Santa Cruz Sc-126, 1:200 dilution) or Anti-actin (I-19) Goat polyclonal IgG (Santa Cruz Sc-1616, 1:4,000 dilution). After washing with *1x PBS (*phosphate-buffered saline) *Tween*, the membrane was incubated for 1 h at 37°C with a fluorophore labeled secondary antibody: Anti-mouse donkey polyclonal IgG 800CW (926-32212, Li-COR, 1:15,000 dilution) or Anti-goat donkey polyclonal IgG 680RD (926-68074, Li-COR, 1:15,000 dilution). Finally, after washing, the membrane was scanned with the *Odyssey Imaging System* (Li-COR). ELISA experiments were performed following the manufacturer's instructions. IL-6 protein was measured in HaCaT, HaCaT-pLVX, HaCaT-16E6, HaCaT-18E6, HaCaT-62E6, HaCaT-84E6, HeLa, and SiHa cells supernatants using the *Human IL-6 ELISA Kit* (Thermo Fisher Scientific).

Cell Transfections

Transfections were conducted in HaCaT cells using the *X-tremeGENE 9 transfection reagent* (Roche), 3 μL of transfection reagent was used for each ug of DNA, all other transfection procedures were as recommended by the manufacturer. Twenty-four hour post-transfection, cells were harvested and RNA was extracted. HaCaT-pLXSN and HaCaT-16E6E7 stable transfectant cells were established as follow: 3×10^5 HaCaT cells were seeded in 6 well plates, and 24 h later, the cells were transfected with 1 μg of pLXSN vector or pLXSN-16E6E7 vector. Twenty-four hour post-transfection, 500 μg/mL of G-418 antibiotic was added to the cells. The cells were maintained growing with antibiotic for 23 days and then RNA was extracted to perform the qPCR assays.

Cervical Sample Collection and Analysis

Cervical samples were collected from women who attended a medical examination at the Clinic of Dysplasia in the

Gynecology and Obstetrics Hospital- Centro Médico Nacional de Occidente (CMNO-IMSS) in Guadalajara, Jalisco, Mexico. Before sampling, all participants were informed about this research protocol and decided to participate voluntarily; all of them signed informed consent. All procedures performed were in accordance with the ethical standards and were approved by the National Scientific Research Committee of IMSS (CNIC) with the Register number: R-2012-785-090. Sample recruitment was done from 2017 to 2018 by gynecologists, with a cytobrush inserted into the endocervical canal and positivity to HPV16 and 18 was determined by the Linear Array Genotyping Test as previously described (7). We recruited 9 HPV negative cervical samples from women without lesion (control), 7 HPV16 positive cervical samples from women with Cervical Intraepithelial Neoplasia grade 1 (CIN1) lesions, and 3 HPV18 positive CIN1 samples, and RNA was extracted from those samples to perform qPCR analyses.

Immunohistochemistry Analysis

Histologically normal cervical epithelium ($n = 3$) and squamous cell carcinoma samples positive to HPV16 ($n = 3$) that were paraffin-embedded were used for automated immunodetection assays using the Ventana BenchMark XT System, (Roche, Mannheim, Germany), the anti-IL-6R antibody (Santa Cruz Biotechnology, sc-373708, 1:100 dilution), and the ultraView Universal DAB Detection Kit (Roche Applied Science), following the manufacturers' instructions. IL-6R expression was evaluated and classified according to their level of positivity.

Statistical Analysis

Statistical significance was determined using the unpaired t Student test assuming same standard deviation and Gaussian distribution. The results that were statistically significant are indicated with * when $p < 0.05$ and with ** when $p < 0.01$ in the corresponding figures.

RESULTS

IL-6 Is Overexpressed in HPV16 and HPV18 Positive CC Cell Lines and CIN1 Samples

Initially, IL-6 expression was evaluated in HaCaT keratinocytes (HPV–) and HeLa (HPV18+) and SiHa (HPV16+) CC derived cell lines showing that IL-6 mRNA and protein is highly expressed in HeLa and SiHa cells compared to HaCaT cells (**Figures 1A,B**). As this result suggests that HR-HPVs may be promoting the overexpression of IL-6, IL-6 mRNA expression was evaluated in CIN1 HPV16 and HPV18 positive samples compared to control HPV negative cervical samples without lesion. The experiment reveals that in CIN1 samples positive for HPV16 or HPV18, IL-6 is upregulated compared to control samples (**Figure 1C**).

IL-6 Expression Increases in Keratinocytes by the Presence of HR-HPV E6 and E7 Oncogenes, Especially E6*

The previous results indicate a possible role of HPV infection on the expression of IL-6, but whether this upregulation is a direct action of the oncoproteins or if oncogenic and non-oncogenic HPVs have the same ability to modulate IL-6, were new questions that needed to be addressed. In order to determine which HPV oncoprotein was involved in the regulation of IL-6 expression, the effect of E5, E6, and E7 oncoproteins from HPV16 and HPV18 compared to non-carcinogenic HPV62 and 84 proteins was evaluated. We decided to use the HaCaT cell line as study model since those cells have an inactive p53 protein and we wanted to evaluate the effect of the oncoproteins on IL-6 independently of its action over p53. It has already been reported that p53 negatively regulates IL-6 expression and that E6 induces the degradation of p53. First, we transduced HaCaT cells with E5, E6, or E7 from HPV16, 18, 62, or 84 individually. To evaluate transduction efficiency, the expression of the viral genes in the transduced cells was assessed with qPCR assay confirming that E5, E6, and E7 genes were expressed in the corresponding cell line compared to the HaCaT-pLVX control cells that do not express any of those genes (**Figure 2A**). Then, to corroborate those results, the qPCR amplification products were visualized in agarose electrophoresis. As observed in **Figure 2B**, E5 gene is expressed in HaCaT-16E5, HaCaT-18E5, HaCaT-62E5, HaCaT-84E5, and in SiHa (HPV16E5) cells, but not in HeLa cell line. E6 gene expression products reveal that HaCaT-16E6 expresses only the spliced isoforms of E6, E6*I, and E6*II, while SiHa cells express fl-E6 and E6*I. Moreover, both HaCaT-18E6 and HeLa cells express E6* but no HPV18 fl-E6. Fl-E6 is expressed in HaCaT-62E6 and HaCaT-84E6 cells as no spliced isoforms of E6 have been reported in non-carcinogenic HPVs. Finally, E7 gene is expressed in the four HaCaT cell lines transduced with HPV16E7, HPV18E7, HPV62E7, or HPV84E7, as well as in HPV16 and HPV18 positive CC cells SiHa and HeLa, respectively.

After this characterization of our study model, IL-6 expression was evaluated in all transduced HaCaT cells compared to HaCaT-pLVX control, revealing an IL-6 mRNA overexpression in HaCaT-E6 cells, especially in HaCaT-16E6* and HaCaT-18E6* (**Figure 2C**). Also, IL-6 expression was around twice in HaCaT-E7 cells compared to HaCaT-pLVX, whereas there was a slight decrease in IL-6 mRNA levels in the presence of HPV16 and 18 E5, and no significant changes with HPV62 and 84 E5 (**Figure 2C**). As the most pronounced overexpression of IL-6 is observed in HaCaT cells that express the different E6 genes, we measured IL-6 protein in HaCaT-E6 supernatants with ELISA test. A higher secretion of IL-6 in HaCaT-E6 cells, especially in HaCaT-16E6* cells was detected (**Figure 2D**).

As HPV16E6* strongly upregulates IL-6 expression, we focused on HPV16 oncoproteins and we did dose dependent transfections of HaCaT cells with pLXSN-HPV16E6E7 plasmid that expresses both HPV16 E6 and E7 oncoproteins. The transfected keratinocytes with 0.5, 1 or 2 ug of vector express E6 and E7 proteins (mainly fl-E6 but also E6*) and their expression levels are proportional to the plasmid dose (**Figure 3Ai**). IL-6 mRNA expression levels are also proportional to the vector dose but IL-6 overexpression in E6E7 transfected cells is not observed with 1 and 2 ug transfection, and is significantly higher with 0.5 ug transfection but not as drastic as in transduced cells (**Figure 3Aii**). Therefore, we established a stable transfectant HaCaT cell line that expresses both HPV16 E6 and E7 genes

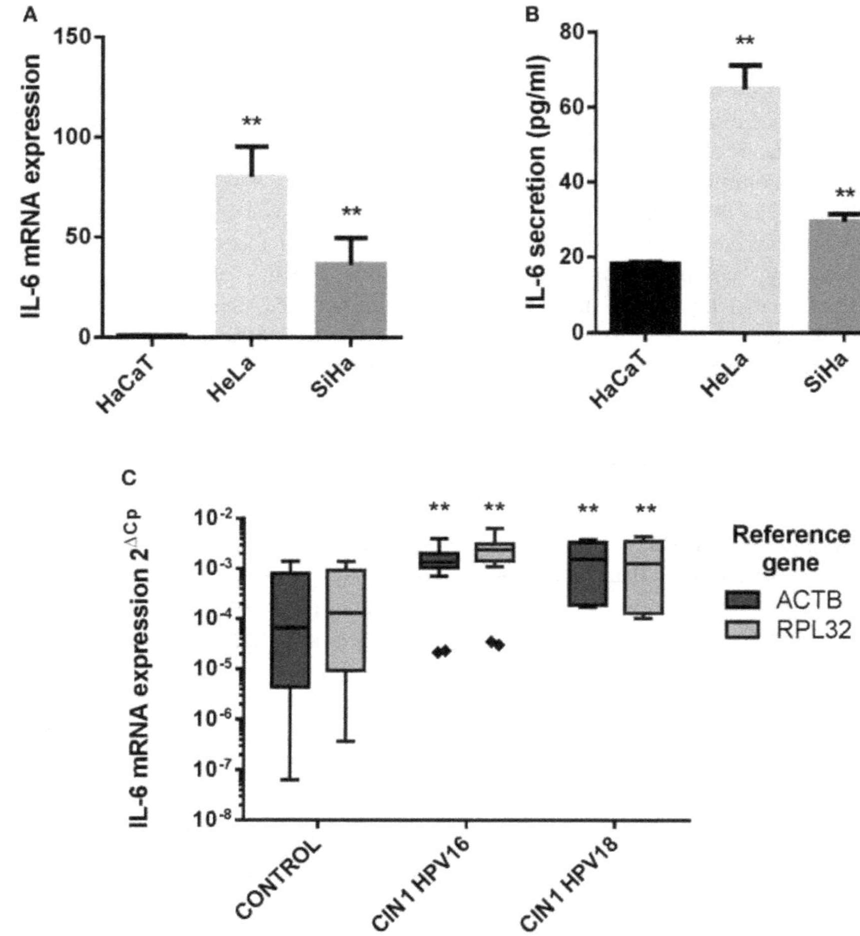

FIGURE 1 | IL-6 expression in HaCaT, HeLa, SiHa cells, and in cervical samples. **(A)** IL-6 mRNA relative expression in HaCaT, HeLa, and SiHa cell lines evaluated by qPCR using actin, RPLPO and RPL32 as reference genes. **(B)** IL-6 protein expression measured by ELISA test in HaCaT, HeLa and SiHa supernatants. Error bars in **(A,B)** represent standard deviation. **(C)** IL-6 mRNA expression in 9 HPV negative cervical samples without lesion (Control), 7 HPV16 positive CIN1 cervical samples (CIN I HPV16) and 3 HPV18 positive CIN1 cervical samples (CIN I HPV18) using actin and RPL32 as reference genes. Values are represented as $2^{\Delta Cp}$ (Cp Reference Gene—Cp Target Gene). The graph displays median (white lines), 25–75th percentile (boxes), interquartile ranges (Whiskers) and outlier data (triangles). Asterisks indicate statistical significance ($^{**}p < 0.01$).

to check if IL-6 overexpression is time dependent and needs a longer exposition to the oncoproteins. E6, E6*I, and E7 oncogene expression is confirmed in HaCaT-16E6E7 stable transfectant cells (**Figure 3Bi**) and IL-6 expression increase in keratinocytes with E6 and E7 is corroborated with this model (**Figure 3Bii**).

IL-6R Is Expressed in the Proliferative Basal Layer of Normal Keratinocytes and in Cervical Tumoral Cells

Considering the previous observations, we wondered if the keratinocytes also have a strong IL-6 receptor (IL-6R) expression so that IL-6 signaling could be autocrine. At mRNA level, HeLa and SiHa CC cells showed higher IL-6 expression compared to non-tumorigenic HaCaT cells (**Figure 4A**). In addition, we observed a modest tendency to increase in the expression of IL6R in HaCaT cells transduced with HPV16-E6* and HPV18-E6* compared to HaCaT-pLVX control cells (**Figure 4B**). Immunohistochemical analysis of cervical samples derived from women without lesion (control) and from women with CC (all CC samples were squamous cell carcinomas positive to HPV16 as confirmed by the Linear Array Genotyping test) showed that control tissues expressed IL-6R mainly in the proliferative basal layer of the epithelium. However, as the cells migrate to the parabasal and intermediate layers, a clear nuclear staining was observed (**Figure 4C**, control). Moreover, all CC tissues were IL-6R positive, especially in the tumor front (**Figure 4C**, CC). These results suggest that IL-6R expression is related to a proliferative phenotype in keratinocytes and is therefore expressed by cervical tumoral cells. The later could indicate a higher receptivity to IL-6 cytokine and its association with cell proliferation.

Regulation of IL-6 by E6/E7 Is in Part p53 Independent

HaCaT immortalized keratinocytes have mutations in p53 that affect its function and E6-targeted degradation (22, 23). It has previously been described that wild type p53 represses IL-6

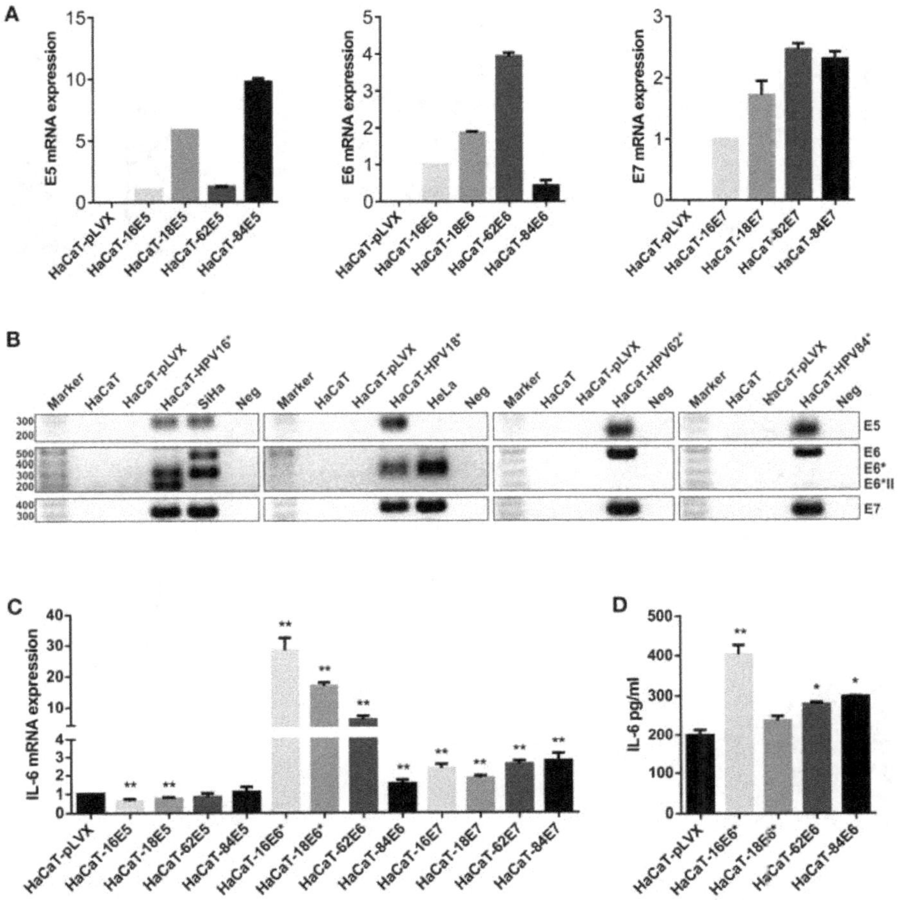

FIGURE 2 | Evaluation of IL-6 expression in E5-, E6-, and E7-transduced HaCaT keratinocytes. **(A)** E5, E6, and E7 expression measured by qPCR in HaCaT transduced cell lines using HaCaT-16E5, HaCaT-16E6, and HaCaT-16E7 as calibrators and actin as reference gene. **(B)** Visualization of E5, E6, E7, and E6 isoforms mRNAs expressed in transduced HaCaT cell lines, HeLa, and SiHa cells. (*) HaCaT-16, HaCaT-18, HaCaT-62, and HaCaT-84 refer to HaCaT cells transduced with one of the 3 genes E5, E6, or E7 separately to check E5, E6, and E7 expression, respectively. The expected amplicon size for each viral gene is indicated in **Table S1**. Water was used as template in the negative controls (Neg). **(C)** IL-6 mRNA expression evaluated by qPCR in E5, E6, or E7 from HPV16, 18, 62, or 84 transduced HaCaT cells, using HaCaT-pLVX cells as calibrator and actin, RPLP0, and RPL32 as reference genes. **(D)** Protein levels of IL-6 measured by ELISA test in HaCaT-pLVX and HaCaT-E6 supernatants. Asterisks indicate statistical significance (*$p < 0.05$ and ** $p < 0.01$).

promoter activity and that mutated p53 increase them (24–26). In order to evaluate p53 participation in E6 regulation of IL-6 expression, we first evaluated p53 protein degradation in HaCaT cells transduced with E6 of HPV-16,−18,−62, and−84. All four HaCaT-E6 transduced cell lines and HaCaT-pLVX control cells express p53 compared to HeLa and SiHa cells, in which p53 protein is degraded (**Figure 5A**). Moreover, despite of mutant p53 presence in HaCaT cells, E6E7 proteins increase almost three times IL-6 expression as already mentioned (**Figure 3Bii**), indicating an additional mechanism independent of p53 function. To corroborate IL-6 regulation by p53, IL-6 expression was evaluated in hTERT immortalized primary keratinocytes that have wt p53 or silenced p53 (hTERT-crisp53). As depicted in **Figure 5B**, there is an increase in IL-6 expression in the absence of p53. Additionally, it is worth mentioning that a previous study assessed IL-6 expression in primary human foreskin keratinocytes (therefore with p53wt) infected with the empty retroviral vector pLXSN (negative control) or with pLXSN vector expressing E6E7 genes from HPV16, and the results indicate a more pronounced induction of IL-6 expression in the presence of HPV16 oncoproteins (20).

DISCUSSION

Cytokines are soluble mediators known to keep immune homeostasis and participate in inflammatory response to infections or injury, they play diverse functions and can show pleiotropic properties. In particular, interleukin 6 participates in many biological processes such as chronic inflammation, autoimmunity, infectious diseases and cancer (27). The link between IL-6 and oncogenic progression has been widely reported and IL-6 overexpression has been observed in a variety of solid tumors, both in the tumor microenvironment and in the serum of affected patients, which explains why this cytokine has been proposed as a prognostic biomarker and a therapeutic target in cancer (28, 29). At early stages of HPV infection,

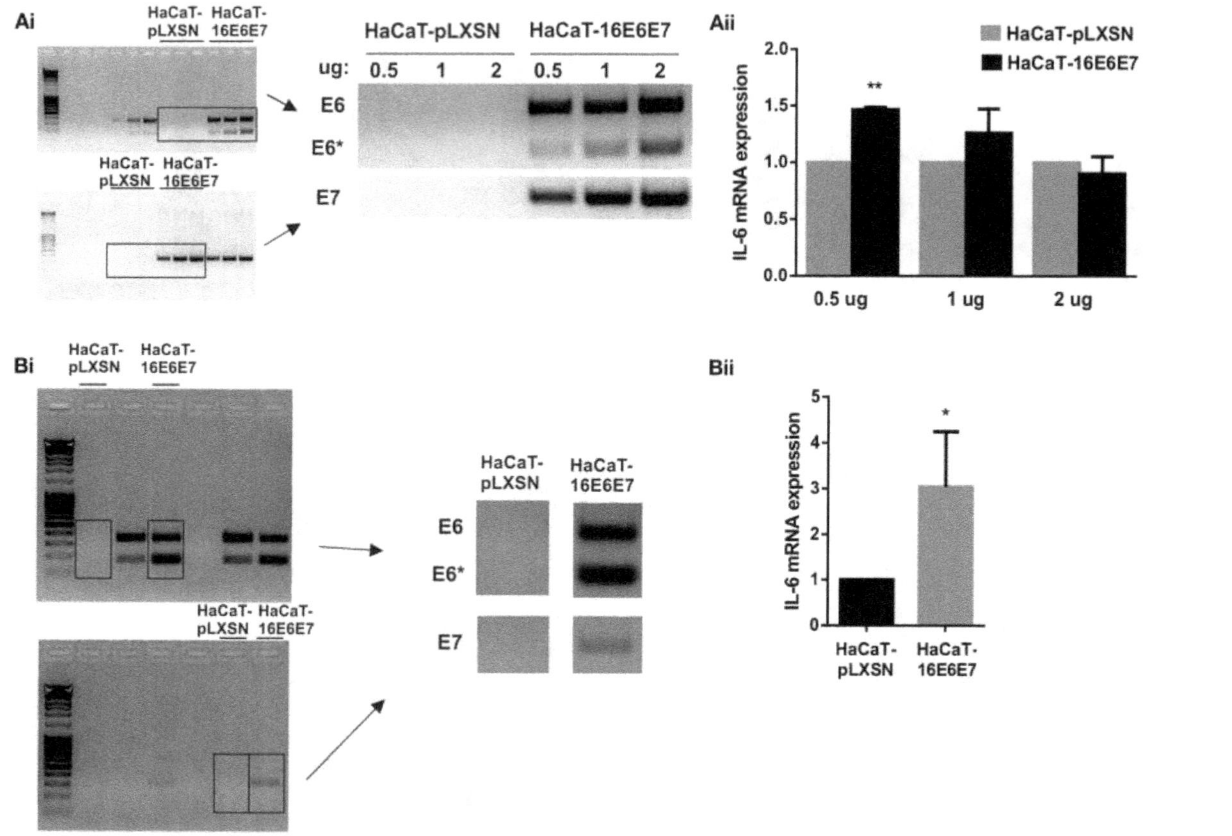

FIGURE 3 | Evaluation of IL-6 expression in the presence of HPV16E6E7. **(Ai)** Expression of E6/E6* and E7 in transiently transfected HaCaT cells with 0.5, 1, or 2 ug of pLXSN or pLXSN-16E6E7 plasmids. Originals blots are shown left and representative pictures right. **(Aii)** IL-6 mRNA expression in those same cells. **(Bi)** E6/E6* and E7 expression in stable transfected HaCaT cells. Original blots left and representative pictures right. **(Bii)** IL-6 expression measured by qPCR in HaCaT and HaCaT transduced with E6/E7 from HPV16 (*$p < 0.05$ and **$p < 0.01$).

a down-modulation of IL-6 expression and other cytokines, like IL-1β and IL-1α, has been reported (30). However, high expression of IL-6 has been related with a bad prognosis for cervical cancer patients and immunohistochemistry experiments demonstrate that tumor cells and stromal cells show high and moderate IL-6 expression respectively, and macrophages showed positive correlation with IL-6 positivity in stroma (31). In fact, different works have reported an upregulation of IL-6 in CC, but whether HPV oncoproteins are involved in this upregulation has been poorly studied. In addition, differences between HR-HPVs and LR-HPVs regarding the modulation or regulation of IL-6 expression has not previously been addressed.

In this work, we report the overexpression of IL-6 in HeLa and SiHa HPV positive CC cell lines compared to non-tumorigenic HaCaT keratinocytes. This result may suggest that CC derived cells have acquired the ability to up-modulate IL-6 expression. Audirac-Chalifour et al. working with samples at various stages of cervical cancer, observed the upregulation of IL-6 in low-grade squamous intraepithelial lesion and CC samples (32). In line with these observations, we report an IL-6 upregulation in HPV16 and HPV18 positive cervical samples from women with CIN1 compared to control cervical samples without lesion and negative to HPV infection. These results strongly suggested that HPV infection could mediate IL-6 regulation. Cheng et al. have observed an up-regulatory effect of HPV16 and HPV18 E6 and E7 to IL-6 expression in E6 and E7 transfected lung cancer cells (33). Also, the repression of HPV18 E6 and E7 in basal cell carcinoma cells reduced IL-6 expression levels (34). In addition, Dell'Oste et al. reported an increase in IL-6 mRNA expression and protein secretion in primary keratinocytes immortalized with both E6E7 genes from HPV16 compared to control keratinocytes (20). In this work we compare the effect of HR vs. LR viral proteins on IL-6 expression in HaCaT transduced cells, revealing an IL-6 upregulation by HR HPV16 and HPV18 E6* and E7 oncoproteins individually, mainly by E6*. LR HPV62 and HPV84 E6 and E7 proteins, that have been barely studied, also induce the increase of IL-6 mRNA expression, even though the effect was not so pronounced as with HR oncoproteins. Interestingly, HPV16 and HPV18 E5 proteins decrease IL-6 expression whereas no significant variations were seen with HPV62 and HPV84 E5. IL-6 protein secretion was similar in HaCaT-18E6*, −62E6, and −84E6, and the higher IL-6 levels were observed in HaCaT-16E6*.

The analysis of viral gene expression in each transduced HaCaT cell line with E5, E6 or E7 from HPV16, 18, 62

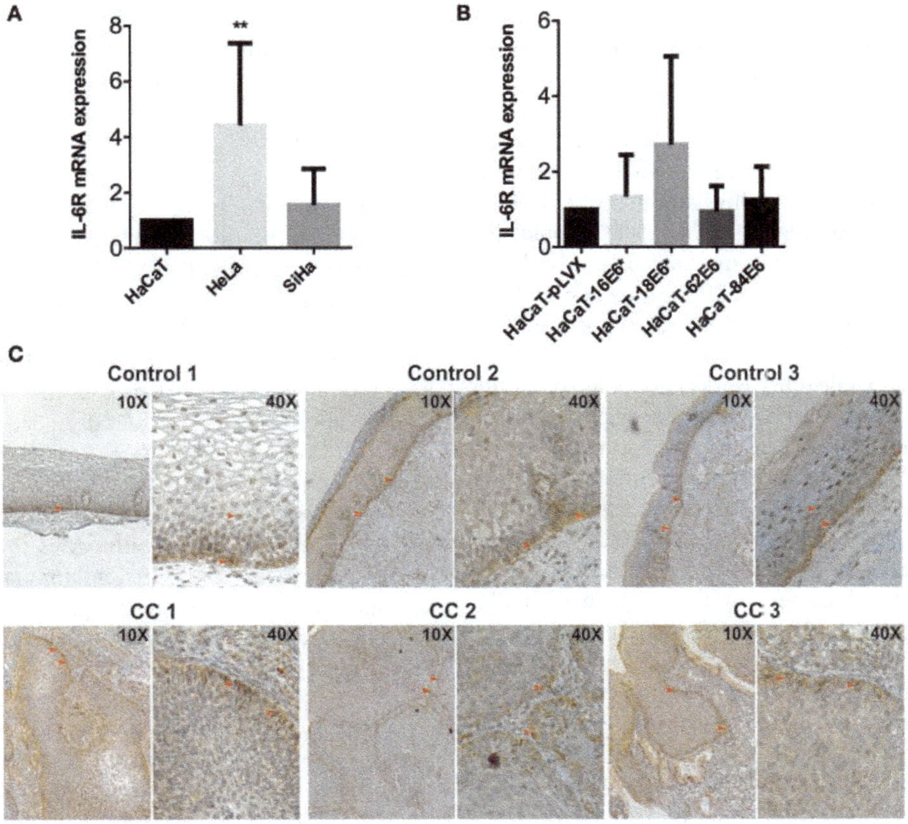

FIGURE 4 | Evaluation of IL-6R expression in cell lines and cervical tissues. **(A)** IL-6R mRNA expression evaluated by qPCR in HaCaT, HeLa, and SiHa cells and **(B)** in E6 transduced HaCaT cells using HaCaT-pLVX as calibrator. Actin and RPL32 were used as reference genes, error bars represent standard deviation and asterisks indicate statistical significance (**$p < 0.01$). **(C)** IL-6R protein expression by immunohistochemical analysis in control and cervical cancer (CC) tissues. Red arrows indicate positive signal to IL-6R.

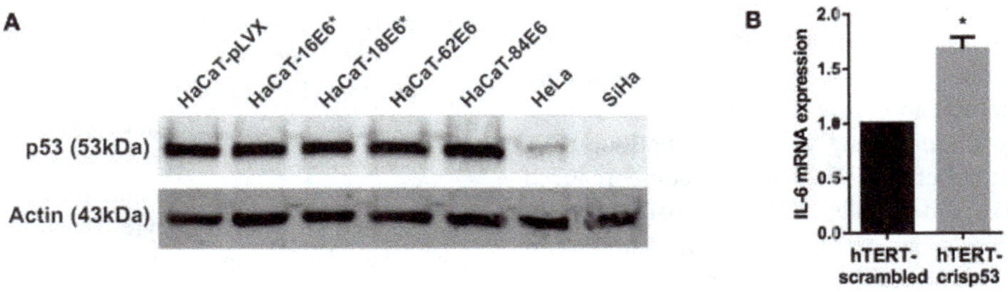

FIGURE 5 | Effect of p53 on IL-6 expression. **(A)** p53 protein levels evaluated by western blot in HaCaT-pLVX, HaCaT-E6, HeLa, and SiHa cells. Boxes in the upper blot include wells relevant for this experiment, lower edited picture shows the same but in a clearer form. **(B)** IL-6 expression in hTERT immortalized keratinocytes silenced for p53 (hTERT-crisp53) compared to the control hTERT-scrambled cells. IL-6 expression was measured by qPCR. Actin was used as reference gene. The asterisk indicates statistical significance ($p < 0.05$).

or 84 demonstrated that exclusively E6* spliced isoforms are expressed in HaCaT-16E6 and HaCaT-18E6 cells. Also, SiHa cells (HPV16+) expressed E5, E6, E6*, and E7 proteins, while HeLa cells (HPV18+) expressed only E6* and E7 proteins and no E5 or fl-E6 expression was observed.

Transiently transfected HaCaT cells with HPV16E6E7 expressed both E6 and low levels of E6* proteins and IL-6 expression was not significantly altered, however, in HaCaT-16E6E7 stable transfectant cells, both E6 and E6* are expressed, predominantly E6*, and IL-6 is now overexpressed. The later suggests that the overexpression of IL-6 is time and E6* expression dependent, and E6* must prevail over fl-E6 to induce IL-6 upregulation. Following the last hypothesis, E6* expression has been reported to be modulated by EGF and EGFR (35), and it is well established that the EGFR is mainly expressed in the basal layer of cervical epithelium (36). At early stages of HPV infection, when the viral genome remains episomal, the E6 mRNA is expressed at low levels and since the microenvironment of the basal layer is rich in EGF and EGFR, the expression of fl-E6 could be favored leading to the negative regulation of IL-6. Thereafter, the expression of E6* could be induced by cell migration into the upper layers where less EGFR expression has been observed. Another possibility is that the loss of E2 regulation and the increment of E6 mRNA levels (37) could also favor E6* expression. Whatever the mechanism involved, the final consequence is the increment of IL-6 expression and the induction of its connate pathway, which has been involved with tumor promotion (28, 38). IL-6 induction suggests E6* as a pro-inflammatory oncogene, while other works have pointed out the alternate E6*I protein as the most abundant oncogene transcript in premalignant or malignant cervical and oropharyngeal tumors (39–41). In addition, the isoform E6*II has been also reported in CC and the association between E6*I/E6*II expression and the grade of cervical lesions are controversial (13). However, there are also studies that propose E6*II expression as an indicator of cervical neoplasia severity (42). Whether HPV16 E6*II by its own also regulates IL-6 expression remains unclear. Further studies need to be performed to better understand the E6 splicing patterns according to lesion severity. Indeed, many works have tried to elucidate the role of those fl-E6 and E6* spliced proteins in carcinogenesis, but there is not a general consensus on their biological significance. Although only HR fl-E6 has the ability to transform its target cell, HPV18 E6* protein binds to fl-E6 preventing p53 degradation (43, 44). Furthermore, contrarily to what is seen with HPV16 E6, binding of E6* to procaspase-8 results in its stabilization and may sensitize cells to apoptosis (45). Also, E6*II sensitizes C33A cell to cisplatin-induced apoptosis (46). Moreover, HPV16 E6* reduces tumor formation in cervical carcinoma xenografts in mice, pointing to anti-oncogenic characteristics of E6* (47). In contrast, Rosenberger et al. propose that during the first stages of viral infection of the basal keratinocytes, HPV might require high levels of fl-E6 to inhibit apoptosis through p53 degradation, and that afterwards with increasing cell differentiation, HPV would express E7, and therefore E6*, to overcome reduced cell proliferation (35). Additionally, E6* may participate in virus-induced mutagenesis by increasing oxidative stress and DNA damage (48). All these studies must be put together and corroborated *in vivo* to understand the mechanisms that regulate the splicing of HPV mRNAs and the biological significance of the switch from one transcript to another.

Although many studies have focused on IL-6 and its involvement in cervical carcinogenesis, there are few reports on IL-6R and its implication in CC. In the present work, we demonstrate that IL-6 receptor expression is increased in CC cell lines and in cervical tissues derived from women with squamous cell carcinoma. Interestingly, IL-6R expression was also positive in the proliferative basal layer of the cervical epithelium in control tissues, suggesting that IL-6R might be expressed in proliferative and tumoral keratinocytes, and that the high IL-6 expression in CC could be acting in an autocrine and paracrine manner in keratinocytes and not only in immune cells. In line with our results, it has been recently demonstrated that IL-6R is overexpressed CC tissue compared to normal control tissue (49). HR HPV infected keratinocytes are therefore capable of secreting high levels of IL-6 due in part to the presence of viral oncoproteins, and also expressing IL-6R and be receptive to IL-6 signaling.

Finally, it is worth mentioning that IL-6 synthesis is strictly regulated both transcriptionally and post-transcriptionally (15). Transcription factors like NF-IL6 and NF-κB activate IL-6 transcription (50). In contrast, Rb and p53 proteins repress IL-6 promoter, and mutant p53 has the opposite effect contributing to IL-6 overexpression (25, 26). HaCaT immortalized keratinocytes have dysfunctional mutated p53 that in our study model is insensitive to E6*-targeted degradation (22, 23). In this regard, IL-6 up-modulation by E6* observed in HaCaT cells is mediated independently of p53 degradation. This conclusion is also supported by the upregulation of IL-6 after silencing wt p53 in immortalized keratinocytes that is not as strong as in the presence of E6E7, in both mutated p53 and wt p53 keratinocytes (20). Therefore, this process could be modulated by E6 trough induction of p53 degradation but also by a mechanism independent of p53.

In conclusion, HPV oncoproteins are multifunctional and in this work we show that IL-6 is one of their multiple targets. Indeed, E5, E6, and E7 are involved by many mechanisms in the development of chronic inflammation associated with cervical carcinogenesis (51). Both HR and LR E6 and E7 proteins upregulate IL-6 expression in keratinocytes, especially HR E6* isoforms, and IL-6 is also overexpressed in CIN1 samples compared to control cervical samples without lesion. IL-6R is also overexpressed in tumoral proliferative keratinocytes in CC tissues which are then receptive to proliferative signals through IL-6 signaling. Since many studies have reported E6* as the predominant transcript in malignant lesions and CC, this E6 truncated form may participate in the maintenance of the chronic inflammatory microenvironment through IL-6 overexpression. Further studies must unravel if upregulation of IL-6 in keratinocytes is correlated with keratinocyte transformation during the first stages of viral infection or with proliferation and malignancy that promote carcinogenesis.

ETHICS STATEMENT

Cervical samples were collected from women who attended a medical examination at the Clinic of Dysplasia in the Gynecology and Obstetrics Hospital- Centro Médico Nacional de Occidente (CMNO-IMSS) in Guadalajara, Jalisco, Mexico. Before sampling, all participants were informed about this research protocol and decided to participate voluntarily; all of them signed informed consent. All procedures performed were in accordance with the ethical standards and were approved by the National Scientific Research Committee of IMSS (CNIC) with the Register number: R-2012-785-090.

AUTHOR CONTRIBUTIONS

CA-I cloned all HPV16, 18, 62, and 84 proteins, developed the HaCaT transduced cell lines, conducted the transient and stable transfections, performed the IL-6 and p53 expression analysis, and wrote the first draft of the manuscript. LL-T, PO-L, and WR-C were involved in patient interviews and cervical sample recruitment. AM-P performed the Linear Array HPV test and qPCR assays with the cervical samples. AP-S was involved in the immunohistochemistry analysis. AA-L and LJ-S designed the study, supervised all experiments and analyses, and completed the manuscript. All authors read and approved the final manuscript.

ACKNOWLEDGMENTS

We would like to thank all members of the Immunology Division of CIBO-IMSS (Guadalajara, Mexico) and the members of the Infections and Cancer Biology Group in IARC-WHO (Lyon, France) for their constant support and help during this research work, especially to Massimo Tommasino, Assunta Venuti, and Maria Grazia Ceraolo. We are also committed to the IMSS Research Network on HPV.

SUPPLEMENTARY MATERIAL

Table S1 | Primers and experimental conditions used for PCR amplifications.

Figure S1 | p53 and IL-6 expression in E6 transduced HaCaT cells compared to HaCaT-pLVX control cells, after p53 wt transfection. **(A)** p53 mRNA relative expression in HaCaT-pLVX, −16E6*, −18E6*, −62E6, and −84E6 cells transfected with pcDNA3-p53wt compared to cells transfected with empty pcDNA3 vector. **(B)** IL-6 mRNA expression in the same cells transfected with pcDNA3-p53wt compared to cells transfected with pcDNA3 empty vector. Actin was used as reference gene and error bars represent standard deviation. Results from three independent experiments are shown in this Figure. pcDNA3 and pcDNA3-p53wt were transfected in the cells using X-tremeGENE HP DNA Transfection Reagent (06365752001, Roche) and RNA was extracted 24 h post-transfection.

REFERENCES

1. Bravo IG, Félez-Sánchez M. Papillomaviruses viral evolution, cancer and evolutionary medicine. *Evol Med Public Health.* (2015) 2015:32–51. doi: 10.1093/emph/eov003
2. Bernard H-U, Burk RD, Chen Z, van Doorslaer K, zur Hausen H, de Villiers EM. Classification of papillomaviruses (PVs) based on 189 PV types and proposal of taxonomic amendments. *Virology.* (2010) 401:70–9. doi: 10.1016/j.virol.2010.02.002
3. Egawa N, Doorbar J. The low-risk papillomaviruses. *Virus Res.* (2017) 231:119–27. doi: 10.1016/j.virusres.2016.12.017
4. GLOBOCAN. *Estimated Cancer Incidence, Mortality and Prevalence Worldwide in 2012.* (2012). Availble online at: http://globocan.iarc.fr/Pages/fact_sheets_cancer.aspx
5. Zur Hausen H. Papillomaviruses and cancer: from basic studies to clinical application. *Nat Rev Cancer.* (2002) 2:342–50. doi: 10.1038/nrc798
6. Artaza-Irigaray C, Flores-Miramontes MG, Olszewski D, Magaña-Torres MT, López-Cardona MG, Leal-Herrera YA, et al. Genetic variability in E6, E7 and L1 genes of human papillomavirus 62 and its prevalence in Mexico. *Infect Agents Cancer.* (2017) 12:15. doi: 10.1186/s13027-017-0125-x
7. Flores-Miramontes MG, Torres-Reyes LA, Alvarado-Ruíz L, Romero-Martínez SA, Ramírez-Rodríguez V, Balderas-Peña LM, et al. Human papillomavirus genotyping by linear array and next-generation sequencing in cervical samples from Western Mexico. *Virol J.* (2015) 12:161. doi: 10.1186/s12985-015-0391-4
8. Moody CA, Laimins LA. Human papillomavirus oncoproteins: pathways to transformation. *Nat Rev Cancer.* (2010) 10:550–60. doi: 10.1038/nrc2886
9. Klingelhutz AJ, Roman A. Cellular transformation by human papillomaviruses: lessons learned by comparing high-and low-risk viruses. *Virology.* (2012) 424:77–98. doi: 10.1016/j.virol.2011.12.018
10. Agatston PW, Kowalski R, Limber S. Students' perspectives on cyber bullying. *J Adolesc Health.* (2007) 41:S59–60. doi: 10.1016/j.jadohealth.2007.09.003
11. Schwartz S. Papillomavirus transcripts and posttranscriptional regulation. *Virology.* (2013) 445:187–96. doi: 10.1016/j.virol.2013.04.034
12. Mesplède T, Gagnon D, Bergeron-Labrecque F, Azar I, Sénéchal H, Coutlée F, et al. p53 degradation activity, expression, and subcellular localization of E6 proteins from 29 human papillomavirus genotypes. *J Virol.* (2012) 86:94–107. doi: 10.1128/JVI.00751-11
13. Olmedo-Nieva L, Muñoz-Bello JO, Contreras-Paredes A, Lizano M. The role of E6 spliced isoforms (E6*) in human papillomavirus-induced carcinogenesis. *Viruses.* (2018) 10:45. doi: 10.3390/v10010045
14. Pim D, Tomaić V, Banks L. The HPV E6* proteins from high-risk, mucosal human papillomaviruses can direct the degradation of cellular proteins in the absence of full-length e6 protein. *J Virol.* (2009) 83:9863–74. doi: 10.1128/JVI.00539-09
15. Tanaka T, Narazaki M, Kishimoto T. IL-6 in inflammation, immunity, and disease. *Cold Spring Harbor Perspect Biol.* (2014) 6:a016295. doi: 10.1101/cshperspect.a016295
16. Hodge DR, Hurt EM, Farrar WL. The role of IL-6 and STAT3 in inflammation and cancer. *Eur J Cancer.* (2005) 41:2502–12. doi: 10.1016/j.ejca.2005.08.016
17. Wei L-H, Kuo M-L, Chen C-A, Cheng W-F, Cheng S-P, Hsieh F-J, et al. Interleukin-6 in cervical cancer: the relationship with vascular endothelial growth factor. *Gynecol Oncol.* (2001) 82:49–56. doi: 10.1006/gyno.2001.6235
18. Song Z, Lin Y, Ye X, Feng C, Lu Y, Yang G, et al. Expression of IL-1α and IL-6 is Associated with progression and prognosis of human cervical cancer. *Med Sci Monit.* (2016) 22:4475–81. doi: 10.12659/MSM.898569
19. Jee S-H, Shen S-C, Chiu H-C, Tsai W-L, Kuo M-L. Overexpression of interleukin-6 in human basal cell carcinoma cell lines increases anti-apoptotic activity and tumorigenic potency. *Oncogene.* (2001) 20:198–208. doi: 10.1038/sj.onc.1204076
20. Dell'Oste V, Azzimonti B, Mondini M, De Andrea M, Borgogna C, Mesturini R, et al. Altered expression of UVB-induced cytokines in human papillomavirus-immortalized epithelial cells. *J Gen Virol.* (2008) 89:2461–6. doi: 10.1099/vir.0.83586-0
21. Pacini L, Ceraolo MG, Venuti A, Melita G, Hasan UA, Accardi R, et al. UV radiation activates toll-like receptor 9 expression in primary human keratinocytes, an event inhibited by human papillomavirus type 38 E6 and E7 oncoproteins. *J Virol.* (2017) 91:e01123-17. doi: 10.1128/JVI.01123-17

22. Shnitman Magal S, Jackman A, Pei XF, Schlegel R, Sherman L. Induction of apoptosis in human keratinocytes containing mutated p53 alleles and its inhibition by both the E6 and E7 oncoproteins. *Int J Cancer.* (1998) 75:96–104.
23. Lehman TA, Modali R, Boukamp P, Stanek J, Bennett WP, Welsh JA, et al. p53 mutations in human immortalized epithelial cell lines. *Carcinogenesis.* (1993) 14:833–9. doi: 10.1093/carcin/14.5.833
24. Santhanam U, Ray A, Sehgal PB. Repression of the interleukin 6 gene promoter by p53 and the retinoblastoma susceptibility gene product. *Proc Natl Acad Sci USA.* (1991) 88:7605–9. doi: 10.1073/pnas.88.17.7605
25. Margulies L, Sehgal P. Modulation of the human interleukin-6 promoter (IL-6) and transcription factor C/EBP beta (NF-IL6) activity by p53 species. *J Biol Chem.* (1993) 268:15096–100.
26. Angelo LS, Talpaz M, Kurzrock R. Autocrine interleukin-6 production in renal cell carcinoma. *Cancer Res.* (2002) 62:932–40.
27. Jones SA, Jenkins BJ. Recent insights into targeting the IL-6 cytokine family in inflammatory diseases and cancer. *Nat Rev Immunol.* (2018) 18:773–89. doi: 10.1038/s41577-018-0066-7
28. Taniguchi K, Karin M. IL-6 and related cytokines as the critical lynchpins between inflammation and cancer. *Semin Immunol.* (2014) 26:54–74. doi: 10.1016/j.smim.2014.01.001
29. Yao X, Huang J, Zhong H, Shen N, Faggioni R, Fung M, et al. Targeting interleukin-6 in inflammatory autoimmune diseases and cancers. *Pharmacol Ther.* (2014) 141:125–39. doi: 10.1016/j.pharmthera.2013.09.004
30. Karim R, Meyers C, Backendorf C, Ludigs K, Offringa R, van Ommen GJ, et al. Human papillomavirus deregulates the response of a cellular network comprising of chemotactic and proinflammatory genes. *PLoS ONE.* (2011) 6:e17848. doi: 10.1371/journal.pone.0017848
31. Srivani R, Nagarajan B. A prognostic insight on in vivo expression of interleukin-6 in uterine cervical cancer. *Int J Gynecol Cancer.* (2003) 13:331–9. doi: 10.1046/j.1525-1438.2003.13197.x
32. Audirac-Chalifour A, Torres-Poveda K, Bahena-Roman M, Tellez-Sosa J, Martinez-Barnetche J, Cortina-Ceballos B, et al. Cervical microbiome and cytokine profile at various stages of cervical cancer: a pilot study. *PLoS ONE.* (2016) 11:e0153274. doi: 10.1371/journal.pone.0153274
33. Cheng Y-W, Lee H, Shiau M-Y, Wu T-C, Huang T-T, Chang Y-H. Human papillomavirus type 16/18 up-regulates the expression of interleukin-6 and antiapoptotic Mcl-1 in non-small cell lung cancer. *Clin Cancer Res.* (2008) 14:4705–12. doi: 10.1158/1078-0432.CCR-07-4675
34. Hsiao YP, Yang JH, Wu WJ, Lin MH, Sheu GT. E6 and E7 of human papillomavirus type 18 and UVB irradiation corporately regulate interleukin-6 and interleukin-8 expressions in basal cell carcinoma. *Exp Dermatol.* (2013) 22:672–4. doi: 10.1111/exd.12223
35. Rosenberger S, De-Castro Arce J, Langbein L, Steenbergen RD, Rosl F. Alternative splicing of human papillomavirus type-16 E6/E6* early mRNA is coupled to EGF signaling via Erk1/2 activation. *Proc Natl Acad Sci USA.* (2010) 107:7006–11. doi: 10.1073/pnas.1002620107
36. Soonthornthum T, Arias-Pulido H, Joste N, Lomo L, Muller C, Rutledge T, et al. Epidermal growth factor receptor as a biomarker for cervical cancer. *Ann Oncol.* (2011) 22:2166–78. doi: 10.1093/annonc/mdq723
37. Romanczuk H, Thierry F, Howley P. Mutational analysis of cis elements involved in E2 modulation of human papillomavirus type 16 P97 and type 18 P105 promoters. *J Virol.* (1990) 64:2849–59.
38. Chang Q, Daly L, Bromberg J. The IL-6 feed-forward loop: a driver of tumorigenesis. *Semin Immunol.* (2014) 26:48–53. doi: 10.1016/j.smim.2014.01.007
39. Walline HM, Komarck CM, McHugh JB, Bellile EL, Brenner JC, Prince ME, et al. Genomic integration of high-risk HPV alters gene expression in oropharyngeal squamous cell carcinoma. *Mol Cancer Res.* (2016) 14:941–52. doi: 10.1158/1541-7786.MCR-16-0105
40. Cornelissen M, Smits H, Briet M, Van Den Tweel J, Struyk A, Van Der Noordaa J, et al. Uniformity of the splicing pattern of the E6/E7 transcripts in human papillomavirus type 16-transformed human fibroblasts, human cervical premalignant lesions and carcinomas. *J Gen Virol.* (1990) 71:1243–6. doi: 10.1099/0022-1317-71-5-1243
41. Smotkin D, Prokoph H, Wettstein F. Oncogenic and nononcogenic human genital papillomaviruses generate the E7 mRNA by different mechanisms. *J Virol.* (1989) 63:1441–7.
42. Pastuszak-Lewandoska D, Bartosińska-Dyc A, Migdalska-Sęk M, Czarnecka KH, Nawrot E, Domańska D, et al. HPV16 E6* II gene expression in intraepithelial cervical lesions as an indicator of neoplastic grade: a pilot study. *Med Oncol.* (2014) 31:842. doi: 10.1007/s12032-014-0842-6
43. Wang H-K, Duffy AA, Broker TR, Chow LT. Robust production and passaging of infectious HPV in squamous epithelium of primary human keratinocytes. *Genes Dev.* (2009) 23:181–94. doi: 10.1101/gad.1735109
44. Pim D, Banks L. HPV-18 E6* I protein modulates the E6-directed degradation of p53 by binding to full-length HPV-18 E6. *Oncogene.* (1999) 18:7403–8. doi: 10.1038/sj.onc.1203134
45. Filippova M, Johnson MM, Bautista M, Filippov V, Fodor N, Tungteakkhun SS, et al. The large and small isoforms of human papillomavirus type 16 E6 bind to and differentially affect procaspase 8 stability and activity. *J Virol.* (2007) 81:4116–29. doi: 10.1128/JVI.01924-06
46. Vaisman CE, Del Moral-Hernandez O, Moreno-Campuzano S, Aréchaga-Ocampo E, Bonilla-Moreno R, Garcia-Aguiar I, et al. C33-A cells transfected with E6* I or E6* II the short forms of HPV-16 E6, displayed opposite effects on cisplatin-induced apoptosis. *Virus Res.* (2018) 247:94–101. doi: 10.1016/j.virusres.2018.02.009
47. Filippova M, Evans W, Aragon R, Filippov V, Williams VM, Hong L, et al. The small splice variant of HPV16 E6, E6, reduces tumor formation in cervical carcinoma xenografts. *Virology.* (2014) 450:153–64. doi: 10.1016/j.virol.2013.12.011
48. Williams VM, Filippova M, Filippov V, Payne KJ, Duerksen-Hughes P. Human papillomavirus type 16 E6* induces oxidative stress and DNA damage. *J Virol.* (2014) 88:6751–61. doi: 10.1128/JVI.03355-13
49. Luan S, An Z, Bi S, Chen L, Fan J. Interleukin 6 receptor (IL-6R) was an independent prognostic factor in cervical cancer. *Histol Histopathol.* (2018) 33:269–76. doi: 10.14670/HH-11-920
50. Matsusaka T, Fujikawa K, Nishio Y, Mukaida N, Matsushima K, Kishimoto T, et al. Transcription factors NF-IL6 and NF-kappa B synergistically activate transcription of the inflammatory cytokines, interleukin 6 and interleukin 8. *Proc Natl Acad Sci USA.* (1993) 90:10193–7. doi: 10.1073/pnas.90.21.10193
51. Georgescu SR, Mitran CI, Mitran MI, Caruntu C, Sarbu MI, Matei C, et al. New insights in the pathogenesis of HPV infection and the associated carcinogenic processes: the role of chronic inflammation and oxidative stress. *J Immunol Res.* (2018) 2018:5315816. doi: 10.1155/2018/5315816

15

Neutrophils as Trojan Horse Vehicles for *Brucella abortus* Macrophage Infection

*Cristina Gutiérrez-Jiménez[1], Ricardo Mora-Cartín[1], Pamela Altamirano-Silva[2], Carlos Chacón-Díaz[2], Esteban Chaves-Olarte[2], Edgardo Moreno[1] and Elías Barquero-Calvo[1]**

[1] *Programa de Investigación en Enfermedades Tropicales, Escuela de Medicina Veterinaria, Universidad Nacional, Heredia, Costa Rica,* [2] *Centro de Investigación en Enfermedades Tropicales, Facultad de Microbiología, Universidad de Costa Rica, San José, Costa Rica*

***Correspondence:**
Elías Barquero-Calvo
elias.barquero.calvo@una.ac.cr

Brucella abortus is a stealthy intracellular bacterial pathogen of animals and humans. This bacterium promotes the premature cell death of neutrophils (PMN) and resists the killing action of these leukocytes. *B. abortus*-infected PMNs presented phosphatidylserine (PS) as "eat me" signal on the cell surface. This signal promoted direct contacts between PMNs and macrophages (Mϕs) and favored the phagocytosis of the infected dying PMNs. Once inside Mϕs, *B. abortus* replicated within Mϕs at significantly higher numbers than when Mϕs were infected with bacteria alone. The high levels of the regulatory IL-10 and the lower levels of proinflammatory TNF-α released by the *B. abortus*-PMN infected Mϕs, at the initial stages of the infection, suggested a non-phlogistic phagocytosis mechanism. Thereafter, the levels of proinflammatory cytokines increased in the *B. abortus*-PMN-infected Mϕs. Still, the efficient bacterial replication proceeded, regardless of the cytokine levels and Mϕ type. Blockage of PS with Annexin V on the surface of *B. abortus*-infected PMNs hindered their contact with Mϕs and hampered the association, internalization, and replication of *B. abortus* within these cells. We propose that *B. abortus* infected PMNs serve as "Trojan horse" vehicles for the efficient dispersion and replication of the bacterium within the host.

Keywords: *Brucella*, neutrophils, macrophages, Trojan horse, phosphatidylserine

INTRODUCTION

Polymorphonuclear neutrophils (PMNs) are the first line of defense of the innate immune system against bacterial pathogens (1–3). Upon contacts with invading bacteria, PMNs activate their killing mechanisms, release cytokines, and may generate PMN extracellular traps (3–5). Although PMNs kill most of the microorganisms they interact with, there are some pathogens capable to resist the microbicidal actions of these leucocytes (6).

Brucella abortus is a Gram-negative bacteria that cause disease in bovines and humans (7). After host invasion, PMNs are the first immune cells to encounter and phagocytize *Brucella* organisms (8, 9). However, *Brucella*-infected-PMNs release negligible amounts of proinflammatory cytokines, generate low levels of reactive oxygen species and seldom show degranulation (10–12). Moreover, *Brucella* pathogens survive inside PMNs for a protracted period of time (10) and induce the premature death of these cells (12, 13). Although the dying *Brucella*-infected PMNs display phosphatidylserine (PS) on the cell surface, they do not show chromatin condensation or signs of necrosis or oncosis (12). Nevertheless, the exposure of PS on the *B. abortus*-infected PMNs resembles that of apoptotic PMNs. As demonstrated (14), non-infected apoptotic PMNs presenting PS on the surface are removed by macrophages (Mϕs) in a non-phlogistic manner (14). Indeed, the removal of apoptotic PMNs is first established by the release of "find me" signals required for recruitment of mononuclear phagocytes. Then, the recognition of PS on the surface of the apoptotic PMNs constitutes an "eat me" signal, which in course induces the regulated suppression of Mϕs activating mechanisms (14, 15).

We have proposed that the premature PMN cell death induced by *Brucella* organisms may promote the selective non-phlogistic removal of these infected cells by the mononuclear phagocytic system (12, 13). In course, *Brucella* infected PMNs may serve as "Trojan horse" vehicles for efficient bacterial dispersion, intracellular replication and establishing chronic infections, as suggested for other pathogens (16). Here we demonstrate that *Brucella*-infected PMNs are readily phagocyted by murine Mϕs in a non-phlogistic manner, and that bacteria delivered through PMNs, extensively replicate inside Mϕs. The experiments shown here, are a proof of concept for the "Trojan horse" proposal, which states that *Brucella*-infected PMNs serve as vehicles for Mϕ infection and subsequent dispersion throughout the organism.

MATERIALS AND METHODS

Bacteria and Mouse Strains

B. abortus 2308 expressing constitutive red fluorescent protein from *Discosoma coral* (*B. abortus*-RFP), provided by Jean-Jacques Letesson (Unité de Recherche en Biologie Moléculaire, Facultés Universitaires Notre-Dame de la Paix, Namur, Belgium), was used in all experiments. Female BALB/c mice (18–21 g) were supplied by the Escuela de Medicina Veterinaria, Universidad Nacional, Costa Rica, and Instituto Clodomiro Picado, Universidad de Costa Rica, Costa Rica.

Ethics

Bone marrow (BM) was obtained from mice following the consent and guidelines established by the "Comité Institucional para el Cuido y Uso de los Animales de la Universidad de Costa Rica" (CICUA- 47-12) and in accordance with the corresponding law, Ley de Bienestar de los Animales, of Costa Rica (law 9458 on animal welfare). All animals were kept in cages with food and water *ad libitum* under biosafety containment conditions.

Infection Protocols

PMNs were obtained from BM and infected *ex vivo* in the presence of anti-*Brucella* antibodies, following previous protocols (13, 17). Briefly, BM cells were isolated from tibia and femur of mice by flushing bones with HBSS (no calcium, no magnesium) or RPMI medium. Then, BM cells were infected with *B. abortus*-RFP (MOI 50) at 37°C for 1.5 h, washed with PBS, suspended in HBSS, and examined by fluorescent microscopy. The composition and proportion of the infected BM cells have been determined in previous work (17). Under the fluorescent microscope, the estimation of infected murine PMNs is a straightforward process due to the unique donut shape of their nuclei. The proportion of infected and non-infected cells were counted by following a meaningful statistical sampling method (18). *B. abortus* PMN infections were confirmed by flow cytometry using *B. abortus*-RFP and PE anti-Ly6G (RB6-8C5) from eBioscience as previously described (17).

Peritoneal Mϕs were harvested and cultured as previously described (19). *B. abortus*-RFP infection (MOI 50) of 2×10^5 RAW 264.7 or peritoneal Mϕ monolayers was performed by using the gentamicin protection assay to avoid extracellular bacteria (20). Additionally, RAW 264.7 or peritoneal Mϕs were infected by co-cultivating with *B. abortus*-infected PMNs as follows. *B. abortus*-infected PMN were washed with PBS to remove extracellular bacteria. Then, *B. abortus*-infected PMNs were suspended in DMEM without gentamicin and added to the Mϕ monolayers at a rate of 1:1 and incubated for one hour at 37°C. After this period, gentamicin was added. Then, cells were cultivated for up to 48 h and CFU counts determined at 3, 7, 24-, and 48-h post-infection. Alternatively, *B. abortus*-infected PMN were pre-treated with 5 μg/cell of Annexin V (Invitrogen) for 15 min (15) before co-cultivation with RAW 264.7 cells. The CFU counts within *B. abortus*-infected PMN added to RAW 264.7 and peritoneal Mϕs monolayers were calculated retroactively by lysing the PMNs and counting bacteria in agar plates. Controls of co-cultivated non-infected PMN with Mϕ monolayers (at rate 1:1) were run in parallel.

Immunofluorescence

The percentage of cell association (direct cell-cell contact) between *B. abortus*-infected PMN and non-infected PMNs with Mϕs was estimated by fluorescent microscopy at different time points. Infected and non-infected PMNs were fixed with 3.5% paraformaldehyde, centrifuged in a Cytospin 2 (Shandon), mounted with ProLong Gold Antifade reagent with DAPI (Thermo Fisher Scientific), and observed under the fluorescence microscope (Nikon ECLIPSE 80i). Mϕ monolayers co-infected with *B. abortus*-infected PMN were stained with DAPI and FITC-phalloidin (Sigma), fixed and mounted with MOWIOL for analysis as described (12). Controls of non-infected PMNs were used along with the corresponding assays. At least 200 PMNs were counted per slide. Cells were photographed under the fluorescence microscope (Nikon ECLIPSE 80i) using the appropriate color filter channel. Images were cut from microscope field, contrasted and saturated using Hue tool to obtain suitable color separation. Images were merged using Adobe Photoshop 8 software. Internalization of *B. abortus*-infected PMN and non-infected PMNs was documented by live-imaging using Cytation 5 Cell Imaging reader.

Cytokine Determination

For the quantitative determination of TNF-α and IL-10, the supernatants of the infected Mϕs monolayers were collected at different time points and the concentration of cytokines measured by ELISA according to the manufacturer's specifications (Invitrogen).

PMNs Cell Death Determination

For cell death analysis, PMNs were stained with Alexa Flour 488 Annexin V (Invitrogen) and PE anti-Ly6G (RB6-8C5) and APC Cy7 anti-CD16/32 antibodies (from eBioscience and BD Bioscience respectively). *B. abortus*-infected PMN cells were analyzed by flow cytometry using a Guava easyCyte (Millipore) and data analyzed using the FlowJo software, version 10.0.7 (Tree Star, Inc.) (13, 21). Evaluation of PMNs cell death assay was carried out as described before (13). Briefly, aliquots of BM were mixed with *B. abortus*-RFP (MOI 50), supplemented with anti-*Brucella* murine serum for opsonization, and incubated under mild agitation at 37°C for up to 4 h. Cells were then suspended in Annexin-binding buffer (Invitrogen) and Annexin V added and incubated for 30 min on ice in the dark. Cells were washed with ice-cold PBS, fixed with 3.2% paraformaldehyde and subjected to flow cytometry analysis.

Statistics

The Wilcoxon signed-rank test was used to compare the proportion of association between non-infected PMNs and *Brucella*-infected PMNs to Mϕs. Analysis of covariance (ANCOVA) was used to determine the effects of time and treatments on statistical the Log_{10} CFU. Two-way analysis of variance (ANOVA) was used to measure the effect of time and treatments on the percentage of Mϕ infection. Shapiro-Wilks test was applied to assess the normal distribution of data obtained in each experiment, and the Kolmogorov-Smirnov test was applied to data that did not adjust to normality. JMP (https://www.jmp.com) and GraphPad Prism software (https://www.graphpad.com) was used for statistical analysis. Data were processed in Microsoft Office Excel 2016 and GraphPad Prism software. For a meaningful counting number of infected cells, a probability index was followed, according to the total number of PMNs and infected PMNs (18).

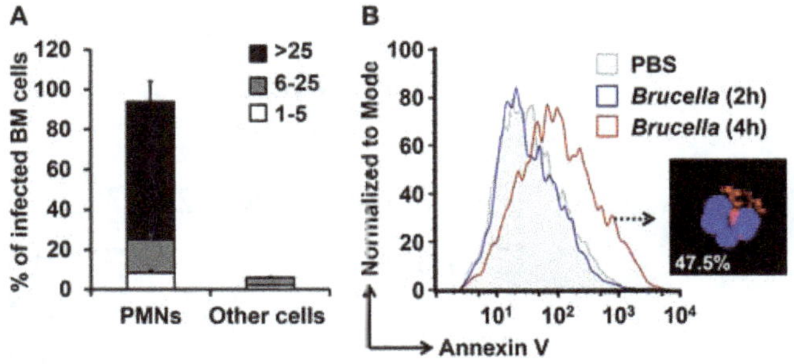

FIGURE 1 | *B. abortus* infect PMNs and promote the exposure of phosphatidylserine. BM cells were incubated with *B. abortus*-RFP (MOI 50) for 4 h. **(A)** Cells were mounted using Frolong Gold containing DAPI (blue nuclei). At least 200 PMNs were counted per sample. The percentage of infection and the number of intracellular bacteria (1–5, 6–25, or >25) per cell was determined by fluorescence microscopy. Cell infections were confirmed by flow cytometry. **(B)** The PMN population analyzed by flow cytometry was gated using anti-Ly6G as PMNs cell marker and analyzed by Annexin V as a cell death marker. These experiments were repeated at least three times.

RESULTS

The limited volume of mouse blood and the low number of PMNs in this fluid, preclude the isolation of a sizeable number of these leukocytes for functional studies. In addition, the extensive manipulation during purification procedures accelerates the cell death of PMNs. In contrast, the number of PMNs in the BM is rather high, comprising between 40 and 50% of all nucleated cells (22). In agreement with previous results (17), close to 94% of the *ex vivo B. abortus* BM-infected cells corresponded to PMNs (**Figure 1A**). We have previously shown that the remaining infected cells are monocytes or progenitor stem cells (17). The distinction between mononuclear infected cells and infected PMNs is straightforward due to the donut shape of the nuclei of the latter cells. Following this, we then tested if *B. abortus* were capable to induce the premature cell death of BM PMNs, as shown before for blood PMNs (13), up to 47.5% of the *B. abortus*-infected PMN were positive for Annexin V at 4 h post-infection (**Figure 1B**).

Then, we explored the association of *Brucella*-PMNs to Mϕs by co-cultivating these two cells *in vitro*. As compared to the non-infected PMN controls, a higher proportion of *Brucella*-infected-PMNs associated with RAW and peritoneal Mϕs was detected (**Figure 2A**). Thereafter, the association between *Brucella*-infected-PMNs and Mϕs, led to the infection of the latter (**Figure 2B**). This phenomenon was completed before 7 h and was specific since non-infected PMNs were not phagocytized by Mϕs (**Figure 3**). However, a strict kinetic analysis was precluded, since Mϕ phagocytosis and the concomitant digestion of PMNs was very fast an uneven event over time.

Then, we tested the rate of bacterial replication after internalization of Mϕs by *Brucella*-infected-PMNs at 1 and 48 h post-infection. As shown in **Figure 4A**, *B. abortus* organisms infected Mϕs at higher rates through phagocytosis of *Brucella*-infected PMNs than when infected with bacteria alone. Moreover, the higher efficiency of Mϕ bacterial infection mediated by *Brucella*-infected-PMNs was evident by the different MOIs delivered in each case. Indeed, in the case of *Brucella*-infected PMNs the number of delivered bacteria corresponded to an MOI of 5; that is, ten times lower than the MOI of 50 used to infect Mϕs with bacteria alone. The efficient internalization process promoted higher kinetics of *B. abortus* replication in Mϕs incubated with *Brucella*-infected-PMNs (**Figure 4B**). In spite of this, the kinetics between RAW and peritoneal Mϕs were different. For instance, RAW Mϕs infected with *B. abortus* alone displayed an initial decline in CFUs at early times of infection, a phenomenon that has been reported before (23). However, after infection of these cells with *Brucella*-infected-PMNs, the initial decline was unnoticeable in these Mϕs; instead, a steady increase in the number of CFUs was observed. In contrast, the kinetic profiles were similar in both, the *Brucella*-PMN infected peritoneal Mϕs and in the controls; though, the number of CFU was always higher in the former infected cells.

The different bacterial replication kinetic observed between the RAW and the peritoneal Mϕs, seemed related to the distinct profiles of cytokines produced during the infection process (**Figure 5**). Except for the regulatory IL-10, which was already

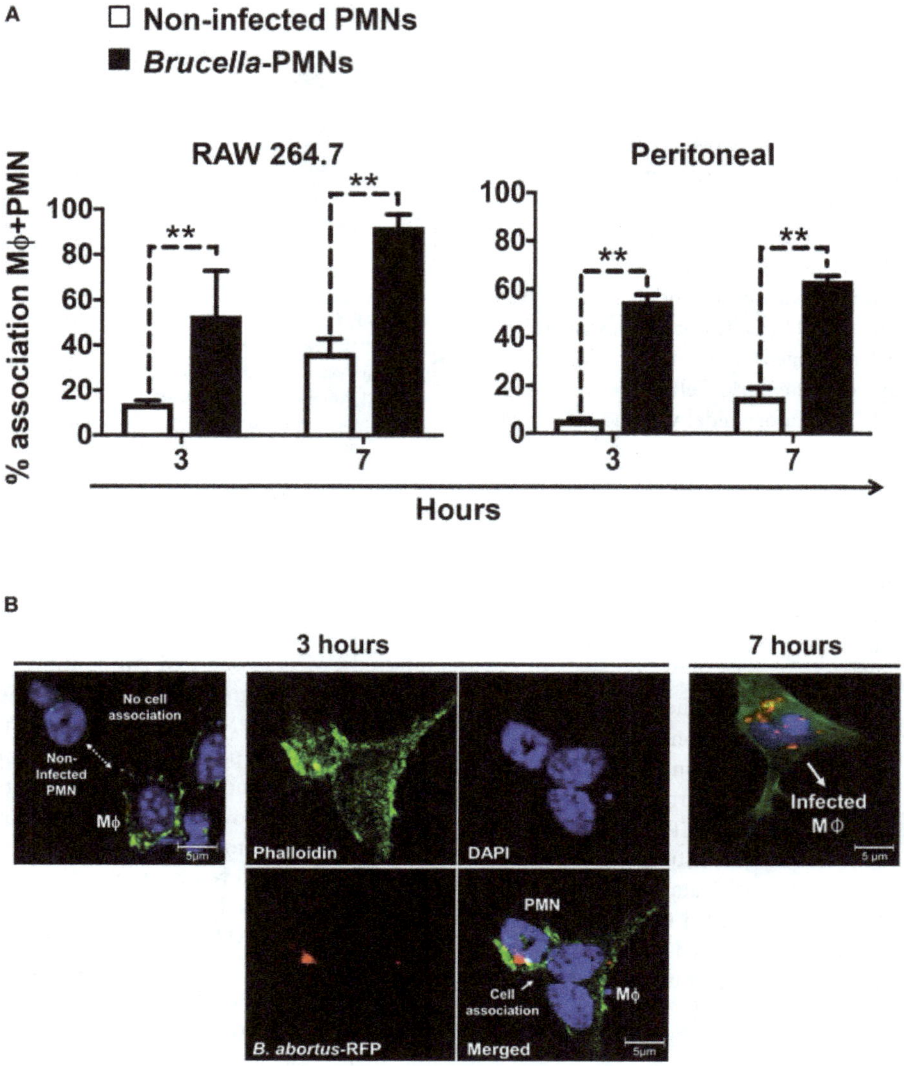

FIGURE 2 | *B. abortus*-infection increase the association of PMN with Mϕs. **(A)** Non-infected or *B. abortus*-RFP-infected PMN were incubated with RAW or peritoneal Mϕs (1:1) at different time points and PMN-Mϕ interactions were quantified. Cells were stained (DAPI, for nuclei; phalloidin-FITC for actin filaments), fixed and mounted with MOWIOL. At least 200 PMNs were counted and the percentage of PMN-Mϕ cell association determined. Values of $p < 0.01$ (**) are indicated in relation to Mϕs incubated with non-infected PMNs. **(B)** RAW Mϕ in the process of association and ingestion *B. abortus*-infected PMN. Infected PMNs are distinguished from other cells by the "donut" shape of their nuclei. Images were photographed under the microscope using the appropriate color filter channel. These experiments were repeated at least three times.

high (>100 μg), the quantities of the TNF-α were under background levels, at early times of the *Brucella*-PMN infected RAW cells. It is worth noting that RAW Mϕs are TNF-α hyperproducers (24). Therefore, it was expected that at later times, once bacteria reached high numbers, the TNF-α increased to very high levels in the *Brucella*-PMNs infected RAW cells, as compared to the controls. Still, the higher amounts of TNF-α at later times of the RAW infected cells did not hamper bacterial replication. Likewise, at early times of *Brucella*-PMN infection of peritoneal Mϕs, the production of TNF-α was low with significant high amounts of the regulatory cytokine IL-10. These differences in cytokine profiles may explain the differences observed between *Brucella*-PMN-infected RAW and peritoneal Mϕs in the replication kinetics. In any case, in both experiments, *Brucella*-PMN-infected Mϕs reached much higher CFU values than the controls infected with bare bacteria alone.

In agreement with our previous reports (13, 21) *Brucella*-infected-PMNs displayed PS on the cell surface (**Figure 1B**). Since this phospholipid is commonly recognized as an "eat me" signal (14), we decided to explore the role of PS in the uptake of *Brucella*-infected PMNs by Mϕs. For this, we used Annexin V to hinder the PS exposed on the *Brucella*-PMN surface. After treatment with Annexin V, the proportion of *Brucella*-PMNs associated with Mϕs significantly diminished (**Figure 6A**). Moreover, bacterial replication was reduced in RAW Mϕs at all-time points (**Figure 6B**), displaying the profile

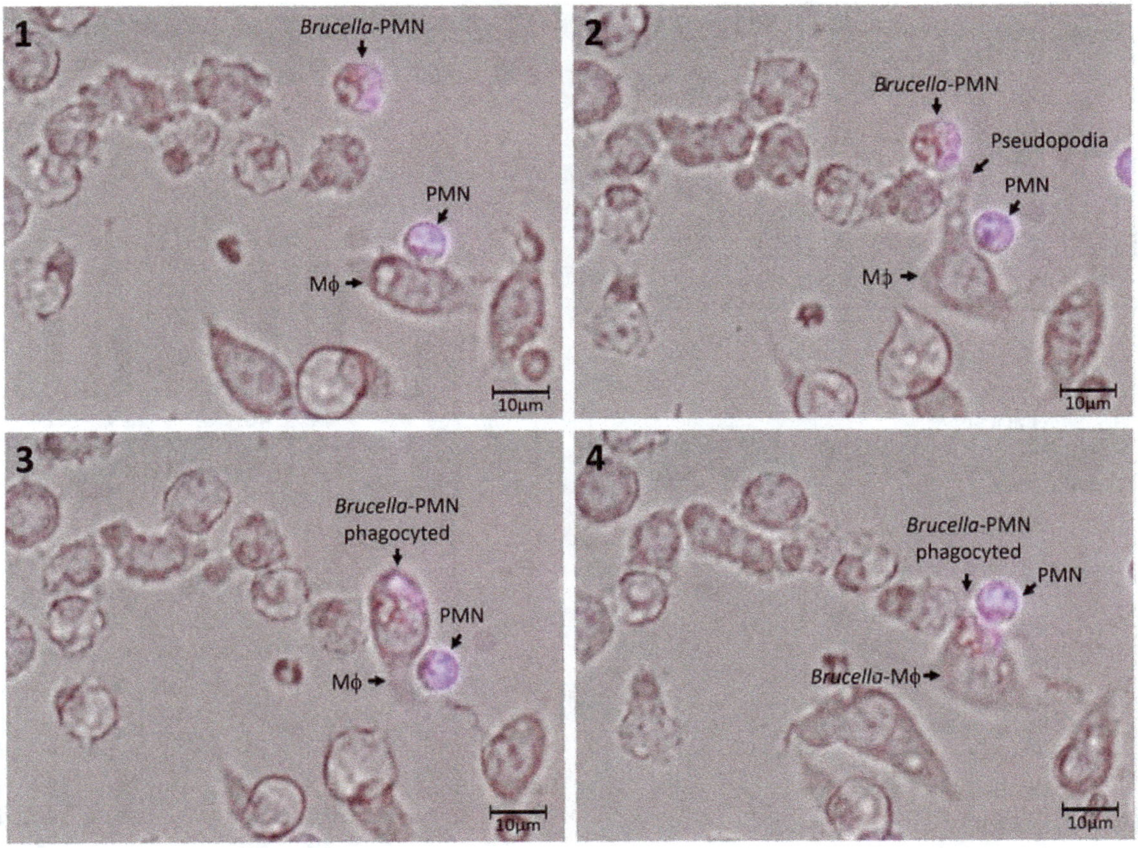

FIGURE 3 | Association and uptake of *B. abortus*-infected PMN by Mϕs. PMNs were incubated with *B. abortus*-RFP (red) (MOI of 50) for 1.5 h; then, cells were pelleted and washed with PBS to remove extracellular bacteria. *Brucella*-infected-PMNs were suspended in DMEM without gentamicin and added to RAW Mϕs monolayers (5×10^3) at a rate of 1:1 and incubated for 10 min at 37°C. After this period, the infected Mϕ monolayers were washed and suspended in DMEM and incubated for up to 5 h. Infected PMNs were stained with Hoescht (blue). Cells were photographed and analyzed under Cytation 3 Cell Imaging Multi-Mode Reader (BioTek) using the appropriate color filter channel. Numbers 1 to 4 correspond to the order in the which images were capture very every 20 min. These experiments were repeated at least three times.

observed after infection with bacteria alone (compare profile with **Figure 4A**). Likewise, the proportion of infected Mϕs was significantly reduced in the *Brucella*-PMNs treated with Annexin V (**Figure 6C**). Thus, PS on the *Brucella*-infected-PMNs surface acted as an "eat me" signal for Mϕs.

DISCUSSION

There are various intracellular pathogens, such as *Chlamydia pneumoniae* and *Leishmania major*, capable to survive within PMNs, kill these cells and use them as vehicles for infecting and colonizing Mϕs (25). This strategy, generally known as the "Trojan horse," serves as a mechanism for microbial dispersion within the host (15). It seems, therefore, that *B. abortus* also follows a Trojan horse strategy by using infected PMNs as vehicles for the dispersion throughout the host mononuclear phagocytic system. A similar strategy to traverse microvascular endothelial cells of the central nervous system via *B. abortus*-infected-monocytes has been proposed (26).

Infecting naïve Mϕs monolayers (such as bone marrow) with bare *Brucella* grown in a bacteriological medium is highly inefficient (23). Infection protocols in cultured Mϕs require high bacterial MOIs (>50) to obtain low numbers (<5 bacteria/cell) of intracellular bacteria. Moreover, a large proportion of these invading bacteria are killed by Mϕs after a few hours (23). Following this, we propose that the common physiological infection of the phagocytic mononuclear system primarily occurs via *Brucella*-infected-PMNs.

There are at least two other pieces of evidence that support this proposal. First, it has been demonstrated that mice depleted of PMNs, eliminate *B. abortus* more readily than their "normal" infected counterparts (21). This is commensurate with the fact that Mϕs kill bare "unprotected" *Brucella* cells more readily than those hidden within PMNs, as shown here. Second, the early internalization of *Brucella*-infected PMNs by Mϕs, seems to occur in a non-phlogistic manner, displaying significant amounts of regulatory IL-10 and low quantities of proinflammatory cytokines, such as TNF-α at early stages of the infection. It is known, that the uptake of apoptotic PMNs by Mϕs,

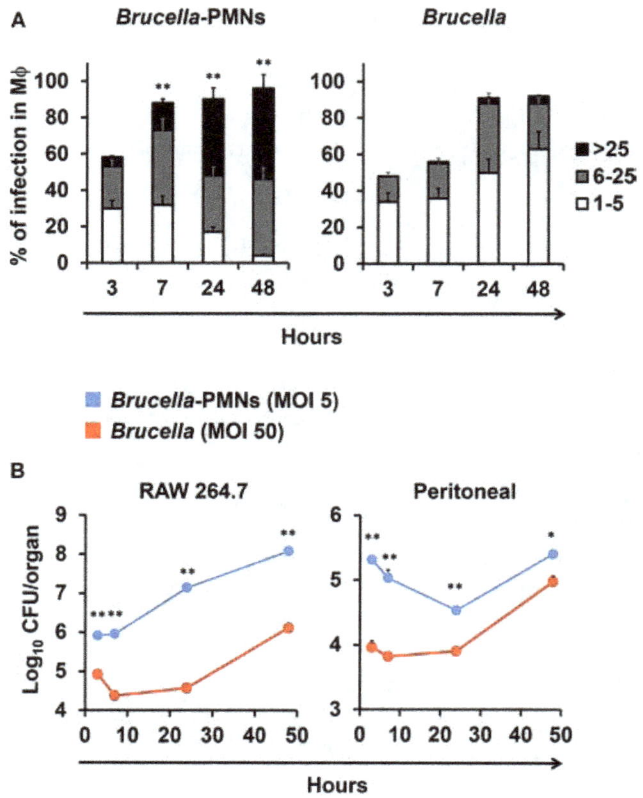

FIGURE 4 | *B. abortus*-infected PMN promote *Brucella* infection of Mϕs. **(A)** RAW Mϕs were incubated with *B. abortus*-RFP alone or with *B. abortus*-infected PMN, then cells were stained (DAPI, for nuclei; phalloidin-FITC for actin filaments), fixed and mounted with MOWIOL, and the number intracellular bacteria (1–5, 6–25, or >25) per Mϕ was determined. The proportion of infection and the number of intracellular bacteria was determined by fluorescence microscopy. At least 200 cells were counted per sample. Values of $p < 0.05$ (*) and $p < 0.01$ (**) are indicated in relation to Mϕs incubated with non-infected PMNs. **(B)** RAW and peritoneal Mϕs were infected with *B. abortus*-RFP alone (MOI 50) or with *B. abortus*-RFP infected PMNs (MOI 5) and CFU determined at different time points. These experiments were repeated at least three times.

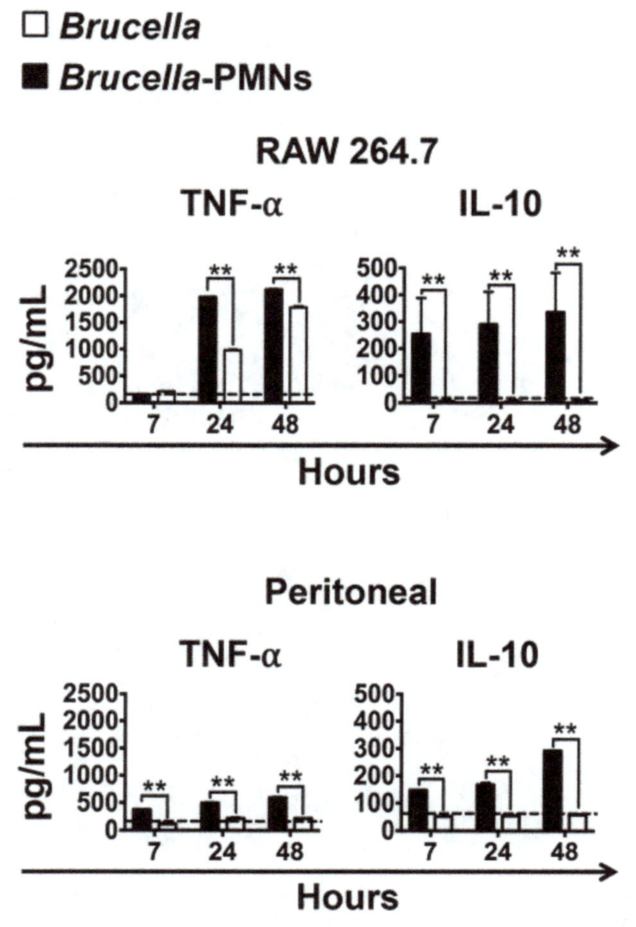

FIGURE 5 | High production of IL-10 and low production of TNF-α in the supernatant of infected Mϕs at initial stages of infection. RAW and peritoneal Mϕs were infected with *B. abortus*-RFP (MOI 50) alone or with *B. abortus*-infected PMNs (MOI 5), and the supernatants collected at different time points. The level of the cytokines was determined by ELISA in the culture supernatants of infected Mϕs. Values of $p < 0.01$ (**) are indicated in relation to Mϕs infected with *Brucella* alone. The backgrounds of the cytokine production by Mϕs co-cultivated with non-infected PMNs are indicated by dashed lines. These experiments were repeated at least three times.

increases the secretion of anti-inflammatory IL-10 cytokine (27). This is relevant since the first 8 h after cell invasion are crucial for pathogenic *Brucella* to redirect its trafficking to its replicating niche within non-activated cells (23). Indeed, previously activated Mϕs display high brucellicidal activity. However, if Mϕs become activated (e.g., through TNF-α or lipopolysaccharide) after 8–24 h of infection, the intracellular bacteria are still capable to replicate extensively (11). The obvious explanation is that at this infection stage, *Brucella* are hidden within vacuoles of the early phagocytic compartment and then protected from Mϕs microbicidal mechanisms. It is worth noting that the overall activation of the immune system in neutropenic *Brucella* infected mice is considerably higher than in the "normal" infected counterparts indicating that PMNs dampen the adaptive immunity in brucellosis (21, 28).

During the early stages of physiological cell death, PS translocates from the cytoplasmic to the extracellular side of the cell membrane (29). The correct redistribution of PS on the outer surface of the plasmatic membrane is a key element for the recognition of dying cells and corresponds a to molecular "eat me" signal that indicates that these dying cells should be engulfed (30). But PS is also a "forget me" signal for the regulated suppression of Mϕs activating mechanisms (14, 15, 31). Within this context, it seems that ingestion of *Brucella*-infected PMNs by Mϕs follows a similar mechanism used to phagocytize apoptotic PMNs. In any case, it is becoming clearer that through evolution *Brucella* organisms are stealth pathogens that have evolved to hamper the activation of the first stages of innate immunity and to establish chronic infections.

In conclusion, the ability of *Brucella* to circumvent the immune response and to replicate within Mϕs are key elements for the pathogen survival and for the establishing long-lasting infections. Here, we showed that *Brucella*-infected PMNs

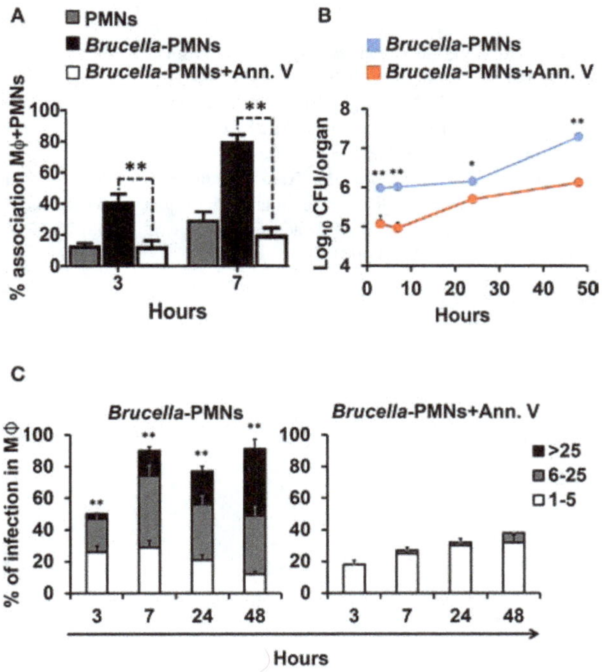

FIGURE 6 | Blockage of PS on the surface of *Brucella*-infected PMNs hampers Mϕ *B. abortus* infection. **(A)** *B. abortus* infected PMNs were pre-treated or not with Annexin V before co-incubation with RAW Mϕs, and cell association estimated. The red dashed line corresponds to the mean value of non-infected PMNs **(B)** *B. abortus* infected PMNs (MOI 5) were pre-treated or not with Annexin V before co-incubation with RAW Mϕs and CFU determined at different time points. **(C)** *B. abortus* infected PMNs were pre-treated or not with Annexin V before co-incubation with RAW Mϕs and the number of infected Mϕs and intracellular bacteria within these cells estimated at different time points. Cells were stained (DAPI for nuclei; phalloidin-FITC for actin filaments), fixed and mounted with MOWIOL. At least 200 cells were counted in each experiment. The percentage of infection and the number of intracellular bacteria (1–5, 6–25, or >25) per Mϕ was determined by fluorescence microscopy. Values of $p < 0.05$ (*) and $p < 0.01$ (**) are indicated in relation to Mϕs incubated with PMNs treated with Annexin V. These experiments were repeated at least three times.

promoted the internalization and replication of *Brucella* within Mϕs using a "Trojan horse" strategy. To reinforce or reject our hypothesis *in vivo* experiments would be necessary.

In this work our main findings are: (i) *Brucella abortus* infected up to 96% of BM-PMNs, inducing a premature death of these cells; (ii) the *Brucella*-infected PMNs displayed PS as "eat me" signal, promoting the association with Mϕs and favoring the bacterial replication within these mononuclear phagocytes; (iii) This phenomenon was specific, since non-infected PMNs were not phagocytized by Mϕs and blockage of PS with Annexin V diminished the Mϕs association and phagocytosis of *Brucella*-infected PMNs; (iv) the low production of proinflammatory cytokines and the high production of the anti-inflammatory IL-10 at the initial stages of infection, correlated with the non-phlogistic Mϕ *Brucella*-PMN uptake and subsequent bacterial replication.

AUTHOR CONTRIBUTIONS

EB-C, EM, and CG-J designed the experiments. CG-J, RM-C, and PA-S performed the experiments. CG-J, RM-C, PA-S, EB-C, EC-O, and EM analyzed the data. CC-D, EC-O, EB-C, and EM contributed reagents, materials, analysis tools. EB-C, EM, and CG-J wrote the paper. All authors revised and approved the manuscript.

FUNDING

This project was supported by the International Centre for Genomic Engineering and Biotechnology (CRP/16/005), Fondo Institucional de Desarrollo Académico de la UNA, FIDA (0087-17), Espacio Universitario de Estudios Avanzados, UCREA (B8762) from the presidency of University of Costa Rica. CG-J and RM-C received a fellowship from Ministerio de Ciencia, Tecnología y Telecomunicaciones, MICITT (PNM-001-2015-1 and PND-014-2015-1 respectively).

ACKNOWLEDGMENTS

We would like to thank Gerardo Ávalos Rodríguez and Ricardo Alvarado for their professional support and discussions of statistical data and Marlen Cordero for her technical assistance in the culture of macrophages.

REFERENCES

1. Colotta F, Re F, Polentarutti N, Sozzani S, Mantovani A. Modulation of granulocyte survival and programmed cell death by cytokines and bacterial products. *Blood.* (1992) 80:2012–20.
2. Kamenyeva O, Boularan C, Kabat J, Cheung GYC, Cicala C, Yeh AJ, et al. Neutrophil recruitment to lymph nodes limits local humoral response to *Staphylococcus aureus*. *PLoS Pathogens.* (2015) 11:e1004827. doi: 10.1371/journal.ppat.1004827
3. Kolaczkowska E, Kubes P. Neutrophil recruitment and function in health and inflammation. *Nat Rev Immunol.* (2013) 13:159–75. doi: 10.1038/nri3399
4. Mantovani A, Cassatella MA, Costantini C, Jaillon S. Neutrophils in the activation and regulation of innate and adaptive immunity. *Nat Rev Immunol.* (2011) 11:519–31. doi: 10.1038/nri3024
5. Gabrilovich D. *The Neutrophils*. London: Imperial College Press (2013).
6. Nathan C. Neutrophils and immunity: challenges and opportunities. *Nat Rev Immunol.* (2006) 6:173–82. doi: 10.1038/nri1785
7. Moreno E, Moriyón I. *The Prokaryotes*. New York, NY: Springer-Verlag (2006).
8. Braude AI. Studies in the pathology and pathogenesis of experimental brucellosis. II. The formation of the hepatic granuloma and its evolution. *J Infect Dis.* (1951) 89:87–94. doi: 10.1093/infdis/89.1.87

9. Ackermann MR, Cheville NF, Deyoe BL. Bovine ileal dome lymphoepithelial cells: endocytosis and transport of *Brucella abortus* strain 19. *Vet Pathol.* (1988) 25:28–35. doi: 10.1177/030098588802500104
10. Kreutzer DL, Dreyfus LA, Robertson DC. Interaction of polymorphonuclear leukocytes with smooth and rough strains of *Brucella abortus. Infect Immunity.* (1979) 23:737–42.
11. Barquero-Calvo E, Chaves-Olarte E, Weiss DS, Guzmán-Verri C, Chacón-Díaz C, Rucavado A, et al. *Brucella abortus* uses a stealthy strategy to avoid activation of the innate immune system during the onset of infection. *PLoS ONE.* (2007) 2:e631. doi: 10.1371/journal.pone.0000631
12. Barquero-Calvo E, Mora-Cartín R, Arce-Gorvel V, de Diego JL, Chacón-Díaz C, Chaves-Olarte E, et al. *Brucella abortus* induces the premature death of human neutrophils through the action of its lipopolysaccharide. *PLoS Pathogens.* (2015) 11:e1004853. doi: 10.1371/journal.ppat.1004853
13. Mora-Cartín R, Chacón-Díaz C, Gutiérrez-Jiménez C, Gurdián-Murillo S, Lomonte B, Chaves-Olarte E, et al. N-formyl-perosamine surface homopolysaccharides hinder the recognition of *Brucella abortus* by mouse neutrophils. *Infect Immunity.* (2016) 84:1712–21. doi: 10.1128/IAI.00137-16
14. Lauber K, Blumenthal SG, Waibel M, Wesselborg S. Clearance of apoptotic cells: getting rid of the corpses. *Mol Cell.* (2004) 14:277–87. doi: 10.1016/S1097-2765(04)00237-0
15. Rupp J, Pfleiderer L, Jugert C, Moeller S, Klinger M, Dalhoff K, et al. *Chlamydia pneumoniae* hides inside apoptotic neutrophils to silently infect and propagate in macrophages. *PLoS ONE.* (2009) 4:e6020. doi: 10.1371/journal.pone.0006020
16. Stark MA, Huo Y, Burcin TL, Morris MA, Olson TS, Ley K. Phagocytosis of apoptotic neutrophils regulates granulopoiesis via IL-23 and IL-17. *Immunity.* (2005) 22:285–94. doi: 10.1016/j.immuni.2005.01.011
17. Gutiérrez-Jiménez C, Hysenaj L, Alfaro-Alarcón A, Mora-Cartín R, Arce-Gorvel V, Moreno E, et al. Persistence of *Brucella abortus* in the bone marrow of infected mice. *J Immunol Res.* 2018:5370414. doi: 10.1155/2018/5370414
18. Viertl R. *Probability and Bayesian Statistics,* 1st edition. New York, NY: Springer US. (1987). doi: 10.1007/978-1-4613-1885-9
19. Lu M, Varley A. Harvest and culture of mouse peritoneal macrophages. *Bio-Protocol.* (2013) 3:e976. doi: 10.21769/BioProtoc.976
20. Chaves-Olarte E, Guzmán-Verri C, Méresse S, Desjardins M, Pizarro-Cerdá J, Badilla J, et al. Activation of Rho and Rab GTPases dissociates *Brucella abortus* internalization from intracellular trafficking. *Cell Microbiol.* (2002) 4:663–76. doi: 10.1046/j.1462-5822.2002.00221.x
21. Barquero-Calvo E, Martirosyan A, Ordoñez-Rueda D, Arce-Gorvel V, Alfaro-Alarcón A, Lepidi H, et al. Neutrophils exert a suppressive effect on Th1 responses to intracellular pathogen *Brucella abortus. PLoS Pathogens.* (2013) 9:e1003167. doi: 10.1371/journal.ppat.1003167
22. Chervenick PA, Boggs DR, Marsh JC, Cartwright GE, Wintrobe MM. Quantitative studies of blood and bone marrow neutrophils in normal mice. *Am Physiol Soc.* (1968) 215:353–60. doi: 10.1152/ajplegacy.1968.215.2.353
23. Celli J, de Chastellier CD, Franchini M, Pizarro-Cerda J, Moreno E, Gorvel J-P. *Brucella* evades macrophage killing via VirB-dependent sustained interactions with the endoplasmic reticulum. *J Exp Med.* (2003) 198:545–56. doi: 10.1084/jem.20030088
24. Rimbach G, Park YC, Guo Q, Moini H, Qureshi N, Saliou C, et al. Nitric oxide synthesis and TNF-alpha secretion in RAW 264.7 macrophages: mode of action of a fermented papaya preparation. *Life Sci.* (2000) 67:679–94. doi: 10.1016/S0024-3205(00)00664-0
25. Laskay T, van Zandbergen G, Solbach W. Neutrophil granulocytes as host cells and transport vehicles for intracellular pathogens: apoptosis as infection-promoting factor. *Immunobiology.* (2008) 213:183–91. doi: 10.1016/j.imbio.2007.11.010
26. Miraglia MC, Rodriguez AM, Barrionuevo P, Rodriguez J, Kim KS, Dennis VA, et al. *Brucella abortus* traverses brain microvascular endothelial cells using infected monocytes as a trojan horse. *Front Cell Infect Microbiol.* (2018) 8:200. doi: 10.3389/fcimb.2018.00200
27. Voll RE, Herrmann M, Roth EA, Stach C, Kalden JR, Girkontaite I. Immunosuppressive effects of apoptotic cells. *Nature.* (1997) 390:350–51. doi: 10.1038/37022
28. Mora-Cartín R, Gutiérrez-Jiménez C, Alfaro-Alarcón A, Chaves-Olarte E, Chacón-Díaz C, Barquero-Calvo E, et al. Neutrophils dampen adaptive immunity in brucellosis. *Infect Immun.* (2019) 87:118–19. doi: 10.1128/IAI.00118-19
29. Vermes I, Haanen C, Steffens-Nakken H, Reutelingsperger C. A novel assay for apoptosis. *Flow cytometric detection of phosphatidylserine expression on early apoptotic cells using fluorescein labelled annexin V. J Immunol Methods.* (1995) 184:39–51. doi: 10.1016/0022-1759(95)00072-I
30. Wu Y, Tibrewal N, Birge RB. Phosphatidylserine recognition by phagocytes: a view to a kill. *Trends Cell Biol.* (2006) 16:189–97. doi: 10.1016/j.tcb.2006.02.003
31. Lauber K, Bohn E, Kröber SM, Xiao Y-J, Blumenthal SG, Lindemann RK, et al. Apoptotic cells induce migration of phagocytes via caspase-3-mediated release of a lipid attraction signal. *Cell.* (2003) 113:717–30. doi: 10.1016/S0092-8674(03)00422-7

16

The Dual Role of the Antibody Response Against the Flavivirus Non-structural Protein 1 (NS1) in Protection and Immuno-Pathogenesis

Arturo Reyes-Sandoval[1] and Juan E. Ludert[2]**

[1] Nuffield Department of Medicine, Jenner Institute, University of Oxford, Oxford, United Kingdom, [2] Department of Infectomics and Molecular Pathogenesis, Center for Research and Advanced Studies (CINVESTAV), Mexico City, Mexico

***Correspondence:**
Arturo Reyes-Sandoval
arturo.reyes@ndm.ox.ac.uk
Juan E. Ludert
jludert@cinvestav.mx

Dengue and Zika viruses are closely related mosquito-borne flaviviruses responsible for major public health problems in tropical and sub-tropical countries. The genomes of both, dengue and zika viruses encodes 10 genes that are translated into three structural proteins (C, prM, and E) and seven non-structural proteins (NS1, NS2A, NS2B, NS3, NS4A, NS4B, and NS5). The non-structural protein 1 (NS1) is a highly conserved glycoprotein of approximately 48–50 KDa. In infected cells, NS1 is found as a homodimer associated with intracellular membranes and replication complexes, serving as a scaffolding protein in virus replication and morphogenesis. NS1 is secreted efficiently from infected cells as a hexamer and is found in patient's sera during the acute phase of the disease. NS1 detection in sera is a valuable diagnostic marker and immunization with NS1 has been shown to protect animal models from lethal challenges with dengue and Zika viruses. Nevertheless, soluble NS1 has been associated with severe dengue and anti-NS1 antibodies have been reported to cross-react with host platelets and endothelial cells and thus presumably contribute to pathogenesis. Due to the implications of NS1 in arbovirus pathogenesis and its relevance as vaccine candidate, we discuss the dual role that anti-NS1 antibodies may play in protection and disease and the challenges that need to be overcome to develop safe and effective NS1-based vaccines against dengue and Zika.

Keywords: dengue, Zika, flavivirus, NS1 protein, arbovirus, vaccines against flavivirus, immuno-pathogenesis, molecular mimicry

INTRODUCTION

Dengue is the most important mosquito-borne viral disease in humans. It is endemic in over 100 countries and it is estimated that nearly 2/3 of the world's population lives in risk areas for this disease. The dengue virus (DENV) is classified as part of the genus *Flavivirus* within the family *Flaviviridae* and is transmitted to humans mainly by two mosquito species, *Aedes aegypti* and *Aedes albopictus* (1). Other mosquito-borne flaviviruses causing disease in humans are the Yellow fever virus, the West Nile virus, the Japanese encephalitis virus and the Zika virus.

There are four DENV serotypes circulating around the world and all can cause disease. Whilst most DENV infections are asymptomatic, they can present clinical signs such as high-degree fever, headache, muscle, joint pain, and rash; clinical signs are usually fully resolved within 5–7 days in dengue fever (DF). However, DF can evolve in a fraction of the patients to a life-threatening form of the disease, severe dengue (SD), characterized by bleeding, plasma leakage and organ impairment (2). DENV infection confers life-long protection against the homologous serotype. However, a secondary infection with a heterologous serotype is a risk factor for the development of severe dengue (3, 4). The antibody-dependent enhancement (ADE) has been pointed as a major mechanism underlying the increased risk of severe dengue during secondary infections (4). Despite the great burden associated with dengue, so far there is no specific treatment for this disease (5) and, unfortunately, the current licensed tetravalent live-attenuated vaccine has been associated with predisposition to severe dengue when applied to DENV-naive people (6).

The DENV virion is enveloped with ~50 nm in diameter and the genome consists of a single-stranded RNA molecule of positive polarity of approximately 11 Kb (7). The DENV genome encodes for 3 structural proteins (capsid, C; precursor membrane and membrane prM/M; envelope, E) and for 7 non-structural proteins (NS1, NS2A, NS2B, NS3, NS4A, NS4B, NS5), all derived from a polyprotein of around 3,400 amino acids by proteolytic processing (7). Viral replication occurs in the cytoplasm in association with the rough endoplasmic reticulum (RER) and involves both viral NS proteins and cellular proteins, for replication, translation, and encapsidation of the genome (7). Finally, in vertebrate cells, mature virions are secreted to the extracellular media, along with the NS1 protein, following a classical secretory route that involves the Golgi complex and the previous cleavage of the prM protein by the host protease furin (8).

THE MULTIPLE PROPERTIES OF THE FLAVIVIRUS NS1 PROTEIN

The DENV NS1 is a glycoprotein of around 46–50 KDa, that shows high conservation among the 4 DENV serotypes and even among various other arthropod-borne flaviviruses (9–11). Mature monomeric NS1 is released into the lumen of the ER after cleavage from E and NS2A. In the infected cell, NS1 is found mainly associated to intracellular membranes and organelles induced by the virus infection. However, a fraction of NS1 can also be found associated with lipid rafts on the plasma membrane or soluble, secreted into the supernatant (12, 13). Membrane-associated NS1 is dimeric, with well-defined hydrophobic and hydrophilic faces, facing the ER membrane and the ER lumen, respectively (14). Secreted NS1 is an open barrel hexamer associated with lipids (14, 15). Three distinct domains have been identified along the structure of NS1; a β-roll domain comprising the first 29 amino-terminal residues, followed by a "wing" domain, comprising positions 30–180 and finally a β-ladder domain, constituted by the carboxy-terminal residues 181–352. While the wing and β-ladder domain are basically hydrophilic in nature, the β-roll domain is hydrophobic and likely to interact with cell membranes (13). NS1 has been found as an organizational protein of the viral replication complexes essential for viral viability, even though its exact role in DENV the replication is not yet fully understood. It has been suggested that intracellular NS1 is a necessary cofactor for viral RNA replication and virion morphogenesis and may also play a role in the modulation of the innate immune response (13, 14).

NS1 is found at high levels (in the order of μ/ml) in the sera of infected patients early during infection and extensive evidence suggests that NS1 is related to SD pathogenesis (9–11). Fundamental characteristics that distinguish SD from the more benign forms of the disease are hemorrhage, coagulopathy, and a sharp increase in vascular permeability (2). Disease severity have been found to correlate with high levels of circulating NS1 in patient's sera (16–18). To explain the direct participation of NS1 in SD, several mechanisms, such as the capacity of NS1 to form complexes with prothrombin/thrombin, have been proposed (17). More recent evidence indicates that DENV NS1 has the capacity to directly induce glycocalyx degradation as well as destabilization of tight junctions in a tissue-specific manner, suggesting a direct participation of NS1 in the endothelial plasma leakage observed in patients with SD (19, 20). Soluble NS1 has also been shown to activate key cell components of vascular homeostasis such as macrophages, mononuclear peripheral cells and platelets via direct interaction with Toll-Like Receptor 4 (TLR4) (21, 22). The NS1-mediated activation of macrophages and mononuclear cells leads to secretion of pro-inflammatory cytokines, known to alter tight junctions (23), while the activation of platelets leads to increased platelet aggregation, adhesion to endothelial cells and phagocytosis by macrophages. In addition, pre-incubation of hepatocytes with soluble NS1 enhances the replicative capacity of these cells for dengue, suggesting a role for NS1 in the modulation of innate immune responses (13). All these results strongly support the notion that soluble NS1 directly participates in the plasma leakage, thrombocytopenia, and hemorrhages associated with SD.

ANTI-NS1 ANTIBODIES CROSS REACTIVITY WITH HOST MOLECULES

Soluble NS1 elicits strong humoral responses in the host. Anti-NS1 antibodies can either be protective or deleterious to the host, as NS1 antibodies can recognize host factors by molecular mimicry to cause tissue damage and impair physiological functions. The notion that anti-NS1 antibodies do participate in dengue pathogenesis resulted from experiments by Falconar, who showed that anti-NS1 monoclonal antibodies cross-react with human fibrinogen, thrombocytes and endothelial cells and produce hemorrhage in a mouse model (24).

Plasma leakage is one of the key clinical manifestations of severe dengue and a major target for anti-NS1 antibodies are endothelial cells, key players in maintaining vascular homeostasis. In a pioneering article on the subject, Lin et al. (25) reported that sera collected from dengue patients contained antibodies able to induce damage to HUVEC endothelial cells via caspase activation and induction of apoptosis. Pre-treatment with recombinant NS1 reduced the damaging capacity of the sera. The same group later reported that binding of anti-NS1 antibodies to HMEC-1 endothelial cells causes the expression of proinflammatory cytokines such as IL-6, IL-8, and MCP-1 and cell activation as indicated by the expression of adhesion molecules such as ICAM-1 (26). The molecular bases of the cross reactivity of anti-NS1 antibodies with endothelial cells have been partially defined. Using HUVEC cells, Liu et al. (27) found that the human protein LYRIC (lysine rich CEACAM1 co-isolated) is a target recognized by anti-NS1 cross-reactive antibodies in endothelial cells. The binding of cross-reactive anti-NS1 monoclonal antibodies (mAbs) to LYRIC enhanced apoptosis and complement-dependent cell cytotoxicity, indicating that the recognition of LYRIC is indeed associated to endothelial cell damage. Finally, an epitope located in a disordered loop of the wing domain of NS1 (116–119) has been deemed responsible for the cross reactivity between NS1 and LYRIC (**Figure 1A**). Of note, LYRIC plays a role in the activation of various signaling pathways, including the NF-κB; in agreement, the reduction of apoptosis and nitric oxide (NO) production of endothelial cells mediated by anti-NS1 antibody binding can be significantly reduced if cells are treated with inhibitors of the NF-κB pathway (29, 30).

Anti-NS1 cross reactive antibodies may also play a role in the liver damage observed in patients with dengue, as suggested by observations using a murine model. Inoculation of mice with recombinant DENV NS1, but not with JEV NS1, resulted in the production of antibodies capable of recognizing naïve mouse liver endothelial cells and interestingly, not kidney endothelial cells. Moreover, mice inoculated with rNS1 or passively immunized with anti-NS1 IgG, showed altered transaminase (AST and ATL) levels, but not indication of kidney damage (31); yet, there is not obvious explanation for the organ specific damage cause by anti-NS1 antibodies.

Coagulopathy and thrombocytopenia are also features associated with SD. Anti-NS1 antibodies have also been reported to target platelets, thrombin and plasminogen. The protein disulfide isomerase (PDI) on platelets is recognized by antibodies that recognize a peptide of DENV NS1 corresponding to amino acid residues 311–330, located in the C terminal region, in the β-ladder domain (**Figure 1B**). These antibodies are present in the sera of naturally infected patients and upon binding to platelets are capable of inhibiting isomerase activity and promote platelet aggregation (32, 33). In addition, platelets opsonized by anti-NS1 antibodies are more readily phagocytosed by macrophages (34). Finally, anti-NS1 antibodies also recognize components of the coagulation pathways, pointing to a role of these antibodies in the hemorrhagic disorders associated with dengue (35). After immunization of mice with DENV rNS1, several mAbs capable of recognizing human plasminogen could be isolated (35). These mAbs not only bind plasminogen but also induce its activation and conversion to plasmin due to catalytic properties. Again, the cross-reactive epitope on NS1 raising the higher affinity mAbs (305–311) is in the β-ladder, C-terminal region of the protein (**Figure 1C**).

THE NS1 PROTEIN AS A VACCINE CANDIDATE

Traditionally, dengue vaccines have been developed using the envelope (E) and pre-membrane proteins (prM) of dengue virus (DENV) as immunogens. This approach has resulted in the first licensed vaccine with regulatory approval in various countries (36). However, alternative strategies are still pursued due to the risk of vaccine-related ADE induction made evident during follow up studies of the CYD-TDV leading vaccine candidate (37). NS1 has been an attractive candidate for many years due to (a) lack of presence on the virion's surface, resulting in lower risk of inducing antibodies with ADE potential; (b) high degree of conservation amongst DENV serotypes; (c) high levels of NS1 protein secretion of up to 50 μg/ml of plasma, which correlates with severity during DHF/DSS (13, 38) and acts as a viral toxin, thus becoming a potential vaccine target; (d) early evidence that recovered patients have high titers of anti-NS1 antibodies; (e) high levels of immunogenicity and evidence of protection against DENV infection in mice upon NS1 vaccination and the involvement of antibodies and $CD4^{+}$ T cells (39). This is in spite of the controversial role that anti-NS1 antibodies can play, such as the cross reactivity with endothelial cell surface proteins leading to apoptosis (25–27, 29, 30), platelet cross reactivity causing dysfunction and tendency to bleed (32, 33) and reactivity with proteins of the coagulation cascade, such as thrombin (40) (**Figures 1A-D**). Initial observations made by Schlesinger et al. during mid 1980s of the protective efficacy of the glycoprotein gp48 (NS1) against Yellow Fever in mice (41) and macaques (42) led to the seminal work showing that immunization with DENV-2 NS1 protein was able to elicit protection against a homologous DENV infection (43). Recombinant viral vectors in the form of vaccinia virus made an early entry in the NS1 vaccine field, and vaccine efficacy was demonstrated using mouse encephalitis DENV models (44). By 2003, DNA vaccines had become a trend in vaccinology and attempts to induce immunity against DENV without risk of ADE prompted the development of DNA vaccines expressing NS1. Co-administration of DNA-NS1 with IL-12 as genetic adjuvant demonstrated efficacy against a DENV-2 challenge (45). Importantly, it became evident for genetic vaccination that leading sequences are of major importance in targeting the protein to the secretory pathway to enhance antibody responses and improve efficacy of DNA-NS1 vaccines (46, 47), an early lesson for future flavivirus vaccine design using DNA or viral vectors (48). NS1 has eventually been produced in bacteria and used as vaccine in presence of adjuvants. Inclusion of *E. coli* ETEC heat-labile toxin (LT_{G33D}) as adjuvant has been shown to yield better efficacy against a DENV-2 challenge than traditional adjuvants like Alum or Freund's adjuvant (49). Vaccinations with NS1, as well as NS1-immune sera or mAbs can protect against a lethal DENV challenge, thus underscoring the potential of NS1-based vaccines. NS1 vaccination may result in cross-reactivity with host proteins of vaccinees, hence making this a challenging approach. However, mAbs have been useful to identify non cross-reactive sequences through epitope mapping using phage display that are yet able to show protective efficacy against a challenge

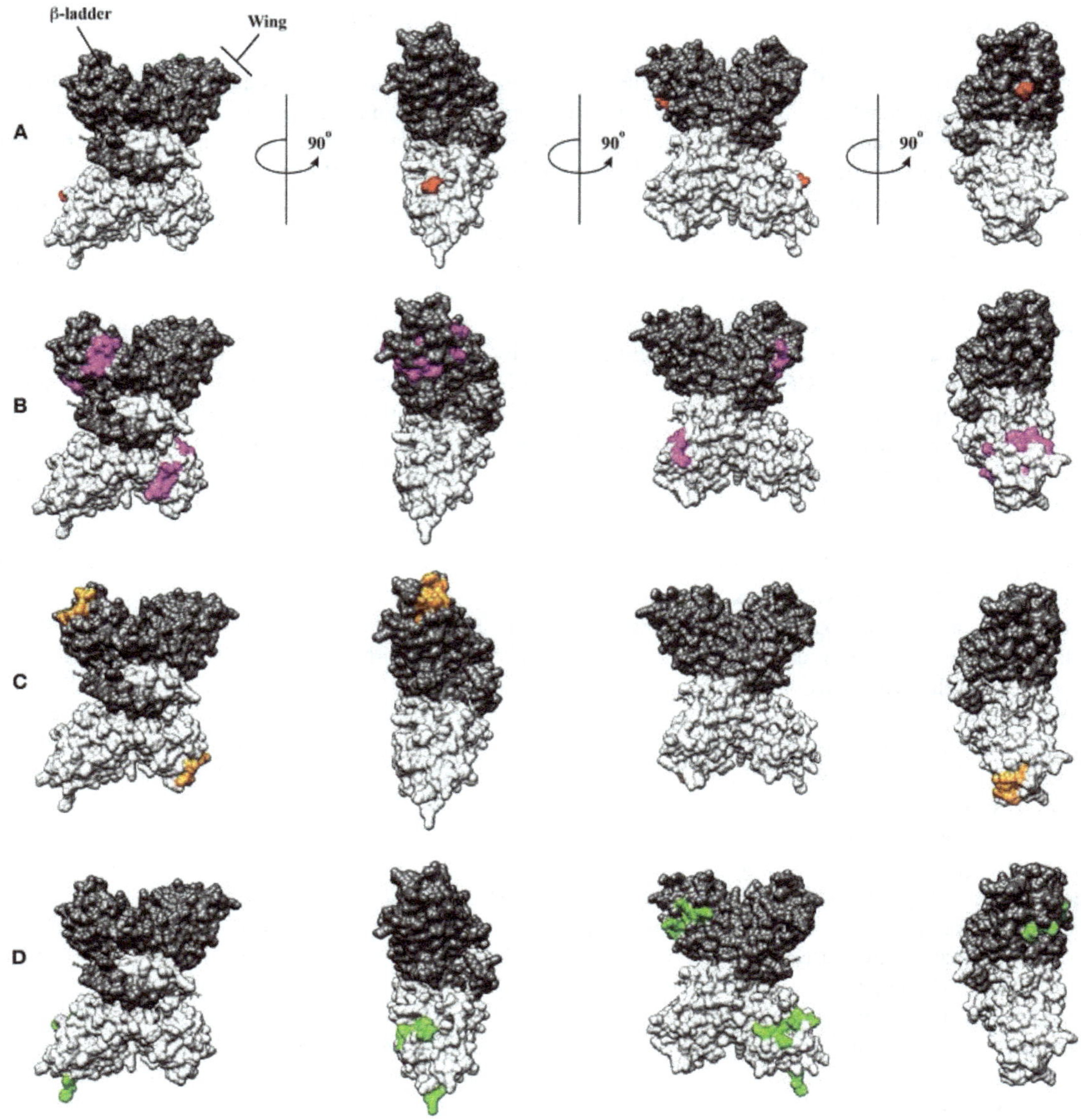

FIGURE 1 | Molecular model of dengue virus NS1 showing regions involved in molecular mimicry with LYRIC in endothelial cells **(A)**, with the protein disulfide isomerase in platelets **(B)** and plasminogen **(C)**. Those two last epitopes overlap in one position (311). An immunodominant epitope presumably involved in protection (28) is also shown **(D)**. Interestingly, this last epitope does not overlap with any of the epitopes related to molecular mimicry. Monomers are shown in gray and white and wing and ladders domain are indicated.

with DENV (50). The latter research highlights the potential of monoclonal antibodies and structural-guided vaccinology to design NS1 vaccines with ability to protect against infection with yet a reduced potential of adverse reactions due to cross reactivity with self-antigens. NS1 has also proven valuable in immunity and vaccine development against Zika virus (ZIKV) in the context of potential increased severity through ADE between the two highly similar ZIKV and DENV. Human monoclonal antibodies against ZIKV NS1 have been isolated and shown protective efficacy in mouse models through the engagement of FcγR without the requirement of virus neutralization (51). These results lead to a subsequent demonstration of protective efficacy of an NS1-based DNA vaccine in a lethal ZIKV challenge model (52).

CONCLUDING REMARKS

The mechanisms underlying severe dengue are not fully understood, but certainly involve a combination of viral virulence, host genetics, and immunopathology. For as long as ADE has been recognized as an immune mechanism that promotes severe dengue (DHF/DSS), efforts have been made to find alternative DENV vaccine strategies to induce immune responses against antigens other than structural components of the DENV virion. The observation that both, structural (prM and Envelope) proteins and the non-structural protein 1 (NS1) elicit strong humoral immune responses in infected individuals has prompted the development of vaccines against both DENV components. Recently, it was shown that IgG anti-NS1 antibodies in sera from a phase II clinical trial were effective in preventing endothelial damage cause by NS1 in an *in vitro* model (53). These antibodies will not only prevent ADE but can confer NS1 cross protection with the other 3 DENV serotypes. Nevertheless, development of NS1 vaccines is yet a challenging approach due to the cross-reactive immune responses between NS1 and self-antigens in endothelia, platelets and clotting factors. NS1 structural studies and availability of monoclonal antibodies are permitting the identification of peptide sequences within NS1 domains that are suitable to generate immunity against DENV with a decrease in cross reactivity to self-antigens. Interestingly, anti-JEV NS1 antibodies, used as controls in various experiments with anti-NS1 antibodies (26, 31) do not cause any cell damage. Structural studies showed differences between the JEV NS1 and the DENV NS1 in the C-terminal, β-ladder domain, where cross-reactive epitopes to platelets and plasminogen are located (54). Indeed, antibodies to chimeric JEV-DENV NS1 protein showed reduced cross-reactivity while still conferring protection in a mouse model (55). Finally, despite the compelling evidence obtained *in vitro* and with animal models, indicating a role for anti-NS1 antibodies in SD pathogenesis, it is wise to keep in mind that plasma leakage, thrombocytopenia, and other vascular clinical signs are all transient and last only for a few days, much shorter than the presumed half-life of any antibody. Thus, additional research is still needed to fully understand the association between anti-NS1 antibodies and dengue pathogenesis in patients and the extent to which molecular mimicry need to be avoided in NS1 based vaccines.

AUTHOR CONTRIBUTIONS

All authors listed have made a substantial, direct and intellectual contribution to the work, and approved it for publication.

ACKNOWLEDGMENTS

The authors like to thank Dr. Jose Luis Zambrano for the elaboration of the figure.

REFERENCES

1. Wilder-Smith A, Gubler DJ, Weaver SC, Monath TP, Heymann DL, Scott TW. Epidemic arboviral diseases: priorities for research and public health. *Lancet Infect Dis.* (2017) 17:e101–6. doi: 10.1016/S1473-3099(16)30518-7
2. Guzman MG, Harris E. Dengue. *Lancet.* (2015) 385b:453–65. doi: 10.1016/S0140-6736(14)60572-9
3. Wahala WM1, Silva AM. The human antibody response to dengue virus infection. *Viruses.* (2011) 12:2374–95. doi: 10.3390/v3122374
4. Halstead SB. Dengue Antibody-dependent enhancement: knowns and unknowns. *Microbiol Spectr.* (2014). doi: 10.1128/microbiolspec.AID-0022-2014
5. Whitehorn J, Simmons CP. The pathogenesis of dengue. *Vaccine.* (2011) 29:7221–8. doi: 10.1016/j.vaccine.2011.07.022
6. Sridhar S, Luedtke A, Langevin E, Zhu M, Bonaparte M, Machabert T, et al. Effect of dengue serostatus on dengue vaccine safety and efficacy. *N Engl J Med.* (2018) 379:327–40. doi: 10.1056/NEJMoa1800820
7. Clyde K, Kyle JL, Harris E. Recent advances in deciphering viral and host determinants of dengue virus replication and pathogenesis. *J Virol.* (2006) 80:11418–31. doi: 10.1128/jvi.01257-06
8. Heinz FX, Stiasny K. Flaviviruses and their antigenic structure. *J Clin Virol.* (2012) 55:289–95. doi: 10.1016/j.jcv.2012.08.024
9. Muller DA, Young PR. The flavivirus NS1 protein: molecular and structural biology, immunology, role in pathogenesis and application as a diagnostic biomarker. *Antiviral Res.* (2013). 98:192–208. doi: 10.1016/j.antiviral.2013.03.008
10. Chen HR, Lai YC, Yeh TM. Dengue virus non-structural protein 1: a pathogenic factor, therapeutic target, and vaccine candidate. *J Biomed Sci.* (2018) 25:58. doi: 10.1186/s12929-018-0462-0
11. Rastogi M, Sharma N, Singh SK. Flavivirus NS1: a multifaceted enigmatic viral protein. *Virol J.* (2016) 13:131. doi: 10.1186/s12985-016-0 590-7
12. Alcalá AC, Medina F, González-Robles A, Salazar-Villatoro L, Fragoso-Soriano RJ, Vásquez C, et al. The dengue virus non-structural protein 1 (NS1) is secreted efficiently from infected mosquito cells. *Virology.* (2016). 488:278–87. doi: 10.1016/j.virol.2015.11.020
13. Alcon-LePoder S, Sivard P, Drouet MT, Talarmin A, Rice C, Flamand M. Secretion of flaviviral non-structural protein NS1: from diagnosis to pathogenesis. *Novartis Found Symp.* (2006) 277:233–47; discussion 247–53.
14. Akey DL, Brown WC, Dutta S, Konwerski J, Jose J, Jurkiw TJ, et al. Flavivirus NS1 structures reveal surfaces for associations with membranes and the immune system. *Science.* (2014) 343:881–5. doi: 10.1126/science.1247749
15. Gutsche I, Coulibaly F, Voss JE, Salmon J, d'Alayer J, Ermonval M, et al. Secreted dengue virus nonstructural protein NS1 is an atypical barrel-shaped high-density lipoprotein. *Proc Natl Acad Sci USA.* (2011) 108:8003–8. doi: 10.1073/pnas
16. Libraty DH, Young PR, Pickering D, Endy TP, Kalayanarooj S, Green S, et al. High circulating levels of the dengue virus nonstructural protein. *J Infect Dis.* (2006) 193:1078–88. doi: 10.1086/343813
17. Avirutnan P1, Punyadee N, Noisakran S, Komoltri C, Thiemmeca S, Auethavornanan K, et al. Vascular leakage in severe dengue virus infections: a potential role for the nonstructural viral protein NS1 and complement. *J Infect Dis.* (2006) 186:1165–8. doi: 10.1086/500949
18. De la Cruz-Hernández SI, Flores-Aguilar H, González-Mateos S, López-Martinez I, Alpuche-Aranda C, Ludert JE, et al. Determination of viremia and concentration of circulating nonstructural protein 1 in patients infected with dengue virus in Mexico. *Am J Trop Med Hyg.* (2013) 88:446–54. doi: 10.4269/ajtmh.12-0023
19. Puerta-Guardo H, Glasner DR, Harris E. Dengue virus NS1 disrupts the endothelial glycocalyx, leading to hyperpermeability. *PLoS Pathog.* (2016) 12:e1005738. doi: 10.1371/journal.ppat.1005738
20. Puerta-Guardo H, Glasner DR, Espinosa DA, Biering SB, Patana M, Ratnasiri K, et al. Flavivirus NS1 triggers tissue-specific vascular endothelial dysfunction reflecting disease tropism. *Cell Rep.* (2019) 26:1598–613.e8. doi: 10.1016/j.celrep.2019.01 036
21. Modhiran N, Watterson D, Muller DA, Panetta AK, Sester DP, Liu L, et al. Dengue virus NS1 protein activates cells via Toll-like receptor 4 and disrupts endothelial cell monolayer integrity. *Sci Transl Med.* (2015) 7:304ra142. doi: 10.1126/scitranslmed.aaa3863
22. Chao CH, Wu WC, Lai YC, Tsai PJ, Perng GC, Lin YS, et al. Dengue virus nonstructural protein 1 activates platelets via Toll-like receptor 4, leading to thrombocytopenia and hemorrhage. *PLoS Pathog.* (2019) 15:e1007625.doi: 10.1371/journal.ppat.1007625
23. Puerta-Guardo H, Raya-Sandino A, González-Mariscal L, Rosales VH, Ayala-Dávila J, Chávez-Mungía B, et al. The cytokine response of U937-derived macrophages infected through antibody-dependent enhancement of dengue virus disrupts cell apical-junction complexes and increases vascular permeability. *J Virol.* (2013) 87:7486–501. doi: 10.1128/JVI.00085-13

24. Falconar AK. The dengue virus nonstructural-1 protein (NS1) generates antibodies to common epitopes on human blood clotting, integrin/adhesin proteins and binds to human endothelial cells: potential implications in haemorrhagic fever pathogenesis. *Arch Virol.* (1997) 142:897–916.
25. Lin CF, Lei HY, Shiau AL, Liu CC, Liu HS, Yeh TM, et al. Antibodies from dengue patient sera cross-react with endothelial cells and induce damage. *J Med Virol.* (2003) 69:82–9. doi: 10.1002/jmv.10261
26. Lin CF, Chiu SC, Hsiao YL, Wan SW, Lei HY, Shiau AL, et al. Expression of cytokine, chemokine, and adhesion molecules during endothelial cell activation induced by antibodies against dengue virus nonstructural protein 1. *J Immunol.* (2005) 174:395–403. doi: 10.4049/jimmunol.174.1.395
27. Liu IJ, Chiu CY, Chen YC, Wu HC. Molecular mimicry of human endothelial cell antigen by autoantibodies to nonstructural protein 1 of dengue virus. *J Biol Chem.* (2011) 286:9726–36. doi: 10.1074/jbc.M110.170993
28. Hertz T, Beatty PR, MacMillen Z, Killingbeck SS, Wang C, Harris E. Antibody epitopes identified in critical regions of dengue virus nonstructural 1 protein in mouse vaccination and natural human infections. *J Immunol.* (2017) 198:4025–35. doi: 10.4049/jimmunol.1700029
29. Chen CL, Lin CF, Wan SW, Wei LS, Chen MC, Yeh TM, et al. Anti-dengue virus nonstructural protein 1 antibodies cause NO-mediated endothelial cell apoptosis via ceramide-regulated glycogen synthase kinase-3β and NF-κB activation. *J Immunol.* (2013) 191:1744–52. doi: 10.4049/jimmunol.1201976
30. Lin CF, Lei HY, Shiau AL, Liu HS, Yeh TM, Chen SH, et al. Endothelial cell apoptosis induced by antibodies against dengue virus nonstructural protein 1 via production of nitric oxide. *J Immunol.* (2002) 169:657–64. doi: 10.4049/jimmunol.169.2.657
31. Lin CF, Wan SW, Chen MC, Lin SC, Cheng CC, Chiu SC, et al. Liver injury caused by antibodies against dengue virus nonstructural protein 1 in a murine model. *Lab Invest.* (2008) 88:1079–89. doi: 10.1038/labinvest.2008.70
32. Chen MC, Lin CF, Lei HY, Lin SC, Liu HS, Yeh TM, et al. Deletion of the C-terminal region of dengue virus nonstructural protein 1 (NS1) abolishes anti-NS1-mediated platelet dysfunction and bleeding tendency. *J Immunol.* (2009) 183:1797–803. doi: 10.4049/jimmunol.0800672
33. Cheng HJ, Lei HY, Lin CF, Luo YH, Wan SW, Liu HS, et al. Anti-dengue virus nonstructural protein 1 antibodies recognize protein disulfide isomerase on platelets and inhibit platelet aggregation. *Mol Immunol.* (2009) 47:398–406. doi: 10.1016/j.molimm.2009.08.033
34. Wan SW, Yang YW, Chu YT, Lin CF, Chang CP, Yeh TM, et al. Anti-dengue virus nonstructural protein 1 antibodies contribute to platelet phagocytosis by macrophages. *Thromb Haemost.* (2016) 115:646-56. doi: 10.1160/TH15-06-0498
35. Chuang YC, Lin J, Lin YS, Wang S, Yeh TM. Dengue virus non-structural protein 1 induced antibodies cross-react with human plasminogen and enhance its activation. *J Immunol.* (2016) 196:1218–26. doi: 10.4049/jimmunol.1500057
36. Prompetchara E, Ketloy C, Thomas SJ, Ruxrungtham K. Dengue vaccine: global development update. *Asian Pac J Allergy Immunol.* (2019) doi: 10.12932/AP-100518-0309
37. Hadinegoro SR, Arredondo-García JL, Capeding MR, Deseda C, Chotpitayasunondh T, Dietze R, et al. Efficacy and long-term safety of a dengue vaccine in regions of Endemic Disease. *N Engl J Med.* (2015) 373:1195–206. doi: 10.1056/NEJMoa1506223
38. Alcon S, Talarmin A, Debruyne M, Falconar A, Deubel V, Flamand M. Enzyme-linked immunosorbent assay specific to Dengue virus type 1 nonstructural protein NS1 reveals circulation of the antigen in the blood during the acute phase of disease in patients experiencing primary or secondary infections. *J Clin Microbiol.* (2002) 40:376–81. doi: 10.1128/jcm.40.02.376-381.2002
39. Gonçalves AJ, Oliveira ER, Costa SM, Paes MV, Silva JF, Azevedo AS, et al. Cooperation between CD4+ T cells and humoral immunity is critical for protection against dengue using a DNA vaccine based on the NS1 antigen. *PLoS Negl Trop Dis.* (2015) 9:e0004277. doi: 10.1371/journal.pntd.0004277
40. Lin SW, Chuang YC, Lin YS, Lei HY, Liu HS, Yeh TM. Dengue virus nonstructural protein NS1 binds to prothrombin/thrombin and inhibits prothrombin activation. *J Infect.* (2012) 64:325–34. doi: 10.1016/j.jinf.2011.11.023
41. Schlesinger JJ, Brandriss MW, Walsh EE. Protection against 17D yellow fever encephalitis in mice by passive transfer of monoclonal antibodies to the nonstructural glycoprotein gp48 and by active immunization with gp48. *J Immunol.* (1985) 135:2805–9.
42. Schlesinger JJ, Brandriss MW, Cropp CB, Monath TP. Protection against yellow fever in monkeys by immunization with yellow fever virus nonstructural protein NS1. *J Virol.* (1986) 60:1153–5.
43. Schlesinger JJ, Brandriss MW, Walsh EE. Protection of mice against dengue 2 virus encephalitis by immunization with the dengue 2 virus non-structural glycoprotein NS1. *J Gen Virol.* (1987) 68:853–7.
44. Falgout B, Bray M, Schlesinger JJ, Lai CJ. Immunization of mice with recombinant vaccinia virus expressing authentic dengue virus nonstructural protein NS1 protects against lethal dengue virus encephalitis. *J Virol.* (1990) 64:4356–63.
45. Wu SF, Liao CL, Lin YL, Yeh CT, Chen LK, Huang YF, et al. Evaluation of protective efficacy and immune mechanisms of using a non-structural protein NS1 in DNA vaccine against dengue 2 virus in mice. *Vaccine.* (2003) 21:3919–29. doi: 10.1016/S0264-410X(03)00310-4
46. Costa SM, Freire MS, Alves AM. DNA vaccine against the non-structural 1 protein (NS1) of dengue 2 virus. *Vaccine.* (2006) 24:4562–4. doi: 10.1016/j.vaccine.2005.08.022
47. Costa SM, Azevedo AS, Paes MV, Sarges FS, Freire MS, Alves AM. DNA vaccines against dengue virus based on the ns1 gene: the influence of different signal sequences on the protein expression and its correlation to the immune response elicited in mice. *Virology.* (2007) 358:413–23. doi: 10.1016/j.virol.2006.08.052
48. López-Camacho C, Abbink P, Larocca RA, Dejnirattisai W, Boyd M, Badamchi-Zadeh A, et al. Rational Zika vaccine design via the modulation of antigen membrane anchors in chimpanzee adenoviral vectors. *Nat Commun.* (2018) 9:2441. doi: 10.1038/s41467-018-04859-5
49. Amorim JH, Diniz MO, Cariri FA, Rodrigues JF, Bizerra RS, Gonçalves AJ, et al. Protective immunity to DENV2 after immunization with a recombinant NS1 protein using a genetically detoxified heat-labile toxin as an adjuvant. *Vaccine.* (2012) 30:837–45. doi: 10.1016/j.vaccine.2011.12.034
50. Lai YC, Chuang YC, Liu CC, Ho TS, Lin YS, Anderson R, et al. Antibodies against modified NS1 wing domain peptide protect against dengue virus infection. *Sci Rep.* (2017) 7:6975. doi: 10.1038/s41598-017-07308-3
51. Bailey MJ, Duehr J, Dulin H, Broecker F, Brown JA, Arumemi FO, et al. Human antibodies targeting Zika virus NS1 provide protection against disease in a mouse model. *Nat Commun.* (2018) 9:4560. doi: 10.1038/s41467-018-07008-0
52. Bailey MJ, Broecker F, Duehr J, Arumemi F, Krammer F, Palese P, et al. Antibodies elicited by an NS1-based vaccine protect mice against zika virus. *MBio.* (2019) 10:e02861-18. doi: 10.1128/mBio.02861-18
53. Sharma M, Glasner DR, Watkins H, Puerta-Guardo H, Kassa Y, Egan MA, et al. Magnitude and functionality of the NS1-specific antibody response elicited by a live-attenuated tetravalent dengue vaccine candidate. *J Infect Dis.* (2019) jiz081. doi: 10.1093/infdis/jiz081
54. Poonsiri T, Wright GSA, Diamond MS, Turtle L, Solomon T, Antonyuk SV. Structural study of the C-terminal domain of nonstructural protein 1 from Japanese encephalitis *Virus. J Virol.* (2018) 92:e01868-17. doi: 10.1128/JVI.01868-17
55. Wan SW, Lu YT, Huang CH, Lin CF, Anderson R, Liu HS, et al. Protection against dengue virus infection in mice by administration of antibodies against modified nonstructural protein 1. *PLoS ONE.* (2014) 9:e92495. doi: 10.1371/journal.pone.0092495

17

The Dual Role of the Immune Response in Reproductive Organs During Zika Virus Infection

*Haruki Arévalo Romero[1], Tania A. Vargas Pavía[2], Manuel A. Velázquez Cervantes[2], Arturo Flores Pliego[2], Addy C. Helguera Repetto[2] and Moises León Juárez[2]**

[1] Laboratory of Immunology and Molecular Microbiology, Multidisciplinary Academic Division of Jalpa de Méndez, Department of Genomics, University Juárez Autonomous of Tabasco, Jalpa de Méndez, Mexico, [2] Laboratory of Perinatal Virology, Department of Immuno-Biochemistry, National Institution of Perinatology "Isidro Espinosa de los Reyes", Mexico City, Mexico

***Correspondence:**
Moises León Juárez
moisesleoninper@gmail.com

Zika virus is a mosquito-borne viral disease that emerged as a significant health problem in the Americas after an epidemic in 2015. Especially concerning are cases where Zika is linked to the development of brain abnormalities in newborns. Unlike other flaviviruses, Zika can be transmitted sexually, increasing the potential for intraspecies infection. Several reports show that the virus can persist for months in the testis of males after clearance of viremia, and that females are highly susceptible to infection via sexual transmission. The most common route of sexual transmission is male-to-female, which suggests that the mechanism driving persistence of Zika in the testis is essential for dissemination. The immune system plays an essential role in Zika infection. In females, a robust response inhibits the virus to control the infection. In males, however, the immunological response to Zika infection correlates with viral persistence. Thus, the immune system may have a dual role in sexually transmitted pathogenesis. The mechanism by which the immune system allows the virus to enter an immune-privileged site while continuing to disseminate is unclear. In this mini-review, we highlight advances in our knowledge of sexually transmitted Zika virus pathogenesis and the possible mechanisms mounted by the immune system that control or exacerbate the infection.

Keywords: Zika virus, sexual transmission, immune response, reproduction, interferon

INTRODUCTION

Zika virus (ZIKV) is a health risk worldwide that is disseminated primarily by insect vectors. Tracking the outbreak of Zika in the Americas in 2015 showed that the virus had been circulating in several countries in Africa and Asia. It is primarily transmitted through *Aedes aegypti* mosquito bites (1, 2). Infection may cause several health complications including microcephaly and congenital Zika syndrome that are associated with vertical transmission (3). This led the World Health Organization to declare the ZIKV outbreak a public health emergency of international concern in 2016 (4). This problem became even more relevant when it was shown that transmission of the pathogen was not exclusive to mosquito bites, similar to that for other flaviviruses. Clinical evidence shows that ZIKV has the potential for human-to-human transmission through sexual routes, including male-to-female, female-to-male, and male-to-male transmission (5–7).

Additionally, ZIKV infiltrates several biological fluids including breastmilk, urine, tears, and saliva (8–10). Thus, it is possible that ZIKV can spread via multiple routes of infection. Several reports suggest that tropism of ZIKV to sexual organs could be a bridge for sexual transmission similar to that employed by human immunodeficiency virus (HIV-1) or human papilloma virus (HPV) (11, 12). Interestingly, the immune response in the male and female reproductive organs could play a role in the spread, persistence, and clearance of ZIKV infection. In this mini-review, we collect the current evidence supporting a dual role of the immune response in the reproductive system organs during ZIKV infection as a promoter of viral dissemination in males and having protective roles in females.

Clinical Reports

Foy et al. reported for the first time that ZIKV might be sexually transmissible. The virus was identified in a woman that had not traveled to an area endemic for ZIKV transmission. She developed symptoms of the disease after sexual contact with her husband in the days after he returned from a trip to Senegal (13). Since this initial finding, several studies have been published indicating sexual transmission of ZIKV in other areas not endemic for mosquito transmission, such as Europe and North America (14, 15). Additionally, these reports show that male-to-female transmission is more frequent than female-to-male transmission (16–18). Interestingly, studies that have reported shedding of ZIKV in genital fluids to suggest a more robust presence in semen, compared to that in vaginal fluids, and a clear persistence of ZIKV for at least 188 days following symptom onset (19). Moreover, the only study focused on detecting the ZIKV in vaginal secretions showed that the virus could persist for 60–180 days after the onset of symptoms (20). However, the assays determining the ZIKV viability were not conducted, in contrast to the studies on semen samples that determined the production of infective virus in Vero cells (21). Additionally, a similar behavior was observed in studies with other viral sexual transmission such as Hepatitis C, Ebola, HIV-1, and Herpes identifying high viral loads in seminal fluid samples (22–25). The studies also showed greater transmission from male-to-female and the viral load was evaluated in vaginal fluids, but the test to detect viral viability in these samples was not performed. Altogether, these data suggest that cells residing in the male reproductive system are highly susceptible to viral infection or that the female reproductive system presents a more effective defense against the pathogen. These hypotheses need to be addressed adequately through further research.

Tropism of ZIKV to Sexual Organs

The male reproductive tract (MRT) constitutes the testis, epididymis, deferens tubules, prostate, seminal vesicle, bulbourethral glands, and penile urethra. These structures are required for the production, maturation, and protection of spermatozoa from immunoreaction and infectious agents (26, 27). The female reproductive tract (FRT) is organized into two functional compartments associated with fetal development (upper FRT) and the external environment (lower FRT). The vagina and ectocervix constitute the lower FRT and are organized by a keratinized stratified squamous epithelium. The endocervix, uterus, and fallopian tubes comprise the upper FRT and consist of a single layer of columnar epithelium (28). Implementation of animal models has been essential to identify the cellular targets of ZIKV within reproductive tracts (29). Results from these models have shown that ZIKV has high tropism in the MRT, infecting cell types that include spermatogonia, primary spermatocytes, Sertoli cells, peritubular myoid cells, Leydig cells, and epithelial cells of the lumen (30). In contrast, in human testis *ex vivo,* ZIKV can infect and replicate in a range of somatic and germ cells, such as testicular macrophages, peritubular cells, Leydig, and Sertoli cells. However, the infection was weaker in human cells than that observed in the mouse model (31). Finally, ZIKV was also found in the spermatozoa from ZIKV-infected men, suggesting that ZIKV could infect the zygote and cause fetal congenital diseases. We propose that the immune response could help ZIKV gain access to spermatozoa in the MRT (32).

In the case of cells within the FRT, few reports have evaluated their susceptibility to ZIKV infection. The experimental evidence from animal model mosquito bite inoculates suggests that ZIKV is present in reproductive tract tissues such as the cervix and vagina (33). Additionally, studies on immunocompetent mice showed that vaginal inoculation of ZIKV lead to productive replication of the virus within the vaginal mucosa and ovarian follicles. Additionally, ZIKV replication in the vaginal tissue of a pregnant mouse was followed by infection of the fetal brain, suggesting vertical transmission (34). Cellular models *in vitro* have shown that human endometrial stromal cells are permissive to ZIKV infection and replication. Interestingly, *in vitro* decidualization of this cellular model increased the replication of ZIKV, suggesting that endometrial cells have an important role during sexual transmission of ZIKV. They might provide a viral reservoir for infection of cells at the maternal-fetal interface during pregnancy (35). Finally, current studies that focus on the use of human tissues or primary cultures of FRT cells need to be performed to evaluate if the behavior of ZIKV infection in animal models is similar to that in humans. The establishment of vaginal and cervical epithelial cells could be an exciting model as they have been used for the study of HIV-1 and Herpes simplex virus (36, 37).

Role of the Immune System in Sexual Transmission of ZIKV

Viral evolution requires development of a mechanism to evade the host immune response and manipulate cells for their own replication, allowing it to spread to other cells (38). ZIKV evades the immune system (IS) by regulating the type I interferon response with its encoded NS5 protein (39). Mice lacking components of IFN pathway are more susceptible to ZIKV infection, highlighting the importance of the IS for the control of the virus (40).

Among flaviviruses, sexual transmission is unique to ZIKV, marking an unusual potential for human-to-human transmission. The immune privileged nature of the testis protects germ cells from immune attack that occurs during infection. While clinical reports clearly identified persistence

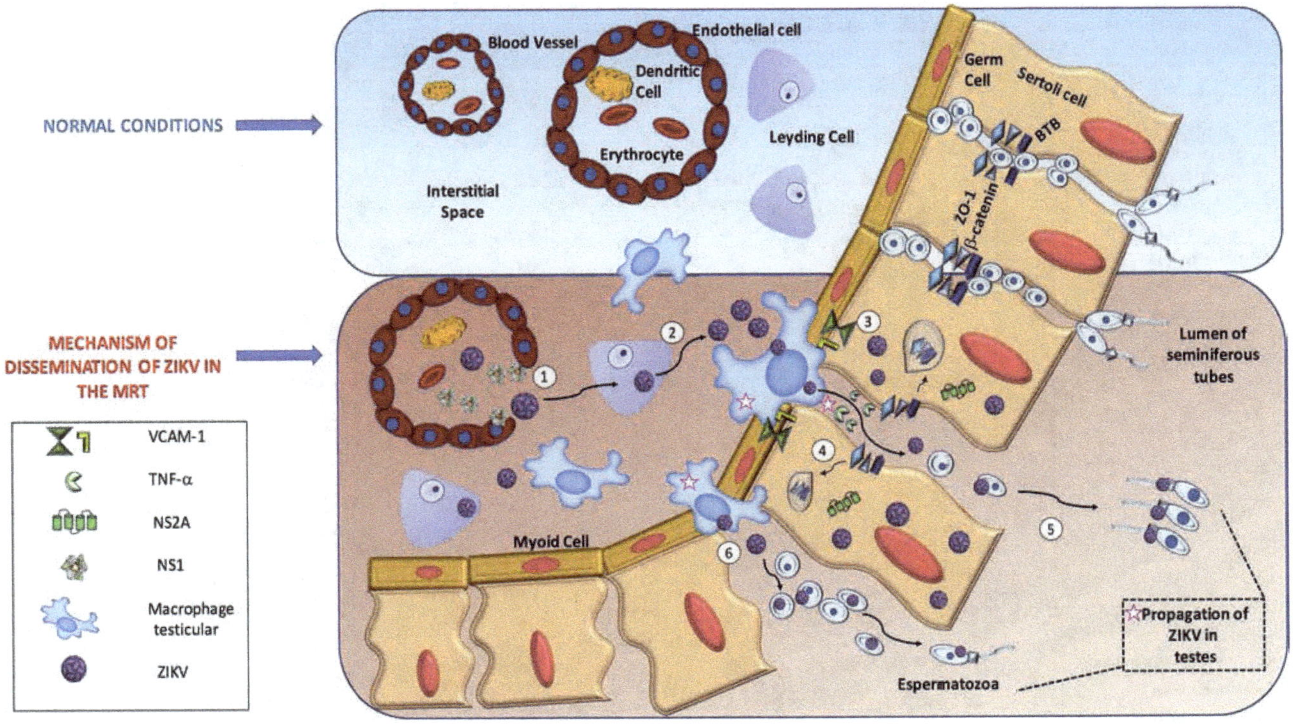

FIGURE 1 | The dissemination process of ZIKV in male reproductive tract. In the male reproductive tract, Immune system mechanism might promote ZIKV dissemination. (1) ZIKV travel in infected immune cells such as Dendritic cells to testis; ZIKV NS1 protein increase the permeability of endothelial cells to allow virus access toward interstitial space, (2) ZIKV infect Leydig cells increase the production of viruses in the zone, (3) ZIKV can infect Sertoli cells and change the immunosuppressive microenvironment to a robust antiviral response. Activated macrophages secrete TNF-α that disrupt the Blood Testicular Barrier by degradation of tight junction proteins such as ZO-1 allowing ZIKV reach and infect germ cells, (4) In parallel, is possible that on infected Sertoli cells the NS2A protein target to degradation proteins of tight junction complexes helping also to reach germ cells, (5) Finally, through adhesion molecules such as VCAM-1 ZIKV infected macrophages can interact with Sertoli cells (6) and direct infiltrate the lumen of seminiferous tubules and ZIKV could infect eventually germinal cells.

of viral RNA in seminal fluid, little is known about how ZIKV passes from blood to the MRT, nor how it persists in the testis. The mechanism seems to involve different cell types, including immune system cells, for transport to target tissues. For example, ZIKV was preferentially found in the cell fraction of blood samples from humans exposed to an endemic area, suggesting that ZIKV could use this mechanism for transport before crossing tissue barriers in the male body (41, 42).

ZIKV seems uses a conserved arboviral strategy for primary infection. Semliki Forest virus (SFV) is an alphavirus that is a close relative to the Chikungunya virus. It was shown that a cutaneous innate immune response involuntarily facilitated viral infection. The mechanism involved neutrophil-dependent inflammation at mosquito bite sites that promoted the recruitment of myeloid cells that are permissive to the virus. These then released new infectious viral particles targeting new cellular targets (43). We hypothesize that the same mechanism may be used by ZIKV to spread its infection. In support of this possibility, human *in vitro*-generated dendritic cells (DCs) are permissive to ZIKV infection (44). Additionally, using a pigtail macaque model it was shown that male animals were more susceptible to ZIKV persistence in peripheral lymph nodes and dissemination to mucosal tissues. The mechanism involves two steps: an inflammatory response that follows ZIKV infection that drives the recruitment of innate cells as early targets of the virus. The infected cells are myeloid DCs, non-classic monocytes, and natural killer (NK) cells. Unlike SFV, the recruitment of cells is driven by plasmocytoid DCs in a MCP-1 dependent manner, which also supports the dissemination and persistence of ZIKV (45). Altogether, these data show that IS inadvertently plays a role in viral tropism, persistence, and pathogenesis of ZIKV.

In general, we consider that there are two routes to reach spermatids in the seminiferous tubules. One is that ZIKV uses the IS to reach the testis and manipulate the antiviral mechanism to disrupt the blood testicular barrier (BTB) junctions. The other possibility is that ZIKV proteins directly destroy the junctions to cross the barrier. We believe these processes are not exclusive, as both are supported by evidence in the literature (45–47). Once ZIKV reaches the testicles, we assume that the virus gains access to germinal cells by three mechanisms. (1) ZIKV can infect or alter the endothelium and pass to the interstitial space, (2) infection of different cells elicits disruption of junctional adhesions in a manner that is dependent on IS antiviral activity or a direct function of ZIKV protein, and (3) direct transmigration of infected immune cells from the blood to the seminiferous tubules.

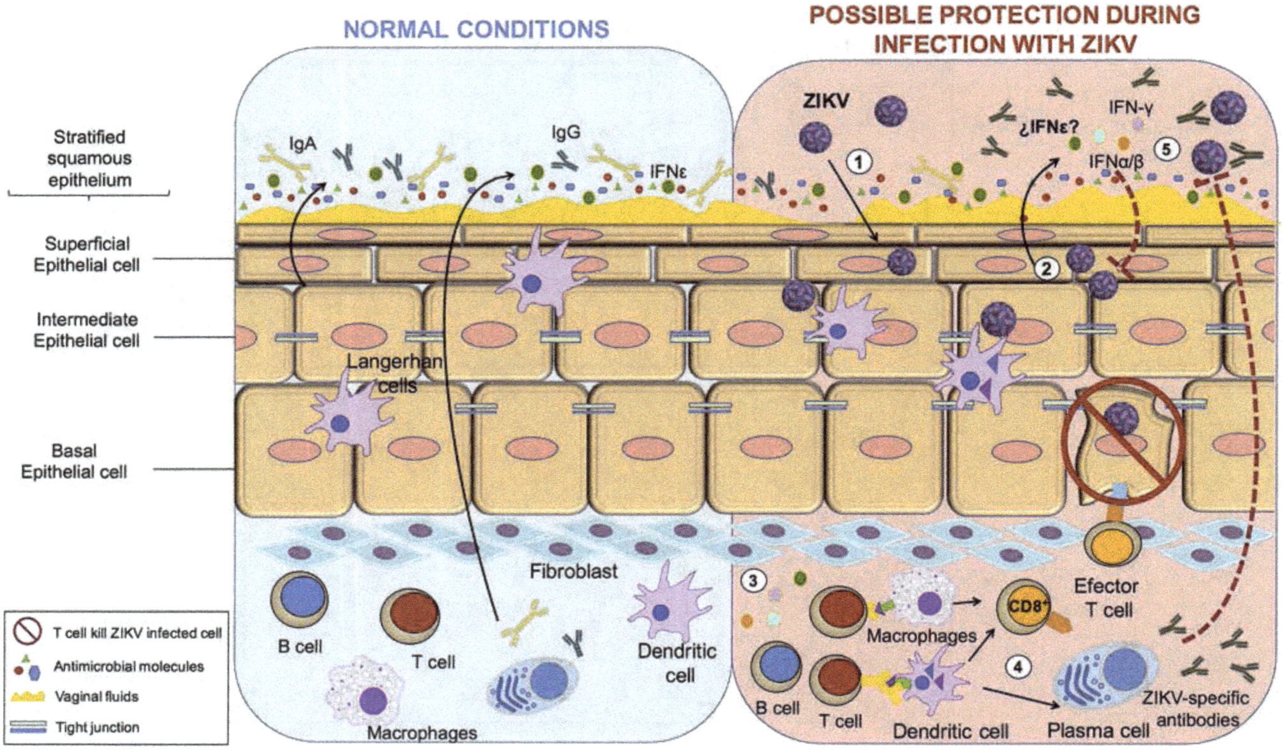

FIGURE 2 | The protection process of ZIKV in female reproductive tract. Immune system mechanism protects against ZIKV infection in female reproductive tract. (1) ZIKV infect vaginal epithelial cells, (2) infected cells produce IFN-α,β,γ, and possibly IFN-ε which initiates the intracellular antiviral state (3) immune cells increases antigen presentation leading to T and B cell activation, (4) effector B cells secrete ZIKV-specific antibodies and effector cytotoxic T cells kill ZIKV infected cells; (5) Finally, the IS mechanism control and protect against ZIKV.

A recent study supported endothelial passage, showing that ZIKV NS1 protein bound specifically to endothelial cells including human umbilical vein endothelial cells (HUVECs) and human brain microvascular endothelial cells (HBMECs), causing a decrease in their permeability. The mechanism implies degradation of the endothelial glycocalyx layer by the activation of sialidase and cathepsin L-heparanase both *in vitro* and *in vivo* (48). Another piece of evidence is indirect but concordant with endothelial passage. ZIKV could persistently infect and replicates in primary HBMECs. Moreover, ZIKV was delivered from both apical and basolateral surfaces suggesting a direct mechanism to cross the blood brain barrier (49). In addition, it was shown that the Sertoli cells that constitute the BTB were highly susceptible to ZIKV infection suggesting that ZIKV may be able to utilize this crossing mechanism directly (46). Finally, a study using the bluetongue virus in a ram model showed testicular damage due to viral replication in the endothelial cells of the peritubular area in the testis, resulting in the destruction of the Sertoli cell barrier associated with type I interferon response raising the possibility that ZIKV may use a similar mechanism of this related arbovirus in humans (50). Overall, these studies suggest that ZIKV can infect and alter endothelial barriers to facilitate virus dissemination into target organs facing other target cells, such as Sertoli cells, and macrophages in the interstitial space. In parallel, the extravasation of fluids can induce inflammation that also helps the virus to disrupt other barriers, such as BTB, to enhance viral infection. However, studies describing this mechanism in human or mouse endothelial testicular cells are lacking and need to be tested.

For the second mechanism, using an *in vitro* BTB model with human Sertoli cells it was observed that ZIKV could infect these cells for a long term without induction of cell death, and that Sertoli cells can mount a robust antiviral response. The virus did not directly alter tight or adherent junctions, but induced the expression of VCAM-1 that provides the interaction for the transmigration of monocytes across the epithelial cell model. More importantly, the inflammatory cytokine TNF-α released from ZIKV-infected macrophages affected the permeability of the BTB by degrading ZO-1 protein suggesting that IS can help ZIKV gain access to developing germ cells (46). Similar results were obtained with the use of a 3-D model of HBMECs. This experiment showed that apical junctions restrict the infection capability of several RNA viruses. However, treatment of the 3-D cultures with TNF-α disrupted the formation of cell-cell junctions and correlated with an increase in ZIKV viral RNA and infectious titers (51). Another study using RNAseq analysis of ZIKV-infected Sertoli cells showed that these cells responded to ZIKV with a diversity of innate antiviral mechanism. Importantly the analysis of upregulated genes on interferon, antigen presentation, and cross-talk between DC and

NK signaling pathways correlated with the downregulation of genes involved in adherent junctions, tubulin α/β complex, and 14-3-3 signaling pathways (52). Interestingly, a clear correlation exists between the peak of the immune response and the downregulation of genes that control cell cycle progression. These data suggest that ZIKV could modulate the change from an immunosuppressive microenvironment in Sertoli cells to a strong antiviral response that alters the permeability of BTB with a concomitant delay in proliferation. This would prolong the time for viral progeny production, ensure persistence, and allow dissemination via sexual transmission.

Direct evidence of the disruption of cell junctions by ZIKV came from the use of the NS2A protein in mouse radial glial cells and human brain organoids. NS2A interacted directly with adherent junction components, such as ZO-1, β-catenin, SMAD7, and NUMBL, targeting them for lysosomal degradation and inducing aberrant cortical layer formation. We hypothesize that the same mechanism could be used by ZIKV in the testis to gain access to seminiferous tubules, but this needs to be tested (47).

Finally, evidence for the third mechanism was shown using 3-D culture HBMECs in transwell assays. ZIKV-infected monocytes crossed the epithelial barrier and infected primary human astrocytes plated in the basolateral chamber (51). Using a similar approach with Sertoli cells it was observed that ZIKV-infected macrophages interacted with and induced the permeability of the cells, suggesting that after induction the leakiness of the barrier allowed infiltration to the lumen of the seminiferous tubules and probably infection of germ cells (46). These studies suggest that the IS, when attempting to control viral infection, actually assists the entry of ZIKV to this immune-privileged site, causing persistence that allows sexual transmission (**Figure 1**).

On the other hand, within the human FRT, protection against sexually transmitted infection is opposed to biological fertility (53). The role of the FRT during ZIKV infection and sexual transmission has not been extensively evaluated. However, the mucosal immune system is the first line of defense against pathogens. The innate and adaptive elements of the mucosal immune system have evolved to meet the special challenges that are associated with the FRT (54). Interestingly, in contrast to that in males, the IS mechanism against ZIKV correlates with protection of the FRT. For example, interferon (IFN)-ε is constitutively expressed by epithelial cells in the FRT and protects against herpes simplex virus-2 infection. This protective role of the IFN-ε may also be prohibitive for ZIKV infection, but this needs to be tested (55). Protection via IFN response was shown by the administration of recombinant IFN-β/λ in primary human vaginal/cervical epithelial cells. This restricted ZIKV replication by induction of canonical IFN-stimulated genes (56). In agreement with this study, the induction of a strong IFN response is necessary to prevent vaginal ZIKV infection in mice because the virus elicits minimal induction of IFN response and seems to regulate the activation of antigen presenting cells (57).

Additionally, it is necessary to consider the regulation of the immune system by sex hormones when evaluating ZIKV infection of the FRT. For example, estradiol and progesterone coordinate unique patterns of epithelial cells, stromal fibroblast, and immune cell functions that optimize the conditions for fetal survival and maternal protection (58). This is supported by the analysis of an immunocompetent animal model infected with ZIKV. Hormonal treatments in the FRT promoted the transmission and replication of virus. This study suggested that women establish correct innate and cellular antiviral mechanisms and hormonal regulation to control the infection (59). In mice, subcutaneous ZIKV inoculation elicited a cellular and humoral response that protected subsequent intravaginal inoculation (60). These studies suggest that in females a robust immune response protects against sexual exposure instead of helping the viral establishment and persistence. In conclusion, these data show that antiviral IS mechanisms in the FRT correlate with protection, the opposite of the response mechanism in the MRT. This is in agreement with clinical data indicating that the female-to-male route of sexual transmission is less frequent than the male-to-female route is. However, is important to consider other factors associated with the sexual transmission of the ZIKV. For example, it was reported that the microtrauma in the epithelial barrier of FTR during intercourse promotes the sexual transmission of HIV-1 or HVB (61, 62). In addition, relevant future studies are needed to understand the role of hormones that regulated the menstrual cycle and the effect on sexual transmission of ZIKV in the FRT. Recently, it has been suggested that estradiol is associated with activation of the innate immune mechanism and initiation of the antiviral responses, and that the modulation by sexual hormones results in alteration of a woman's susceptibility to HIV-1 and other infections (61, 63). The understanding about the role of hormones in different stages of menstrual cycle or pregnancy may help to resolve question on the mechanism of ZIKV to persist in the FRT (**Figure 2**).

Finally, whether sexual transmission (STx) has any influence on vertical transmission (Vtx) of ZIKV is yet unanswered. Until now, the literature shows that the mechanisms of immune response in FRT can control ZIKV infection via STx, and in humans, to our knowledge, data indicating Vtx after sexual transmission does not exist. However, a mouse model with suppressed IFN response showed that males have infectious viruses in the testicles and can transmit sexually to females during the early phase of infection. Importantly, in the few cases of pregnancy with STx of ZIKV, there was only evidence of infection in cells of the uterus and placenta, but there was no clear evidence of Vtx in the fetuses. In contrast, Vtx was clear after peripheral ZIKV infection, since 26% of brains of the fetuses/pups were positive for ZIKV RNA (64).

In the context of peripheral infection, the mechanisms described to alter BTB could be used by ZIKV to infect the placenta. A study shows that placental macrophages can be infected by ZIKV and respond to the infection by inflammatory and antiviral signaling pathways. The authors propose that placental macrophages support efficient ZIKV replication, and this may result in the subsequent infection of neural progenitor cells (65). However, a report showing Vtx without breakdown of the placental barrier also exists. The discordance in these studies show the complexity of the ZIKV infection and argue that these mechanisms may have a role during the Vtx, but more studies are needed to evaluate them correctly.

CONCLUSIONS

ZIKV can infect and regulate different cells, including immune system cells, to ensure survival and persistence. In the MRT, the activation of different immunological events in response to ZIKV infection correlate with viral persistence that, conversely, in females, are necessary to inhibit the virus and control the infection. We highlight some important aspects of the immune system that assist ZIKV dissemination into the reproductive organs, thus showing that IS can have a dual role in the pathogenesis of sexual transmission. However, the molecular mechanism used by ZIKV in human cells to guarantee infection has not been investigated thoroughly. Understanding the molecular mechanisms utilized by the virus for dissemination will be invaluable to develop new targets for therapeutic intervention.

AUTHOR CONTRIBUTIONS

ML and HA designed the concept and completed the final editing of the manuscript. All authors contributed to writing of the manuscript. MV and TV prepared the figures. All authors read approved the manuscript for publication.

REFERENCES

1. Baud D, Musso D, Vouga M, Alves MP, Vulliemoz N. Zika virus: a new threat to human reproduction. *Am. J. Reprod. Immunol.* (2017) 77:e12614. doi: 10.1111/aji.12614
2. Gutierrez-Bugallo G, Piedra LA, Rodriguez M, Bisset JA, Lourenco-de-Oliveira R, Weaver SC, et al. Vector-borne transmission and evolution of Zika virus. *Nat Ecol Evol.* (2019) 3:561–9. doi: 10.1038/s41559-019-0836-z
3. Pomar L, Musso D, Malinger G, Vouga M, Panchaud A, Baud D. Zika virus during pregnancy: from maternal exposure to congenital Zika virus syndrome. *Prenat Diagn.* (2019) 39:420–30. doi: 10.1002/pd.5446
4. *WHO Director-General Summarizes the Outcome of the Emergency Committee regarding clusters of microcephaly and Guillain-Barré Syndrome.* (2016). Available online at: http://www.who.int/mediacentre/news/statements/2016/emergency-committee-zika-microcephaly/en/
5. Arsuaga M, Bujalance SG, Diaz-Menendez M, Vazquez A, Arribas JR. Probable sexual transmission of Zika virus from a vasectomised man. *Lancet Infect Dis.* (2016) 16:1107. doi: 10.1016/S1473-3099(16)30320-6
6. Hills SL, Russell K, Hennessey M, Williams C, Oster AM, Fischer M, et al. Transmission of Zika virus through sexual contact with travelers to areas of ongoing transmission - continental United States, 2016. *Morb Mortal Wkly Rep.* (2016) 65:215–6. doi: 10.15585/mmwr.mm6508e2
7. Turmel JM, Abgueguen P, Hubert B, Vandamme YM, Maquart M, Le Guillou-Guillemette H, et al. Late sexual transmission of Zika virus related to persistence in the semen. *Lancet.* (2016) 387:2501. doi: 10.1016/S0140-6736(16)30775-9
8. Basarab M, Bowman C, Aarons EJ, Cropley I. Zika virus. *BMJ.* (2016) 352:i1049. doi: 10.1136/bmj.i1049
9. Walczynska A, Sobczyk L. The underestimated role of temperature-oxygen relationship in large-scale studies on size-to-temperature response. *Ecol Evol.* (2017) 7:7434–41. doi: 10.1002/ece3.3263
10. Niedrig M, Patel P, El Wahed AA, Schadler R, Yactayo S. Find the right sample: a study on the versatility of saliva and urine samples for the diagnosis of emerging viruses. *BMC Infect Dis.* (2018) 18:707. doi: 10.1186/s12879-018-3611-x
11. Craigo JK, Gupta P. HIV-1 in genital compartments: vexing viral reservoirs. *Curr Opin HIV AIDS.* (2006) 1:97–102. doi: 10.1097/01.COH.0000200507.27578.26
12. Foresta C, Patassini C, Bertoldo A, Menegazzo M, Francavilla F, Barzon L, et al. Mechanism of human papillomavirus binding to human spermatozoa and fertilizing ability of infected spermatozoa. *PLoS ONE.* (2011) 6:e15036. doi: 10.1371/journal.pone.0015036
13. Foy BD, Kobylinski KC, Chilson Foy JL, Blitvich BJ, Travassos da Rosa A, Haddow AD, et al. Probable non-vector-borne transmission of Zika virus, Colorado, USA. *Emerg Infect Dis.* (2011) 17:880–2. doi: 10.3201/eid1705.101939
14. Matsumura N, Robertson IM, Hamza SM, Soltys CM, Sung MM, Masson G, et al. A novel complex I inhibitor protects against hypertension-induced left ventricular hypertrophy. *Am J Physiol Heart Circ Physiol.* (2017) 312:H561–70. doi: 10.1152/ajpheart.00604.2016
15. Frank C, Cadar D, Schlaphof A, Neddersen N, Gunther S, Schmidt-Chanasit J, et al. Sexual transmission of Zika virus in Germany, April 2016. *Euro Surveill.* (2016) 21: 30252. doi: 10.2807/1560-7917.ES.2016.21.23.30252
16. Deckard DT, Chung WM, Brooks JT, Smith JC, Woldai S, Hennessey M, et al. Male-to-male sexual transmission of Zika virus–Texas, January 2016. *Morb Mortal Wkly Rep.* (2016) 65:372–4. doi: 10.15585/mmwr.mm6514a3
17. Freour T, Mirallie S, Hubert B, Splingart C, Barriere P, Maquart M, et al. Sexual transmission of Zika virus in an entirely asymptomatic couple returning from a Zika epidemic area, France, April 2016. *Euro Surveill.* (2016) 21:30254. doi: 10.2807/1560-7917.ES.2016.21.23.30254
18. Hamer DH, Wilson ME, Jean J, Chen LH. Epidemiology, prevention, and potential future treatments of sexually transmitted Zika virus infection. *Curr Infect Dis Rep.* (2017) 19:16. doi: 10.1007/s11908-017-0571-z
19. Gornet ME, Bracero NJ, Segars JH. Zika virus in semen: what we know and what we need to know. *Semin Reprod Med.* (2016) 34:285–92. doi: 10.1055/s-0036-1592312
20. Reyes Y, Bowman NM, Becker-Dreps S, Centeno E, Collins MH, Liou GA, et al. Prolonged shedding of Zika virus RNA in vaginal secretions, Nicaragua. *Emerg Infect Dis.* (2019) 25:808–10. doi: 10.3201/eid2504.180977
21. Mansuy JM, Dutertre M, Mengelle C, Fourcade C, Marchou B, Delobel P, et al. Zika virus: high infectious viral load in semen, a new sexually transmitted pathogen? *Lancet Infect Dis.* (2016) 16:405. doi: 10.1016/S1473-3099(16)00138-9
22. Wejstal R. Sexual transmission of hepatitis C virus. *J Hepatol.* (1999) 31:92–5.
23. Vetter P, Fischer WA II, Schibler M, Jacobs M, Bausch DG, Kaiser L. Ebola virus shedding and transmission: review of current evidence. *J Infect Dis.* (2016) 214:S177–84. doi: 10.1093/infdis/jiw254
24. Sutthent R, Chaisilwattana P, Roongpisuthipong A, Wirachsilp P, Samrangsarp K, Chaiyakul P, et al. Shedding of HIV-1 subtype E in semen and cervico-vaginal fluid. *J Med Assoc Thai.* (1997) 80:348–57.
25. Aryee EA, Bailey RL, Natividad-Sancho A, Kaye S, Holland MJ. Detection, quantification and genotyping of Herpes Simplex virus in cervicovaginal secretions by real-time PCR: a cross sectional survey. *Virol J.* (2005) 2:61. doi: 10.1186/1743-422X-2-61
26. Li N, Wang T, Han D. Structural, cellular and molecular aspects of immune privilege in the testis. *Front Immunol.* (2012) 3:152. doi: 10.3389/fimmu.2012.00152

27. Chen Q, Deng T, Han D. Testicular immunoregulation and spermatogenesis. *Semin Cell Dev Biol.* (2016) 59:157–65. doi: 10.1016/j.semcdb.2016.01.019
28. Hafez ES. Structural and ultrastructural parameters of the uterine cervix. *Obstet Gynecol Surv.* (1982) 37:507–16.
29. da Silva LRC. Zika virus trafficking and interactions in the human male reproductive tract. *Pathogens.* (2018) 7:51. doi: 10.3390/pathogens7020051
30. Govero J, Esakky P, Scheaffer SM, Fernandez E, Drury A, Platt DJ, et al. Zika virus infection damages the testes in mice. *Nature.* (2016) 540:438–42. doi: 10.1038/nature20556
31. Matusali G, Houzet L, Satie AP, Mahe D, Aubry F, Couderc T, et al. Zika virus infects human testicular tissue and germ cells. *J Clin Invest.* (2018) 128:4697–710. doi: 10.1172/JCI121735
32. Salam AP, Horby P. Isolation of viable Zika virus from spermatozoa. *Lancet Infect Dis.* (2018) 18:144. doi: 10.1016/S1473-3099(18)30020-3
33. Dudley DM, Newman CM, Lalli J, Stewart LM, Koenig MR, Weiler AM, et al. Infection via mosquito bite alters Zika virus tissue tropism and replication kinetics in rhesus macaques. *Nature Commun.* (2017) 8:2096. doi: 10.1038/s41467-017-02222-8
34. Yockey LJ, Varela L, Rakib T, Khoury-Hanold W, Fink SL, Stutz B, et al. Vaginal exposure to Zika virus during pregnancy leads to fetal brain infection. *Cell.* (2016) 166:1247–56.e4. doi: 10.1016/j.cell.2016.08.004
35. Pagani I, Ghezzi S, Ulisse A, Rubio A, Turrini F, Garavaglia E, et al. Human endometrial stromal cells are highly permissive to productive infection by Zika virus. *Sci Rep.* (2017) 7:44286. doi: 10.1038/srep44286
36. Kinlock BL, Wang Y, Turner TM, Wang C, Liu B. Transcytosis of HIV-1 through vaginal epithelial cells is dependent on trafficking to the endocytic recycling pathway. *PLoS ONE.* (2014) 9:e96760. doi: 10.1371/journal.pone.0096760
37. Ayehunie S, Wang YY, Landry T, Bogojevic S, Cone RA. Hyperosmolal vaginal lubricants markedly reduce epithelial barrier properties in a three-dimensional vaginal epithelium model. *Toxicol Rep.* (2018) 5:134–40. doi: 10.1016/j.toxrep.2017.12.011
38. Leon-Juarez M, Martinez-Castillo M, Gonzalez-Garcia LD, Helguera-Repetto AC, Zaga-Clavellina V, Garcia-Cordero J, et al. Cellular and molecular mechanisms of viral infection in the human placenta. *Pathog Dis.* (2017) 75:ftx093. doi: 10.1093/femspd/ftx093
39. Grant A, Ponia SS, Tripathi S, Balasubramaniam V, Miorin L, Sourisseau M, et al. Zika virus targets human STAT2 to inhibit type I interferon signaling. *Cell Host Microbe.* (2016) 19:882–90. doi: 10.1016/j.chom.2016.05.009
40. Li H, Saucedo-Cuevas L, Regla-Nava JA, Chai G, Sheets N, Tang W, et al. Zika virus infects neural progenitors in the adult mouse brain and alters proliferation. *Cell Stem Cell.* (2016) 19:593–8. doi: 10.1016/j.stem.2016.08.005
41. Joguet G, Mansuy JM, Matusali G, Hamdi S, Walschaerts M, Pavili L, et al. Effect of acute Zika virus infection on sperm and virus clearance in body fluids: a prospective observational study. *Lancet Infect Dis.* (2017) 17:1200–8. doi: 10.1016/S1473-3099(17)30444-9
42. Murray KO, Gorchakov R, Carlson AR, Berry R, Lai L, Natrajan M, et al. Prolonged detection of Zika virus in vaginal secretions and whole blood. *Emerg Infect Dis.* (2017) 23:99–101. doi: 10.3201/eid2301.161394
43. Pingen M, Bryden SR, Pondeville E, Schnettler E, Kohl A, Merits A, et al. Host inflammatory response to mosquito bites enhances the severity of arbovirus infection. *Immunity.* (2016) 44:1455–69. doi: 10.1016/j.immuni.2016.06.002
44. Hamel R, Dejarnac O, Wichit S, Ekchariyawat P, Neyret A, Luplertlop N, et al. Biology of Zika virus infection in human skin cells. *J Virol.* (2015) 89:8880–96. doi: 10.1128/JVI.00354-15
45. O'Connor MA, Tisoncik-Go J, Lewis TB, Miller CJ, Bratt D, Moats CR, et al. Early cellular innate immune responses drive Zika viral persistence and tissue tropism in pigtail macaques. *Nature Commun.* (2018) 9:3371. doi: 10.1038/s41467-018-05826-w
46. Siemann DN, Strange DP, Maharaj PN, Shi PY, Verma S. Zika virus infects human sertoli cells and modulates the integrity of the *in vitro* blood-testis barrier model. *J Virol.* (2017) 91:e00623-17. doi: 10.1128/JVI.00623-17
47. Yoon KJ, Song G, Qian X, Pan J, Xu D, Rho HS, et al. Zika-virus-encoded NS2A disrupts mammalian cortical neurogenesis by degrading adherens junction proteins. *Cell Stem Cell.* (2017) 21:349–58.e6. doi: 10.1016/j.stem.2017.07.014
48. Puerta-Guardo H, Glasner DR, Espinosa DA, Biering SB, Patana M, Ratnasiri K, et al. Flavivirus NS1 triggers tissue-specific vascular endothelial dysfunction reflecting disease tropism. *Cell Rep.* (2019) 26:1598–613.e8. doi: 10.1016/j.celrep.2019.01.036
49. Mladinich MC, Schwedes J, Mackow ER. Zika virus persistently infects and is basolaterally released from primary human brain microvascular endothelial cells. *MBio.* (2017) 8:e00952-17. doi: 10.1128/mBio.00952-17
50. Puggioni G, Pintus D, Melzi E, Meloni G, Rocchigiani AM, Maestrale C, et al. Testicular degeneration and infertility following arbovirus infection. *J Virol.* (2018) 92:e01131-18. doi: 10.1128/JVI.01131-18
51. Bramley JC, Drummond CG, Lennemann NJ, Good CA, Kim KS, Coyne CB. A three-dimensional cell culture system to model RNA virus infections at the blood-brain barrier. *mSphere.* (2017) 2:e00206-17. doi: 10.1128/mSphere.00206-17
52. Strange DP, Green R, Siemann DN, Gale M Jr, Verma S. Immunoprofiles of human Sertoli cells infected with Zika virus reveals unique insights into host-pathogen crosstalk. *Sci Rep.* (2018) 8:8702. doi: 10.1038/s41598-018-27027-7
53. Nguyen PV, Kafka JK, Ferreira VH, Roth K, Kaushic C. Innate and adaptive immune responses in male and female reproductive tracts in homeostasis and following HIV infection. *Cell Mol Immunol.* (2014) 11:410–27. doi: 10.1038/cmi.2014.41
54. Culshaw A, Mongkolsapaya J, Screaton G. The immunology of Zika Virus. *F1000Res.* (2018) 7:203. doi: 10.12688/f1000research.12271.1
55. Fung KY, Mangan NE, Cumming H, Horvat JC, Mayall JR, Stifter SA, et al. Interferon-epsilon protects the female reproductive tract from viral and bacterial infection. *Science.* (2013) 339:1088–92. doi: 10.1126/science.1233321
56. Caine EA, Scheaffer SM, Arora N, Zaitsev K, Artyomov MN, Coyne CB, et al. Interferon lambda protects the female reproductive tract against Zika virus infection. *Nature Commun.* (2019) 10:280. doi: 10.1038/s41467-018-07993-2
57. Khan S, Woodruff EM, Trapecar M, Fontaine KA, Ezaki A, Borbet TC, et al. Dampened antiviral immunity to intravaginal exposure to RNA viral pathogens allows enhanced viral replication. *J Exp Med.* (2016) 213:2913–29. doi: 10.1084/jem.20161289
58. Wira CR, Rodriguez-Garcia M, Patel MV. The role of sex hormones in immune protection of the female reproductive tract. *Nat Rev Immunol.* (2015) 15:217–30. doi: 10.1038/nri3819
59. Tang WW, Young MP, Mamidi A, Regla-Nava JA, Kim K, Shresta S. A mouse model of Zika virus sexual transmission and vaginal viral replication. *Cell Rep.* (2016) 17:3091–8. doi: 10.1016/j.celrep.2016.11.070
60. Scott JM, Lebratti TJ, Richner JM, Jiang X, Fernandez E, Zhao H, et al. Cellular and humoral immunity protect against vaginal Zika virus infection in mice. *J Virol.* (2018) 92:e00038-18. doi: 10.1128/JVI.00038-18
61. Ghosh M, Rodriguez-Garcia M, Wira, CR. Immunobiology of genital tract trauma: endocrine regulation of HIV acquisition in women following sexual assault or genital tract mutilation. *Am J Reprod Immunol.* (2013) 69:51–60. doi: 10.1111/aji.12027
62. Reiner NE, Judson FN, Bond WW, Francis DP, Petersen NJ. Asymptomatic rectal mucosal lesions and hepatitis B surface antigen at sites of sexual contact in homosexual men with persistent hepatitis B virus infection. *Ann Intern Med.* (1982) 96:170–3. doi: 10.7326/0003-4819-96-2-170
63. Patel MV, Shen Z, Rossoll RM, Wira CR. Estradiol-regulated innate antiviral responses of human endometrial stromal fibroblasts. *Am J Reprod Immunol.* (2018) 80:e13042. doi: 10.1111/aji.13042
64. Winkler CW, Woods TA, Rosenke R, Scott DP, Best SM, Peterson KE. Sexual and vertical transmission of Zika virus in anti-interferon receptor-treated Rag1-deficient mice. *Sci Rep.* (2017) 7:7176. doi: 10.1038/s41598-017-07099-7
65. Quicke KM, Bowen JR, Johnson EL, McDonald CE, Ma H, O'Neal JT, et al. Zika virus infects human placental macrophages. *Cell Host Microbe.* (2016) 20:83–90. doi: 10.1016/j.chom.2016.05.015

18

Klebsiella pneumoniae ST258 Negatively Regulates the Oxidative Burst in Human Neutrophils

Luis A. Castillo[1]*, Federico Birnberg-Weiss[1], Nahuel Rodriguez-Rodrigues[1], Daiana Martire-Greco[1], Fabiana Bigi[2], Veronica I. Landoni[1], Sonia A. Gomez[3] and Gabriela C. Fernandez[1]

[1] Laboratorio de Fisiología de los Procesos Inflamatorios, Instituto de Medicina Experimental (IMEX)- Consejo Nacional de investigaciones Científicas y Tecnológicas (CONICET)/Academia Nacional de Medicina de Buenos Aires, Buenos Aires, Argentina, [2] Instituto de Agrobiotecnología y Biología Molecular (IABIMO), Instituto Nacional de Tecnología Agropecuaria (INTA), Consejo Nacional de investigaciones Científicas y Tecnológicas (CONICET), Buenos Aires, Argentina, [3] Servicio de Antimicrobianos, Instituto Nacional de Enfermedades Infecciosas Dr. Carlos G. Malbrán (INEI), Administración Nacional de Laboratorios e Institutos de Salud (ANLIS), Buenos Aires, Argentina

****Correspondence:***
Luis A. Castillo
luiscastillo718@gmail.com

The epidemic clone of *Klebsiella pneumoniae* (Kpn), sequence type 258 (ST258), carbapenamase producer (KPC), commonly infects hospitalized patients that are left with scarce therapeutic option since carbapenems are last resort antibiotics for life-threatening bacterial infections. To improve prevention and treatment, we should better understand the biology of Kpn KPC ST258 infections. Our hypothesis was that Kpn KPC ST258 evade the first line of defense of innate immunity, the polymorphonuclear neutrophil (PMN), by decreasing its functional response. Therefore, our aim was to evaluate how the ST258 Kpn clone affects PMN responses, focusing on the respiratory burst, compared to another opportunistic pathogen, *Escherichia coli* (Eco). We found that Kpn KPC ST258 was unable to trigger bactericidal responses as reactive oxygen species (ROS) generation and NETosis, compared to the high induction observed with Eco, but both bacterial strains were similarly phagocytized and cause increases in cell size and CD11b expression. The absence of ROS induction was also observed with other Kpn ST258 strains negative for KPC. These results reflect certain selectivity in terms of the functions that are triggered in PMN by Kpn, which seems to evade specifically those responses critical for bacterial survival. In this sense, bactericidal mechanisms evasion was associated with a higher survival of Kpn KPC ST258 compared to Eco. To investigate the mechanisms and molecules involved in ROS inhibition, we used bacterial extracts (BE) and found that BE were able to inhibit ROS generation triggered by the well-known ROS inducer, fMLP. A sequence of experiments led us to elucidate that the polysaccharide part of LPS was responsible for this inhibition, whereas lipid A mediated the other responses that were not affected by bacteria, such as cell size increase and CD11b up-regulation. In conclusion, we unraveled a mechanism of immune evasion of Kpn KPC ST258, which may contribute to design more effective strategies for the treatment of these multi-resistant bacterial infections.

Keywords: immune evasion, *Klebsiella pneumoniae*, neutrophils, respiratory burst, LPS

INTRODUCTION

Klebsiella pneumoniae (Kpn) is a Gram-negative pathogen causing a wide range of infections from urinary tract infections to pneumonia. Kpn is a member of the so-called ESKAPE group of microorganisms, a term that emphasizes the fact that they effectively "escape" the effects of antibacterial drugs (1). Antimicrobial resistance is a significant problem for the treatment of infectious diseases caused by resistant bacteria worldwide. Specifically, resistance to carbapenems, the antibiotics of last resort for life-threatening bacterial infections, has significantly increased mortality and morbidity in patients hospitalized in intensive care units or in long-term care facilities (2). As an example, mortality in patients suffering from bacteriemia or pulmonary infections caused by carbapenem-resistant Kpn strains ranges between ~30 and 70% (3). A clinically relevant Kpn clone has been genetically classified as multilocus sequence type 258 (ST258), which is a hyper-epidemic clone responsible for the global dispersion of carbapenem resistance. This resistance is conferred by an enzyme known as Kpn-Carbapenemase (KPC) (3), and the strains belonging to the ST258 are also resistant to all β-lactam antibiotics and generally contain additional resistance genes that confer resistance to aminoglycosides and quinolones (3). In Argentina, since 2010, the entry of ST258 into the country has altered our health system, since today this clone has been detected in most health institutions of the country (4). Although the ST258 clone is the most extended Kpn KPC lineage, the basis of its success, outside of antibiotic resistance, remains unknown.

In this sense, our hypothesis is that evasion strategies of the ST258 clone could allow it to escape the immune system. This could favor a rapid transmission and persistence within the community, and particularly, in the intra-hospital environment. In fact, some mechanisms of immune evasion in other not-ST258 not-KPC+ Kpn strains have been described, such as the resistance and down-regulation of β-defensins in the lung, the resistance to complement, and a reduction in their phagocytosis. These strategies have been associated with components of the polysaccharide capsule of Kpn, and to mucoviscosity phenotypes (5–8). In particular, the infection biology of Kpn KPC ST258 is poorly understood. The exact consequences of Kpn KPC ST258-PMN interaction need to be elucidated, in order to establish the success of KPC and to start delineating new possible therapeutic approaches.

PMN are the first cell line of antibacterial host defense. During the first steps of PMN activation, an increment in their forward scatter (FSC) flow cytometry parameter occurs. This has been associated with the spreading process itself, but also to the translocation and fusion of easily mobilized granules with the cytoplasmatic membrane (exocytosis), exposing the interior membrane surface of the granules to the exterior, therefore increasing the total surface area of the cell and, in consequence, the FSC (9, 10). Additionally, exocytosis causes the up-regulation in the plasmatic membrane of molecules and receptors involved in PMN adhesion to endothelial cells, such as CD11b.

Upon encountering bacteria, PMN capture, ingest, and kill them by the production of reactive oxygen species (ROS) within intracellular phagosomes (11). ROS are produced by a multicomponent oxidase complex, named the NADPH oxidase, which is unassembled and inactive in resting cells but assembles at the plasma or phagosomal membrane upon PMN activation. Critical elements of the oxidase components are segregated in the membrane and cytosol. Upon activation, these components translocate, in order to interact with the membrane components of the complex, where a functional oxidase is assembled and becomes active. Additionally, PMN were shown to generate web-like extracellular fibers known as neutrophil extracellular traps (NETs), composed of deoxyribonucleic acid (DNA), histones, and antimicrobial granule proteins, which are highly effective at trapping and killing invasive bacteria (12). NETosis is usually dependent on ROS generation, although ROS-independent NETosis has also been reported (13). Moreover, ROS-independent mechanisms are also important in PMN-mediated killing. These mechanisms include the delivery of proteolytic enzymes stored in PMN granules into the phagosome.

Considering the clinical relevance and rapid dissemination of Kpn KPC ST258, it is necessary to better understand the interaction PMN-bacteria in order to design new strategies that might contribute in the treatment of infections with this multi-resistant bacterial strain. Therefore, our aim was to study whether Kpn KPC ST258 is able to actively evade the first line of defense of the immune response, the PMN. For this purpose, we challenged human PMN with Kpn KPC ST258 and measured different PMN responses. For comparison, we used another Gram-negative opportunistic bacillus, *Escherichia coli* (Eco). Moreover, as we found that Kpn KPC ST258 was a poor inducer of ROS generation, the mechanisms and molecules involved in this phenomenon were also investigated.

MATERIALS AND METHODS

Ethics Statement

Human normal samples were obtained from voluntary donors. This study was performed according to institutional guidelines (National Academy of Medicine, Buenos Aires, Argentina) and received the approval of the institutional ethics committee (No. 12524/17/X), and written informed consent was provided by all the subjects.

Blood Samples

Blood samples were obtained from healthy volunteer donors who had not taken any medication for at least 10 days before the day of sampling. Blood was obtained by venipuncture of the forearm vein and was drawn directly into citrated plastic tubes.

Polymorphonuclear Neutrophil (PMN) Isolation

Neutrophils were isolated by Ficoll-Hypaque gradient centrifugation (Ficoll Pharmacia, Uppsala; Hypaque, Wintthrop Products, Buenos Aires, Argentina) and dextran sedimentation, as previously described (14). Contaminating erythrocytes were removed by hypotonic lysis. After washing, the cells (96% neutrophils on May Grünwald/Giemsa-stained Cyto-preps) were suspended in RPMI 1640 supplemented with 2% heat-inactivated fetal calf serum (FCS) and used immediately after.

Bacterial Strains and Cultures

The experiments were performed using two types of Gram-negative bacteria: *E. coli* (ATCC® 25922™) and a local clinical isolate of *Klebsiella pneumoniae* KPC carbapenemase producer, belonging to sequence type 258 (Kpn KPC ST258, Strain ID: M9885. See also **Supplementary Material 1**). Other bacterial strains used were: Kpn ATCC 700603 (not-ST258), three Kpn ST258 KPC negative (M19091, M19216, and M19145), and three Kpn ST258 KPC positive (M22738, M22810, and M22910) strains. For details see **Supplementary Material 1**. Bacteria were grown in Tryptic Soy Broth (TSB) (Britania) for 18 h at 37°C. 100 μL of the culture was added into 10 mL of fresh TSB, and grown for another 4 h with agitation, until the organism reached log phase. Bacteria was pelleted by centrifugation at 9,600 g for 15 min, washed twice in phosphate buffered saline (PBS) 1x, and resuspended at the desired concentration. Bacteria concentration was determined by measuring O.D. at 600 nm, and adjusting to 0.09 absorbance units, that is equivalent to 1×10^8 colony forming units (CFU)/mL; CFU concentration was confirmed by counting on Tryptic Soy Agar (TSA).

Recombinant Bacterial Strains Expressing Green Fluorescent Protein (GFP)

Fifty milliliters of Eco and Kpn KPC ST258 were cultured on LB until O.D. 600 nm = 0.6, harvested by centrifugation at 10,000 g for 10 min and washed four times with one volume of 10% glycerol and finally resuspended in 500 μl of 10% glycerol. These bacteria (50 μl) were electroporated with 1 μg of plasmid pML1335, kindly provided by Dr. Michael Niederweis, at 200 ohms, 2.5 V and 25 μFa. Plasmid pML1335 (15) contains the GFP gene under mycobacterial promotor (Psmyc). This vector carries ColE1 for replication and a hygromycin resistance gene. After electroporation bacteria were cultivated in 1 ml of SOC medium during 1 h and then plated on LB agar with hygromycin (200 μg/ml). Plates were incubated overnight at 37°C. The presence of GFP in individual colonies was evaluated by microscopy, irradiating the bacteria with ultraviolet light. Only colonies containing "green" bacteria were selected and used in further experiments.

Phagocytosis Studies

Flow Cytometry

PMN (1×10^6) were incubated with 1×10^7 CFU of GFP-Kpn KPC ST258 or GFP-Eco for 1 h at 37°C (total bacteria-PMN interaction) or 4°C (for bacterial adhesion) in 5% CO_2. After incubation, GFP+ PMN were evaluated by flow cytometry and expressed as the percentage of PMN associated to GFP-bacteria (37°C) or the percentage of PMN with bacteria attached (4°C). The percentage of phagocytosis was calculated subtracting the percentage of adhesion to the total interaction.

Confocal Laser Scanning Microscopy

PMN (3×10^5) were mixed with 3×10^6 CFU of GFP-Kpn KPC ST258 or GFP-Eco in cold RPMI with 2% FCS and seeded gently onto glass coverslips coated with 0.001% poly-L-lysine in a 24-well plate. Assay plates were centrifuged at 524 g during 5 min at 4°C to synchronize phagocytosis. Samples were incubated at 37°C in 5% CO_2 during 1 h, fixed with 4% PFA, permeabilized with Triton X-100 0.25%, and stained with 1 μg/mL TRIT-C Phalloidin (Sigma-Aldrich) in order to observe PMN actin, and 1 μg/mL TOPRO-3 (ThermoFisher Scientific) for DNA staining, during 1 h. High resolution images were acquired using a FluoView FV1000 confocal microscope (Olympus, Tokyo, Japan) equipped with a Plapon 60x/1·42 objective lens and processed using Olympus Flow view software. First, to perform a random acquisition of images, PMN were focused on TRIT-C Phalloidin staining only, and 10 fields were observed, with at least 5 cells/field. The acquisition of each field was performed in Z-Stack mode, acquiring one frame every 1.2 μm from the upper focal plane to the lower plane. Images were analyzed using the Fiji software with the aid of the orthogonal view, in order to distinguish between internalized and adhered bacteria. Phagocytized bacterium were defined as a GFP+ particle surrounded by PMN actin, observed in both XZ and YZ planes of the orthogonal view. Values were expressed as the percentage of PMN with GFP+ bacteria internalized or adhered. The number of bacteria internalized *per* PMN was also quantified.

Bactericidal Activity Assays

Killing of bacteria by PMNs was determined using PMNs (1×10^6) combined with 1×10^6 of bacteria in 24-well tissue culture plate. One hour after incubation PMN were lysed with H_2O. The resultant solution was plated on TSA in serial dilutions. CFU were enumerated the following day, and the relative CFU was calculated with the following equation: (CFU + PMN/CFU – PMN) × 100, where CFU + PMN was the number of CFU in the presence of PMN and CFU – PMN was the number of CFU in the absence of PMN.

Bacterial Extracts

Mechanical disruption of bacteria was performed using 0.1 mm Zirconia beads as described previously (16). Briefly, bacterial strains were cultured in 10 mL of TSB until log phase. Bacteria was pelleted by centrifugation at 9,600 g for 15 min, washed twice in PBS 1x, resuspended in 500 μL of PBS 1x with 300 mg of Zirconia beads, and then strongly vortexed during 5 min. The suspension was centrifuged at 9,600 g for 15 min and the supernatant (bacterial extract, BE) was stored.

Protein Quantification

Protein concentration in bacteria or BE was determined using the Bradford Method (17). A standard curve using bovine serum albumin ranging from 50 to 250 μg/ml was used.

Polysaccharide Quantification

The amount of polysaccharides was determined using the phenol-sulfuric method. Briefly, 100 μL of the BE was mixed with phenol 6% and sulfuric acid 98%, incubated during 1 h and the resultant yellow-gold color was read at 490 nm.

Assay for Degradation of Hydrogen Peroxide (H_2O_2)

H_2O_2 degradation was evaluated over time using a DeNovix DS-11spectrophotometer (DeNovix Inc.), by means of the property of peroxide to absorb at 240 nm. H_2O_2 0.036% v/v absorbance was evaluated during 240 s, with or without BE (10 µg/mL of protein). A decay control was performed by the addition of 10 Units of catalase.

Evaluation of the Importance of Protein Content in BE

Heat Treatment

BE were treated for 60 min at 60°C for protein denaturalization and enzyme inactivation.

Trichloroacetic Acid Precipitation (TCA)

In order to precipitate proteins, TCA (15% v/v) was added to BE. The solution was incubated 30 min at −4°C and centrifuged at 9,600 g for 15 min. The supernatant was discarded, the pellet (protein fraction) was resuspended in PBS 1x and precipitated once again with pure acetone during 2 h at −4°C. After that, suspension was centrifuged and acetone was evaporated by dried air incubation. Dried protein fraction (PF) was resuspended in PBS 1x and adjusted to pH = 7.0 with NaOH 0.5 N. Final protein concentration was measured using the Bradford Method and adjusted to 100 µg/mL. TCA precipitated 97% of total proteins measured as stated in section Protein Quantification.

Evaluation of the Importance of Polysaccharides Content in BE

Concanavalin a (Con A) Precipitation

Depletion of molecules containing mannose was performed by precipitation with 10 µg/mL Con A (Sigma-Aldrich) in the presence of 10 mM Ca^2 (Merck) for 30 min at 37°C. After incubation, the solution was centrifuged at 9,600 g for 30 min. and the supernatant, free of containing mannose molecules, was reserved. Con A precipitates 75% of total carbohydrates, measured as stated in Polysaccharide Quantification.

Oxidation With Periodic Acid (PA)

When treated with PA, glycols are oxidized to aldehydes, losing their biological effect. In this sense, BE were oxidized with PA (Sigma-Aldrich) at a 0.1% final concentration, and stirred during 1 h. After oxidation, the solution was neutralized with NaOH 0.5 N until pH = 7.0.

LPS Depletion and Isolation

Depletion of LPS was performed using a Polymyxin B-Agarose column (Sigma-Aldrich). The column was washed with endotoxin-free 0.1 M ammonium bicarbonate buffer (pH = 8.0), in order to remove the glycerol storage solution; then it was centrifuged at 9,600 g for 5 min and resuspended with an equal volume of BE. The polymyxin B-Agarose-BE suspension was stirred for 30 min at 37°C, and then it was centrifuged at 9,600 g for 10 min and the supernatant (BE-LPS) was reserved.

LPS was eluted from the column using 1% sodium deoxycholate (Sigma-Aldrich) and then the solution was dialyzed to eliminate the salt and resuspended in endotoxin-free water.

Flow Cytometry Studies

5×10^5 PMN were incubated with a specific mouse anti-human CD11b antibody conjugated with phycoerythrin (PE) (Dako, Santa Clara, CA, USA). Debris was excluded by FSC-SSC, and the increase on FSC or CD11b expression was analyzed within the gated-viable PMN. Mean fluorescence intensity of the CD11b was determined on 50.000 events.

Measurement of Fluctuations in Intracellular Ca^{2+}

Changes in intracellular Ca^{2+} were monitored using Fluo-3AM (Sigma Aldrich), as previously described (18). Briefly, neutrophils suspended at a concentration of 5×10^6 cells/ml in RPMI 1640 were incubated with 4 mM Fluo-3AM for 20 min at 30°C. Then loaded cells were washed twice and suspended at 5×10^6 cells/ml in RPMI 1640 supplemented with 1% FCS. Aliquots of 15 µl of this cell suspension were added to 300 µl of RPMI 1640 medium containing 1% FCS and warmed at 37°C. The samples were immediately loaded onto the flow cytometer, and the basal fluorescence (FL-1) was recorded during 15 s. Then cells were stimulated with fMLP (10^{-7} M), and the fluorescence was recorded during an additional 150 s. Acquisition of samples was performed at 37°C. Fluctuations in cytoplasmatic free calcium concentrations were recognized as alterations in Fluo-3AM fluorescence intensity over time.

Reactive Oxygen Species (ROS) Generation

To determine the production of ROS by flow cytometry DHR-123, a derivative of rhodamine 123, was used following the protocol described by Leech et al. (19). Briefly, isolated PMN (5×10^5) were incubated 15 min at 37°C with 1 µM DHR-123. Subsequently, the cells were incubated with or without the stimuli for 30 min at 37°C 5% CO_2 in a humidified atmosphere. Immediately after, the green fluorescence was determined.

Neutrophil Extracellular Traps (NETs) Formation

PMN (5×10^5) were seeded gently onto glass coverslips coated with 0.001% poly-L-lysine in a 24-well plate in triplicate, allowed to settle, and incubated in the presence of bacteria (bacteria:PMN ratio 20:1). Cells were incubated for 3 h at 37°C 5% CO_2. After the incubation period, samples were gently fixed with 4% PFA, then washed with PBS 1x, and stained for DNA with propidium iodide (Vector Laboratories) and elastase using a specific antibody anti-PMN elastase (Merk Millipore, Darmstadt, Germany). Images for NETs evaluation were acquired using a FluoView FV1000 confocal microscope (Olympus, Tokyo, Japan) equipped with a Plapon 60x/1·42 objective lens and processed using Olympus. At least 10 different fields were observed in each triplicate (×200). NETs areas were determined as previously reported (20) in at least five pictures obtained in ×200 using the wand tool of the

FIJI software (21). The scale for the measurement was obtained from the data given in the confocal microscope image.

Chemotaxis

Chemotaxis was quantified using a modification of the Boyden chamber technique (22). A cell suspension (50 μl) containing 2 × 10^6 cells/ml in RPMI with 2% FCS, was placed in the top wells of a 48-well micro-chemotaxis chamber. A PVP-free polycarbonate membrane (3 μm pore size; Neuro Probe Inc. Gaithersburg MD, USA) separated the cells from lower wells containing either RPMI or the stimulus. The chamber was incubated for 30 min at 37°C in a 5% CO_2 humidified atmosphere. After incubation, the filter was stained with TINCION-15 (Biopur SRL, Rosario, Argentina), and the number of PMN on the undersurface of the filter was counted in a five random high-power fields (HPF) ×400 for each of triplicate filters.

Statistical Analysis

Results were expressed as the mean ± SEM. Statistical analysis of the data was performed using the analysis of variance (ANOVA), applying Tukey's post-test. $P < 0.05$ were considered significant.

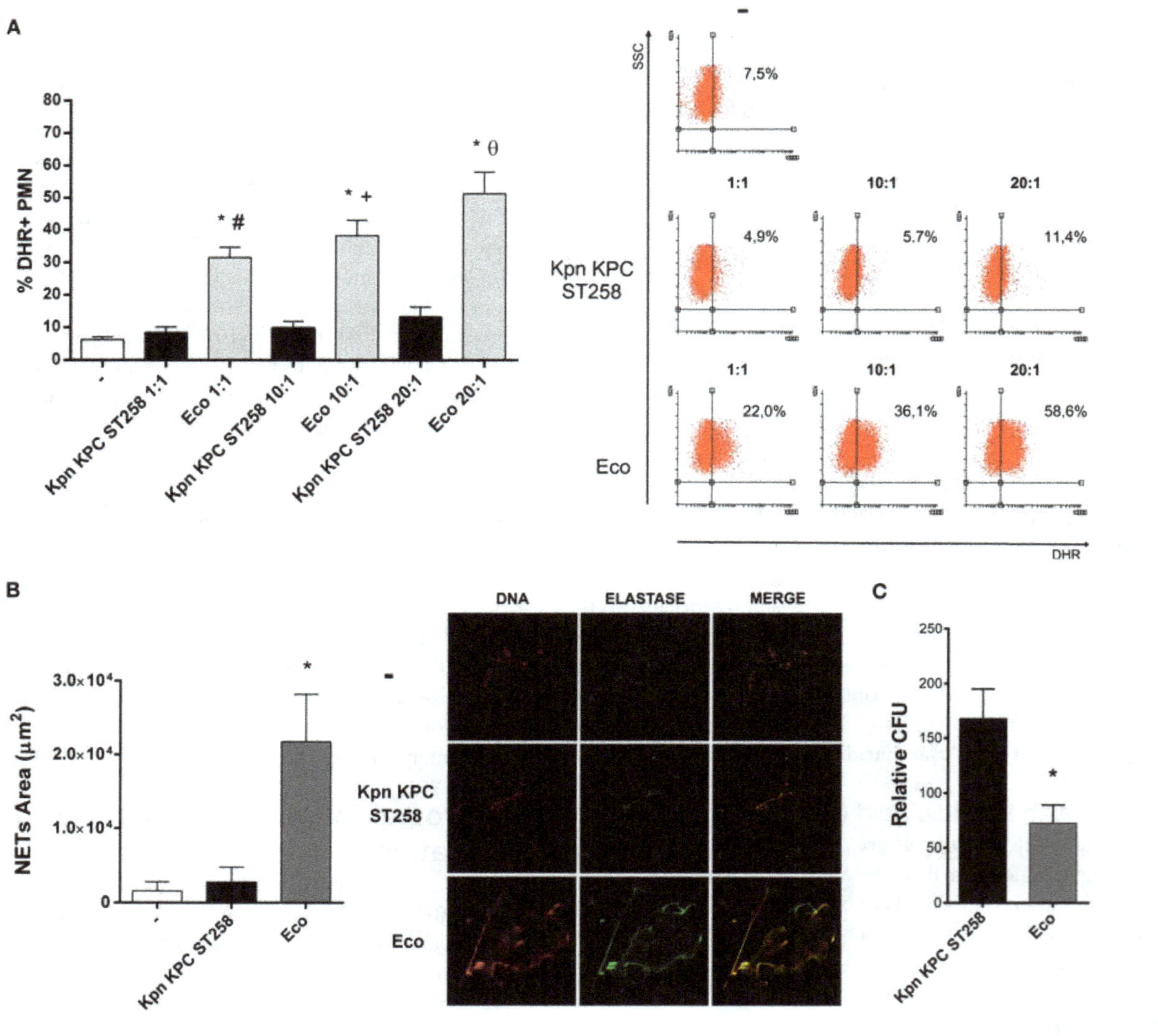

FIGURE 1 | Kpn KPC ST258 is a poor inducer of ROS generation. Kpn KPC ST258 and Eco were incubated with isolated human PMN in different Bacteria:PMN ratios for 30 min. ROS was measured by flow cytometry using DHR. **(A)** Percentage (%) of DHR + PMN. Right panel: Representative dot-plots showing the SSC vs. DHR profiles. $n = 10$; $^*p < 0.05$ vs. untreated (-); # $p < 0.05$ vs. Kpn KPC ST258 1:1, $+p < 0.05$ vs. Kpn KPC ST258 10:1; $\theta\ p < 0.05$ vs. Kpn KPC ST258 20:1. **(B)** Isolated PMN were incubated with Kpn KPC ST258 and Eco in a Bacteria:PMN ratio of 20:1 for 3 h. NETs were stained for DNA and elastase and were visualized by confocal microscopy. NETs area (μm^2) was measured using the FIJI software as described in material and methods. $n = 10$. $^*p < 0.05$ vs. untreated (-) and vs. Kpn KPC ST258. Right panel: Representative microphotographs of confocal images showing PMN from the untreated (-), Kpn KPC ST258, and Eco groups stained for DNA or elastase visualization and the merge of the images (x 200). **(C)** Kpn KPC ST258 or Eco were incubated for 1 h with PMN and the remaining viable colony forming units (CFU) were evaluated using TSA plates. Relative CFU was calculated as indicated in material and methods. $n = 9$. $^*p < 0.05$ vs. Kpn KPC ST258. In all cases, results are expressed as the mean ± SEM.

RESULTS

Kpn KPC ST258 Triggers a Poor Respiratory Burst in PMN

Considering the clinical importance of the hyper-epidemic clone of Kpn producer of carbapenemase (KPC) that belongs to the ST258 (Kpn KPC ST258), we focused our study on this bacterial clone. We first investigated the respiratory burst, which plays an important role in innate immunity against invading microorganisms using different bacteria:PMN ratios. The fluorogenic dye, dihydrorhodamine 123 (DHR), was used for detection of reactive oxygen species (ROS). As shown in **Figure 1A**, ROS generation was strongly induced after 30 min when PMN were challenged with Eco. However, Kpn KPC ST258 was not able to induce a respiratory burst in PMN in any of the ratios assayed. The possibility that Kpn KPC ST258 was a slower inducer of ROS was ruled out as the percentages of ROS-producing PMN at 1 and 2 h were 8.8 and 10.8%, respectively,

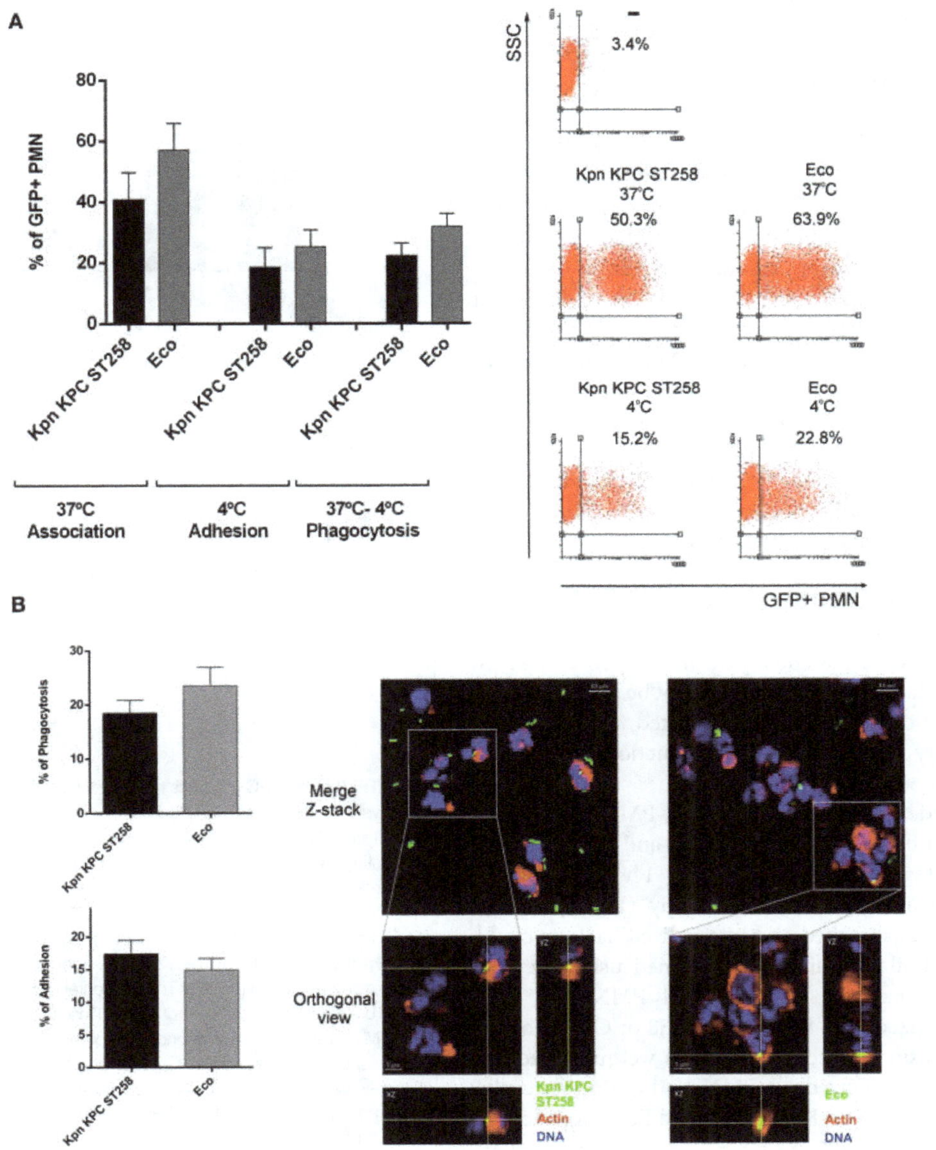

FIGURE 2 | Kpn KPC ST258 and Eco are similarly phagocytized by PMN. Percentage of phagocytosis and bacterial attachment were evaluated by both flow cytometry **(A)** and confocal microscopy **(B)** techniques. GFP-Kpn KPC ST258 and GFP-Eco were incubated with isolated human PMN as described in material and methods. **(A)** Percentage of association and adhesion of GFP-bacteria to PMN were measured at 37°C and 4°C, respectively. Percentage of PMN that have phagocytized GFP-Bacteria was calculated by subtraction (37°C–4°C). $n = 8$. Right panel: Representative Dot-Plots. **(B)** Percentage of PMN with phagocytized or adhered GFP-Bacteria evaluated by confocal microscopy. $n = 5$. Right panel: representative Z-Stack merged microphotographs and orthogonal view, showing PMN with phagocytized GFP-Bacteria. Actin was stained with TRIT-C phalloidin (red) and DNA with TOPRO-3 (blue). Images were analyzed using Fiji software as described in materials and methods. In all cases results were expressed as the mean ± SEM.

and were not different from the percentage observed at 30 min (data not shown).

The viability of PMN was measured in parallel by flow cytometry using propidium iodide, and none of the conditions assayed induced cell death (**Supplementary Material 2**). We decided to use a bacteria:PMN ratio of 20:1 to perform all the experiments that followed.

We next wanted to address the importance of carrying KPC in the lack of ROS induction by Kpn. We performed the assay using other Kpn strains: one ATCC, not ST258, three other clinical isolates of Kpn ST258 but negative for KPC, and three other clinical isolates of Kpn ST258 positive for KPC. We found that all ST258 clinical isolated of Kpn were unable to induce a respiratory burst in PMN independently of the presence of KPC (**Supplementary Material 3**). Moreover, the ATCC strain was also a poor inducer of ROS in PMN.

As the production of ROS has been associated with the capacity of PMN to form NETs (23), we also evaluated NETosis triggered by Kpn KPC ST258. **Figure 1B** shows that Kpn KPC ST258 was also a poor inducer of NETosis after 3 h of incubation, whereas Eco induced a significant amount of NETs.

Next, to evaluate whether the poor induction of ROS and NETs by Kpn results in increased bacterial survival, PMN were incubated with Kpn KPC ST258 or Eco for 1 h. Then, cells were lysed and total colony formation units (CFU) were determined on agar plates. As shown in **Figure 1C**, the CFU count for Kpn KPC ST258 was higher compared to Eco.

Altogether, these results indicate that Kpn KPC ST258 is a poor inducer of important PMN bactericidal mechanisms, and this is associated with higher bacterial survival.

PMN Are Able to Sense Kpn KPC ST258

Taking into account the results found in the previous section, we next asked if Kpn KPC ST258 could be sense by PMN. If PMN recognizes Kpn, the lack of response would not be due to the lack of interaction/ingestion, and could be associated with some type of active modulatory mechanism of PMN functionality fulfilled by the bacterium.

Therefore, in order to investigate bacteria-PMN interaction, we used GFP-recombinant Kpn KPC ST258 and GFP-Eco and analyze the percentage of phagocytosis after 1 h of incubation by flow cytometry and confocal microscopy (**Figures 2A,B**). Using both techniques, attached and internalized bacteria could be distinguished. Similar results were obtained using the two different techniques and the percentage of PMN that have attached or phagocytized GFP-Kpn KPC ST258 or GFP-Eco was similar. Moreover, using the confocal images we quantified the number of bacteria internalized *per* PMN, and again the results obtained were similar for Kpn KPC ST258 and Eco (No. bacteria internalized *per* PMN: Kpn KPC ST258 = 1.17 ± 0.18, Eco = 1.20 ± 0.04, $n = 5$).

To determine whether this bacteria-PMN interaction leads to PMN activation, we measured the increase in their FSC, a rapid and sensitive parameter related to initial sensing of inflammatory/infectious stimuli. Kpn KPC ST258 was equally capable of inducing an FSC increase in PMN compared to Eco (**Figure 3A**). Moreover, initial steps in PMN activation involve

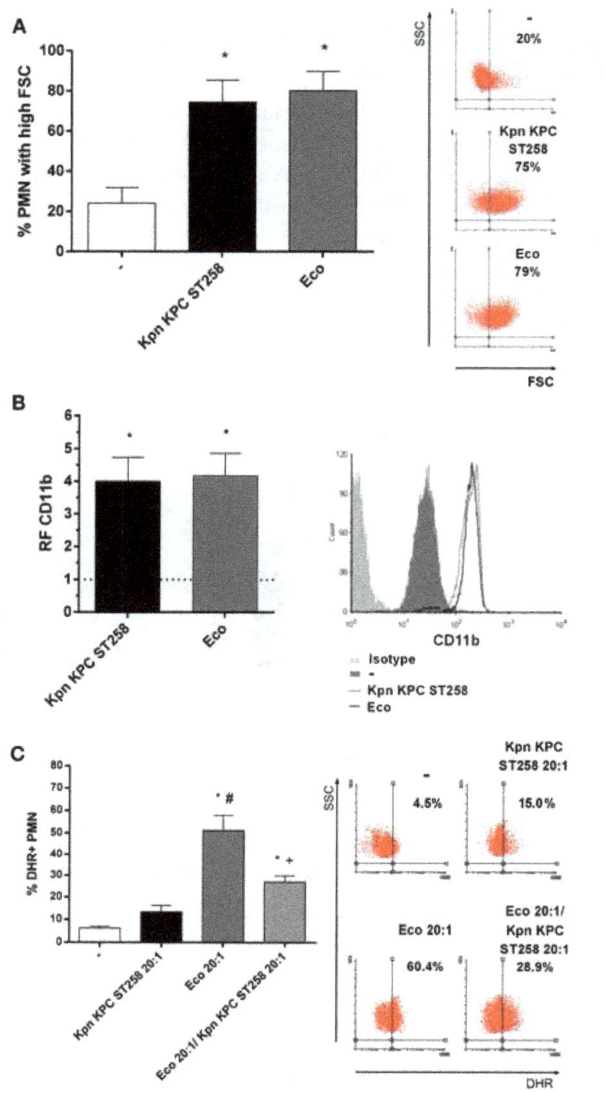

FIGURE 3 | Kpn KPC ST258 is recognized by PMN. Kpn KPC ST258 and Eco were incubated with isolated human PMN in a Bacteria:PMN ratio of 20:1 for 30 min. **(A)** The % of PMN that increased their Forward Size Scatter (FSC) after stimulation with Kpn KPC ST258 or Eco, or left untreated (-) was determined by flow cytometry. Results were expressed as the mean ± SEM, $n = 8$. $^*p < 0.05$ vs. (-). Right panel: representative dot-plots showing SSC vs. FSC profiles of PMN with no treatment (-), Kpn KPC ST258 or Eco. **(B)** Expression of CD11b. The MFI of the adhesion marker CD11b was determined by flow cytometry. The horizontal dashed-line represents the CD11b expression of the control group. Results were expressed as the mean ± SEM of the relative fluorescence (RF) of the MFI of the different treatments with respect to untreated PMN. $n = 5$. $^*p < 0.05$ vs. (-). Right panel: Representative histogram of the expression of CD11b in the different experimental groups. **(C)** % of DHR+ PMN of Kpn KPC ST258-Eco co-cultures. Results were expressed as the mean ± SEM. $n = 5$. $^*p < 0.05$ vs. untreated (-); # $p < 0.05$ vs. Kpn KPC ST258 20:1, +$p < 0.05$ vs. Eco 20:1. Right panel: representative dot-plots showing SSC vs. DHR profiles.

the mobilization of intracellular granules, resulting in the up-regulation in the plasma membrane of molecules that were present in the membrane of intracellular granules. This is the case of CD11b that was measured on the surface of PMN after incubation with the different bacterial strains. As depicted in **Figure 3B**, the up-regulation of CD11b in PMN was similar for Kpn KPC ST258 and Eco. Altogether, these results indicate that Kpn KPC ST258 was interacting with PMN, and although PMN was similarly sensing Kpn KPC ST258 and Eco, for Kpn, this sensing caused dual effects on PMN, modulating some functions positively, but negatively regulating others.

Moreover, in order to investigate whether Kpn KPC ST258 was able to interfere with ROS induced by other bacteria, we co-cultured PMN with Kpn KPC ST258 and Eco and found that Kpn KPC ST258 was able to decrease the respiratory burst triggered by Eco (**Figure 3C**). Again, the diminished ROS generation was not due to PMN death caused by bacterial mixture (**Supplementary Material 2**). This result indicates that Kpn KPC ST258 is delivering a negative signal in PMN that also affects the response to other stimuli.

A Bacterial Cell Wall Component of Kpn KPC ST258 Inhibits ROS Generation Triggered by fMLP

In order to study which component was involved in the regulation of ROS by Kpn KPC ST258, we performed bacterial extracts (BE) enriched in bacterial cell wall components and used these BE in a ROS production assay, triggering ROS with fMLP, a well-known ROS inducer. The use of strong positive inducer is critical to evidence an active inhibitory mechanism. Moreover, we also used Eco BE to determine whether ROS modulation was exclusive for Kpn. The concentration of BE used was approximately equivalent to the amount of protein found in 1 $\times 10^7$ CFU, corresponding to a bacteria:PMN ratio of 20:1. Even though none of the BE by themselves were able to trigger ROS in PMN, when we evaluated the modulation of ROS generation induced with fMLP by BE (**Figure 4A**), we observed a statistically significant reduction in the % of ROS-producing PMN by Kpn KPC ST258 BE, whereas Eco BE did not affect the percentage of ROS-producing PMN.

As the main components of BE are proteins and polysaccharides, we quantified both types of molecules in BE from Kpn KPC ST258 and Eco and performed the ROS generation measurements normalizing Kpn KPC ST258 and Eco BE according to their protein or polysaccharide content. The inhibition of ROS generation caused by Kpn KPC ST258 BE was similar when BE concentrations were normalized according to their protein or polysaccharide content (**Supplementary Material 4**).

In contrast to the inhibition observed for ROS generation, and similarly to what was observed with the whole bacteria, BE from Kpn KPC ST258 and Eco were equally able to increase the FSC of PMN and their CD11b expression (**Figures 4B,C**). When incubated together with fMLP, none of the BE negatively modulated the FSC and CD11b expression increases induced by fMLP.

Considering the above result, the first issue we wanted to exclude was that BE from Kpn KPC ST258 may contain components that were able to scavenge or directly degrade hydrogen peroxide (H_2O_2), the product detected in the ROS generation assay used in this study. For this purpose, we measured H_2O_2 degradation over time, by means of the property of H_2O_2 to absorb at 240 nm. As shown in **Figure 4D**, the addition of catalase, used as a positive control, caused a rapid decrease in the absorbance of H_2O_2, whereas Kpn KPC ST258 BE did not affect H_2O_2 levels over time. This result indicates that the component responsible for fMLP-induced ROS inhibition is not scavenging H_2O_2.

Mechanisms Involved in Kpn KPC ST258 BE-Mediated Inhibition of fMLP-Induced ROS

PMN's fMLP receptor belongs to the family of G-protein-coupled seven-transmembrane receptors (24). We wanted to address if Kpn KPC ST258 BE may be also affecting ROS generation triggered in response to other stimuli that signal by a different receptor of the same family of seven-transmembrane receptors. As shown in **Figure 5A**, leukotriene B_4 (LB_4) was able to induce ROS, and the presence of Kpn KPC ST258 BE partially abolished this induction. Therefore, the inhibition of ROS by BE is not specific for fMLP, and it may affect a common signaling pathway triggered by other G-protein-coupled seven-transmembrane receptors.

Then, we asked whether Kpn KPC ST258 could also modulate other PMN functions triggered by fMLP. We evaluated chemotaxis toward fMLP using a Boyden chamber in the presence or absence of Kpn KPC ST258 BE and found that, similarly to what was observed in ROS generation, the presence of Kpn KPC ST258 BE partially decreased the number of PMN that migrate toward fMLP (**Figure 5B**).

We next wanted to study the mechanism involved in the inhibition of fMLP-induced ROS production mediated by Kpn KPC ST258. One of the first steps in fMLP signaling is the mobilization of Calcium (Ca^{2+}) from intracellular stores (24). In order to evaluate whether the inhibitory component present in Kpn KPC ST258 BE was affecting Ca^{2+} mobilization, we used a Fluo 3-AM probe and evaluated intracellular variations in Ca^{2+} levels by flow cytometry measuring the increase in the fluorescence of this reactive over time, in the presence or absence of Kpn KPC ST258 BE, using fMLP as the stimulus. As depicted in **Figure 6A**, the intracellular Ca^{2+} mobilization induced by fMLP was not affected by the presence of Kpn KPC ST258 BE. These results indicate that Kpn KPC ST258 BE is not inhibiting fMLP-induced ROS by affecting Ca^{2+} mobilization.

Another possibility was that Kpn KPC ST258 BE could be interfering with the final steps necessary for ROS induction, that is, NADPH oxidase assembly. PMA is often used to bypass cell surface receptors and induce a more direct activation of the NADPH oxidase via a direct protein kinase C-mediated phosphorylation of $p47^{phox}$ (25). Therefore, we evaluated ROS production using PMA as a stimulus in the presence or absence of Kpn KPC ST258 BE (**Figure 6B**). We found that PMA induced a strong respiratory burst in PMN, and the presence of Kpn KPC ST258 BE was not able to modulate it, indicating that the component/s of Kpn KPC ST258 BE that are inhibiting ROS production are not acting at the NADPH oxidase assembly level.

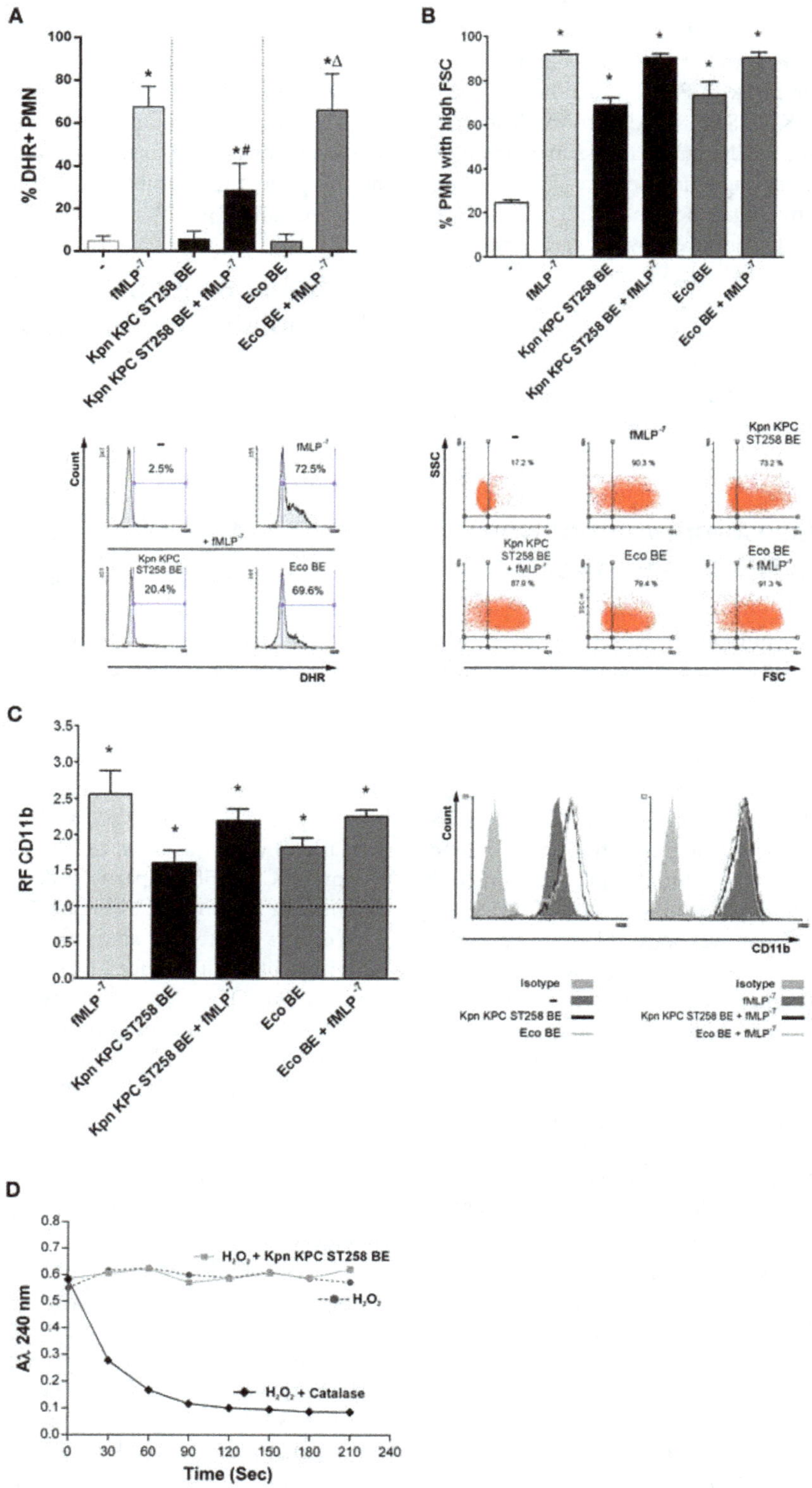

FIGURE 4 | A bacterial cell wall component of Kpn KPC ST258 inhibits ROS generation. Bacterial extracts (BE) from Kpn KPC ST258 or Eco were obtained and PMN were incubated for 30 min with these BE (10 μg/mL of total protein) in the presence or absence of fMLP (10^{-7} M). **(A)** ROS generation. The percentage of DHR+ PMN was determined by flow cytometry. $n = 10$. Results were expressed as the mean ± SEM. *$p < 0.05$ vs. untreated (-); # $p < 0.05$ vs. fMLP^{-7}; Δ$p < 0.05$ vs. Kpn KPC ST258 BE + fMLP^{-7}. Lower panel: Representative histograms of SSC vs. DHR. **(B)** FSC increase. The percentage of PMN that increased their FSC was determined by flow cytometry. $n = 10$. Results were expressed as the mean ± SEM. *$p < 0.05$ vs. (-). Lower panel: Representative dot-plots of SSC vs. FSC profiles.

(Continued)

FIGURE 4 | (C) CD11b expression. The MFI of the adhesion marker CD11b was determined by flow cytometry and expressed as the relative fluorescence (RF) of the MFI of the different treatments with respect to untreated PMN. $n = 10$. Results were expressed as the mean ± SEM; *$p < 0.05$ vs. (-). Right panel: Representative histograms of CD11b expression. **(D)** H_2O_2 degradation over time. The absorbance at 240 nm was recorded for H_2O_2 (0.036% v/v) in the presence of catalase (10 U) or Kpn KPC ST258 BE (10 µg/mL of total protein). $n = 3$.

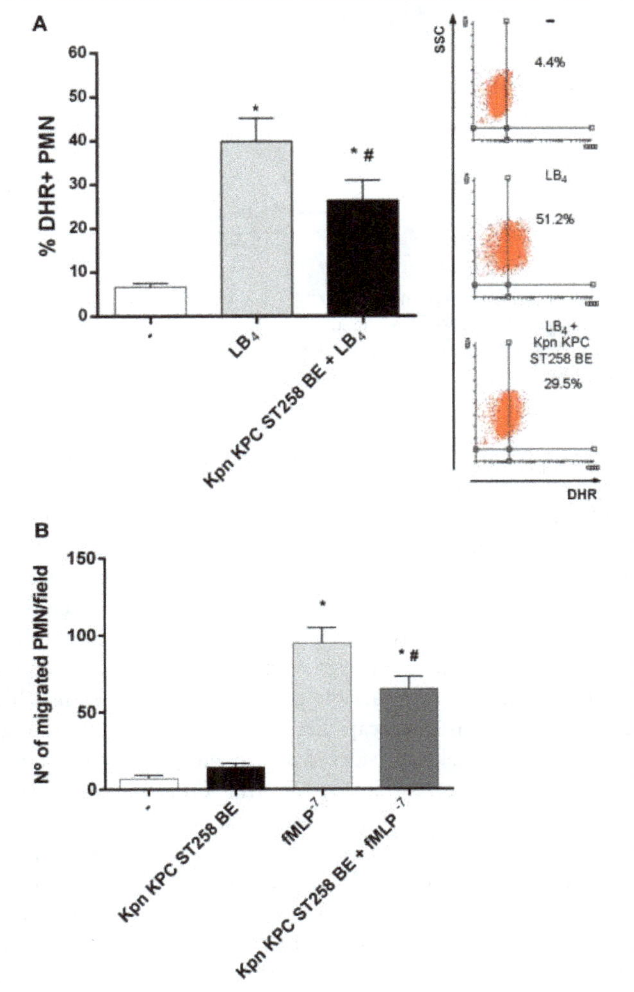

FIGURE 5 | BE from Kpn KPC ST258 inhibits ROS mediated by leukotriene B_4 (LB_4), and also negatively modulates other functions mediated by fMLP. **(A)** ROS was triggered by LB_4 (0.1 µg/mL) in the presence or absence of Kpn KPC ST258 BE and the % of DHR+ PMN was measured by flow cytometry. Results were expressed as the mean ± SEM. Right panel: Representative dot-plot showing SSC vs. DHR profiles. $n = 7$; *$p < 0.05$ vs. untreated (-); # $p < 0.05$ vs. LB_4. **(B)** Chemotactic response using a Boyden chamber. The number of PMN that have migrated toward fMLP (10^{-7} M) through a 3 µm-pore membrane in the presence or absence of Kpn KPC ST258 BE is shown. Results were expressed as the mean ± SEM, $n = 6$; *$p < 0.05$ vs. (-); # $p < 0.05$ vs. fMLP^{-7}.

The Inhibitory Component of Kpn KPC ST258 BE Is a Polysaccharide

In order to investigate the nature of the component that mediates the inhibition of fMLP-induced ROS generation, we first evaluated the possible contribution of proteins in this phenomenon. We performed a heat treatment of Kpn KPC ST258 BE (60 min at 60°C) to denature proteins and abolish any enzymatic activity. As **Figure 7A** shows, the ability of Kpn KPC ST258 BE to inhibit ROS generation by fMLP was not modified by heat treatment. Moreover, to exclude the possible participation of a structural component of proteins, independently of their enzymatic activity, protein precipitation was performed, and this precipitated fraction (PF) was used to evaluate its direct inhibitory potential. We found that precipitated proteins from BE were not able to inhibit fMLP-induced ROS production.

Polysaccharides are the other major component of bacterial cell walls. Taking into account that mannose is a usual polysaccharide residue found in bacterial walls, and considering that concanavalin A (Con A) binds mannose residues and is able to precipitate mannose-containing molecules (26), we incubate Kpn KPC ST258 BE with Con A, and then centrifuged this Con A-treated Kpn KPC ST258 BE in order to deplete mannose-containing molecules from these BE. As depicted in **Figure 7B**, Con A treatment abolished the ability of Kpn KPC ST258 BE to inhibit fMLP-induced ROS generation. Moreover, polysaccharides can be oxidized by periodic acid (PA) losing their native conformation (27). Treatment of Kpn KPC ST258 BE with PA also abolished Kpn KPC ST258 BE's ability to inhibit fMLP-induced ROS generation (**Figure 7C**).

Altogether, these results indicate that the inhibitory ability of Kpn KPC ST258 BE is not dependent on a protein but is mediated by a mannose-containing molecule. More specifically, we could identify the direct participation of a polysaccharide in the inhibitory phenomenon.

The Polysaccharide Part of LPS of Kpn KPC ST258 Inhibits fMLP-Induced ROS

Lipopolysaccharide (LPS) is a major component of Gram-negative bacteria membranes. LPS is localized in the outer layer of the membrane and is, in non-capsulated strains as Kpn KPC ST258, exposed on the cell surface. LPS is comprised of a hydrophilic polysaccharide and a hydrophobic component known as lipid A. The antibiotic Polymyxin B (PMX) interacts with the lipid A of LPS and it can be used, when conjugated to agarose beads, to deplete the entire LPS molecule from solutions. When Kpn KPC ST258 BE were depleted using this PMX column, and the depleted fraction (-LPS) was used in ROS production triggered by fMLP, we found that depletion of LPS completely abolished BE's ability to inhibit ROS (**Figure 8A**). In accordance, when LPS was recovered from the column by elution with sodium deoxycholate, dialyzed and this purified LPS was evaluated for its inhibitory properties, we observed a direct inhibition of LPS on fMLP-induced ROS. Moreover, we used the PMX ability to neutralize lipid A-mediating effects to confirm the involvement of the polysaccharide part of LPS in the inhibition of

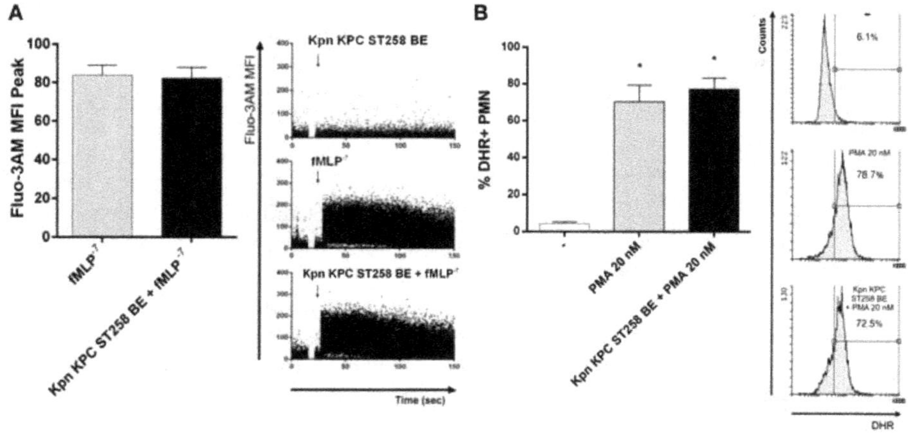

FIGURE 6 | (A) Intracellular Ca^{2+} mobilization. PMN were incubated with Fluo 3-AM and Ca^{2+} mobilization was triggered by fMLP in the presence or absence of Kpn KPC ST258 BE and the mean ± SEM of the peak MFI of Fluo 3-AM is shown. $n = 6$. Right panel: Representative dot-plots profiles of one representative experiment out of three showing the Fluo 3-AM fluorescence over time. **(B)** ROS triggered by PMA in the presence or absence of KPC ST258 BE. Results were expressed as the mean ± SEM of the % of DHR+ PMN. $n = 7$. $^*p < 0.05$ vs. (-). Right panel: Representative histograms showing SSC vs. DHR profiles.

ROS generation. For this purpose, soluble PMX was added to BE and the mixture Kpn KPC ST258 BE+PMX was added to PMN for evaluation. In this case, the addition of PMX in BE did not reverse the inhibitory effect mediated by Kpn KPC ST258 BE, ruling out any role of lipid-A in the inhibitory effect of LPS.

LPS-depleted fractions of Kpn KPC ST258 BE also lost their PMN stimulating properties, measured by the increase in the % of FSC and CD11b, whereas Kpn KPC ST258 BE+PMX directly added to PMN abolished the capacity of BE to induce an increase in the FSC and CD11b expression (**Figures 8B,C**).

Altogether, these results account for the polysaccharide part of LPS as responsible for the inhibition of fMLP-induced ROS.

DISCUSSION

Infections caused by KPC-producing Kpn ST258 are a major cause of healthcare-associated infections worldwide, including ventilator-associated pneumonia and catheter-related bloodstream infections (28, 29), and have been associated with increased cost and length of stay as well as frequent treatment failures and death (30–32). KPC producers are multidrug resistant (especially to all β-lactams), and therapeutic options for treating KPC-related infections remain limited. In parallel with their adaptation to antimicrobial exposure, some studies have demonstrated that these microorganisms have evolved mechanisms to evade host innate immune clearance. Evasion strategies are dangerous as persistence and chronic colonization not only select for more fit organisms, as previously demonstrated (33), but also increase the potential for invasive infection and further development of antibiotic resistance, particularly in vulnerable patient populations. Considering the clinical relevance of Kpn KPC ST258, in this study, we were interested in analyzing the interaction of this clone of Kpn with human PMN, a key cell of the innate immune response, in an effort to better understand the infection biology of this pathogen, a necessary aspect for the potential design of new strategies to treat Kpn infections.

Our results indicate that Kpn KPC ST258 is a poor inducer of the main bactericidal responses of PMN, ROS generation, and NETs formation compared to another opportunistic Gram-negative bacillus, like *E. coli*. ST258 is the most common sequence type of antibiotic resistant Kpn in our country and others (4, 34). However, these bacteria readily undergo recombination events and have highly variable plasmid content, antimicrobial resistance patterns, and capsular composition (35). Although Kpn may be typically considered as a single entity, even among the ST258 strains very different patterns of infection are elicited in model systems (36). Therefore, it was important to analyze local clinical isolates of the ST258 that varied in different aspects (**Supplementary Materials 1, 3**). Our results indicate that the lack of ROS induction was present in all ST258 strains analyzed, including isolates obtained from distant geographical cities within our country; this mechanism has been present since the year 2008, and was not exclusive for KPC producers, indicating that the absence of ROS represents an advantageous mechanism for the ST258 independently of the antibiotic resistant. Moreover, it is possible that our results can be extended to other not-ST258, as the ATCC clone used in this study showed a similar evasion strategy.

The lack of ROS induction could be explained if Kpn KPC ST258 was not being ingested by PMN. However, our results showed that the percentage of PMN that have phagocytized Kpn KPC ST258 and the number of Kpn KPC ST258 internalized *per* PMN were similar compared to Eco. In this regard, the amount of bacteria internalized *per* PMN is in line with the results shown by Kobayashi et al., who reported similar values for another ST258 strain (37). We have chosen *Eco* for comparison, as this bacterium is also a Gram negative bacillus from the *Enterobacteriaceae* family, with a similar size as Kpn, and therefore a good reference for comparison. Even though Kpn is considered as an example of a poor phagocytized organism, the percentages of phagocytosis

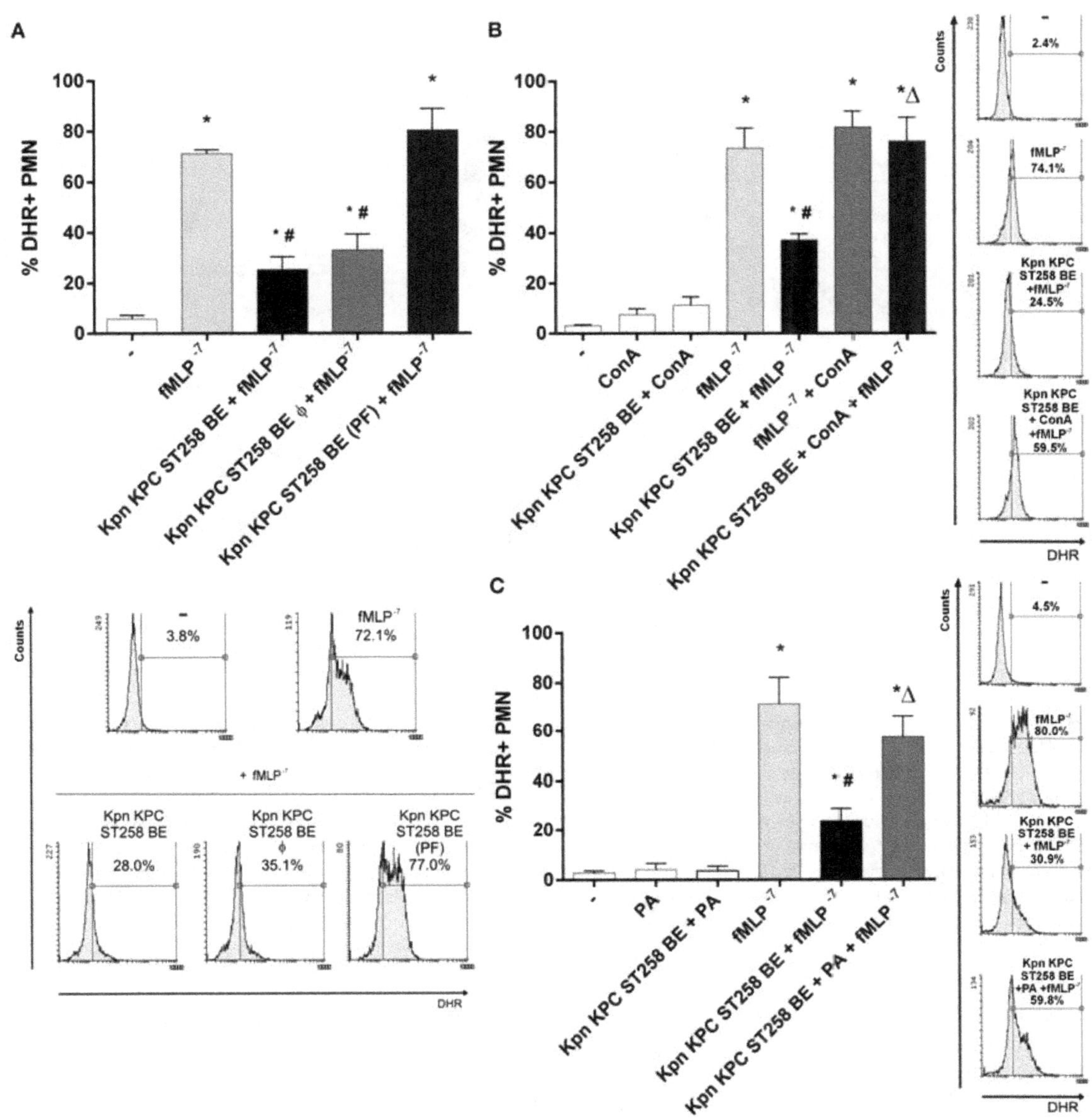

FIGURE 7 | Unraveling the nature of the inhibitory component in KPC ST258 BE. **(A)** fMLP-triggered ROS was measured in PMN in the presence of heat-treated (Φ) KPC ST258 BE or in protein-precipitated fractions (PF). Results of the % of DHR+ PMN were expressed as the mean ± SEM. Lower panel: representative histogram showing SSC vs. DHR. $n = 7$. $^{*}p < 0.05$ vs. untreated (-); # $p < 0.05$ vs. fMLP^{-7}. **(B)** Mannose-containing molecules in KPC ST258 BE were depleted by precipitation with Concanavalin A (Con A) and this depleted fraction was assayed for its inhibitory potential in fMLP-induced ROS. The % of DHR+ PMN is shown and results were expressed as the mean ± SEM, $n = 7$. $^{*}p < 0.05$ vs. untreated (-); # $p < 0.05$ vs. fMLP^{-7}; $\Delta p < 0.05$ vs. Kpn KPC ST258 BE + fMLP^{-7}. Right panel: Representative histograms showing SSC vs. DHR. **(C)** Oxidation of polysaccharides in KPC ST258 BE was performed by periodic acid (PA) treatment and ROS was triggered by fMLP in the presence of these oxidized-BE. Results (% of DHR+ PMN) were expressed as the mean ± SEM. $n = 5$. $^{*}p < 0.05$ vs. untreated (-); # $p < 0.05$ vs. fMLP^{-7}; $\Delta p < 0.05$ vs. Kpn KPC ST258 BE + fMLP^{-7}. Right panel: Representative histograms showing SSC vs. DHR.

of Kpn throughout the literature are variable and depend on the particular bacterial strain (38). However, what is consistent is that the amount of capsule (associated to hyermucoviscocity phenotypes) is crucial for being phagocytized and is usually correlated with resistance to complement killing (7). Our local strain ST258 of Kpn is not resistant to complement killing (our unpublished results) and is not phenotypically a mucoid strain, two characteristics that are aligned with a bacterium that is capable of being phagocytized.

What is important to highlight is that although phagocytosis was similar for both Kpn and Eco, Eco was able to trigger a high respiratory burst and Kpn KPC ST258 was not. Moreover, when we measured the overall result of PMN-Kpn interaction by measuring the remaining colony formation units (CFU), Kpn showed a higher survival compared to Eco. These results can be explained by different possibilities. It is possible, that Kpn is less sensitive to non-oxidative killing, or may be impairing mobilization to the phagosome of different NADPH subunits, as

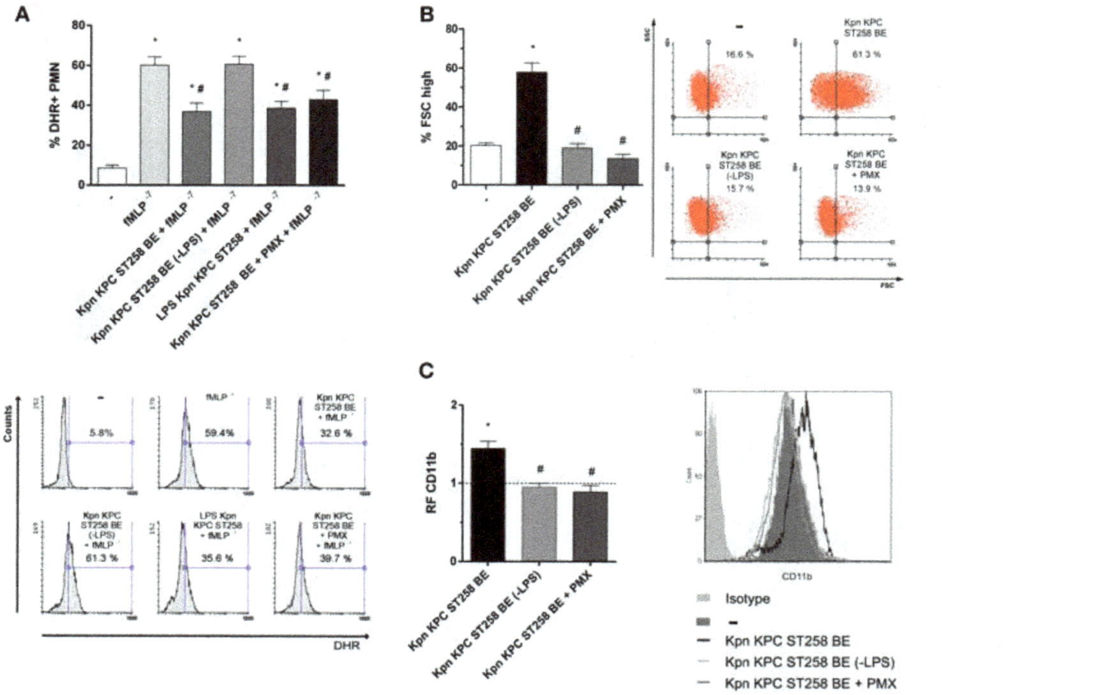

FIGURE 8 | Depletion of LPS in KPC ST258 BE reversed the inhibition of ROS. **(A)** LPS from KPC ST258 BE was depleted using a polymyxin b (PMX)-agarose columns. LPS-depleted fractions (-LPS) were used to assay fMLP-induced ROS generation. Additionally, incubation of KPC ST258 BE with soluble PMX was performed and the mixture KPC ST258 BE+PMX was also used. Results were expressed as the mean ± SEM of the % of DHR+ PMN. $n = 10$. $^*p < 0.05$ vs. untreated (-); # $p < 0.05$ vs. fMLP^{-7}. Lower panel: Representative histograms showing SSC vs. DHR. **(B)** The percentage of PMN that increased their FSC (% FSC high) was measured by flow cytometry in KPC ST258 BE depleted from LPS (-LPS) and in KPC ST258 BE+PMX. Results were expressed as the mean ± SEM. $n = 10$. $^*p < 0.05$ vs. untreated (-); # $p < 0.05$ vs. Kpn KPC ST258 BE. Right panel: Representative dot-plots showing SSC vs. FSC profiles. **(C)** CD11b expression was measured in the different groups by flow cytometry and results were expressed as the relative fluorescence (RF) of the MFI with respect to untreated PMN. The horizontal dashed-line represents the CD11b expression of the control group. Results were expressed as the mean ± SEM. $n = 6$. $^*p < 0.05$ vs. untreated (-); # $p < 0.05$ vs. Kpn KPC ST258 BE. Right panel: Representative histogram showing MFI expression of CD11b for the different experimental groups.

reported for other bacteria (39). We are currently investigating which of these mechanisms could be operating in Kpn KPC ST258-mediated ROS inhibition.

The widely held belief is that Kpn is a stealth pathogen, which fails to stimulate innate immune responses (40), shielding its pathogen-associated molecular patterns from detection by the immune system, thereby avoiding the interaction with hematopoietic and non-hematopoietic cells to prevent the activation of host antimicrobial responses. This belief is in contrast with our results that have shown that Kpn is being sensed by PMN, at least similarly to Eco, but for Kpn this leads to a lack of ROS induction. Additionally, our work described for the first time that Kpn KPC ST258 was able to modulate ROS triggered by Eco, indicating that the interaction of Kpn KPC ST258 with PMN was, in fact, negatively regulating ROS generation. This may also have clinical implications as the presence of Kpn may favor the survival and dissemination of other bacteria in cases of co-infections in hospitalized patients (41, 42).

Using BE we have demonstrated that Kpn was actively subverting host defenses. To evidence the absence of vs. an inhibitory phenomenon, a positive inducer, as was fMLP in our work, had to be used. Using this experimental approach, the inhibitory effect on ROS production mediated by a structural bacterial wall component of Kpn KPC ST258 was revealed. This was not surprising as capsule components or LPS have been reported as the responsible mediators of several evasion mechanisms of Kpn (43). In an attempt to elucidate the intracellular pathway affected by Kpn KPC ST258 in the cascade of events triggered by the ROS inducer fMLP, we performed several experiments using BE but, unfortunately, our results were not conclusive in this way, as Ca^{2+}mobilization or NADPH oxidase assembly were not affected by the presence of BE. However, BE-mediated inhibition of ROS generation was also found for LB_4, another classical ROS inducer that interacts with a seven-transmembrane receptor, indicating that Kpn KPC ST258 BE may be interfering with a common downstream pathway of this type of receptors.

LPS is a major component of the bacterial wall of Gram negative organisms. LPS consists of three different parts, in the following order, from inside the membrane to the outside: lipid A (also known as endotoxin), a core sugar consisting of 3-deoxy-D-manno-oct-2-ulosonic acid (Kdo) moieties, and the O-antigen, which consists of repeating oligosaccharide units. The lipid A component of LPS is recognized by Toll-like receptor 4 (TLR4) and its co-receptor MD-2 on host cells (44). Carbohydrates are usually recognized by other type of receptors, e.g., C-type lectin receptors, sometimes associated to inhibitory functions (45). Inhibitory receptors play key roles in regulating aspects of the immune response mainly by blocking activating pathways (46). Several inhibitory receptors have been described in PMN and are usually composed of a cytoplasmic tail that contains at least one immune-receptor tyrosine-based inhibitory motif (ITIM) (47). Some of these receptors have been shown to bind a diverse array of glycan ligands of endogenous or microbial origin. Our experiments using LPS-depleted and purified LPS clearly demonstrated that ROS inhibition triggered by fMLP was mediated by the LPS molecule of Kpn KPC ST258, and more specifically, by the polysaccharide portion. Moreover, LPS seems to play a dual role in its interaction with PMN. Whereas, the polysaccharide part of the molecule was found to be involved in ROS inhibition, neutralization of lipid A by PMX in the BE annulled the stimulation of cell size increase and CD11b expression, indicating that these effects were dependent on lipid A of Kpn's LPS. This is an interesting observation, as the same molecule can exert selectivity in its suppressive properties, avoiding bactericidal functions that are critical for bacterial survival. A certain functional selectivity was also found with the entire bacteria, which was able to affect specifically ROS and NETs generation but did not affect the increase in FSC and CD11b up-regulation. It should be noted that ROS inhibition mediated by LPS was partial, although the lack of induction caused by the whole bacteria was absolute. This indicates either that the native conformation of LPS could be more efficient compared to its form adopted after partial purification, or it could also be possible that more than one evasive molecule/strategy may be coexisting in Kpn.

Considering all this, it can be speculated that LPS can be delivering positive signals via TLR4 receptors by the lipid A portion (48), and, at the same time, negative signals through its interaction with another yet-unidentified receptor by the polysaccharide part. Supporting our findings of Kpn delivering negative signals, other authors have found that LPS O-polysaccharide of Kpn, although not ST258, abrogates the activation of inflammatory responses in the human lung alveolar epithelial A549 cells line by targeting NF-κB and MAPK signaling pathways (49, 50). We are currently investigating the identity of the putative inhibitory receptor involved in the phenomenon described in this work, as we believe that targeting inhibitory receptors that regulate the threshold activation of PMN would be beneficial in other clinical scenarios, as for the treatment of some inflammatory diseases.

In summary, our work describes new insights in the biology of Kpn KPC ST258, revealing active mechanisms of innate immune evasion. Moreover, the relevance of our findings can be extended to other pathophysiological contexts, but specifically, for Kpn infections, understanding the pathways involved in Kpn KPC ST258-mediated inhibition of ROS might provide the basis to delineate selective complementary alternatives for the management of this wide-spread, multi-resistant pathogen.

AUTHOR CONTRIBUTIONS

LC, GF, VL, and SG conceived and designed the experiments. LC, FB-W, NR-R, and FB performed the experiments. LC, VL, DM-G, and GF analyzed and interpreted the data. GF and DM-G contributed with reagents, materials, and analysis tools. GF and LC wrote the manuscript. VL, DM-G, and SG revised the manuscript. LC, FB-W, NR-R, DM-G, FB-W, VL, SG, and GF approved the version to be published, and agreed to be accountable for all aspects of the work in ensuring that questions related to the accuracy or integrity of any part of the work are appropriately investigated and resolved.

ACKNOWLEDGMENTS

The authors want to thank Dr. Mirta Giordano for providing Fluo 3-AM and for technical assistance, Dr. Federico Fuentes for confocal microscopy assistance, and Tomas Falzone for providing reagents necessary for some experiments.

REFERENCES

1. Boucher HW, Talbot GH, Bradley JS, Edwards JE, Gilbert D, Rice LB, et al. Bad bugs, nodrugs: no ESKAPE! An update from the Infectious Diseases Society of America. *Clin Infect Dis.* (2009) 48:1–12. doi: 10.1086/595011
2. Munoz-Price LS, Poirel L, Bonomo RA, Schwaber MJ, Daikos GL, Cormican M, et al. Clinical epidemiology of the global expansion of *Klebsiella pneumoniae* carbapenemases. *Lancet Infect Dis.* (2013) 13:785–96. doi: 10.1016/S1473-3099(13)70190-7
3. Deleo FR, Chen L, Porcella SF, Martens CA, Kobayashi SD, Porter AR, et al. Molecular dissection of the evolution of carbapenem-resistant multilocus sequence type 258 *Klebsiella pneumoniae*. *Proc Natl Acad Sci USA.* (2014) 111:4988–93. doi: 10.1073/pnas.1321364111
4. Gomez SA, Pasteran FG, Faccone D, Tijet N, Rapoport M, Lucero C, et al. Clonal dissemination of *Klebsiella pneumoniae* ST258

harbouring KPC-2 in Argentina. *Clin Microbiol Infect.* (2011) 17:1520–4. doi: 10.1111/j.1469-0691.2011.03600.x

5. Domenico P, Salo RJ, Cross AS, Cunha BA. Polysaccharide capsule-mediated resistance to opsonophagocytosis in *Klebsiella pneumoniae. Infect Immun.* (1994) 62:4495–9.
6. Moranta D, Regueiro V, March C, Llobet E, Margareto J, Larrarte E, et al. *Klebsiella pneumoniae* capsule polysaccharide impedes the expression of beta-defensins by airway epithelial cells. *Infect Immun.* (2010) 78:1135–46. doi: 10.1128/IAI.00940-09
7. Lee CH, Chang CC, Liu JW, Chen RF, Yang KD. Sialic acid involved in hypermucoviscosity phenotype of *Klebsiella pneumoniae* and associated with resistance to neutrophil phagocytosis. *Virulence.* (2014) 5:673–9. doi: 10.4161/viru.32076
8. Gomez-Simmonds A, Uhlemann AC. Clinical implications of genomic adaptation and evolution of carbapenem-resistant *Klebsiella pneumoniae. J Infect Dis.* (2017) 215(Suppl. 1):S18–27. doi: 10.1093/infdis/jiw378
9. Cole AT, Garlick NM, Galvin AM, Hawkey CJ, Robins RA. A flow cytometric method to measure shape change of human neutrophils. *Clin Sci.* (1995) 89:549–54. doi: 10.1042/cs0890549
10. Lacy P. Mechanisms of degranulation in neutrophils. *Allergy Asthma Clin Immunol.* (2006) 2:98–108. doi: 10.1186/1710-1492-2-3-98
11. El-Benna J, Hurtado-Nedelec M, Marzaioli V, Marie JC, Gougerot-Pocidalo MA, Dang PM. Priming of the neutrophil respiratory burst: role in host defense and inflammation. *Immunol Rev.* (2016) 273:180–93. doi: 10.1111/imr.12447
12. Amulic B, Hayes G. Neutrophil extracellular traps. *Curr Biol.* (2011) 21:R297–8. doi: 10.1016/j.cub.2011.03.021
13. Kenny EF, Herzig A, Krüger R, Muth A, Mondal S, Thompson PR, et al. Diverse stimuli engage different neutrophil extracellular trap pathways. *Elife.* (2017) 6:e24437. doi: 10.7554/eLife.24437
14. Böyum A. Separation of leukocytes from blood and bone marrow. Introduction. *Scand J Clin Lab Invest Suppl.* (1968) 97:7.
15. Huff J, Czyz A, Landick R, Niederweis M. Taking phage integration to the next level as a genetic tool for mycobacteria. *Gene.* (2010) 468:8–19. doi: 10.1016/j.gene.2010.07.012
16. Vandeventer PE, Weigel KM, Salazar J, Erwin B, Irvine B, Doebler R, et al. Mechanical disruption of lysis-resistant bacterial cells by use of a miniature, low-power, disposable device. *J Clin Microbiol.* (2011) 49:2533–9. doi: 10.1128/JCM.02171-10
17. Bradford MM. A rapid and sensitive method for the quantitation of microgram quantities of protein utilizing the principle of protein-dye binding. *Anal Biochem.* (1976) 72:248–54. doi: 10.1016/0003-2697(76)90527-3
18. Kao JP, Harootunian AT, Tsien RY. Photochemically generated cytosolic calcium pulses and their detection by fluo-3. *J Biol Chem.* (1989) 264:8179–84.
19. Leech M, Hutchinson P, Holdsworth SR, Morand EF. Endogenous glucocorticoids modulate neutrophil migration and synovial P-selectin but not neutrophil phagocytic or oxidative function in experimental arthritis. *Clin Exp Immunol.* (1998) 112:383–8. doi: 10.1046/j.1365-2249.1998.00601.x
20. Rodriguez-Rodrigues N, Castillo LA, Landoni VI, Martire-Greco D, Milillo MA, Barrionuevo P, et al. Prokaryotic RNA associated to bacterial viability induces polymorphonuclear neutrophil activation. *Front Cell Infect Microbiol.* (2017) 7:306. doi: 10.3389/fcimb.2017.00306
21. Schindelin J, Arganda-Carreras I, Frise E, Kaynig V, Longair M, Pietzsch T, et al. Fiji: an open-source platform for biological-image analysis. *Nat Methods.* (2012) 9:676–82. doi: 10.1038/nmeth.2019
22. Betsuyaku T, Liu F, Senior RM, Haug JS, Brown EJ, Jones SL, et al. A functional granulocyte colony-stimulating factor receptor is required for normal chemoattractant-induced neutrophil activation. *J Clin Invest.* (1999) 103:825–32. doi: 10.1172/JCI5191
23. Stoiber W, Obermayer A, Steinbacher P, Krautgartner WD. The Role of Reactive Oxygen Species (ROS) in the formation of Extracellular Traps (ETs) in humans. *Biomolecules.* (2015) 5:702–23. doi: 10.3390/biom5020702
24. Cattaneo F, Parisi M, Ammendola R. Distinct signaling cascades elicited by different Formyl Peptide Receptor 2 (FPR2) agonists. *Int J Mol Sci.* (2013) 14:7193–230. doi: 10.3390/ijms14047193
25. Castagna M, Takai Y, Kaibuchi K, Sano K, Kikkawa U, Nishizuka Y. Direct activation of calcium-activated, phospholipid-dependent protein kinase by tumor-promoting phorbol esters. *J Biol Chem.* (1982) 257:7847–51.
26. Bhattacharyya L, Brewer CF. Precipitation of concanavalin A by a high mannose type glycopeptide. *Biochem Biophys Res Commun.* (1986) 137:670–4. doi: 10.1016/0006-291X(86)91130-7
27. Malinin GI. Oxidation of tissue polysaccharides by periodic acid dimethyl sulfoxide and its anhydrous and aqueous mixtures. *J Histochem Cytochem.* (1977) 25:188–92. doi: 10.1177/25.3.190311
28. Gomez-Simmonds A, Greenman M, Sullivan SB, Tanner JP, Sowash MG, Whittier S, et al. Population structure of *Klebsiella pneumoniae* causing bloodstream infections at a New York City Tertiary Care Hospital: diversification of multidrug-resistant isolates. *J Clin Microbiol.* (2015) 53:2060–7. doi: 10.1128/JCM.03455-14
29. Tumbarello M, Trecarichi EM, De Rosa FG, Giannella M, Giacobbe DR, Bassetti M, et al. Infections caused by KPC-producing *Klebsiella pneumoniae*: differences in therapy and mortality in a multicentre study. *J Antimicrob Chemother.* (2015) 70:2133–43. doi: 10.1093/jac/dkv086
30. Lee GC, Burgess DS. Treatment of *Klebsiella pneumoniae* carbapenemase (KPC) infections: a review of published case series and case reports. *Ann Clin Microbiol Antimicrob.* (2012) 11:32. doi: 10.1186/1476-0711-11-32
31. Tuon FF, Rocha JL, Toledo P, Arend LN, Dias CH, Leite TM, et al. Risk factors for KPC-producing *Klebsiella pneumoniae* bacteremia. *Braz J Infect Dis.* (2012) 16:416–9. doi: 10.1016/j.bjid.2012.08.006
32. Jiao Y, Qin Y, Liu J, Li Q, Dong Y, Shang Y, et al. Risk factors for carbapenem-resistant *Klebsiella pneumoniae* infection/colonization and predictors of mortality: a retrospective study. *Pathog Glob Health.* (2015) 109:68–74. doi: 10.1179/2047773215Y.0000000004
33. Ahn D, Peñaloza H, Wang Z, Wickersham M, Parker D, Patel P, et al. Acquired resistance to innate immune clearance promotes *Klebsiella pneumoniae* ST258 pulmonary infection. *JCI Insight.* (2016) 1:e89704. doi: 10.1172/jci.insight.89704
34. Kitchel B, Rasheed JK, Patel JB, Srinivasan A, Navon-Venezia S, Carmeli Y, et al. Molecular epidemiology of KPC-producing *Klebsiella pneumoniae* isolates in the United States: clonal expansion of multilocus sequence type 258. *Antimicrob Agents Chemother.* (2009) 53:3365–70. doi: 10.1128/AAC.00126-09
35. Diago-Navarro E, Chen L, Passet V, Burack S, Ulacia-Hernando A, Kodiyanplakkal RP, et al. Carbapenem-resistant *Klebsiella pneumoniae* exhibit variability in capsular polysaccharide and capsule associated virulence traits. *J Infect Dis.* (2014) 210:803–13. doi: 10.1093/infdis/jiu157
36. Xiong H, Carter RA, Leiner IM, Tang YW, Chen L, Kreiswirth BN, et al. Distinct contributions of neutrophils and CCR2+ monocytes to pulmonary clearance of different *Klebsiella pneumoniae* strains. *Infect Immun.* (2015) 83:3418–27. doi: 10.1128/IAI.00678-15
37. Kobayashi SD, Porter AR, Dorward DW, Brinkworth AJ, Chen L, Kreiswirth BN, et al. Phagocytosis and killing of carbapenem-resistant ST258 *Klebsiella pneumoniae* by human neutrophils. *J Infect Dis.* (2016) 213:1615–22. doi: 10.1093/infdis/jiw001
38. Heinzelmann M, Gardner SA, Mercer-Jones M, Roll AJ, Polk HC. Quantification of phagocytosis in human neutrophils by flow cytometry. *Microbiol Immunol.* (1999) 43:505–12. doi: 10.1111/j.1348-0421.1999.tb02435.x
39. Gallois A, Klein JR, Allen LA, Jones BD, Nauseef WM. Salmonella pathogenicity island 2-encoded type III secretion system mediates exclusion of NADPH oxidase assembly from the phagosomal membrane. *J Immunol.* (2001) 166:5751–8. doi: 10.4049/jimmunol.166.9.5741
40. Paczosa MK, Mecsas J. *Klebsiella pneumoniae*: going on the offense with a strong defense. *Microbiol Mol Biol Rev.* (2016) 80:629–61. doi: 10.1128/MMBR.00078-15
41. Okada F, Ando Y, Honda K, Nakayama T, Ono A, Tanoue S, et al. Acute *Klebsiella pneumoniae* pneumonia alone and with concurrent infection: comparison of clinical and thin-section CT findings. *Br J Radiol.* (2010) 83:854–60. doi: 10.1259/bjr/28999734
42. Giovane RAS, Brooks S. Carbapenem-resistant enterobacteriaceae co-infections with klebsiella; a retrospective study. *Int Arch Med.* (2015) 8:1–15. doi: 10.3823/1738
43. Bengoechea JA, Sa Pessoa J. *Klebsiella pneumoniae* infection biology: living to counteract host defences. *FEMS Microbiol Rev.* (2019) 43:123–44. doi: 10.1093/femsre/fuy043

44. Maeshima N, Fernandez RC. Recognition of lipid A variants by the TLR4-MD-2 receptor complex. *Front Cell Infect Microbiol.* (2013) 3:3. doi: 10.3389/fcimb.2013.00003
45. Redelinghuys P, Brown GD. Inhibitory C-type lectin receptors in myeloid cells. *Immunol Lett.* (2011) 136:1–12. doi: 10.1016/j.imlet.2010.10.005
46. Fernandes MJ, Naccache PH. The role of inhibitory receptors in monosodium urate crystal-induced inflammation. *Front Immunol.* (2018) 9:1883. doi: 10.3389/fimmu.2018.01883
47. Pyz E, Marshall AS, Gordon S, Brown GD. C-type lectin-like receptors on myeloid cells. *Ann Med.* (2006) 38:242–51. doi: 10.1080/07853890600608985
48. Park BS, Lee JO. Recognition of lipopolysaccharide pattern by TLR4 complexes. *Exp Mol Med.* (2013) 45:e66. doi: 10.1038/emm.2013.97
49. Regueiro V, Moranta D, Frank CG, Larrarte E, Margareto J, March C, et al. *Klebsiella pneumoniae* subverts the activation of inflammatory responses in a NOD1-dependent manner. *Cell Microbiol.* (2011) 13:135–53. doi: 10.1111/j.1462-5822.2010.01526.x
50. Tomás A, Lery L, Regueiro V, Pérez-Gutiérrez C, Martínez V, Moranta D, et al. Functional genomic screen identifies *Klebsiella pneumoniae* factors implicated in blocking Nuclear Factor kappaB (NF-kappaB) signaling. *J Biol Chem.* (2015) 290:16678–97. doi: 10.1074/jbc.M114.621292

Permissions

All chapters in this book were first published by Frontiers; hereby published with permission under the Creative Commons Attribution License or equivalent. Every chapter published in this book has been scrutinized by our experts. Their significance has been extensively debated. The topics covered herein carry significant findings which will fuel the growth of the discipline. They may even be implemented as practical applications or may be referred to as a beginning point for another development.

The contributors of this book come from diverse backgrounds, making this book a truly international effort. This book will bring forth new frontiers with its revolutionizing research information and detailed analysis of the nascent developments around the world.

We would like to thank all the contributing authors for lending their expertise to make the book truly unique. They have played a crucial role in the development of this book. Without their invaluable contributions this book wouldn't have been possible. They have made vital efforts to compile up to date information on the varied aspects of this subject to make this book a valuable addition to the collection of many professionals and students.

This book was conceptualized with the vision of imparting up-to-date information and advanced data in this field. To ensure the same, a matchless editorial board was set up. Every individual on the board went through rigorous rounds of assessment to prove their worth. After which they invested a large part of their time researching and compiling the most relevant data for our readers.

The editorial board has been involved in producing this book since its inception. They have spent rigorous hours researching and exploring the diverse topics which have resulted in the successful publishing of this book. They have passed on their knowledge of decades through this book. To expedite this challenging task, the publisher supported the team at every step. A small team of assistant editors was also appointed to further simplify the editing procedure and attain best results for the readers.

Apart from the editorial board, the designing team has also invested a significant amount of their time in understanding the subject and creating the most relevant covers. They scrutinized every image to scout for the most suitable representation of the subject and create an appropriate cover for the book.

The publishing team has been an ardent support to the editorial, designing and production team. Their endless efforts to recruit the best for this project, has resulted in the accomplishment of this book. They are a veteran in the field of academics and their pool of knowledge is as vast as their experience in printing. Their expertise and guidance has proved useful at every step. Their uncompromising quality standards have made this book an exceptional effort. Their encouragement from time to time has been an inspiration for everyone.

The publisher and the editorial board hope that this book will prove to be a valuable piece of knowledge for researchers, students, practitioners and scholars across the globe.

List of Contributors

Nuriban Valero-Pacheco
Unidad de Investigación Médica en Inmunoquímica, Hospital de Especialidades del Centro Médico Nacional Siglo XXI, Instituto Mexicano del Seguro Social, Mexico City, Mexico
Departamento de Inmunología, Escuela Nacional de Ciencias Biológicas, Instituto Politécnico Nacional, Mexico City, Mexico
Nuffield Department of Medicine, The Henry Wellcome Building for Molecular Physiology, The Jenner Institute, University of Oxford, Oxford, United Kingdom

Joshua Blight, Phillip Kemlo and Arturo Reyes-Sandoval
Nuffield Department of Medicine, The Henry Wellcome Building for Molecular Physiology, The Jenner Institute, University of Oxford, Oxford, United Kingdom

Gustavo Aldapa-Vega and Marisol Pérez-Toledo
Unidad de Investigación Médica en Inmunoquímica, Hospital de Especialidades del Centro Médico Nacional Siglo XXI, Instituto Mexicano del Seguro Social, Mexico City, Mexico
Departamento de Inmunología, Escuela Nacional de Ciencias Biológicas, Instituto Politécnico Nacional, Mexico City, Mexico

Isabel Wong-Baeza and Luvia E. Sánchez-Torres
Departamento de Inmunología, Escuela Nacional de Ciencias Biológicas, Instituto Politécnico Nacional, Mexico City, Mexico

Ayako Kurioka and Paul Klenerman
Peter Medawar Building for Pathogen Research, University of Oxford, Oxford, United Kingdom

Christian Perez-Shibayama and Cristina Gil-Cruz
Institute of Immunobiology, Kantonsspital St. Gallen, St. Gallen, Switzerland

Rodolfo Pastelin-Palacios
Facultad de Química, Universidad Nacional Autónoma de México, Mexico City, Mexico

Armando Isibasi
Unidad de Investigación Médica en Inmunoquímica, Hospital de Especialidades del Centro Médico Nacional Siglo XXI, Instituto Mexicano del Seguro Social, Mexico City, Mexico

Constantino López-Macías
Unidad de Investigación Médica en Inmunoquímica, Hospital de Especialidades del Centro Médico Nacional Siglo XXI, Instituto Mexicano del Seguro Social, Mexico City, Mexico
Visiting Professor of Immunology, Nuffield Department of Medicine, University of Oxford, Oxford, United Kingdom
Mexican Translational Immunology Research Group, FOCIS Centres of Excellence, Cuernavaca, Mexico

M. Ayelén Milillo, Aldana Trotta, Agustina Serafino, José Luis Marin Franco, Julieta Alcain, Melanie Genoula, Luciana Balboa and Paula Barrionuevo
Instituto de Medicina Experimental (CONICET-Academia Nacional de Medicina), Buenos Aires, Argentina

Fábio V. Marinho and Sergio Costa Oliveira
Departamento de Bioquímica e Imunologia, Universidade Federal de Minas Gerais, Belo Horizonte, Brazil

Guillermo H. Giambartolomei
Instituto de Inmunología, Genética y Metabolismo, Hospital de Clínicas "José de San Martín" (CONICET-UBA), Buenos Aires, Argentina

L. Paulina Maldonado-Ruiz
Medical/Veterinary Entomology Laboratory, Department of Entomology, Kansas State University, Manhattan, KS, United States

Lidia Montenegro-Cadena, Brittany Blattner, Sapna Menghwar and Berlin Londono-Renteria
Vector Biology Laboratory, Department of Entomology, Kansas State University, Manhattan, KS, United States

Ludek Zurek
Department of Pathology and Parasitology, CEITEC Center for Zoonoses, University of Veterinary and Pharmaceutical Sciences, Brno, Czechia

Yoatzin Peñaflor-Téllez, Adrian Trujillo-Uscanga, Jesús Alejandro Escobar-Almazán and Ana Lorena Gutiérrez-Escolano
Departamento de Infectómica y Patogénesis Molecular, Centro de Investigación y de Estudios Avanzados, IPN, Mexico City, Mexico

Rubén López-Santiago, Ana Beatriz Sánchez-Argáez, Liliana Gabriela De Alba-Núñez and Martha Cecilia Moreno-Lafont
Departamento de Inmunología, Escuela Nacional de Ciencias Biológicas, Instituto Politécnico Nacional, Mexico City, Mexico

Shantal Lizbeth Baltierra-Uribe
Departamento de Microbiología, Escuela Nacional de Ciencias Biológicas, Instituto Politécnico Nacional, Mexico City, Mexico

María F. Ferrer and Pablo Thomas
Laboratorio de Virus Animales, Instituto de Biotecnología y Biología Molecular, CONICET-Universidad Nacional de La Plata, La Plata, Argentina

Aída O. López Ortiz
Laboratorio de Virus Animales, Instituto de Biotecnología y Biología Molecular, CONICET-Universidad Nacional de La Plata, La Plata, Argentina
Laboratorio de Trombosis Experimental, Instituto de Medicina Experimental, CONICET-Academia Nacional de Medicina, Buenos Aires, Argentina

Andrea E. Errasti
Facultad de Medicina, Instituto de Farmacologia, University of Buenos Aries, Buenos Aires, Argentina,

Nancy Charo and Eugenio A. Carrera Silva
Laboratorio de Trombosis Experimental, Instituto de Medicina Experimental, CONICET-Academia Nacional de Medicina, Buenos Aires, Argentina

Victor Romanowski and Ricardo M. Gómez
Laboratorio de Virus Animales, Instituto de Biotecnología y Biología Molecular, CONICET-Universidad Nacional de La Plata, La Plata, Argentina
Global Viral Network, Baltimore, MD, United States

Juan Gorgojo and María E. Rodriguez
Centro de Investigación y Desarrollo en Fermentaciones Industriales, CONICET-Universidad Nacional de La Plata, La Plata, Argentina

Carmem Beatriz Wagner Giacoia-Gripp, Andressa da Silva Cazote, Tatiana Pereira da Silva and Mariza Gonçalves Morgado
Laboratory of AIDS and Molecular Immunology, Oswaldo Cruz Institute (FIOCRUZ), Rio de Janeiro, Brazil

Flávia Marinho Sant'Anna, Carolina Arana Stanis Schmaltz, Aline Benjamin and Valeria Cavalcanti Rolla
Clinical Research Laboratory on Mycobacteria, National Institute of Infectious Diseases Evandro Chagas (FIOCRUZ), Rio de Janeiro, Brazil

Tania de Souza Brum
HIV Clinical Research Center, Nova Iguaçu General Hospital (HGNI), Rio de Janeiro, Brazil

Juliana Arruda de Matos
Clinical Research Laboratory on Health Surveillance and Immunization, National Institute of Infectious Diseases Evandro Chagas (FIOCRUZ), Rio de Janeiro, Brazil

Júlio Silva
Platform for Clinical Research, National Institute of Infectious Diseases Evandro Chagas (FIOCRUZ), Rio de Janeiro, Brazil

José Henrique Pilotto
Laboratory of AIDS and Molecular Immunology, Oswaldo Cruz Institute (FIOCRUZ), Rio de Janeiro, Brazil
HIV Clinical Research Center, Nova Iguaçu General Hospital (HGNI), Rio de Janeiro, Brazil

Daniel Scott-Algara
Unit of Lymphocyte Cell Biology, Pasteur Institute, Paris, France

Natalia Alvarez, Wbeimar Aguilar-Jimenez and Maria T. Rugeles
Grupo Inmunovirología, Facultad de Medicina, Universidad de Antioquia (UdeA), Medellín, Colombia

Armando Alfredo Mateos-Chávez, Luis Fernando Flores-Martínez, Guillermina Juliana Baay-Guzmán and Rosendo Luria-Pérez
Unit of Investigative Research on Oncological Diseases, Children's Hospital of Mexico Federico Gomez, Mexico City, Mexico

Paola Muñoz-López and Elayne Irene Becerra-Báez
Unit of Investigative Research on Oncological Diseases, Children's Hospital of Mexico Federico Gomez, Mexico City, Mexico
Posgrado en Biomedicina y Biotecnología Molecular, Escuela Nacional de Ciencias Biológicas, Instituto Politécnico Nacional, Mexico City, Mexico

Diego Prada-Gracia and Liliana Marisol Moreno-Vargas
Research Unit on Computational Biology and Drug Design, Children's Hospital of Mexico Federico Gomez, Mexico City, Mexico

Uriel Juárez-Hernández
Unit of Investigative Research on Oncological Diseases, Children's Hospital of Mexico Federico Gomez, Mexico City, Mexico
Department of Molecular Biomedicine, Center for Research and Advanced Studies of the National Polytechnic Institute, Mexico City, Mexico

Bibiana Chávez-Munguía
Department of Infectomics and Molecular Pathogenesis, Center for Research and Advanced Studies of the National Polytechnic Institute, Mexico City, Mexico

Lourdes Cabrera-Muñóz
Department of Clinical and Experimental Pathology, Children's Hospital of Mexico Federico Gomez, Mexico City, Mexico

Karina A. Pasquevich, Marianela V. Carabajal, Francisco F. Guaimas, Laura Bruno, Mara S. Roset, Lorena M. Coria, Diego A. Rey Serrantes, Diego J. Comerci and Juliana Cassataro
Consejo Nacional de Investigaciones Científicas y Técnicas (UNSAM-CONICET), Instituto de Investigaciones Biotecnológicas Dr. Rodolfo A. Ugalde, Universidad Nacional de San Martín, Buenos Aires, Argentina

Federico Perdomo-Celis and Maria T. Rugeles
Grupo Inmunovirología, Facultad de Medicina, Universidad de Antioquia, Medellin, Colombia

Natalia A. Taborda
Grupo Inmunovirología, Facultad de Medicina, Universidad de Antioquia, Medellin, Colombia
Grupo de Investigaciones Biomédicas Uniremington, Programa de Medicina, Facultad de Ciencias de la Salud, Corporación Universitaria Remington, Medellin, Colombia

Lomeli-Martinez
Department of Wellbeing and Sustainable Development, Centro Universitario del Norte, University of Guadalajara, Colotlán, Mexico
Biological and Agricultural Sciences Ph.D. Program, Centro Universitario de la Ciénega, University of Guadalajara, Ocotlán, Mexico

Eulogio Valentin-Goméz
GMCA Research Unit, Department of Microbiology and Ecology, University of Valencia, Valencia, Spain
Severe Infection Group, Health Research Institute "La Fe," Valencia, Spain

Juan J. Varela-Hernández and Silvia Y. Martinez-Salazar
Department of Medical and Life Sciences, Centro Universitario de la Ciénega, University of Guadalajara, Ocotlán, Mexico

Monserrat Alvarez-Zavala, Karina Sanchez-Reyes, Moises Ramos-Solano and Rodolfo I. Cabrera-Silva
HIV and Immunodeficiencies Research Institute, Clinical Medicine Department, Centro Universitario de Ciencias de la Salud-University of Guadalajara, Guadalajara, Mexico

Victor M. Ramirez-Anguiano
Department of Integrated Dentistry Clinics, Centro Universitario de Ciencias de la Salud, University of Guadalajara, Guadalajara, Mexico

Manuel A. Lomeli-Martinez
Department of Wellbeing and Sustainable Development, Centro Universitario del Norte, University of Guadalajara, Colotlán, Mexico

Luz A. González-Hernández and Jaime F. Andrade-Villanueva
HIV and Immunodeficiencies Research Institute, Clinical Medicine Department, Centro Universitario de Ciencias de la Salud-University of Guadalajara, Guadalajara, Mexico
HIV Unit Department, University Hospital "Fray Antonio Alcalde," University of Guadalajara, Guadalajara, Mexico

Gaurav Shrivastava, Giovani Visoso-Carvajal, Julio Garcia-Cordero, Nicolás Villegas-Sepulveda and Leticia Cedillo-Barron
Departmento de Biomedicina Molecular Centro de Investigación y Estudios Avanzados-Instituto Politécnico Nacional, Mexico City, Mexico

Moisés Leon-Juarez
Departamento de Inmunobioquímica, Instituto Nacional de Perinatología, Mexico City, Mexico

Bibiana Chavez-Munguia
Departamento de Infectomica y Biologia Molecular, Centro de Investigación y Estudios Avanzados-Instituto Politécnico Nacional, Mexico City, Mexico

Tomas Lopez
Departamento de Genética del Desarrollo y Fisiología Molecular, Instituto de Biotecnología, UNAM Cuernavaca, Cuernavaca, Mexico

Porfirio Nava
Departamento de Fisiologia, Biofisica y Neurociencias, Cinvestav Zacatenco, Mexico City, Mexico

Artaza-Irigaray, Adriana Aguilar-Lemarroy, Pablo Ortiz-Lazareno and Luis F. Jave-Suárez
Centro de Investigación Biomédica de Occidente, Instituto Mexicano del Seguro Social, Guadalajara, Mexico

Andrea Molina-Pineda
Centro de Investigación Biomédica de Occidente, Instituto Mexicano del Seguro Social, Guadalajara, Mexico
Programa de Doctorado en Ciencias Biomédicas, Centro Universitario de Ciencias de la Salud, Universidad de Guadalajara, Guadalajara, Mexico

Laura P. Limón-Toledo
Centro Médico Nacional de Occidente, Instituto Mexicano del Seguro Social, Hospital de Ginecología y Obstetricia, Guadalajara, Mexico

Ana L. Pereira-Suárez
Departamento de Fisiología, Centro Universitario de Ciencias de la Salud, Universidad de Guadalajara, Guadalajara, Mexico

Wendoline Rojo-Contreras
Instituto Mexicano del Seguro Social, Hospital General Regional 110, Guadalajara, Mexico

Cristina Gutiérrez-Jiménez, Ricardo Mora-Cartín, Edgardo Moreno and Elías Barquero-Calvo
Programa de Investigación en Enfermedades Tropicales, Escuela de Medicina Veterinaria, Universidad Nacional, Heredia, Costa Rica

Pamela Altamirano-Silva, Carlos Chacón-Díaz and Esteban Chaves-Olarte
Centro de Investigación en Enfermedades Tropicales, Facultad de Microbiología, Universidad de Costa Rica, San José, Costa Rica

Reyes-Sandoval
Nuffield Department of Medicine, Jenner Institute, University of Oxford, Oxford, United Kingdom

Juan E. Ludert
Department of Infectomics and Molecular Pathogenesis, Center for Research and Advanced Studies (CINVESTAV), Mexico City, Mexico

Tania A. Vargas Pavía, Manuel A. Velázquez Cervantes, Arturo Flores Pliego, Addy C. Helguera Repetto and Moises León Juárez
Laboratory of Perinatal Virology, Department of Immuno-Biochemistry, National Institution of Perinatology "Isidro Espinosa de los Reyes", Mexico City, Mexico

Luis A. Castillo, Federico Birnberg-Weiss, Nahuel Rodriguez-Rodrigues, Daiana Martire-Greco, Veronica I. Landoni and Gabriela C. Fernandez
Laboratorio de Fisiología de los Procesos Inflamatorios, Instituto de Medicina Experimental (IMEX)- Consejo Nacional de investigaciones Científicas y Tecnológicas (CONICET)/Academia Nacional de Medicina de Buenos Aires, Buenos Aires, Argentina

Fabiana Bigi
Instituto de Agrobiotecnología y Biología Molecular (IABIMO), Instituto Nacional de Tecnología Agropecuaria (INTA), Consejo Nacional de investigaciones Científicas y Tecnológicas (CONICET), Buenos Aires, Argentina

Sonia A. Gomez
Servicio de Antimicrobianos, Instituto Nacional de Enfermedades Infecciosas Dr. Carlos G. Malbrán (INEI), Administración Nacional de Laboratorios e Institutos de Salud (ANLIS), Buenos Aires, Argentina

Index